W9-BRY-325

Eli Lilly and Company is pleased to present you with this complimentary copy of *Recent Advances in Otitis Media with Effusion*.

Proceedings of the
Third International Symposium

RECENT ADVANCES IN OTITIS MEDIA WITH EFFUSION

May 17-20, 1983
Fort Lauderdale, Florida

Editorial Committee
David J. Lim, M.D., *Editor-in-Chief*
Charles D. Bluestone, M.D.
Jerome O. Klein, M.D.
John D. Nelson, M.D.

Presented by

Department of Otolaryngology
Ohio State University College of Medicine

Sponsored by

The Center for Continuing Medical Education
Ohio State University College of Medicine

B.C. Decker Inc • Philadelphia • Toronto

Publisher: **B.C. Decker Inc.**
3228 South Service Road
Burlington, Ontario L7N 3H8

B.C. Decker Inc.
P.O. Box 30246
Philadelphia, PA 19103

Recent Advances in Otitis Media with Effusion ISBN 0-941158-18-7

Library of Congress catalog card number: 83-72419

10 9 8 7 6 5 4 3 2 1

IN MEMORIAM

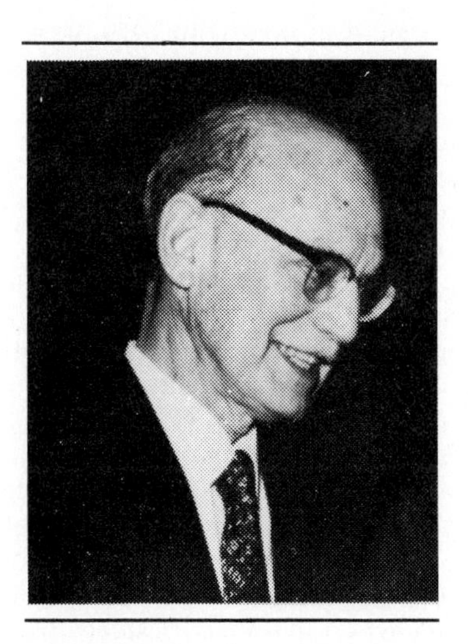

Ben H. Senturia, M.D.
1910-1982

It is with deep sadness that we dedicate this Third International Symposium on Recent Advances in Otitis Media with Effusion to the memory of Ben Harlan Senturia. Dr. Senturia was intimately involved in planning and organizing the first and second International Symposia on Otitis Media with Effusion. He edited and oversaw publication of the proceedings of those meetings as supplements in his beloved *Annals of Otology, Rhinology & Laryngology*. He somehow sensed that he might not be here to enjoy this symposium which reflects the increasing interest and advanced knowledge of otitis media throughout the world. Unfortunately, he died just when we were in the planning stages for this meeting. We are sure, had he been here this week, he would have been proud of the progress made in the past four years. We miss his presence; we know he would want all of us to strive for the further advancement of knowledge of otitis media with effusion.

Charles D. Bluestone, M.D.
David J. Lim, M.D.

OBITUARY*

Ben Harlan Senturia was born in St. Louis, was graduated from Washington University in 1931 with an A.B. degree, and received an M.D. from Washington University School of Medicine in 1935 with membership in the Alpha Omega Alpha honorary medical society. On completion of his residency in Otolaryngology at McMillan Hospital (1935-1938), he was appointed to the faculty of Washington University School of Medicine and to the staffs of Jewish, Barnes and Children's Hospitals in St. Louis.

During his service in the U.S. Air Force (1942-1945), Dr. Senturia was assigned to the Research Section of the School of Aviation Medicine where he conducted major investigations in infections of the external ear and in noise-induced hearing loss. His research in external otitis resulted in two textbooks. Following his military service, he returned to Washington University. At the McMillan Hospital Department of Otolaryngology, Dr. Senturia taught medical students and graduate students; and he conducted major research programs, including a number of significant studies on secretory otitis media (OME) which helped to establish the role of bacteria and inflammation as one important pathogenic factor. At the first International Symposium on Recent Advances in Otitis Media with Effusion, held in Columbus, Ohio, in 1974, he was honored as the first guest of honor. In 1979, he was named Professor Emeritus of Clinical Otolaryngology at Washington University.

Dr. Senturia assumed the directorship of the Department of Otolaryngology at The Jewish Hospital of St. Louis in 1952, and retained this post until 1972, when he was named Director Emeritus.

In 1958, Dr. Senturia was selected by Dr. Arthur Proetz to be the Associate Editor of the *Annals of Otology, Rhinology and Laryngology*, a position he held until Dr. Proetz' death in 1966, when Dr. Senturia became Editor.

From 1963 to 1973, Dr. Senturia served as Chairman of the Committee on Otolaryngic Pathology of the American Academy of Ophthalmology and Otolaryngology. In this capacity, he organized the Symposium on Histopathology and Pathophysiology of the Middle Ear in 1970. He was the Academy's First Vice-President from 1971 to 1972, a member of its Council, and inspired a teaching collaboration between the Academy and the Armed Forces Institute of Pathology.

Dr. Senturia was President of the American Otological Society from 1972 to 1973 and also served as Secretary and Chairman of the Board of Trustees of the Research Fund of the Society, the special committee responsible for distributing funds for otological research. In 1976, Dr. Senturia was the Society's Guest of Honor, and in 1980 he received its prestigious Award of Merit.

Dr. Senturia had been ill for some time but insisted on continuing his clinical activities. Not surprisingly, the cardiac arrest leading to his final illness occurred in the clinic while he was examining the ears of a 16-month-old child. Dr. Senturia, the beloved, kind, caring physician, the brilliant research scientist, the dedicated, meticulous editor of the *Annals of Otology, Rhinology & Laryngology*, and cofounder of this prestigious symposium, died on July 7, 1982. His wife Nancy, whom he married in December 1942, his son, Ben H. Jr.; and his daughter, Alice survive him.

---

*Modified from the obituary by Victor Goodhill, M.D. Reprinted with permission from the *Annals of Otology, Rhinology & Laryngology*.

CONTRIBUTORS

SUDHIR P. AGARWAL, M.D.

University of Minnesota Medical School, Minneapolis, Minnesota
Silent Otitis Media

PER E. ALM, M.D.

National Defense Research Institute, Umeå, Sweden
Provoking Effusion in Experimental Otitis Media with Effusion

H. AMANO, M.D.

Kansai Medical University, Osaka, Japan
Adrenergic Innervation of Eustachian Tube in Guinea Pigs

ROBERT G. ANDERSON, M.D.

University of Texas Health Science Center at Dallas, Texas
Inflammatory Effects of Otic Drops on the Middle Ear

BENGT ANDERSSON, M.D.

University of Göteborg, Sweden
Molecular Mechanisms of Adhesion of Streptococcus Pneumoniae *to Human Oropharyngeal Epithelial Cells*
Children with Frequent Attacks of Acute Otitis Media: A Re-Examination After Eight Years Concerning Middle Ear Changes, Hearing, Tubal Function, and Bacterial Adhesion to Pharyngeal Epithelial Cells

ULRIK KOKS ANDREASSEN, M.D.

Gentofte University Hospital, Hellerup, Denmark
Natural History of Secretory Otitis Media

CLAUDIA S. ANDREWS, M.D.

Vanderbilt University School of Medicine, Nashville, Tennessee
Natural History of Acute and Serious Otitis Media During the First Two Years of Life

WOLFGANG ARNOLD, M.D.

Kantonsspital, Luzern, Switzerland
Proteinases and Proteinase Inhibitors in Middle Ear Effusions

NOBUO AYANI, M.D.

Kansai Medical University, Osaka, Japan
Fluid Clearance of the Eustachian Tube

LEONA W. AYERS, M.D.

Ohio State University College of Medicine, Columbus, Ohio
Biotypes of Serologically Nontypable H. influenzae *Isolated from the Middle Ear and Pharynx of Patients with Otitis Media with Effusion*

JEAN BARNISHAN, M.S.

Ohio State University College of Medicine, Columbus, Ohio
Biotypes of Serologically Nontypable H. influenzae *Isolated from the Middle Ear and Pharynx of Patients with Otitis Media with Effusion*

PAUL B. BATALDEN, M.D.

St. Louis Park Medical Center, Minneapolis, Minnesota
Cefaclor Versus Amoxicillin in the Treatment of Acute Otitis Media
A Case-control Study Exploring Possible Risk Factors for Childhood Otitis Media

SHARON BATCHER, B.S.

University of California Medical Center, San Diego, California
Local Antibody in a Model of Otitis Media with Effusion

GILEAD BERGER, M.D.

University of Toronto, Ontario, Canada
Histamine Levels in Middle Ear Effusions

JOEL M. BERNSTEIN, M.D., Ph.D.

State University of New York at Buffalo, New York
The Clinical Significance of Coagulase-Negative Staphylococci in Otitis Media with Effusion
Defective Phagocytic and Antibacterial Activity of Middle Ear Neutrophils
Lymphocyte-Macrophage Interaction in Otitis Media with Effusion

FRED H. BESS, Ph.D.

Vanderbilt University School of Medicine, Nashville, Tennessee
Natural History of Acute and Serous Otitis Media During the First Two Years of Life
Audiologic and Speech Evaluation of a Prospectively Followed Cohort of Normal Children

C. WARREN BIERMAN, M.D.

University of Washington, Seattle, Washington
Prevalence of Middle Ear Dysfunction and Otitis Media with Effusion in Atopic Children

HERBERT G. BIRCK, M.D.

Ohio State University College of Medicine, Columbus, Ohio
Endotoxin in Middle Ear Effusions from Patients with Chronic Otitis Media with Effusion
Biotypes of Serologically Nontypable H. influenzae *Isolated from the Middle Ear and Pharynx with Otitis Media with Effusion*
Ventilation Tubes in the Pediatric Population

VIRGINIA BLACK

University of California Medical Center, San Diego, California
Local Antibody in a Model of Otitis Media with Effusion

MARK M. BLATTER, M.D.

* University of Pittsburgh, Pittsburgh, Pennsylvania
Clinical Profile of Children with Acute Otitis Media Caused by Branhamella Catarrhalis

GUNNAR D. BLOOM, M.D., Ph.D.

University of Umeå, Sweden
Provoking Effusion in Experimental Otitis Media with Effusion

CHARLES D. BLUESTONE, M.D.

* University of Pittsburgh, Pittsburgh, Pennsylvania
Prevalence and Incidence of Otitis Media in a Group of Preschool Children in the United States
Definitions and Classifications: State of Knowledge

* School of Medicine

Eustachian Tube Function in Infants and Children with Down's Syndrome

Panel Discussion

Surgical Management of Otitis Media with Effusion

Efficacy of Myringotomy With and Without Tympanostomy Tube Insertion in the Treatment of Chronic Otitis Media in Infants and Children

The Effects of Otitis Media with Effusion ("Secretory" Otitis Media) on Hearing Sensitivity in Children

TORBEN BRASK, M.D. Ph.D.

Odense University Hospital, Denmark
Sonotubometry

BRUCE R. BRIGGS, B.S.

Ohio State University College of Medicine, Columbus, Ohio
Experimental Otitis Media with Effusion Induced by Nonviable H. influenzae
Endotoxin in Middle Ear Effusions from Patients with Chronic Otitis Media with Effusion

JACK E. BRINN, Ph.D.

East Carolina University School of Medicine, Greenville, North Carolina
The Mongolian Gerbil as an Animal Model of Otitis Media

SOLGUN BYGDEMAN, M.D.

Huddinge University Hospital, Sweden
The Nasopharyngeal Microflora of Otitis-Prone Children

ANITA BYLANDER, M.D.

University of Lund, Malmö, Sweden
Eustachian Tube Function in Children With and Without Otologic History

ERDEM I. CANTEKIN, Ph.D.

University of Pittsburgh School of Medicine, Pittsburgh, Pennsylvania
Eustachian Tube Function in Children with Unrepaired Cleft Palates
A Primate Model of Cleft Palate and Middle Ear Disease: Results of a One-Year Postcleft Follow-up
Efficacy of Myringotomy With and Without Tympanostomy Tube Insertion in the Treatment of Chronic Otitis Media in Infants and Children
State of the Art: Physiology and Pathophysiology of the Eustachian Tube
The Effects of Otitis Media with Effusion ("Secretory" Otitis Media) on Hearing Sensitivity in Children

BARBARA A. CARLSON, B.S.

University of Minnesota Medical School, Minneapolis, Minnesota
Contributions of Bacteria and Polymorphonuclear Leukocytes to Middle Ear Inflammation in Chronic Otitis Media with Effusion

BRITT E. M. CARLSSON, M.D., Ph.D.

Södersjukhuset, Stockholm, Sweden
Protease—Protease Inhibitor Balance in Otitis Media with Effusion

MARGARETHA L. CASSELBRANT, M.D., Ph.D.

University of Pittsburgh School of Medicine, Pittsburgh, Pennsylvania
Prevalence and Incidence of Otitis Media in a Group of Preschool Children in the United States

ANTONINO CATANZARO, M.D.

University of California Medical Center, San Diego, California
Local Antibody in a Model of Otitis Media with Effusion

POUL CHRISTENSEN, M.D.

University Hospital, Lund, Sweden
Effect of Pneumococcal Vaccination on Acute Otitis Media in Children Attending Day Care Nurseries

C. CIOCE, M.D.

Ospedale dei Bambini V. Buzzi, Milan, Italy
Otitis Media in Newborns

J. C. COOPER, Jr., Ph.D.

University of Texas Health Science Center at San Antonio, Texas
The Efficacy of School Screening for Otitis Media

J. CUMELLA, M.D.

State University of New York at Buffalo, New York
Lymphocyte-Macrophage Interaction in Otitis Media with Effusion

HAL J. DANIEL III, Ph.D.

East Carolina University School of Medicine, Greenville, North Carolina
The Mongolian Gerbil as an Animal Model of Otitis Media

L. DE LUCA

Ospedale dei Bambini V. Buzzi, Milan, Italy
Otitis Media in Newborns

THOMAS F. DeMARIA, Ph.D.

Ohio State University College of Medicine, Columbus, Ohio
Endotoxin in Middle Ear Effusions from Patients with Chronic Otitis Media with Effusion
Biotypes of Serologically Nontypable H. influenzae *Isolated from the Middle Ear and Pharynx of Patients with Otitis Media with Effusion*
Experimental Otitis Media with Effusion Induced by Nonviable H. influenzae

WARREN F. DIVEN, Ph.D.

University of Pittsburgh, Pennsylvania
Hydrolase Activity in Otitis Media with Effusion

WILLIAM J. DOYLE, Ph.D.

* University of Pittsburgh, Pennsylvania
Prevalence and Incidence of Otitis Media in a Group of Preschool Children in the United States
Eustachian Tube Function in Children with Unrepaired Cleft Palates
Eustachian Tube Function in Infants and Children with Down's Syndrome
Histopathology of Otitis Media in Infants with Cleft and High Arched Palates
A Primate Model of Cleft Palate and Middle Ear Disease

DIANE DRYJA

State University of New York at Buffalo and Children's Hospital of Buffalo, New York
Clinical Significance of Coagulase-Negative Staphylococci in Otitis Media with Effusion

JAMES EDLIN, M.D.

University of Minnesota Medical School, Minneapolis, Minnesota
Factors Involved in the Alteration of Middle Ear Effusion Composition

JOHN A. EICHLER, B.Sc.

University of Pittsburgh, School of Public Health, Pittsburgh, Pennsylvania
Effect of Otitis Media with Effusion ("Secretory" Otitis Media) on Hearing Sensitivity in Children

SHIRO ESAKI, M.D.

Jikei University School of Medicine, Tokyo, Japan
Secretory Otitis Media and Middle Ear Cholesteatoma

M. FACCHINI, D.S.

Ospedale dei Bambini V. Buzzi, Milan, Italy
Otitis Media in Newborns

* School of Medicine

BERNT FALK, M.D.

University Hospital, Linköping, Sweden
New Techniques for Measuring Eustachian Tube Responses

JENS ULRIK FELDING, M.D.

Hjørring Hospital, Denmark
Adenoidectomy for Eustachian Tube Dysfunction
Impedance as an Indicator in Irreversible Otopathology and Hearing Loss in Nine-Year-Olds

MICHAEL R. FELDMAN, Ph.D.

Children's Hospital of Pittsburgh, Pittsburgh, Pennsylvania
Prevalence and Incidence of Otitis Media in a Group of Preschool Children in the United States

HAROLD PETER FERRER, M.D., F.F.C.M., D.P.H.

Worcester & District Health Authority, Worcester, U.K.
Impedance Measurements in the Diagnosis of Otitis Media with Effusion

MOGENS FIELLAU-NIKOLAJSEN, M.D., Ph.D.

Hjørring Hospital, Denmark
Influence of Early Otitis Media with Effusion on Reading Achievement
Adenoidectomy for Eustachian Tube Dysfunction
Tympanometric Prediction of Hearing Loss in Secretory Otitis Media
Impedance as an Indicator in Irreversible Otopathology and Hearing Loss in Nine-Year-Olds

HANS HENRIK FISCHER, M.D.

Hjørring Hospital, Denmark
Adenoidectomy for Eustachian Tube Dysfunction

MILDRED R. FLAHERTY, R.N., M.N., P.N.P.

Children's Hospital of Pittsburgh, Pittsburgh, Pennsylvania
Prevalence and Incidence of Otitis Media in a Group of Preschool Children in the United States

ANDERS FREIJD, M.D.

Huddinge University Hospital, Sweden
The Nasopharyngeal Microflora of Otitis-Prone Children
IgG Subclass Levels in Otitis-Prone Children

THOMAS J. FRIA, Ph.D.

University of Pittsburgh School of Medicine, Pittsburgh, Pennsylvania
Efficacy of Myringotomy With and Without Tympanostomy Tube Insertion in the Treatment of Chronic Otitis Media with Effusion in Infants and Children
The Effects of Otitis Media with Effusion ("Secretory" Otitis Media) on Hearing Sensitivity in Children

DORIS FULTON, B.S.

Case Western Reserve University, Cleveland, Ohio
Susceptibility of Beta-Lactamase-Producing Strains of Branhamella Catarrhalis *to Selected, Orally Administered Antimicrobial Agents*

TATSUYA FUJIYOSHI, M.D.

Medical College of Oita, Japan
Secretory IgA, Serum IgA, and Free Secretory Component in Middle Ear Effusion

ROBERT S. FULGHUM, Ph.D.

East Carolina University School of Medicine, Greenville, North Carolina
The Mongolian Gerbil as an Animal Model of Otitis Media

CLIFTON T. FURUKAWA, M.D.

University of Washington, Seattle, Washington
Prevalence of Middle Ear Dysfunction and Otitis Media with Effusion in Atopic Children

GEORGE A. GATES, M.D.

University of Texas Health Science Center at San Antonio, Texas
The Efficacy of School Screening for Otitis Media
History of Treated Persistent Otitis Media with Effusion

SYDNEY S. GELLIS, M.D.

New England Medical Center Hospital, Boston, Massachusetts
Panel Discussion

G. SCOTT GIEBINK, M.D.

University of Minnesota Medical School, Minneapolis, Minnesota
Contributions of Bacteria and Polymorphonuclear Leukocytes to Middle Ear Inflammation in Chronic Otitis Media with Effusion
The Pathogenesis of Experimental Pneumococcal Otitis Media During Respiratory Virus Infection in Chinchillas
A Case-control Study Exploring Possible Risk Factors for Childhood Otitis Media
Comparative Histopathology of Animal Models in Otitis Media in Chinchillas
Epidemiology and Natural History of Otitis Media
Factors Involved in the Alteration of Middle Ear Effusion Composition
Cefaclor Versus Amoxicillin in the Treatment of Acute Otitis Media
Sensorineural Hearing Loss in an Animal Model of Purulent Otitis Media
Effects of Ibuprofen, Corticosteroid, and Penicillin on the Pathogenesis of Experimental Pneumococcal Otitis Media

ROBERT H. GLEW, Ph.D.

* University of Pittsburgh, Pennsylvania
Hydrolase Activity in Otitis Media with Effusion

MARCOS V. GOYCOOLEA, M.D., M.S., Ph.D.

Santiago, Chile
Is There a Normal Microflora in the Middle Ear Cavity?

JOHN W. GREENE, M.D.

Vanderbilt University School of Medicine, Nashville, Tennessee
Natural History of Acute and Serous Otitis Media During the First Two Years of Life

PAUL GRÖNROOS, M.D., Ph.D.

Central Hospital of Tampere, Finland
Pneumococci and Their Capsular Polysaccharide Antigens in Middle Ear Effusion in Acute Otitis Media
Pneumococcal Vaccination and Otitis Media in Infants and Children

VELI-MIES HÄIVÄ, M.S.

National Public Health Institute, Oulu, Finland
Pneumococci and Their Capsular Polysaccharide Antigens in Middle Ear Effusion in Acute Otitis Media

TERRY HANLEY, M.A.

Riverview Children's Center, Verona, Pennsylvania
Prevalence and Incidence of Otitis Media in a Group of Preschool Children in the United States

JEFFREY HARRIS, M.D.

University of California Medical Center, San Diego, California
Local Antibody in a Model of Otitis Media with Effusion

YOSHIE HASHIDA, M.D.

* University of Pittsburgh, Pennsylvania
Histopathology of Otitis Media in Infants with Cleft and High Arched Palates

* School of Medicine

S. HASHIMOTO, M.D.

Tohoku University School of Medicine, Sendai, Japan
Experimental Otitis Media with Effusion

MICHAEL HAWKE, M.D., F.R.C.S.(C)

University of Toronto, Ontario, Canada
Histamine Levels in Middle Ear Effusions

GERALD B. HEALY, M.D.

Children's Hospital Medical Center, Boston, Massachusetts
Antimicrobial Therapy for Chronic Otitis Media with Effusion

ERWIN M. HEARNE III, Ph.D.

University of Texas Health Science Center at San Antonio, Texas
The Efficacy of School Screening for Otitis Media
History of Treated Persistent Otitis Media with Effusion

STEN HELLSTRÖM, M.D., Ph.D.

University of Umeå, Sweden
Provoking Effusion in Experimental Otitis Media with Effusion
Appearance of Effusion Material in the Attic Space Correlated With an Impaired Eustachian Tube Function

ELJA HERVA, M.D., Ph.D.

National Public Health Institute, Oulu, Finland
Pneumococci and Their Capsular Polysaccharide Antigens in Middle Ear Effusion in Acute Otitis Media
Pneumococcal Vaccination and Otitis Media in Infants and Children

SETH V. HETHERINGTON, M.D.

University of Minnesota Medical School, Minneapolis, Minnesota
Contributions of Bacteria and Polymorphonuclear Leukocytes to Middle Ear Inflammation in Chronic Otitis Media with Effusion

JAMES C. HILL, Ph.D.

National Institute of Allergy and Infectious Diseases, NIH, Bethesda, Maryland
Immunization Against Pneumococcal Otitis Media

KARL HOCHSTRASSER, M.D.

University of Munich (München), West Germany
Proteinases and Proteinase Inhibitors in Middle Ear Effusions

POUL ERIK HØJSLET, M.D.

Hjørring Hospital, Denmark
Impedance as an Indicator in Irreversible Otopathology and Hearing Loss in Nine-Year-Olds

SVEND HOLM-JENSEN, M.D.

Gentofte University Hospital, Hellerup, Denmark
Natural History of Secretory Otitis Media

G. RICHARD HOLT, M.D.

University of Texas Health Science Center at San Antonio, Texas
History of Treated Persistent Otitis Media with Effusion

YOSHIO HONDA, M.D.

Jikei University School of Medicine, Tokyo, Japan
Secretory Otitis Media and Middle Ear Cholesteatoma

SATORU HONGO, M.D.

St. Luke's International Hospital, Tokyo, Japan
Complications of Otitis Media with Effusion in Japanese Children

IWAO HONJO, M.D.

Kochi Medical School, Kochi, Japan
Endoscopic Observation of the Eustachian Tube in Otitis Media with Effusion

RONALD P. HOOGMOED, B.A.

East Carolina University School of Medicine, Greenville, North Carolina
The Mongolian Gerbil as an Animal Model of Otitis Media

MARGARET K. HOSTETTER, M.D.

University of Minnesota Medical School, Minneapolis, Minnesota
Contributions of Bacteria and Polymorphonuclear Leukocytes to Middle Ear Inflammation in Chronic Otitis Media with Effusion

BIRGITTA HOVELIUS, M.D.

Community Health Sciences Center, Dalby, Sweden
Effect of Pneumococcal Vaccination on Acute Otitis Media in Children Attending Day Care Nurseries

VIRGIL M. HOWIE, M.D.

University of Texas Medical Branch, Galveston, Texas
Bactericidal Antibody to Antigenically Distinct Nontypable Strains of H. influenzae *Isolated from Acute Otitis Media*

K. HOZAWA, M.D.

Tohoku University School of Medicine, Sendai, Japan
Experimental Otitis Media

EGBERT H. HUIZING, M.D.

University Hospital, Utrecht, The Netherlands
In Vivo Immunology

BURKHARD HUSSL, M.D.

University of Innsbruck, Austria
Fine Morphology of Tympanosclerosis

GERD HVID, M.D.

Gentofte University Hospital, Hellerup, Denmark
Natural History of Secretory Otitis Media

Y. IBATA, M.D.

Kyoto Prefectural University of Medicine, Japan
Adrenergic Innervation of Eustachian Tube in Guinea Pigs

AMY INGRAHAM, B.A.

Children's Hospital of Pittsburgh, Pittsburgh, Pennsylvania
A Primate Model of Cleft Palate and Middle Ear Disease

LEIF INGVARSSON, M.D.

University of Lund, Malmö, Sweden
Eustachian Tube Function in Children With and Without Otologic History
Epidemiology of Acute Otitis Media in Children—A Cohort Study in an Urban Population
Epidemiologic Aspects in Children with Recurrent Acute Otitis Media

ALF IVARSSON, Ph.D.

University of Lund, Malmö, Sweden
Eustachian Tube Function in Children With and Without Otologic History

THERESA JABALEY, M.A.

Michael Reese Hospital and Medical Center, Chicago, Illinois
A Comparative Trial of Steroids Versus Placebos for Treatment of Chronic Otitis Media with Effusion

NIELS JON JOHNSEN, M.D.

University of Copenhagen, Denmark
Penicillin Treatment for Acute Otitis Media in Children

CANDICE E. JOHNSON, M.D., Ph.D.

Case Western Reserve University School of Medicine, Cleveland, Ohio
Twice Daily Antimicrobial Therapy for Acute Otitis Media

FINN JØRGENSEN, M.D.

Sahlgren's Hospital, Göteborg, Sweden
Molecular Mechanisms of Adhesion of Streptococcus Pneumoniae *to Human Oropharyngeal Epithelial Cells*

JAMES H. JORGENSEN, Ph.D.

University of Texas Health Science Center at San Antonio, Texas
Molecular Mechanisms of Adhesion of Streptococcus Pneumoniae *to Human Oropharyngeal Epithelial Cells*

S. K. JUHN, M.D.

University of Minnesota Medical School, Minneapolis, Minnesota
Contributions of Bacteria and Polymorphonuclear Leukocytes to Middle Ear Inflammation in Chronic Otitis Media with Effusion
Factors Involved in the Alteration of Middle Ear Effusion Composition
Biochemistry of Middle Ear Effusion
Comparative Histopathology of Animal Models of Otitis Media in Chinchillas
Effects of Ibuprofen, Corticosteroid, and Penicillin on the Pathogenesis of Experimental Pneumococcal Otitis Media

TIMOTHY T. K. JUNG, M.D., Ph.D.

University of Minnesota Medical School, Minneapolis, Minnesota
Silent Otitis Media
Comparative Histopathology of Animal Models of Otitis Media in Chinchillas
Factors Involved in the Alteration of Middle Ear Effusion Composition
Effects of Ibuprofen, Corticosteroid, and Penicillin on the Pathogenesis and Experimental Pneumococcal Otitis Media

Y. KAKU, M.D.

Tohoku University School of Medicine, Sendai, Japan
Experimental Otitis Media

OLOF KALM, M.D.

University of Lund, Sweden
Complement and Pneumococcal Antibodies During and After Recurrent Otitis Media

CARL KAMME, M.D.

University Hospital, Lund, Sweden
Effect of Pneumococcal Vaccination on Acute Otitis Media in Children Attending Day Care Nurseries

Y. KANEKO, M.D.

Tohoku University School of Medicine, Sendai, Japan
Experimental Otitis Media

RAYMOND B. KARASIC, M.D.

Boston University School of Medicine, Boston, Massachusetts
Serologic Response in Experimental Otitis Media due to Nontypable H. influenzae

PEKKA KARMA, M.D., Ph.D.

University of Tampere, Finland
Pneumococci and Their Capsular Polysaccharide Antigens in Middle Ear Effusion in Acute Otitis Media
Transformation Response of Lymphocytes to Phytohemagglutinin and Pokeweed Mitogen in Patients with Secretory Otitis Media
Pneumococcal Vaccination and Otitis Media in Infants and Children

FREDDY KARUP PEDERSEN, M.D.

Statens Seruminstitut, Copenhagen, Denmark
Complement and Pneumococcal Antibodies During and After Recurrent Otitis Media

K. KAWAMOTO, M.D.

Tohoku University School of Medicine, Sendai, Japan
Experimental Otitis Media

CHEE HOON KIM

Case Western Reserve University, Cleveland, Ohio
Susceptibility of Beta-Lactamase-Producing Strains of Branhamella Catarrhalis *to Selected, Orally Administered Antimicrobial Agents*

CORALIE KIRKLAND, Dip.H.Sc.

University of Otago Medical School, Dunedin, New Zealand
Some Factors of Possible Etiological Significance
Some Developmental Characteristics Associated with Otitis Media with Effusion

MASANORI KITAJIRI, M.D.

Kansai Medical University, Osaka, Japan
Autonomic Innervation of the Tubotympanum
Adrenergic Innervation of Eustachian Tube in Guinea Pigs
Histopathology of Otitis Media in Infants with Cleft and High Arched Palates

JEROME O. KLEIN, M.D.

Boston University School of Medicine, Boston, Massachusetts
Otitis Media with Effusion During the First Three Years of Life and Development of Speech and Language
Antimicrobial Management and Prevention of Otitis Media with Effusion

PAUL M. KLUYSENS, M.D., Ph.D.

State University Hospital, Ghent, Belgium
Some Predisposing Factors in Otitis Media with Effusion

LINDA J. KNAPP, M.D.

Case Western Reserve University School of Medicine, Cleveland, Ohio
Twice Daily Antimicrobial Therapy for Acute Otitis Media

YOKO KODA, M.D.

Kansai Medical University, Osaka, Japan
Fluid Clearance of the Eustachian Tube

MARKKU KOSKELA, M.Sc.

Oulu University, Oulu, Finland
Recurrent Pneumococcal Otitis Media
Pneumococci and Their Capsular Polysaccharide Antigens in Middle Ear Effusion in Acute Otitis Media

ANTHONY L. KOVATCH, M.D.

* University of Pittsburgh, Pennsylvania
Clinical Profile of Children with Acute Otitis Media Caused by Branhamella Catarrhalis

W. KUIJPERS, Ph.D.

University of Nijmegen, The Netherlands
Experimental Occlusion of the Eustachian Tube
The Short- and Long-Term Effects of Tubal Occlusion in a Germ-Free Animal Model

WIETSE KUIS, M.D.

University Children's Hospital, Utrecht, The Netherlands
In Vivo Immunology

TADAMI KUMAZAWA, M.D.

Kansai Medical University, Osaka, Japan
Fluid Clearance of the Eustachian Tube
Adrenergic Innervation of Eustachian Tube in Guinea Pigs

* School of Medicine

YUICHI KURONO, M.D.

Medical College of Oita, Japan
Secretory IgA, Serum IgA, and Free Secretory Component in Middle Ear Effusion

KAREN L. LaMARCO, M.S.

* University of Pittsburgh, Pennsylvania
Hydrolase Activity in Otitis Media with Effusion

SVEN LARSSON, M.D.

University of Göteborg, Sweden
Molecular Mechanisms of Adhesion of Streptococcus Pneumoniae *to Human Oropharyngeal Epithelial Cells*

PER L. LARSEN, M.D.

Gentofte University Hospital, Hellerup, Denmark
Experimental Long-Term Tubal Occlusion in Cats

CHAP T. LE, M.D., Ph.D.

University of Minnesota School of Public Health, Minneapolis, Minnesota
Contributions of Bacteria and Polymorphonuclear Leukocytes to Middle Ear Inflammation in Chronic Otitis Media with Effusion
Cefaclor Versus Amoxicillin in the Treatment of Acute Otitis Media

HAKON LEFFLER, M.D., Ph.D.

University of Göteborg, Sweden
Molecular Mechanisms of Adhesion of Streptococcus Pneumoniae *to Human Oropharyngeal Epithelial Cells*

MAIJA LEINONEN, Ph.D.

National Public Health Institute, Helsinki, Finland
Pneumococci and Their Capsular Polysaccharide Antigens in Middle Ear Effusion in Acute Otitis Media
Pneumococcal Vaccination and Otitis Media in Infants and Children

TORBEN LILDHOLDT, M.D.

Odense University Hospital, Denmark
Sonotubometry

DAVID J. LIM, M.D.

Ohio State University College of Medicine, Columbus, Ohio
Fine Morphology of Tympanosclerosis
Anatomy, Morphology, Cell biology and Pathology of the Tubotympanium
Biotypes of Serologically Nontypable H. influenzae *Isolated from the Middle Ear and Pharynx of Patients with Otitis Media with Effusion*
Endotoxin in Middle Ear Effusions from Patients with Chronic Otitis Media with Effusion
Experimental Otitis Media with Effusion Induced by Nonviable H. influenzae

LINDA L. LOPEZ, B.S.N., R.N.

University of Texas Health Science Center at San Antonio, Texas
The Efficacy of School Screening for Otitis Media

JØRGEN LOUS, M.D.

School Health Service of the Municipality of Hirtshals, Hjørring, Denmark
Influence of Early Otitis Media with Effusion on Reading Achievement

KAJ LUNDGREN, M.D.

University of Lund, Malmö, Sweden
Epidemiology of Acute Otitis Media in Children—A Cohort Study in an Urban Population
Epidemiologic Aspects in Children with Recurrent Acute Otitis Media

JUKKA LUOTONEN, M.D.

University of Oulu, Finland
Recurrent Pneumococcal Otitis Media

SHOICHI MAEDA, M.D.

Medical College of Oita, Japan
Secretory IgA, Serum IgA, and Free Secretory Component in Middle Ear Effusion

BENGT MAGNUSON, M.D.

University Hospital, Linköping, Sweden
New Techniques for Measuring Eustachian Tube Responses

GÖRAN MAGNUSSON, Ph.D.

Swedish Sugar Company, Arlöv, Sweden
Molecular Mechanisms of Adhesion of Streptococcus Pneumoniae *to Human Oropharyngeal Epithelial Cells*

P. HELENA MÄKELÄ, M.D., Ph.D.

National Public Health Institute, Helsinki, Finland
Pneumococci and Their Capsular Polysaccharide Antigens in Middle Ear Effusion in Acute Otitis Media
Pneumococcal Vaccination and Otitis Media in Infants and Children

AURORA B. MALDONALDO

Santiago, Chile
Is There a Normal Microflora in the Middle-Ear Cavity?

FERNANDO MANCINI, M.D.

University of Minnesota Medical School, Minneapolis, Minnesota
Silent Otitis Media

ELLEN M. MANDEL, M.D.

University of Pittsburgh School of Medicine, Pennsylvania
Efficacy of Myringotomy With and Without Tympanostomy Tube Insertion in the Treatment of Chronic Otitis Media With Effusion in Infants and Children
The Effect of Otitis Media with Effusion ("Secretory" Otitis Media) on Hearing Sensitivity in Children

JACK S. MANDEL, M.D., Ph.D.

University of Minnesota School of Public Health, Minneapolis, Minnesota
A Case-control Study Exploring Possible Risk Factors for Childhood Otitis Media

RONNI MANNOS, M.A.

Boston University Medical Center, Boston, Massachusetts
Otitis Media with Effusion During the First Three Years of Life and Development of Speech and Language

COLIN D. MARCHANT, M.D.

Case Western Reserve University School of Medicine, Cleveland, Ohio
Detection of Asymptomatic Otitis Media in Early Infancy
Susceptibility of Beta-Lactamase-Producing Strains of Branhamella Catarrhalis *to Selected, Orally Administered Antimicrobial Agents*
Bactericidal Antibody to Antigenically Distinct Nontypable Strains of H. influenzae *Isolated from Acute Otitis Media*
Twice Daily Antimicrobial Therapy for Acute Otitis Media

GABRIEL MARSHAK, M.D.

University of Pittsburgh School of Medicine, Pennsylvania
Efficacy of Myringotomy With and Without Tympanostomy Tube Insertion in the Treatment of Chronic Otitis Media with Effusion in Infants and Children

SUSAN G. MARSHALL, M.D.

University of Washington, Seattle, Washington
Prevalence of Middle Ear Dysfunction and Otitis Media with Effusion in Atopic Children

GUMARO C. MARTINEZ, M.D.

Santiago, Chile
Is There a Normal Microflora in the Middle-Ear Cavity?

A. RICHARD MAW, M.B., B.S., F.R.C.S.

Bristol Royal Infirmary, Bristol, U.K.

* School of Medicine

Chronic Otitis Media with Effusion and Adenotonsillectomy

KATHRYN B. McCONNELL, B.A.

Vanderbilt University School of Medicine, Nashville, Tennessee
Natural History of Acute and Serous Otitis Media During the First Two Years of Life
Audiologic and Speech Evaluation of a Prospectively Followed Cohort of Normal Children

KAREN-INGER MEISTRUP-LARSEN, M.D.

Kommunehospitalet, Copenhagen, Denmark
Penicillin Treatment for Acute Otitis Media in Children

PAULA MENYUK, Ph.D.

Boston University School of Education, Boston, Massachusetts
Otitis Media with Effusion During the First Three Years of Life and Development of Speech and Language

WILLIAM LEE MEYERHOFF, M.D., Ph.D.

University of Texas Health Science Center at Dallas, Texas
Inflammatory Effects of Otic Drops on the Middle Ear

RICHARD H. MICHAELS, M.D.

* University of Pittsburgh, Pennsylvania
Clinical Profile of Children with Acute Otitis Media Caused by Branhamella Catarrhalis

TOKICHIRO MITOMA, M.D.

Kochi Medical School, Kochi, Japan
Endoscopic Observation of the Eustachian Tube in Otitis Media with Effusion

TADAHITO MIZOROGI, M.D.

Jikei University School of Medicine, Tokyo, Japan
Secretory Otitis Media and Middle Ear Cholesteatoma

MOTOHIRO MOCHIZUKI, M.D.

St. Luke's International Hospital, Tokyo, Japan
Complications of Otitis Media with Effusion in Japanese Children

GORO MOGI, M.D.

Medical College of Oita, Japan
Secretory IgA, Serum IgA, and Free Secretory Component in Middle Ear Effusion

LINDA L. MOORE, Ph.D.

State University of New York at Buffalo, New York
Defective Phagocytic and Antibacterial Activity of Middle Ear Neutrophils

TETSUO MORIZONO, M.D.

University of Minnesota Medical School, Minneapolis, Minnesota
Sensorineural Hearing Loss in an Animal Model of Purulent Otitis Media

NIELS MYGIND, M.D., Ph.D.

University of Copenhagen, Denmark
Penicillin Treatment for Acute Otitis Media in Children

R. NAUMANN, M.D.

University of Munich (München), Germany
Proteinases and Pronteinase Inhibitors in Middle Ear Effusions

JOHN D. NELSON, M.D.

University of Texas Health Science Center at Dallas, Texas
Microbiology of Acute Otitis Media with Effusion
Panel Discussion

ERWIN NETER, M.D.

State University of New York at Buffalo, New York
The Clinical Significance of Coagulase-Negative Staphylococci in Otitis Media with Effusion

LEO G. NIEDERMAN, M.D., M.P.H.

Michael Reese Hospital and Medical Center, Chicago, Illinois
A Comparative Trial of Steroids Versus Placebos for Treatment of Chronic Otitis Media with Effusion

TSUNEKI NOZOE, M.D.

Kansai Medical University, Osaka, Japan
Fluid Clearance of the Eustachian Tube

OLLE NYLÉN, M.D., Ph.D.

University of Göteborg, Sweden
Molecular Mechanisms of Adhesion of Streptococcus Pneumoniae *to Human Oropharyngeal Epithelial Cells*
Children with Frequent Attacks of Acute Otitis Media

PEARAY L. OGRA, M.D.

State University of New York at Buffalo, New York
Defective Phagocytic and Antibacterial Activity of Middle Ear Neutrophils
Lymphocyte-Macrophage Interaction in Otitis Media with Effusion

TOSHIO OHNISHI, M.D.

St. Luke's International Hospital, Tokyo, Japan
Complications of Otitis Media in Japanese Children

PHILLIP A. OKEOWO, M.D., F.R.C.S.

Lagos University Teaching Hospital, Lagos, Nigeria
Prevalence and Incidence of Otitis Media in a Group of Preschool Children in the United States

T. OKITSU, M.D.

Tohoku University School of Medicine, Sendai, Japan
Incidence of Secretory Otitis Media

BERTIL OLOFSSON, Ph.D.

University of Lund, Malmö, Sweden
Epidemiology of Acute Otitis Media in Children—A Cohort Study in an Urban Population
Epidemiologic Aspects in Children with Recurrent Acute Otitis Media

NOBUHIRO OKAZAKI, M.D.

Ohio State University College of Medicine, Columbus, Ohio
Fluid Clearance of the Eustachian Tube
Experimental Otitis Media with Effusion Induced by Nonviable H. influenzae

ERVIN OSTFELD, M.D., M.Sc.

Weizmann Institute of Science, Rehovot, Israel
Mass Spectrometric Analysis of Gas Composition in the Guinea Pig Middle Ear-Mastoid System

VIVIANNE OXELIUS, M.D.

University of Lund, Sweden
IgG Subclass Levels in Otitis-Prone Children

E. PACIFICO, D.S.

Ospedale dei Bambini V. Buzzi, Milan, Italy
Otitis Media in Newborns

ANTTI PALVA, M.D.

University of Oulu, Finland
Transformation Response of Lymphocytes to Phytohemagglutinin and Pokeweed Mitogen in Patients with Secretory Otitis Media

* School of Medicine

MICHAEL M. PAPARELLA, M.D.

University of Minnesota Medical School, Minneapolis, Minnesota
Silent Otitis Media
Sensorineural Hearing Loss in an Animal Model of Purulent Otitis Media
Complications and Sequelae of Otitis Media

JACK L. PARADISE, M.D.

* University of Pittsburgh, Pennsylvania
Nonantimicrobial Management and Prevention of Otitis Media with Effusion
Panel Discussion
Efficacy of Myringotomy With and Without Tympanostomy Tube Insertion in the Treatment of Chronic Otitis Media with Effusion in Infants and Children

STEPHEN I. PELTON, M.D.

Boston University School of Medicine, Boston, Massachusetts
Serologic Response in Experimental Otitis Media due to Nontypable H. influenzae

G. PESTALOZZA, M.D.

Ospedale dei Bambini V. Buzzi, Milan, Italy
Otitis Media in Newborns

WILLIAM E. PIERSON, M.D.

University of Washington, Seattle, Washington
Prevalence of Middle Ear Dysfunction and Otitis Media with Effusion in Atopic Children

SEPPO PÖNTYNEN, M.D.

University of Tampere, Finland
Pneumococcal Vaccination and Otitis Media in Infants and Children

KARIN PRELLNER, M.D.

University of Lund, Sweden
Complement and Pneumococcal Antibodies During and After Recurrent Otitis Media
Effect of Pneumococcal Vaccination on Acute Otitis Media in Children Attending Day Care Nurseries

RICHARD B. PRIOR, Ph.D.

Ohio State University College of Medicine, Columbus, Ohio
Endotoxin in Middle Ear Effusions from Patients with Chronic Otitis Media with Effusion

DAVID W. PROOPS, B.D.S., M.B., F.R.C.S.

University of Toronto, Ontario, Canada
Histamine Levels in Middle Ear Effusions

JUHANI PUKANDER, M.D.

University of Tampere, Finland
Pneumococcal Vaccination and Otitis Media in Infants and Children

NARENDRANATH S. RANADIVE, Ph.D.

University of Toronto, Ontario, Canada
Histamine Levels in Middle Ear Effusions

JAMES S. REILLY, M.D.

* University of Pittsburgh, Pennsylvania
Eustachian Tube Function in Children with Unrepaired Cleft Palates

KEITH S. REISINGER, M.D.

* University of Pittsburgh, Pennsylvania
Clinical Profile of Children with Acute Otitis Media Caused by Branhamella Catarrhalis

ULF RENVALL, M.D.

University of Göteborg, Sweden
Reduction of Artificially Increased Middle Ear Air Pressure

HOWARD E. ROCKETTE, Ph.D.

University of Pittsburgh School of Public Health, Pennsylvania
Effect of Otitis Media with Effusion ("Secretory" Otitis Media) on Hearing Sensitivity in Children
Efficacy of Myringotomy With and Without Tympanostomy Tube Insertion in the Treatment of Chronic Otitis Media in Infants and Children

KENNETH F. ROGERS, M.D.

* University of Pittsburgh, Pennsylvania
Prevalence and Incidence of Otitis Media in a Group of Preschool Children in the United States

M. ROMAGNOLI, M.D.

Ospedale dei Bambini V. Buzzi, Milan, Italy
Otitis Media in Newborns

JOHN J. ROORD, M.D.

University Children's Hospital, Utrecht, The Netherlands
In Vivo Immunology

CHRISTER ROSÉN, M.D.

University Hospital, Lund, Sweden
Effect of Pneumococcal Vaccination on Acute Otitis Media in Children Attending Day Care Nurseries

BERNARD A. ROSNER, Ph.D.

Harvard Medical School, Boston, Massachusetts
Otitis Media During the First Three Years of Life and Development of Speech and Language

NOEL ROYDHOUSE, Ch.M., F.R.C.S., F.R.A.C.S.

Middlemore Hospital, Auckland, New Zealand
Bromhexine in the Treatment of Otitis Media with Effusion

HANS RUNDKRANTZ, M.D.

Central Hospital, Skövde, Sweden
Panel Discussion

JOYCE N. RUSS, R.N.

St. Louis Park Medical Center, Minneapolis, Minnesota
A Case-control Study Exploring Possible Risk Factors for Childhood Otitis Media
Cefaclor Versus Amoxicillin in the Treatment of Acute Otitis Media

ALLEN F. RYAN, Ph.D.

UCSD School of Medicine, La Jolla, California
Complement Depletion by Cobra Venom Factor

PAULI RYHÄNEN

University of Oulu, Finland
Transformation Response of Lymphocytes to Phytohemagglutinin and Pokeweed Mitogen in Patients with Secretory Otitis Media

BRITTA RYNNEL-DAGÖÖ, M.D.

Huddinge University Hospital, Sweden
The Nasopharyngeal Microflora of Otitis-Prone Children
IgG Subclass Levels in Otitis-Prone Children

MOHAMED M. SAAD, M.D., Ph.D.

* University of Pittsburgh, Pennsylvania
A Primate Model of Cleft Palate and Middle Ear Disease

JACOB SADÉ, M.D.

Meir Hospital, Kfar Saba, Israel
Mass Spectrometric Analysis of Gas Composition in the Guinea Pig Middle Ear-Mastoid System

M. SAKUMA, M.D.

Tohoku University School of Medicine, Sendai, Japan
Incidence of Secretory Otitis Media

* School of Medicine

BENGT SALÉN, M.D., Ph.D.

University of Umeå, Sweden
Provoking Effusion in Experimental Otitis Media with Effusion
Appearance of Effusion Material in the Attic Space Correlated With An Impaired Eustachian Tube Function

ISAMU SANDO, M.D., D.M.S.

* University of Pittsburgh, Pennsylvania
Histopathology of Otitis Media in Infants with Cleft and High Arched Palates

PATRICIA A. SCHACHERN

University of Minnesota Medical School, Minneapolis, Minnesota
Complications and Sequelae of Otitis Media

JØRGEN SEDERBERG-OLSEN, M.D.

University of Copenhagen, Denmark
Penicillin Treatment for Acute Otitis Media in Children

JACOB SEGAL, M.D.

Hillel Jaffe Memorial Hospital, Hadera, Israel
Mass Spectrometric Analysis of Gas Composition in the Guinea Pig Middle Ear-Mastoid System

SARAH H. SELL, M.D.

Vanderbilt University School of Medicine, Nashville, Tennessee
Natural History of Acute and Serous Otitis Media During the First Two Years of Life

GAIL G. SHAPIRO, M.D.

University of Washington, Seattle, Washington
Prevalence of Middle Ear Dysfunction and Otitis Media with Effusion in Atopic Children

DONALD SHEA, M.A.

University of Minnesota Medical School, Minneapolis, Minnesota
Silent Otitis Media
Comparative Histopathology of Animal Models of Otitis Media in Chinchillas

Y. SHIBAHARA, M.D.

Tohoku University School of Medicine, Sendai, Japan
Experimental Otitis Media with Effusion

PAUL A. SHURIN, M.D.

Case Western Reserve University, Cleveland, Ohio
Detection of Asymptomatic Otitis Media in Early Infancy
Bactericidal Antibody to Antigenically Distinct Nontypable Strains of H. influenzae *Isolated from Acute Otitis Media*
Susceptibility of Beta-Lactamase-Producing Strains of Branhamella Catarrhalis *to Selected, Orally Administered Antimicrobial Agents*
Twice Daily Antimicrobial Therapy for Acute Otitis Media

MICHAEL A. SIKORA

University of Minnesota Medical School, Minneapolis, Minnesota
Sensorineural Hearing Loss in an Animal Model of Purulent Otitis Media

ALEXANDER SILBERBERG, Ph.D.

Weizmann Institute of Science, Rehovot, Israel
Mass Spectrometric Analysis of Gas Composition in the Guinea Pig Middle Ear-Mastoid System

PHIL SILVA, M.A., Ph.D.

University of Otago Medical School, Dunedin, New Zealand
Some Developmental Characteristics Associated with Otitis Media with Effusion
Some Factors of Possible Etiological Significance

ANNE SIMPSON, M.B., Ch.B.

University of Otago Medical School, Dunedin, New Zealand
Some Developmental Characteristics Associated with Otitis Media with Effusion
Some Factors of Possible Etiological Significance

MARKKU SIPILÄ, M.D.

University of Tampere, Finland
Pneumococci and Their Capsular Polysaccharide Antigens in Middle Ear Effusion in Acute Otitis Media

PEKKA SIPILÄ, M.D.

University of Oulu, Finland
Transformation Response of Lymphocytes to Phytohemagglutinin and Pokeweed Mitogen in Patients with Secretory Otitis Media

ANN SITTON, M.S.

Vanderbilt University School of Medicine, Nashville, Tennessee
Natural History of Acute and Serous Otitis Media During the First Two Years of Life
Audiologic and Speech Evaluation of a Prospectively Followed Cohort of Normal Children

A. MASON SMITH, Ph.D.

East Carolina University School of Medicine, Greenville, North Carolina
The Mongolian Gerbil as an Animal Model of Otitis Media

OVE SÖDERBERG, M.D.

University of Umea, Sweden
Appearance of Effusion Material in the Attic Space Correlated with an Impaired Eustachian Tube Function

CHR. HJORT SØRENSEN, M.D.

Gentofte University, Hellerup, Denmark
IgD and Secretory Immunoglobulins in Secretions from the Upper Respiratory Tract of Children with Secretory Otitis Media

HENNING SØRENSON, M.D.

University of Copenhagen, Denmark
Penicillin Treatment for Acute Otitis Media in Children

SVEN-ERIC STANGERUP, M.D.

Gentofte University Hospital, Hellerup, Denmark
Natural History of Secretory Otitis Media

LARS-ERIC STENFORS, M.D., Ph.D.

University of Umeå, Sweden
Appearance of Effusion Material in the Attic Space Correlated with an Impaired Eustachian Tube Function
Provoking Effusion in Experimental Otitis Media with Effusion

IAN STEWART, M.B., Ch.B., F.R.C.S.

University of Otago Medical School, Dunedin, New Zealand
Some Developmental Characteristics Associated with Otitis Media with Effusion
Some Factors of Possible Etiological Significance

SYLVAN E. STOOL, M.D.

* University of Pittsburgh, Pennsylvania
Eustachian Tube Function in Children with Unrepaired Cleft Palates
Efficacy of Myringotomy With and Without Tympanostomy Tube Insertion in the Treatment of Chronic Otitis Media in Infants and Children

JAN W. STOOP, M.D.

University Children's Hospital, Utrecht, The Netherlands
In vivo Immunology: Serous Otitis Media in Children with Immunodeficiency Disorders

* School of Medicine

FRANK SUNDLER, M.D.

University of Lund, Malmö, Sweden
Autonomic Innervation of the Tubotympanum

CATHARINA SVANBORG EDÉN, M.D., Ph.D.

University of Göteborg, Sweden
Molecular Mechanisms of Adhesion of Streptococcus Pneumoniae *to Human Oropharyngeal Epithelial Cells*

F. TACCONE, M.D.

Ospedale dei Bambini V. Buzzi, Milan, Italy
Otitis Media in Newborns

TOMONORI TAKASAKA, M.D.

Tohoku University School of Medicine, Sendai, Japan
Experimental Otitis Media with Effusion: An Immunoelectron Microscopic Study

M. TAKEYAMA, M.D.

Tohoku University School of Medicine, Sendai, Japan
Experimental Otitis Media with Effusion

C. TANAKA, M.D.

Kobe University School of Medicine, Japan
Adrenergic Innervation of Eustachian Tube in Guinea Pigs

DAVID W. TEELE, M.D.

Boston University School of Medicine, Boston, Massachusetts
Detection of Middle Ear Effusion by Acoustic Reflectometry
Otitis Media with Effusion During the First Three Years of Life and Development of Speech and Language

JOHN TEELE, M.S.

Boston University School of Medicine, Boston, Massachusetts
Detection of Middle Ear Effusion by Acoustic Reflectometry

JULIETTE THOMPSON, M.S.N.

Vanderbilt University School of Medicine, Nashville, Tennessee
Natural History of Acute and Serous Otitis Media During the First Two Years of Life
Audiologic and Speech Evaluation of a Prospectively Followed Cohort of Normal Children

JENS THOMSEN, M.D.

Gentofte Hospital, Hellerup, Denmark
Natural History of Secretory Otitis Media
Penicillin Treatment for Acute Otitis Media in Children
Panel Discussion

MATTI TIMONEN, M.D.

University of Tampere, Finland
Pneumococcal Vaccination and Otitis Media in Infants and Children

ÖRJAN TJERNSTRÖM, M.D.

University of Lund, Malmö, Sweden
Eustachian Tube Function in Children With and Without Otologic History

JOHN S. TODHUNTER, Ph.D.

* University of Pittsburgh, Pennsylvania
Computer Generated Eustachian Tube Shape Analysis: A Preliminary Report

KOICHI TOMODA, M.D.

University of Tennessee Center for the Health Sciences, Memphis, Tennessee
Type II Collagen-Induced Autoimmune Salpingitis in Rats

MIRKO TOS, M.D.

Gentofte University Hospital, Hellerup, Denmark
Natural History of Secretory Otitis Media
Experimental Long-Term Tubal Occlusion in Cats

VIRGINIA A. TURCZYK, R.N., P.N.A.

Case Western Reserve University School of Medicine, Cleveland, Ohio
Detection of Asymptomatic Otitis Media in Early Infancy
Twice Daily Antimicrobial Therapy for Acute Otitis Media

MIMI A. TUTIHASI, M.D.

Case Western Reserve University School of Medicine, Cleveland, Ohio
Detection of Asymptomatic Otitis Media in Early Infancy
Twice Daily Antimicrobial Therapy for Acute Otitis Media

ROLF UDDMAN, M.D.

University of Lund, Malmö, Sweden
Autonomic Innervation of the Tubotympanum

TOYOHARU UMEHARA, M.D.

Medical College of Oita, Japan
Secretory IgA, Serum IgA, and Free Secretory Component in Middle Ear Effusion

KOICHI USHIRO, M.D.

Kochi Medical School, Kochi, Japan
Endoscopic Observation of the Eustachian Tube in Otitis Media with Effusion

EUGENIA M. VALENZUELA

Santiago, Chile
Is There A Normal Microflora in the Middle Ear Cavity?

F. L. VAN BUCHEM, M.D.

St. Elisabeth Ziekenhuis, Tilburg, The Netherlands
Panel Discussion

PAUL B. van CAUWENBERGE, M.D.

State University Hospital, Ghent, Belgium
Some Predisposing Factors in Otitis Media With Effusion

J. M. H. van der BEEK, M.D.

University of Limburg, The Netherlands
The Short- and Long-term Effects of Tubal Occlusion in a Germfree Animal Model
Experimental Occlusion of the Eustachian Tube

WILLIAM K. VAUGHN, Ph.D.

Vanderbilt University School of Medicine, Nashville, Tennessee
Natural History of Acute and Serous Otitis Media During the First Two Years of Life

JAN E. VELDMAN, M.D.

University Hospital, Utrecht, The Netherlands
In Vivo Immunology

WENDY VISSCHER, M.P.H.

University of Minnesota School of Public Health, Minneapolis, Minnesota
A Case-Control Study Exploring Possible Risk Factors for Childhood Otitis Media

CARL-WILHELM VOGEL, Ph.D.

Georgetown University School of Medicine, Washington, D.C.
Complement Depletion by Cobra Venom Factor

MARK W. VOGELGESANG, M.D.

Ohio State University College of Medicine, Columbus, Ohio
Ventilation Tubes in the Pediatric Population

* School of Medicine

CHRISTINE A. WACHTENDORF, M.D.

University of Texas Health Science Center at San Antonio, Texas

The Efficacy of School Screening for Otitis Media

History of Treated Persistent Otitis Media with Effusion

ELLEN R. WALD, M.D.

* University of Pittsburgh, Pennsylvania

Clinical Profile of Children with Acute Otitis Media Caused by Branhamella Catarrhalis

VALRE WALTER-BUCHHOLTZ, M.S.N.

Michael Reese Hospital and Medical Center, Chicago, Illinois

A Comparative Trial of Steroids Versus Placebos for Treatment of Chronic Otitis Media with Effusion

DIANA E. WASIKOWSKI, R.N., P.N.A.

Case Western Reserve University School of Medicine, Cleveland, Ohio

Detection of Asymptomatic Otitis Media in Early Infancy

Twice Daily Antimicrobial Therapy for Acute Otitis Media

STEVE WASSERMAN, M.D.

University of California Medical Center, San Diego, California

Local Antibody in a Model of Otitis Media with Effusion

DOUGLAS B. WEBSTER, Ph.D.

Louisiana State University Medical Center, New Orleans, Louisiana

Conductive Loss Affects Auditory Neuronal Soma Size Only During a Sensitive Postnatal Period

BENJAMIN LeM. WHITE, M.D.

* University of Pittsburgh, Pennsylvania

Eustachian Tube Function in Infants and Children with Down's Syndrome

LOUISE WIDEMAR, M.D.

Huddinge University Hospital, Sweden

Provoking Effusion in Experimental Otitis Media with Effusion

MICHAEL WIEDERHOLD, M.D.

University of Texas at San Antonio, Texas

Experimental Long-Term Tubal Occlusion in Cats

SHEILA WILLIAMS, B.Sc.

University of Otago Medical School, Dunedin, New Zealand

Some Developmental Characteristics Associated with Otitis Media with Effusion

Some Factors of Possible Etiological Significance

JOAN C. WILTSHIRE, R.N., P.N.A.

Case Western Reserve University School of Medicine, Cleveland, Ohio

Detection of Asymptomatic Otitis Media in Early Infancy

Twice Daily Antimicrobial Therapy for Acute Otitis Media

DAVID WONG, B.Sc.

University of Toronto, Ontario, Canada

Histamine Levels in Middle Ear Effusions

CHARLES G. WRIGHT, Ph.D.

University of Texas Health Science Center at Dallas, Texas

Inflammatory Effects of Otic Drops on the Middle Ear

PETER F. WRIGHT, M.D.

Vanderbilt University School of Medicine, Nashville, Tennessee

The Pathogenesis of Experimental Pneumococcal Otitis Media During Respiratory Virus Infection in Chinchillas

Natural History of Acute and Serous Otitis Media During the First Two Years of Life

Audiologic and Speech Evaluation of a Prospectively Followed Cohort of Normal Children

FREDERICK P. WUCHER, M.D.

* University of Pittsburgh, Pennsylvania

Clinical Profile of Children with Acute Otitis Media Caused by Branhamella Catarrhalis

T. YAMANAKA, M.D.

State University of New York at Buffalo, New York

Lymphocyte-Macrophage Interaction in Otitis Media with Effusion

T. YAMASHITA, M.D.

Kansai Medical University, Osaka, Japan

Adrenergic Innervation of Eustachian Tube in Guinea Pigs

JEHUDAH YINON, Ph.D.

Weizmann Institute of Science, Rehovot, Israel

Mass Spectrometric Analysis of Gas Composition in the Guinea Pig Middle Ear-Mastoid System

TAI JUNE YOO, M.D.

University of Tennessee Center for the Health Sciences, Memphis, Tennessee

Type II Collagen-Induced Autoimmune Salpingitis in Rats

R. YUASA, M.D.

Tohoku University School of Medicine, Sendai, Japan

Incidence of Secretory Otitis Media

* School of Medicine

FOREWORD

During the past twenty or thirty years there has been a dramatic expansion of research on otitis media involving not only an increase in the number of active investigators but also an increase in the variety of scientific disciplines those investigators represent. That this has occured is the result of a number of factors: in many scientific areas recent technological advances have opened up new approaches to and new techniques for the study of otitis media; otitis media has been highlighted as a clinical problem of major significance, particularly in children, well justifying increased research attention; investigators have been attracted to the problem because it is now recognized as one whose solution is feasible, using state-of-the-art investigational tools; and symposia such as this have provided forums for the rapid exchange of new ideas and developments—a feature of critical importance in any field where research and technological advance are so rife.

Despite this increase of attention, otitis media still constitutes a major clinical problem; but at the risk of being described as pollyannaish we can now point confidently to the light at the end of the otitis media tunnel—or at least to several half lights. Encouraging progress is being made on a variety of fronts, and it seems likely that research interest and productivity have reached the point where continued progress toward the goal of enhanced prevention and improved treatment of otitis media is assured.

One word of caution, in the form of a question, may be appropriate. Otitis media research is on the move, thanks to the persistence of highly trained individuals such as those who have organized this conference and who have contributed to it and to its predecessors. Has the time come now to highlight the need for training young physician–investigators in each of the many scientific disciplines represented at this meeting, in order to insure that the dramatic advances we have seen recently will continue for years to come? An additional advantage of stressing research training for young physicians will be an increase in clinician–basic scientific collaboration, an important consideration in maintaining the strength of biomedical research in years to come.

Ralph F. Naunton, M.D., F.A.C.S.
Director Communicative Disorders Program
National Institute of Neurological and
Communicative Disorders and Stroke

PREFACE

The first international symposium on otitis media with effusion was held in Columbus, Ohio from May 29 through May 31, 1975. Those of us who participated in that meeting felt a great camaraderie, excitement and enthusiasm, and it became clear that there was a need to maintain an international forum for dealing with the basic and clinical aspects of OME. This led to the second symposium, held from May 9 through May 11, 1979, in Columbus. The proceedings of these meetings, published as supplements to the *Annals of Otology, Rhinology & Laryngology**, have become important reference books in our field.

In organizing the third symposium, it became clear that the worldwide research community had dramatically increased since 1975, and changes were made to the meeting format in order to accommodate a maximum number of papers. We had two panel discussions, 11 state-of-the-art reviews, 104 free papers, and 29 poster presentations. There were about 250 participants from 21 countries. We decided to include as many of these papers as possible in this book; however, format restrictions have limited the space allotted to each. Many authors are publishing full-length papers on these topics in professional journals of their choice.

A meeting of this magnitude could not have been successful without the help of the many people who helped organize the symposium. We thank Michael Paparella for serving on the organizing committee at short notice. Ben Senturia, who had been intimately involved in the planning of this symposium, died before completion of the program; we missed him sorely. We also very much missed Sven Ingelstedt, of Malmö, one of the guiding lights of the symposia, who had died soon after the second symposium.

We also would like to thank the companies who made generous contributions to aid this symposium: Eli Lilly and Company, Beecham Laboratories, Ross Laboratories, Roerig (Pfizer), Merrell Dow Pharmaceuticals, Richards Manufacturing Company, Inc., Grason-Stadler, Inc., and Miles Pharmaceuticals. We are grateful to Eli Lilly and Company for their financial support for the publication of the proceedings and their dissemination, with particular thanks to Ernest Glaser and Robert Kruse. We are grateful to the National Institute of Neurological and Communicative Disorders and Stroke and the National Institute of Allergy and Infectious Diseases of the U.S. National Institutes of Health and to Ohio State University for their support of postsymposium research conferences.

Finally, we thank Jon Hollett, Director of the Center for Continuing Medical Education, Ohio State University College of Medicine, Sharma Hipkiss and Donna Peterson of American Express, and Katherine Adamson, assistant to David Lim. We also thank Brian Decker and his editors, who provided expert editorial assistance in preparing these proceedings.

---

*Supplement 25, Vol. 85, 1976 and Supplement 68, Vol. 89, 1980.

David J. Lim, M.D.
Charles D. Bluestone, M.D.
Jerome O. Klein, M.D.
John D. Nelson, M.D.

GUEST OF HONOR

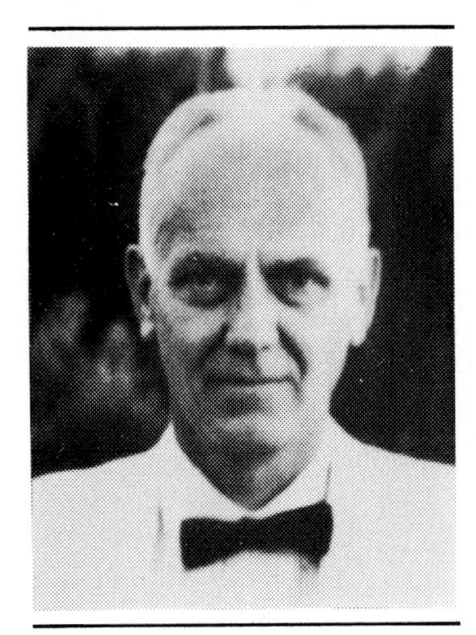

Gunnar O. Proud, M.D.

Gunnar O. Proud, M.D., was born August 6, 1914, in Oregon, Missouri. He received his M.D. degree from Washington University in 1939 and completed his residency in Otolaryngology there in 1942. Following military service in the Pacific, he joined the Department of Otolaryngology at Washington University as an instructor, and remained there as assistant professor until 1950, when he became Chairman of the Department at Kansas University Medical Center. He was promoted to Professor of Otolaryngology in 1952. He is now Professor Emeritus at KUMC.

At KUMC, he and his associates developed an animal model for otitis media with effusion, a contribution which resulted in a number of important papers. He is a dedicated clinician who took clinical questions to the laboratory and inspired many young investigators who were interested in eustachian tube function and middle-ear pathology.

He has served on many important committees and boards, including the Board of Trustees of the Research Fund of the American Otological Society, the Research Committee of the American Academy of Ophthalmology and Otolaryngology (chairman), the American Academy of Ophthalmology and Otolaryngology (first vice-president), the Triological Society (vice-president), the Otosclerosis Study Group (president) of the American Academy of OORL, and the Board of Directors of the American Board of Otolaryngology.

Because of his outstanding contributions and leadership, he was unanimously selected to be the guest of honor at this symposium.

David J. Lim, M.D.

SPECIAL PRESENTATION

OBSERVATIONS ON MIDDLE EAR EFFUSION

The purpose of this report is to bring to your attention a few clinical findings and some results of basic investigative projects, all conducted in an effort to foster a better understanding of the problem of serous otitis media and its ultimate complications. The questions to be addressed are: "What areas are involved by the disease process?"; "How does spontaneous resolution occur?"; "What delivers the initial insult?"; "What factors may be responsible for a predisposition to the condition?"; and "What incites the formation of the retraction pocket?"

Location of the Disease Process

Careful, repeated examination of patients with middle ear effusion lead one to the conclusion that the bulk of the inflammatory reaction is in the epitympanum, the mastoid antrum, and the mastoid air cells, for x-ray studies of the mastoid process almost inevitably demonstrate clouding of the air cells. In addition, most of the fluid is to be found in the posterior portion of the mesotympanum when myringotomy is performed. Moreover, when the attack resolves without surgical intervention, the posterior half of the middle ear cavity is the last to be free of fluid, and the hearing remains depressed after the fluid is no longer apparent. Perhaps during this period the inflammatory process around the ossicles has not abated and their motion may be impeded. During mastoidectomy and epitympanotomy with removal and replacement of the posterior wall of the external auditory canal in patients with refractory effusion, one finds the most inflamed mucosa and exuberant granulation tissue in the antrum and epitympanum and the least in the anterior portion of the mesotympanum.[1] The latter becomes so involved only in the most advanced cases; thus, it may be that the mesotympanum serves merely as an overflow basin to hold the fluid that has actually been secreted by diseased tissue in the mastoid process. Additional proof of this thesis is presented in the section on the retraction pocket.

Spontaneous Resolution

Bortnick obstructed the eustachian tubes of animals, instilled radioactive material into the posterior bullar compartment, and was able to demonstrate this material in the venous blood.[2] This strongly suggests that the fluid may depart through absorption rather than through the eustachian tube in humans.

The Initial Insult

If, indeed, the secreting tissue is largely located in the epitympanum and antrum, perhaps the term "serous otitis media" is a misnomer, and one should speak rather of "epitympanomastoiditis." If so, what provokes the inflammation? Eustachian tube obstruction is frequently incriminated, but one can occasionally see serous fluid behind the tympanic membrane in the presence of a patulous eustachian tube. Numerous investigators have been able to provide an experimental model of effusion by cauterization, packing the lumen, or ligation of the eustachian tube, but the complications of retraction pocket, perforation of the tympanic membrane, and cholesteatoma have not been simulated.[3,4]

Infection has been postulated as the inciting factor,[5] but although positive cultures are reported by some investigators others have failed to obtain them.

Predisposing Factors

Many have noted a strong family history of middle ear disease, even relating to unilaterality. Perhaps some sort of primitive, infection-sensitive tissue present at birth persists in the epitympanum in these patients, and the slightest upper respiratory infection may extend to this area and serve to prod this tissue to misbehavior. During the aging and maturation process this tissue could disappear or become more resistant to infection resulting in a cessation of the problem in some instances when the patient enters his teens.

Observation of subjects with cleft palate will convince one that the incidence of middle ear effusion is far greater among them than in a noncleft-palate population of the same age group. In fact, the experimental model of effusion has been produced by palate division in cats.[6] The frequency of middle ear effusion among victims of Down's and Hurler's syndromes is so great that one is led to wonder why middle ear effusion is not included as a feature of each of them. Accidental or intentional excision of the eustachian cushion when adenoidectomy is performed all too frequently invites the appearance of effusion into the middle ear, but it is inevitably serous in character and not attended by retraction pocket, cholesteatoma formation, or tympanic membrane perforation.

Zimmerman recently presented a series of patients seen initially as examples of middle ear effusion, and each was found to have a primary cyst of the mastoid process in the absence of middle ear cystic extension or drumhead perforation.[7]

As time goes on one may see that a veritable farrago of other hitherto unrecognized phenomena may be responsible for middle ear effusion as we encounter it today.

The Retraction Pocket

The all but inevitable appearance of the pocket in the posterior-superior quadrant of the pars tensa lends additional credibility to the tenet that the largest share of the inflammatory process in so-called serous otitis media is epitympanic and antral, and it serves as a litmus test for further complication. It is assumed that diminished tympanic pressure is responsible for the pocket, and although it has been shown that bullar pressures did indeed fall when the cat's auditory tube was ligated, in no instance did tympanic membrane retraction ensue.[8] One is led to believe that cicatrix between the long crus of the incus and the tympanic membrane is to be blamed for the phenomenon of retraction, which eventually may move anteriorly and involve the entire tympanum, and the area of the eustachian orifice is the last to become affected. In time the adhesions thicken and reduction of the pocket by middle ear inflation becomes impossible. Probably periossicular scar tissue resulting from the inflammation in those areas leads to the state of ossicular fixation.

The Unanswered Questions

A number of other arcane features remain to be explained. For example, the mysterious disappearance of the lenticular process of the incus is a strange occurrence. Perhaps the inflammatory process has compromised the vascular supply of this structure, or erosive microcholesteatoma may be at work. The latter may arise in the retraction pocket because the dynamic migratory pattern of the tympanomeatal epithelium has been disturbed, and entrapment and moisture may lead to infection. Why are cleft palate and Down's and Hurler's syndrome victims more vulnerable to attacks of serous otitis media than those who are not so afflicted?

Obviously only a few unanswered queries have been aired here, and others too numerous to mention are awaiting your answers.

Gunnar O. Proud, M.D.

CONTENTS

Definitions and Classifications

Epidemiology and Natural History

Physiology and Pathophysiology

Anatomy and Pathology

Microbiology

Immunology

Biochemistry

Animal Models

Identification and Diagnosis

Prevention and Management

Medical Treatment Without Antibiotics

Medical Treatment Using Antibiotics

Surgical Management

Complications and Sequelae

DEFINITIONS AND CLASSIFICATIONS

STATE OF THE ART: DEFINITIONS AND CLASSIFICATIONS

CHARLES D. BLUESTONE, M.D.

On July 13, 1978, Dr. Ben Senturia convened a task force on definitions and classification in St. Louis, Missouri. The results of that meeting were presented at the Second International Symposium on Otitis Media with Effusion (1979) and were subsequently published in the proceedings of that meeting (Senturia et al, 1980). Immediately following the symposium, a workshop, sponsored by the National Institute of Neurological and Communicative Disorders and Stroke, was convened to identify the important research questions that arose following the presentations (Lim et al, 1980). An international group of authorities reviewed the recommendations of the task force. Their recommendations were the following.

DEFINITION OF TERMS

Otitis media: An *inflammation* of the middle ear (which may or may not be of infectious origin, in contrast to *infection,* which implies a microbiologic origin).

Effusion: Collection of fluid in the middle ear cavity.

Otorrhea: A discharge through a perforated tympanic membrane.

CLASSIFICATION OF TEMPORAL SEQUENCE

Acute: May include three phases: (1) Onset—may be short and rapid, or signs and symptoms may be subtle and onset slow and insidious; (2) full expression; and (3) resolution.

Chronic: Persistent beyond the expected course.

Subacute: The interval between the end of the acute phase and the beginning of the chronic process.

For our purposes, we arbitrarily consider the acute process to be the initial three weeks, the chronic process to begin at the ninth week following onset, and the subacute phase to be from the fourth week through the eighth week after onset.

CLASSIFICATION OF OTITIS MEDIA AND PERTINENT FACTORS INVOLVED

The diagnosis of otitis media is usually a presumptive one and clinically is usually made on the basis of history and otoscopic examination. A more complete diagnosis is possible if one obtains answers to the following seven questions; some of the answers will be available while others will not.

1. Is effusion or discharge (otorrhea) present and what are its characteristics?

First, the characteristics of the effusion or discharge may be evaluated by ocular inspection of the tympanic membrane and examination of the middle ear through the intact tympanic membrane, which will establish presumptive characterization. For example, in clinical diagnosis based on examination of the eardrum alone (without paracentesis), it is advantageous to characterize effusions presumptively as follows: (1) probably serous, (2) probably purulent, (3) probably mucoid, or (4) probably other.

Second, effusions can be classified and defined as: (1) Serous—a thin watery fluid, (2) purulent—puslike fluid, (3) mucoid—a thick, viscid, mucuslike fluid, (4) other—blood, cerebrospinal fluid, and so on.

Although most effusions may be mixed, for example, seromucoid or mucopurulent, for the purpose of simplicity of classification, physicians are expected to make a decision by gross examination as to which of the above categories is appropriate. Otherwise, the classification becomes so complex that it loses its practicality.

2. Is the tympanic membrane intact or perforated?

3. What is the time frame—acute (0 to 21 days), subacute (22 days to eight weeks), or chronic (over eight weeks).

4. What are the functional characteristics of the ear as determined by audiometry, tympanometry, or other means?

5. What are the microbiologic findings? In the case of positive cultures one needs to know whether only the usual laboratory techniques for bacterial growth and identification were employed or if more sophisticated techniques for anaerobic bacteria, viruses, mycoplasma, or chlamydia were also utilized.

6. What are the pathologic findings? It is generally true that the pathologic characteristics of acute otitis media can be distinguished from those of chronic otitis media, that is, in the acute state there are extensive leukocytic infiltrations and edematous swelling of the submucosa, whereas in chronic inflammation there is more round cell infiltration, extensive fibrosis, proliferation of the mucous membrane, and increased gland formation. It is also known that the middle ear mucosa from ears with mucoid effusions contains more secretory elements than those with serous effusions. However, the histopathologic and cytologic changes related to the specific infecting organisms are poorly established. Information from biopsy materials and from well-documented temporal bones with otitis media with effusion is still sketchy, particularly in the area of temporal sequence of the pathologic changes. Classification based on pathology or cytology alone cannot readily be used for clinical classification at this time.

7. What are the biochemical and immunochemical findings? It is difficult to determine the biochemical and immunochemical characteristics of the effusions without elaborate laboratory examination. These areas are in the investigative stage at this time.

GENERAL CATEGORIES OF OTITIS MEDIA

Some general categories of otitis media are as follows:

1. Otitis media without effusion or perforation of the tympanic membrane: acute, subacute, or chronic.

2. Otitis media with effusion, without perforation of the tympanic membrane: acute (serous, purulent, or other); subacute (serous, purulent, mucoid, or other); or chronic (serous, purulent, mucoid, or other).

3. Otitis media with perforation: acute (with discharge—purulent, serous, or other—or without discharge; subacute (with discharge—purulent, mucoid, serous, or other—or without discharge; or chronic (with discharge—purulent, mucoid, serous, or other).

IMPACT OF THE RECOMMENDATIONS

During the four years since these recommendations were made, there has been a great deal of controversy concerning the definition of the various clinical types and stages of otitis media. One of the major problems is the term "acute" which can refer to the severity or time of onset of the disease. Also, when there is acute infection in the middle ear, the term "acute otitis media with effusion" is not correct when acute otitis media presents without an effusion or when there is an acute perforation and discharge. Also, the terms "secretory," "serous," "nonsuppurative," and "mucoid" otitis media are still used when the middle ear effusion cannot be clinically determined due to an opaque tympanic membrane.

We should be more precise in the use of our terms. What is meant by the term "persistent" otitis media? Some authors use this term to mean chronic otitis media with effusion, while others use it to describe the subacute stage. It is proper to describe an effusion as being persistent for a certain duration, such as "persistent otitis media with effusion of two months' duration." What is meant by the term "impacted" fluid? Should we use the term "fluid" or "effusion"? Does "middle ear effusion" mean the same as "otitis media with effusion''? Some authors use these terms interchangeably. A middle ear effusion is the collection of a liquid in the middle ear secondary to inflammation. What is catarrh? Should this be the term or should it be rhinorrhea? Should we still consider eight weeks' duration of a middle ear effusion as chronic? Should we extend this to three months, since we have new data on natural history? At this time it is imperative that all investigators and authors specifically define the disease they are studying or describing.

RECOMMENDED CLINICAL CLASSIFICATION

The following broad classification is an attempt to resolve this controversy while maintaining the concepts of the previous recommendations.

Otitis Media without Effusion

In certain cases only inflammation of the middle ear mucous membrane and tympanic membrane will be present, without any evidence of a middle ear effusion (Table 1). Clinically, the pneumatic otoscopic appearance of the tympanic membrane will reveal *myringitis,* in which there is usually erythema and opacification of the eardrum but relatively normal mobility to applied positive and negative pressure. Blebs or bullae may be present when the disease is acute. Otitis media without effusion is usually present in the early stages of acute otitis media but may also be found in the stage of resolution of acute otitis media or may even be chronic. Evidence for the existence of this type of otitis media has been provided by the observations of temporal bone histopathologic specimens. The absence of a middle ear effusion when a myringotomy is performed in the presence of otitis media has provided clinical proof that this condition exists in certain cases.

TABLE 1 Clinical Classification of Otitis Media

	Synonyms
Otitis media without effusion	Myringitis
Acute otitis media	Suppurative Purulent Bacterial
Otitis media with effusion	Secretory Nonsuppurative Serous Mucoid
Chronic otitis media	Suppurative Purulent

Acute Otitis Media

The rapid and short onset of signs and symptoms of inflammation in the middle ear is termed acute otitis media. Synonyms such as acute *suppurative* or *purulent* otitis media are acceptable. One or more of the following are present: otalgia (or pulling of the ear in the young infant), fever, or the recent onset of irritability. The tympanic membrane is full or bulging, is opaque, and has limited or no mobility to pneumatic otoscopy—indicative of a middle ear effusion. Erythema of the eardrum is an inconsistent finding. The acute onset of ear pain, fever, and a purulent discharge (otorrhea) through a perforation of the tympanic membrane (or tympanostomy tube) would also be evidence of acute otitis media. Following an episode of acute otitis media, a middle ear effusion that persists for longer than three months is termed chronic otitis media with effusion.

Otitis Media with Effusion

The presence of a relatively asymptomatic middle ear effusion has many synonyms, such as ''secretory,'' ''nonsuppurative,'' or ''serous'' otitis media, but the most acceptable term is ''otitis media with effusion.'' Since the effusion may be serous (transudate), the term ''secretory'' may not be correct in all cases. Likewise, the term ''nonsuppurative'' may not be correct, since a middle ear effusion may contain bacteria and may even be purulent. The term ''serous otitis media'' is appropriate if an amber or bluish effusion can be visualized through a translucent tympanic membrane; however, the most frequent otoscopic finding is opacification of the tympanic membrane that makes assessment of the type of effusion—that is, serous, mucoid, or purulent—impossible. Pneumatic otoscopy will frequently reveal either a retracted or convex tympanic membrane in which the mobility is impaired. However, fullness or even bulging may be visualized. In addition, an air-fluid level, or bubbles, or both may be observed through a translucent tympanic membrane. The duration (not the severity) of the effusion can be divided into acute (less than three weeks), subacute (three weeks to three months) and chronic (greater than three months). The most important distinction between this type of disease and acute otitis media (acute ''suppurative'' otitis media) is that the signs and symptoms of acute infection, for example, otalgia or fever, are lacking in otitis media with effusion, but hearing loss may be present in both conditions. This distinction is important because the management plan may be different.

TABLE 2 Intratemporal Complications and Sequelae of Otitis Media

Hearing loss
Perforation of the tympanic membrane
acute
chronic
Chronic suppurative otitis media
Retraction pocket
Cholesteatoma
Adhesive otitis media
Tympanosclerosis
Ossicular discontinuity
Ossicular fixation
Mastoiditis
acute
chronic
Petrositis
Labyrinthitis
acute
chronic
Facial paralysis
Cholesterol granuloma

TABLE 3 Intracranial Suppurative Complications of Otitis Media and Mastoiditis

Meningitis
Extradural abscess
Subdural empyema
Focal otitic encephalitis
Brain abscess
Lateral sinus thrombosis
Otitic hydrocephalus

A classification of complications and sequelae of otitis media should also be agreed upon. Tables 2 and 3 show a proposed classification. It is important to classify these terms, since these conditions are directly related to otitis media with effusion.

Supported in part by grant #NS16337 from the National Institute of Neurological and Communicative Disorders and Stroke.

BIBLIOGRAPHY

Senturia BH, Bluestone CD, Lim DJ, Saunders WH: Proceedings of the Second International Symposium: Recent advances in otitis media with effusion. Ann Otol Rhinol Laryngol 89(Suppl 68), 1980

Lim DJ, Bluestone CD, Saunders WH, Senturia BH: Report of research conference: Recent advances in otitis media with effusion. Ann Otol Rhinol Laryngol 89(Suppl 69), 1980

EPIDEMIOLOGY AND NATURAL HISTORY

EPIDEMIOLOGY AND NATURAL HISTORY OF OTITIS MEDIA

G. SCOTT GIEBINK, M.D.

Otitis media is a worldwide child health problem, particularly among infants and young children. The magnitude of this problem has been estimated from point-prevalence studies, from retrospective audits in certain populations, and from a few large prospective studies. Over the past ten years we have become increasingly familiar with the frequencies and distribution, that is, the epidemiology, of otitis media, and our understanding of the natural history of otitis media is increasing. This knowledge has caused us to ask specific questions regarding pathogenic mechanisms. An understanding of the epidemiology and natural history of otitis media provides a cornerstone for building solid research designs in clinical and basic science studies of otitis media.

FACTORS IN OTITIS MEDIA

Age

Otitis media is predominantly a disease of infants and young children. Heller was one of the first to point out the predilection of otitis media for affecting young children: 35 percent of 1031 children with otitis media in his practice had experienced their first episode before age 2, and 60 percent had experienced an episode by their fourth birthday.[1] In an extensive survey of otitis media in Alaskan Eskimo children, Kaplan and colleagues reported that 60 percent experienced their first episode of otitis media with otorrhea by age 2.[2] In a study of 488 private practice patients in Alabama, Howie and associates reported that 49 percent had their first otitis media episode by age 1 and 61 percent by age 2.[3] Most recently, Teele and colleagues reported their experience in following more than 2500 children from birth to age 3 in Boston; 47 percent had their first otitis media episode by 1 year and 71 percent by 3 years.[4]

As might be expected, the impact of this disease on medical practice is staggering. In the Boston study, approximately one physician visit in three for children during the first three years of life was for middle ear disease, and three-fourths of follow-up visits were for middle ear disease.[5] After the preschool years, the frequency of otitis media reaches a plateau during the elementary school years at 4 to 5 per year.[3,6] The greater susceptibility of young children to otitis media may be due to the increased frequency of respiratory infection at this age; to an immature immune response to respiratory pathogens; postural feeding practices, such as night-time bottles; or to less competent eustachian tube function.

Sex

Most studies indicate a somewhat greater frequency of otitis media among males (61 to 70 percent of acute otitis media cases), although a few studies have reported no sex difference.[7] Similarly, the prevalence of recurrent acute otitis media and chronic otitis media with effusion (OME) has been reported to be higher in males (59 to 72 percent). The basis for the male predilection has not been investigated and may relate to an overall sex difference in the rate of childhood infection.

Race

A great deal of information has been accumulated on the prevalence of this disease in American blacks, American Indians, Eskimos, and whites. Eskimos, American Indians, and Hispanic children have an incidence even higher than American whites, and otorrhea has been particularly prevalent in Eskimos and American Indians; blacks have a lower incidence than white.[4,8–10] These racial differences may be explained by differences in the length, width, and angle of the bony eustachian tube in American blacks, whites, and Indians.[11]

However, other sociocultural factors may also explain differences in type and severity of otitis media.

Socioeconomic and Cultural

Certainly, factors that cause a delay in seeking medical attention, crowding, suboptimal nutrition, poor hygiene, inadequate treatment compliance, and inattention to symptoms may increase the incidence, type, and severity of otitis media. A number of studies have provided data to support these speculations. In the Boston study of urban children, the incidence of otitis media was greater in homes with many members than in those with few members.[4] Also, children of a lower socioeconomic class, who attended a neighborhood health clinic, had more visits for otitis media during the first year (32 percent) than did upper socioeconomic class children in a private practice (21 percent).[5] However, Wiet and associates reported no correlation between family size or sanitary conditions and incidence of otitis media in Eskimos.[1] Yet Beal found that increased living standards and medical care in an Alaskan native community were associated with a reduction in the rate of chronic otitis media.[2] Similar socioeconomic factors would be expected to contribute to the high incidence of otitis media in American Indians, yet Spivey and Hirschhord reported that the prevalence of otitis media did not change when American Indian children were adopted into middle class foster homes, suggesting that race and genetic risk factors outweigh socioeconomic factors.[13]

Genetic

Three studies have identified family history of middle ear disease as a risk factor for otitis media. Teele and colleagues found that children with a positive sibling or parent history of otitis media had a higher incidence of the disease than children from families with negative family histories.[4] Kraemer and associates recently confirmed this association in a case-control study: the risk of persistent OME was nearly two times higher for children with a positive history than for those with a negative family history of middle ear disease.[14] In this volume, Visscher and associates report similar results that show an association between occurrence of acute otitis media and positive family history of middle ear disease using the case-control design (page 15). Clearly, studies are needed to clarify the apparent genetic predisposition to otitis media.

Season

It has been evident from clinical descriptions of otitis media for over 40 years that this disease follows a seasonal distribution in cold climates which peaks between October and April and declines remarkably during the summer months.[1,7,15] Although the epidemiologic association between otitis media and upper respiratory infection has been apparent for some time, only recently have Henderson and coworkers shown a clear association between certain viral respiratory pathogens, notably respiratory syncytial virus, influenza, and adenovirus, and acute otitis media.[16] These infections also impair eustachian tube function and alter middle ear ventilation, suggesting that this epidemiologic observation may provide a clue to the pathogenesis of otitis media. Unfortunately, careful studies of the prevalence and severity of otitis media have not been performed in warm climates while controlling for other variables, such as respiratory virus infection.

Environment

Socioeconomic, cultural, seasonal, and age factors may independently affect a child's environment, which may in turn influence the prevalence of otitis media. Kraemer and associates have shown that the presence of cigarette smokers in a child's household increases the risk of persistent otitis media with effusion 2.8 times.[14] In addition, the study by Visscher and colleagues (page 14) indicates that day care exposure, considering both hours of exposure and number of children in the center, significantly influences the risk of acute otitis media. Certainly, a group environment for preschool children might intensify exposure to respiratory pathogens, confounding the analysis of several possible interdependent risk factors.

Nutrition

Nutrition, age, socioeconomic and cultural factors are interrelated. Nonetheless, among Eskimo infants, Schaefer reported that the incidence of chronic otitis media was lower in breast- than in bottle-fed babies.[17] However, a similar relationship was not observed by Cunningham in American whites.[18] More information is required on both nutritional content and feeding practices to evaluate these entities as risk factors for otitis media.

RELATED DISORDERS

Paradise and colleagues have emphasized the universality of otitis media with effusion among children with cleft palate,[19] and Schwartz and Schwartz reported an extremely high prevalence of OME in children with Down's syndrome.[20] American Indians experience an increased incidence of cleft palate (2.5 percent versus 1.3 percent in whites), adding another confounding variable to considerations of race and socioeconomic status as risk factors.

Many clinicians have suspected that allergy is a risk factor for otitis media, yet few biochemical investigations of middle ear effusion from patients with OME demonstrate biochemical or histologic evidence of an allergic response in the middle ear. Clinical studies also report conflicting results. Virolainen and coworkers found no correlation between a personal or family history of allergy and OME.[6] Yet the case-control studies reported by Kraemer and associates[14] and Visscher and associates (page 14) both suggest that the allergic or atopic child is at increased risk of otitis media. The answer to this question awaits large, carefully conducted case-control studies in different populations with strict attention to documenting allergy as well as OME and biochemical and immunologic studies of allergic children with OME designed to investigate the middle ear response of these subjects.

COMPLICATIONS AND SEQUELAE

Whether persistent otitis media with effusion represents a complication of acute otitis media or merely the natural history of the acute episode remains largely undetermined. Clearly, the ability to document OME objectively using the pneumatic otoscope and screening tympanometry has become available to all practitioners at a reasonable cost during the past several years.[21] Teele and associates and Schwartz and associates have documented the natural history of effusion disappearance after an acute episode.[4,22] After the first episode of acute otitis media, 70 percent of children still had OME at two weeks, 40 percent at four weeks, 20 percent at eight weeks, and 10 percent at 12 weeks.[4] Among an unselected sample of children with acute otitis media, Schwartz and associates reported a very similar rate of effusion disappearance: 51 percent with OME at two weeks, 23 percent at four weeks, 15 percent at six weeks, 13 percent at eight weeks, 9.5 percent at 12 weeks, and 6 percent at 16 weeks.[22] According to the classification scheme adopted at the second International Symposium, these data indicate that 10 percent of children develop chronic OME (that is, OME persisting for at least 12 weeks) after an episode of acute otitis media.[23]

The timing and number of previous otitis media episodes seem to be two important factors in identifying the child who develops recurrent and chronic OME. In 1957, the British Medical Research Council's report on otitis media noted that recurrent otitis media attacks were increased with each successive attack.[24] Howie and colleagues reported that children who experienced two or more otitis media episodes during the first year of life had twice as many subsequent episodes as the child who had one or no episodes in the first year.[3] Wiet and colleagues also observed that the risk of recurrent otitis media was increased among American Indian children who had their first episode before age 1 year.[10]

Shurin and associates reported that the risk of persistent OME was nearly four times higher in children less than 2 years old with otitis media compared with older children.[25] However, sex, bacterial origin of the otitis episode, type of antibiotic therapy, and history of prior otitis were not risk factors for persistence of OME in this study. In contrast, Kraemer and coworkers reported a striking association between prior otitis history and risk for persistent OME: The risk of persistent disease was increased 6.9 times in children with one to two prior episodes, 8.1 times in children with three to six episodes, and 165.7 times in children with more than six episodes.[14] Birth weight, early feeding patterns, and exposure to other children did not emerge as risk factors for chronic OME.

The incidence of chronic otitis media in the population has also been investigated from prevalence studies of tympanic membrane pathology. A study of 767 elderly men in Gothenburg, Sweden, revealed 5 percent with chronic otitis media, 13 percent with atrophic membrane scars, and 19 percent with tympanosclerosis; 63 percent had normal ear examinations.[26] The prevalence of tympanic membrane perforation in the American Indian population is 8 to 10 percent.[27]

We have investigated the effusion characteristics of children with chronic OME. Among 898 children with clinically manifest chronic OME, 48 percent had mucoid effusion, 10 percent had serous effusion, and 7 percent had seromucoid effusion at operation; 36 percent had no effusion, although middle ear mucosal pathologic findings were evident.[28] Mucoid effusion was more common in younger than older children, and serous effusion was more common in older children. Mucoid otitis media was more often bilateral than serous or seromucoid disease, and mucoid otitis media persisted longer.

The most frequent suppurative complication of otitis media, acute mastoiditis, has largely disappeared with the introduction and widespread use of effective antimicrobial regimens. Yet it is worthwhile to recall that the prevalence of this complication before the introduction of antibiotics was on the order of 3 to 20 percent.[1,29,30] At present, the incidence of acute mastoiditis complicating acute otitis media has been reported to be 0.2 to 2 percent.[24,31] Thus, the considerable decline in the use of myringotomy in cases of acute otitis media has not been accompanied by an increase in the occurrence of mastoiditis. Whether early myringotomy might alter the rate of disappearance of effusion in antibiotic children has not been tested. The sequelae of greatest concern to physicians, parents, and educators is the apparent association between frequent otitis media during early childhood and impaired speech and language development. The current thinking on this subject has been summarized by Menyuk[32]; suffice it to say here that children who experience recurrent otitis media or chronic OME during their early years show language development that differs from children not experiencing this disease. The precise nature of this development in these children must be carefully documented, an explanation must be sought, and information regarding compensatory or "catch-up" development must be obtained.

SUMMARY

We have learned a great deal about the epidemiology and natural history of otitis media since the first international symposium on otitis media was convened in 1975. The problem of understanding factors that affect frequency and distribution of this disease is immense, owing to the multifactorial etiologic factors in the disease. Because of this multifactorial nature, otitis media is not an easy disease to describe. Most reports to date have suffered from certain design inadequacies, including variation in completeness of record audit, in the definition of otitis media, in differentiating acute from recurrent and chronic disease, in the application of adequate epidemiologic methods, in the description of populating characteristics, and in the validation of physician examiners. Statistical design has for the most part been inadequate in these studies; multivariate analysis and controls for confounding variables have rarely been used. Nonetheless, our epidemiologic colleagues have become increasingly interested in otitis media, and their participation in future studies will be essential to bringing us a fuller understanding of otitis media.

This study was supported in part by grant numbers NS-14538 from the National Institute of Neurological and Communicative Disorders and Stroke and AI-17160 from the National Institute of Allergy and Infectious Diseases.

REFERENCES

1. Heller G: A statistical study of otitis media in children. II. The antibiotic era. J Pediatr 42:185, 1953
2. Kaplan CJ, Fleshman JK, Bender TR: Long-term effects of otitis media: A ten-year cohort study of Alaskan Eskimo children. Pediatr 52:577, 1973
3. Howie VM, Ploussard JG, Sloyer J: The "otitis-prone" condition. Am J Dis Child 129:676, 1975
4. Teele DW, Rosner BA, Klein JO: Epidemiology of otitis media in children. Ann Otol Rhinol Laryngol 89(Suppl 68):5, 1980
5. Teele DW, Klein, JO, Rosner B, et al: Middle ear disease and the practice of pediatrics: Burden during the first five years of life. JAMA 249:1026, 1983
6. Virolainen E, Puhakka H, Aantaa E, et al: Prevalence of secretory otitis media in seven to eight-year-old school children. Ann Otol Rhinol Laryngol 89(Suppl 68):7, 1980
7. Paradise JL: Otitis media in infants and children. Pediatr 65:917, 1980
8. Griffith T: Epidemiology of otitis media: An interracial study. Laryngoscope 89:22, 1979
9. Bush PJ, Rabin DL: Racial differences in encounter rates for otitis media. Pediatr Res 14:1115, 1980
10. Wiet RJ, DeBlanc GB, Stewart J, Weider DJ: Natural history of otitis media in the American Native. Ann Otol Rhinol Laryngol 89(Suppl 68):14, 1980
11. Doyle WJ: A functiono-anatomic description of eustachian tube vector relations in four ethnic populations: An osteologic study. Doctoral dissertation, University of Pittsburgh, Pittsburgh, PA, 1977
12. Beal DD: Prevention of otitis media in the Alaska native. In Glorig A, Gerwin KS (eds): *Otitis Media: Proceedings of the National Conference.* Callier Hearing and Speech Center, Dallas, 1970. Springfield, IL: Charles C Thomas, 1972, pp 158–162

13. Spivey G, Hirschhord N: A migrant study of adopted Apache children. Johns Hopkins Med J 40:43, 1977
14. Kraemer MJ, Richardson MA, Weiss NS, et al: Risk factors for persistent middle ear effusions: Otitis media, catarrh, cigarette smoke exposure, and atopy. JAMA 249:1022, 1983
15. Brownlee RC Jr, DeLoache WR, Cowarn CC Jr: Otitis media in children: Incidence, treatment and prognosis in pediatric practice. J Pediatr 75:636, 1969
16. Henderson FW, Collier AM, Sanyal MA, et al: A longitudinal study of respiratory viruses and bacteria in the etiology of acute otitis media with effusion. N Engl J Med 306:1377, 1982
17. Schaefer O: Otitis media and bottle feeding: An epidemiological study of infant feeding habits and incidence of recurrent and chronic middle ear disease in Canadian Eskimos. Can J Public Health 62:478, 1971
18. Cunningham AS: Morbidity in breast-fed and artificially fed infants. J Pediatr 90:726, 1977
19. Paradise JL, Bluestone CD, Felder H: The universality of otitis media in 50 infants with cleft palate. Pediatr 44:35, 1969
20. Schwartz DM, Schwartz RH: Acoustic impedance and otoscopic findings in young children with Down's syndrome. Arch Otolaryngol 104:652, 1978
21. Paradise JL: Tympanometry. N Engl J Med 307:1074, 1982
22. Schwartz RH, Schwartz DM, Rodriguez WJ: Otitis media with effusion (OME): Natural course in untreated children. Pediatr Res 15:556, 1981 (Abstr 687)
23. Senturia BH, Bluestone CD, Klein JO, et al: Report of the ad hoc committee on definition and classification of otitis media and otitis media with effusion. Ann Otol Rhinol Laryngol 89(Suppl 68):3, 1980
24. Medical Research Council of Great Britain: Acute otitis media in general practice. Lancet II:510, 1957
25. Shurin PA, Pelton SI, Donner A: Persistence of middle ear effusion after acute otitis media in children. N Engl J Med 300:1121, 1979
26. Rudin R, Holmquist J: Frequency of pathologic changes in the middle ear. Ann Otol Rhinol Laryngol 89(Suppl 68):11, 1980
27. Zonis RD: Chronic otitis media in the southwestern American Indian. Arch Otolaryngol 88:361, 1968
28. Giebink GS, Le CT, Paparella MM: Epidemiology of otitis media with effusion in children. Arch Otolaryngol 108:563, 1982
29. Bakwin H, Jacobziner H: Prevention of purulent otitis media in infants. J Pediatr 14:730, 1939
30. Hamberger CA: Uber die behandlung der otitis media acuta und gewisser otoganer komplikationen mit sulfonilamid-derivaten. Acta Otolarynol 46(Suppl):1, 1942
31. Diamant M, Diamant B: Abuse and timing of use of antibiotics in acute otitis media. Arch Otolaryngol 100:226, 1974
32. Menyuk P: Design factors in the assessment of language development in children with otitis media. Ann Otol Rhinol Laryngol 88(Suppl 60):78, 1979

OCCURRENCE OF AND RISK FACTORS IN ACUTE OTITIS MEDIA

JUHANI PUKANDER, M.D., MARKKU SIPILÄ, M.D.,
and PEKKA KARMA, M.D.

Acute otitis media (AOM) is one of the most frequent infections in children and has been found to account for every third office visit in pediatric practice.[1] The total number of otitis attacks seems to be continually increasing, and a high incidence of recurrence, especially during the first few years of life, is typical of the disease.[2]

The aim of this study was to evaluate the present occurrence of acute otitis media in Finland on the basis of visits to doctors' offices and to analyze the risk factors that predispose to the disease.

MATERIALS AND METHODS

All cases of AOM seen by a doctor were documented in different areas in Finland over a 12-month period, from June 1, 1978, to May 31, 1979. The total population of all the areas on December 31, 1978, was 146,822.

For a diagnosis of AOM there had to be both acute symptoms (at least one of the following: earache, ear-rubbing, restless sleep, irritability, fever, or other acute respiratory symptoms) and suggestive otoscopic signs (redness and/or outward bulging of the drum or, when pneumatic otoscopy was done, suspicion of effusion). Acute otorrhea alone (through a spontaneously perforated drum or via a tympanostomy tube) was also sufficient to make the diagnosis.

From these otitis patients, 134 children up to 4 years of age were chosen for closer inspection of the risk indicators of AOM. A randomized, age-adjusted, nonotitis control (a child without experience of AOM during his or her life) was located for every child with otitis. The parents of the 268 children in the study were given a questionnaire asking about possible risk indicators. Statistical significance of the results was analyzed against the 0.1 normal standard distribution.

RESULTS

Incidence

During the one-year study period 4582 patients suffered from 6518 episodes of AOM, giving an annual incidence rate of 4.44 percent of the population at risk. The residence-adjusted incidence rate for the whole Finnish population was 4.08 percent. Among children under 16 years of age the incidence rate was 16.6 percent and among children under 10 it was 25.3 percent.

A striking seasonal variation was found in the occurrence of AOM, in that the frequency of attacks was highest in January (13.3 percent) and lowest (3.5 percent) in July.

Age of Otitis Patients

The highest annual incidence (51.4 percent) was during the second year of life. However, when incidence was estimated at ages less than 2 years, in half-year periods, the highest incidence—73.5 per 100 child-years—was found in the age group of 6 to 11 months (Table 1). The mean age of otitis patients was 4 years 9 months and the median age was 2 years 9 months.

TABLE 1 Annual Incidence of Acute Otitis Media by Age

	Annual Incidence Rate per 100 Person-Years		
Age (mo/yrs)	*Males*	*Females*	*Total*
0–5	18.1	18.1	18.1
6–11	92.5	58.1	75.5
12–17	47.6	50.2	48.9
18–23	55.4	42.6	49.1
2	35.4	37.6	36.5
3	30.5	27.2	28.9
4	21.6	26.5	23.9
5	15.5	19.2	17.2
6	13.3	11.2	12.2
7	10.5	9.7	10.1
8	8.9	5.6	7.3
9	5.3	6.3	5.8
10	3.0	3.0	3.0
11	2.4	4.3	3.2
12	1.8	2.7	2.3
13	2.6	1.1	1.9
14	2.6	2.9	2.8
15	2.6	1.9	2.3
≥16	0.19	0.30	0.25

Age at the Primary Attack and Cumulative Incidence

The proportion of children without previous attacks prior to the index attack (that is, the first documented attack during the study year) declined sharply with increasing age, especially during the first two years of life. The proportion of children without previous experience of AOM and the cumulative incidence are inversely related. In the present study only 15 percent of the index attacks were the primary ones among 9-year-old children. This means that 85 percent of the otitis children had experienced AOM before their tenth birthday. When the whole population of children at risk was taken into account, the cumulative incidence was 75 percent before the tenth, 50 percent before the third, and 28 percent before the second birthday (Table 2).

TABLE 2 Cumulative Incidence of AOM by Age

Age (mo/yrs)	*Without Experience of AOM (%)*	*With Experience of AOM (%)*
0–5	94	6
6–11	72	28
12–17	63	37
18–23	56	44
2	50	50
3	43	57
4	38	62
5	34	66
6	31	69
7	27	73
8	26	74
9	25	75

Recurrent Attacks

Among 4337 children 15 years of age or younger, the mean number of recurrent attacks per child-year was 0.88. This denotes a mean interval of 1.14 years from the index attack to the recurrence. The highest tendency to recurrence was during the second year of life (about 1.5 recurrent attacks per child-year), with a subsequent decrease by increasing age. Twenty-eight percent of children with otitis developed additional episodes within the study year: 18 percent once, 7 percent twice, and 3 percent three or more times.

Risk Factors

Sex

The total incidence of 4.84 percent among males was higher than the 4.07 percent among females ($p < 0.001$). Boys under age 2 accounted for this sex difference. Boys experienced multiple episodes significantly more often ($p < 0.001$) than girls during the first two years of life, and boys experienced their primary attacks significantly earlier ($p < 0.001$) than girls. The mean age and the median age were also significantly lower ($p < 0.001$) among boys.

Place of Residence and Type of Housing

Children living in urban areas contracted AOM significantly more often than children living in rural areas, especially during the first five years of life. The type of housing affected the likelihood of contracting AOM. Episodes, especially recurrent episodes, were more numerous ($p < 0.001$) among children living in apartments than those living in houses.

Day Care

The type of day care arrangements had a marked influence on the liability of a child to contract AOM. The risk increased ($p < 0.001$) in the following order: It was lowest among children cared for in their own homes with only their own siblings; intermediate among children cared for in family day care homes with children from other families; and highest among children attending community day care centers.

Breast-feeding

The duration of breast-feeding showed a negative correlation ($p < 0.05$) with the child's liability to contract AOM; this was especially true with recurrent attacks. Fewer recurrences were found among those who had been breast-fed longer than six months.

Miscellaneous

Atopic diathesis predisposed a child significantly ($p < 0.001$) to AOM. Those who suffered most often from repeated respiratory infections were also more liable ($p < 0.001$) to contract AOM. No correlation was found between the otitis history or smoking habits of the parents and the occurrence of AOM in their children.

CONCLUSIONS

Incidence

The annual incidence of AOM seems to have been increasing during the last decades. The incidence rate of 4.44 percent in the present study is higher than rates reported earlier from Great Britain.[3] This alteration might well be a real change in the occurrence of AOM in different times, but bias in study designs might also affect the result. Moreover, the bacteriology of AOM has changed considerably during the last 25 years,[4] and this might also be reflected in the incidence figures.

Age of Otitis Patients and Cumulative Incidence

Most attacks of AOM nowadays are concentrated very strikingly in the youngest age groups. In the present study there was a distinct period from 6 to 11 months of age when otitis was most prevalent by far. Many other recent studies indicate a similar age distribution of AOM patients.[5,6] The most obvious reason for this peak in incidence at about the first birthday is the relatively low concentration of anti-infective immunoglobulins of an infant during the first years of life, with the exception of the first 6 months, owing to the intrauterine transmission of these protecting agents.[7]

The probability that a child has had an experience of AOM increases very sharply during the first years of life. Most children in many studies have had at least one ear infection before their teens,[2,8] confirming that there are only a few children who escape an episode of AOM during childhood.

Recurrent Attacks

In the present study 28 percent of children with index attack experienced an additional attack during the study year; the highest recurrence rate was the second year of life, and the mean number of otitis attacks per child-year was 0.88. Very similar figures (0.7 to 0.9) have been presented previously,[9,10] and the conclusion is that AOM tends to recur very easily, especially among the youngest children.

Risk Factors

Consistent with the results of the present study, boys are found to be more susceptible than girls to AOM.[11] The reason for this is not known at present.

Most episodes occurred in winter. The most obvious reason for this is that AOM very often is a sequela of a viral respiratory infection, and the occurrence of respiratory infections is highest during the cold months of the year. Thus, season plays a very important role in occurrence of AOM.[3,9]

Children in the present study living in urban areas contracted AOM significantly more often than those living in the country. The reason for this is considered to be greater population density, since more people (and especially those who live in apartments) are exposed to the respiratory infections that may precede AOM, and urban children also attend day care centers more often than rural children.[12]

Atopic children have been found to suffer more often from viral upper respiratory infections,[13] which are known to precede AOM very often.[9,14] Furthermore, swelling of the mucous membranes and the accumulation of leukocytes in the lumen of the eustachian tube may disturb its drainage, thus promoting retention of effusion inside the middle ear cleft.[15]

Breast-feeding is found to protect a baby against infections,[16] and this is believed to happen by the transmission of specific immunoglobulins.[17] Opinions on the protective effect of breast-feeding against AOM are contradictory, however; some reports found no correlation between the duration of breast-feeding and the frequency of AOM,[12,18] whereas Schaefer[19] reported the lowest occurrence among those breast-fed longest, which is consistent with the results of our study.

Finally, it has been shown that children attending day care nurseries contract AOM more often than children cared for in their own homes.[12] In addition, Strangert[20] reported about equal frequencies of AOM in family day care and community day care centers. These findings, with the results of the present study indicating the lowest frequency of AOM among home-care children, altogether confirm the conclusion that the larger the number of children in the day care location, the higher the risk of contracting AOM.

REFERENCES

1. Schwartz RH, Schwartz DM: Acute otitis media: Diagnosis and drug therapy. Drugs 19:107, 1980.
2. Teele DW, Klein JO, Rosner BA: Epidemiology of otitis media in children. Ann Otol Rhinol Laryngol 89 (Suppl 68): 5, 1980.
3. Medical Research Council's Working-party for Research in General Practice: Acute otitis media in general practice. Lancet 510, 1957.
4. Herberts G, Jeppsson P-H, Nylén O, Branefors-Helander P: Acute otitis media. Pract Otorhinolaryngol 33:191, 1971.
5. Howie VM: Natural history of otitis media. Ann Otol Rhinol Laryngol 84:67, 1975.
6. Biles RW, Buffler PA, O'Donnell AA: Epidemiology of otitis media: A community study. Am J Publ Health 70 (6):593, 1980.
7. Janeway CA: The immunologic system, allergy and related diseases. In Nelson, WE (ed): *Textbook of Pediatrics*. WB Saunders Company, Philadelphia: pp 473–480.
8. Virolainen E, Puhakka H, Aantaa E, et al: Prevalence of secretory otitis media in seven to eight year old school children. Ann Otol Rhinol Laryngol 89 (Suppl 68): 7, 1980.
9. Reed D, Brody J: Otitis media in urban Alaska. Alaska Medicine 8:64, 1966.
10. Bäckström-Järvinen L, Tiisala R, Kantero R-L, Hallman H: Illness among normal Finnish children during the first five years of life. Ann Paediatr Fenn 12:13, 1966.
11. McEldowney D, Kessner DM: Review of the literature: Epidemiology of otitis media. In Glorig A, Kenneth, GS (eds): *Otitis Media. Proceedings of the National Conference*. Dallas, Tx: Callier Hearing and Speech Center, pp 11–48
12. Vinther B, Elbrønd CB: A population study of otitis media in childhood. Acta Otolaryngol (Stockh) Suppl 360:135, 1979.
13. Minor TE, Baker JW, Dick EC, et al: Greater frequency of viral respiratory infections in asthmatic children compared with their nonasthmatic siblings. J Pediatr 85:472, 1974.
14. Klein JO, Teele DW: Isolation of viruses and mycoplasmas from middle ear effusions: a review. Ann Otol Rhinol Laryngol 75 (Suppl 26): 140, 1976.

15. Yamashita T, Okazaki N, Kumazawa T: Relation between nasal and middle ear allergy. Experimental study. Ann Otol (Suppl 68): 147, 1980.
16. Cunningham AS: Morbidity in breast-fed and artificially fed infants. J Pediatr 90:726, 1977.
17. Welsh JK, May JT: Anti-infective properties of breast milk. J Pediatr 94:1, 1979.
18. Kjellman J-J: Atopic diseases in seven-year-old children. Incidence in relation to family history. Acta Paediatr 66:465, 1977.
19. Schaefer O: Otitis media and bottle-feeding. Can J Public Health 62:478, 1971.
20. Strangert K: Otitis media in young children in different types of day-care. Scand J Infect Dis 9:119, 1977.

A CASE-CONTROL STUDY EXPLORING POSSIBLE RISK FACTORS FOR CHILDHOOD OTITIS MEDIA

WENDY VISSCHER, M.P.H., JACK S. MANDEL, Ph.D., M.P.H.,
PAUL B. BATALDEN, M.D., JOYCE N. RUSS, R.N., and G. SCOTT GIEBINK, M.D.

Otitis media is an extremely common childhood disease. Its recurrent nature and the fact that it may lead to surgery or to central nervous system infection make it "the largest single cause of morbidity with possible sequelae in children."[1] In addition, repeated episodes of otitis media in early life may lead to developmental or educational delays due to transient or permanent hearing loss.[2]

Despite the impact of otitis media on the health of children, few analytic epidemiologic studies have been done to examine possible etiologic factors in this disease. Studies to date have been primarily descriptive, giving characteristics of children with otitis media but using no control group for comparison. Most of these studies have been incidence studies in which the number of episodes of otitis media per child over a specified period of time was determined, often broken down by age, sex, or race. Incidence rates were obtained either by retrospective record review[3–5] or by following a group of children over time.[6–8]

The analytic epidemiologic studies that have been done include one cohort study in which children in day care and home care situations were followed and their rates of otitis media compared over an eight-month period,[9] and two case-control studies, one that looked only at supine bottle feeding[10] and another that looked at family size, day care, and socioeconomic status.[11] The current study was designed to assess the relative importance of a number of potential risk factors for otitis media, including recent upper respiratory tract infection, bottle-feeding, day care exposure, allergies, large family size, and a positive family history of ear infections. The case-control approach was utilized, and various problems encountered in the use of this design in the study of otitis media will be discussed.

MATERIALS AND METHODS

The study population consisted of patients who visited a large pediatrics group practice in the Minneapolis area for their usual medical care. This pediatrics clinic is staffed by 16 pediatricians and four pediatric nurse practitioners who see approximately 1000 children each week. During a two-week period in February 1982, every parent who brought a child into the clinic for any reason was asked to fill out a questionnaire that elicited information on the postulated risk factors. The child was then examined and the pediatrician indicated on the back of the questionnaire whether the child (1) had acute otitis media, (2) was being seen to follow up a previous episode of otitis media, or (3) did not have otitis media that day. The definition of otitis media used in this study was *inflammation of the tympanic membrane or significant effusion by inspection or pneumatic otoscopy.*

The study nurse collected the questionnaires and reviewed them to determine which of the children were eligible as cases or controls. A case was defined as any child presenting with acute otitis media on a study day, regardless of past history of otitis. A control was defined as any child receiving a diagnosis other than otitis media on a study day and who had no prior history of otitis. Otitis media history for potential controls was verified both by the study nurse, who reviewed the child's entire clinic record, and by the parent, who completed a section on ear infections on the questionnaire.

A total of 1744 children were examined during the two weeks (Table 1). Of these, 1055 children were not eligible as either cases or controls because they did not have otitis media on a study day but did have prior histories of ear infections. The status of another 88 children was unknown owing to incomplete clinic records, and there were three refusals. The remaining 598 children were eligible as study subjects: 331 were potential cases and 267 were potential controls. Questionnaires were completed for 300 cases and 240 controls for a combined response rate of 90.3 percent. The fact that the control group was smaller than the case group illustrates how difficult it was to find children who had no past or present history of otitis media.

The age distributions of the case and control groups differed markedly. While the cases were fairly evenly distributed over the preschool years, the majority of the controls were under the age of 2 years. Many of these very young controls may not have had a chance to experience their first episode of otitis media, so one year later (February 1983) the charts of these 166 controls were reviewed, and it was found that 94 of these children had developed otitis in the year since the study had been conducted. Since these 94 children were no longer otitis free, they were excluded from the control group, as they were considered to be misclassified.

The 300 cases and the remaining 146 controls were used in the final analysis. Although the age distribution of the controls had become more similar to that of the cases after the misclassified controls were excluded, the potential effects of age differences on the results could not be ignored. Since matching of cases and controls was impossible because of the different sizes of the groups, the Mantel-Haenszel age-adjusted *chi*-square method[12] was used to control for age differences. This is a widely used technique when a confounding factor is to be controlled by stratification during analysis. The Mantel-Haenszel *chi*-square with one degree of freedom tests the overall association and is calculated by taking a weighted average of the proportions across the strata. The strata used in this analysis were one-year age intervals; the *chi*-squares presented are the weighted averages for ages 0 to 19.

TABLE 1 Study Population

Total children examined		1744
Not eligible		1055
Unknown status		88
Refusals		3
Eligible		598
Cases	331	
Controls	267	
Completed questionnaire		
Cases	300 (90.6%)	
Controls	240 (89.9%)	

RESULTS

The demographic composition of the two groups was similar. There was a slight preponderance of males but the difference was not significant. Both groups were primarily white.

A number of risk factors for otitis media were identified (Table 2). A cold in the past week and the symptoms of fever, ear pain, and decreased hearing were prominent in the case group, as expected. Cases showed more allergies, especially to milk and drugs, than did the controls. In addition, the allergic-type symptoms of runny nose and watery eyes were more common in the cases. It was much more likely that a case would currently be attending a day care facility than a control. Otitis risk also seemed to increase with the number of other children at the day care facility. That is, the cases were more likely to be attending a large day

TABLE 2 Risk Factors

	Cases (%)	*Controls* (%)	χ^2_{MH}	p *Value*
Cold in past week	77.2	38.2	42.54	0.001
Any allergies	16.8	8.6	6.85	0.05
Milk allergies	2.8	0	5.89	0.05
Drug allergy	9.8	2.9	6.39	0.05
Runny nose	15.5	7.1	4.30	0.05
Watery eyes	6.1	1.4	5.26	0.05
Attends day care center	69.4	28.6	24.04	0.001
Use of humidifier in infant's room	68.3	46.9	4.10	0.05
Family history of ear infections	55.1	22.6	16.43	0.001

TABLE 3 Protective Factors

	Cases (%)	*Controls* (%)	χ^2_{MH}	p *Value*
Premature birth	8.7	15.3	5.53	0.05*
Frequent sneezing	9.1	18.6	3.82	0.05*

*Denotes inverse relationship

care center (at least ten children) than were the controls. The use of a humidifier in an infant's (under the age of 1 year) room was also more common among the cases. Finally, after controlling for sibship size (by using only subjects with one sibling), cases were much more likely to show a positive family history (in parents or siblings) of ear infections than were controls.

Two protective factors against otitis media were also identified (Table 3). Premature birth (defined as at least two weeks early) was reported more often in controls than in cases, perhaps reflecting more aggressive antibiotic treatment of premature infants, thus preventing the occurrence of otitis. Frequent sneezing when the child did not have a cold was also more common in the controls. Perhaps sneezing opens the eustachian tube and prevents the establishment of an infection in the middle ear.

Factors that did not appear to be related to the risk of otitis media in children included bottle-feeding; allergic conditions (hay fever, asthma or eczema); number of hours spent at a day care facility per week; type of heating system and carpeting; the use of air filters; exposure to pets, smokers, and stuffed animals; increased family size; and a family history of allergy.

DISCUSSION

The results of this study are limited by the self-administered, nonvalidated nature of the questionnaire and possibly by differential recall of certain items by parents of cases and controls. In addition, the use of a single source for cases and controls may have resulted in a study group that was not representative of the community. Although age was controlled using the Mantel-Haenszel procedure, our original intention was to use the matched pair design. Owing to the ubiquitous nature of the disease, it was impossible to find age-matched controls for the cases. For this reason, perhaps the cohort design is better suited for an epidemiologic study of otitis media.

However, we conclude that four factors deserve further study as bona fide risk factors for childhood otitis media: recent upper respiratory tract infection, allergy, day care exposure, and family history of ear infection.

REFERENCES

1. Howie VM, Ploussard JH, Sloyer JL: Immunization against recurrent otitis media. Ann Otol Rhinol Laryngol 85 (Suppl 25): 254, 1976
2. Kaplan GJ, Fleshman JK, Bender TR, et al: Long-term effects of otitis media in a ten-year cohort study of Alaskan Eskimo children. Pediatrics 52:577, 1973
3. Brownlee RC, DeLoache WR, Cowan CC, Jackson HP: Otitis media in children. J Ped 75:636, 1969
4. Howie VM, Ploussard JH, Sloyer JL: The otitis prone condition. Am J Dis Child 129:676, 1975
5. Froom J, Mold J, Culpepper L, Boisseau V: The spectrum of otitis media in family practice. J Fam Pract 10:599–605, 1980
6. Teele DW, Klein JO, Rosner BA: Epidemiology of otitis media in children. Ann Otol Rhinol Laryngol 89 (Suppl 68):5, 1980
7. Henderson FW, Collier AM, Sanyal MA, et al: A longitudinal study of respiratory viruses and bacteria in the etiology of acute otitis media with effusion. New Engl J Med 306:1377, 1982
8. Hoekelman RA: Infectious illness during the first year. Pediatrics 59:119, 1977
9. Strangert K: Otitis media in young children in different types of day-care. Scand J Infect Dis 9:119–123, 1977
10. Beauregard WG: Positional otitis media. J Ped 79: 294–296, 1971
11. Patterson JE, MacLean DW: Acute otitis media in children. Scot Med J 15:289–296, 1970
12. Mantel N, Haenszel W: Statistical aspects of the analysis of data from retrospective studies of disease. J Natl Cancer Inst 22:719, 1959

PREVALENCE AND INCIDENCE OF OTITIS MEDIA IN A GROUP OF PRESCHOOL CHILDREN IN THE UNITED STATES

MARGARETHA L. CASSELBRANT, M.D., Ph.D., P. A. OKEOWO, M.D., F.R.C.S., M. R. FLAHERTY, R.N., M.N., P.N.P., R. M. FELDMAN, Ph.D., W. J. DOYLE, Ph.D., C. D. BLUESTONE, M.D., K. D. ROGERS, M.D., and T. HANLEY, M.A.

Past epidemiologic studies of otitis media with effusion (OME) have reported a seasonal influence in the prevalence of OME and high negative pressure (HNP).[1–3] Etiologic factors such as age, sex, climate, and race may possibly influence the course of the disease. To define the contribution of each of these factors adequately, thorough natural history studies have to be performed. The purpose of the present study was to define the natural history of OME and HNP by monthly evaluations of a population of preschool children.

MATERIALS AND METHODS

Sixty-six of 85 children, aged 2 to 5 years, attending a day care center in a suburb of Pittsburgh, Pennsylvania, were selected for the study of incidence and prevalence of OME and HNP. Of the children who were excluded from the study, seven already had tympanostomy tubes and one had a known sensorineural hearing loss. Consent for study could not be obtained from the parents of eight children. Three children were enrolled initially but they left the school before they reached a six-month follow-up and thus were excluded from the data presentation. Of the 66 children, 36 were boys and 30 were girls. Sixty-four were white and two were black.

A team consisting of an otolaryngologist, a nurse-coordinator, a nurse trained in tympanometric screening, and an audiologist visited the day care center 1½ days a month between September 1981 and August 1982 to carry out a program of physical examination, otoscopy, and tympanometry for detecting OME, and audiologic screening for documenting hearing loss.

The following observations were recorded for every child present at each monthly examination conducted at the day care center.

First, an ear, nose, and throat examination with detailed otoscopy was performed by an otoscopist validated as described by Bluestone and Cantekin.[4] The children were evaluated for signs and symptoms of OME, upper respiratory infections (URI), and throat infection.

Second, bilateral impedance studies were done including (1) automatic plotting of the tympanogram using the Madsen Z073 electroacoustic impedance bridge with the Hewlett-Packard XY plotter (test frequency 220 Hz, pressure range from −400 to +200 mm water over 16 sec); and (2) automatic plotting of the ipsilateral acoustic reflex.

The tympanograms were classified according to a scheme reported by Paradise and colleagues[5] and were combined with the findings of acoustic reflex and otoscopy into the algorithm of Cantekin and associates to determine the presence or absence of OME. HNP was considered as a tympanometric measure less than −200 mm H_2O. The children were classified according to the middle ear status of the worst ear into four categories: normal, HNP, OME, and tympanostomy tube due to persistent OME.

If the child had not had OME on the previous examination, the presence of OME was counted as a new episode. The duration of the OME episode was assessed when it occurred and resolved during a period of continuous study (that is, no missing monthly observations during the period).

RESULTS

Sixty-six percent of the children were examined 11 or 12 times. Twenty-three percent were examined nine or ten times and the remaining children at least six times. Thirty-four of the 66 children (52 percent) developed OME in at least one ear during the course of the year. Twenty-two children had bilateral disease and 12 had unilateral disease. Sixty-four percent of the boys and 37 percent of the girls developed OME ($p < 0.06$). The incidence of the disease decreased with age for both boys and girls; 69 percent of the children in the 2-year age group developed OME, compared with only 25 percent of the 5-year-olds ($p < 0.10$).

Figure 1 shows the distribution of the children according to middle ear status during the 12 months of follow-up. The monthly incidence of OME and HNP showed a strong seasonal dependence. In September 1981, about 90 percent of the children had normal ears, in contrast to findings during winter months. For example, in February 1982 only 41 percent of the children had normal ears. The months of January through March showed the highest prevalence of HNP and OME. During the spring the prevalence of OME decreased and in August none of the children had OME.

A summary of the frequency and duration of OME and HNP for the one-year observation period is shown in Figure 2. Of the 75 episodes of OME experienced by the 34 children, 73 percent were single episodes, 20 percent had two episodes, and only a few children developed three episodes of OME. The 114 episodes of HNP in 42 children had a similar frequency distribution: 52 percent were single episodes and 40 percent had two episodes. Most children recovered from a new episode of

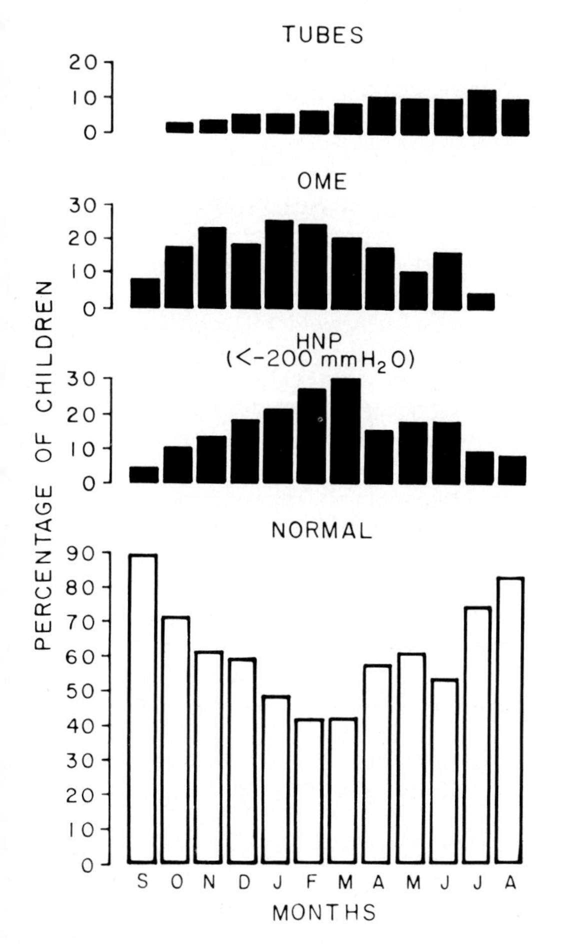

Figure 1 Monthly distribution of children according to the middle ear status of their worst ear. The data shown are from September 1981 through August 1982.

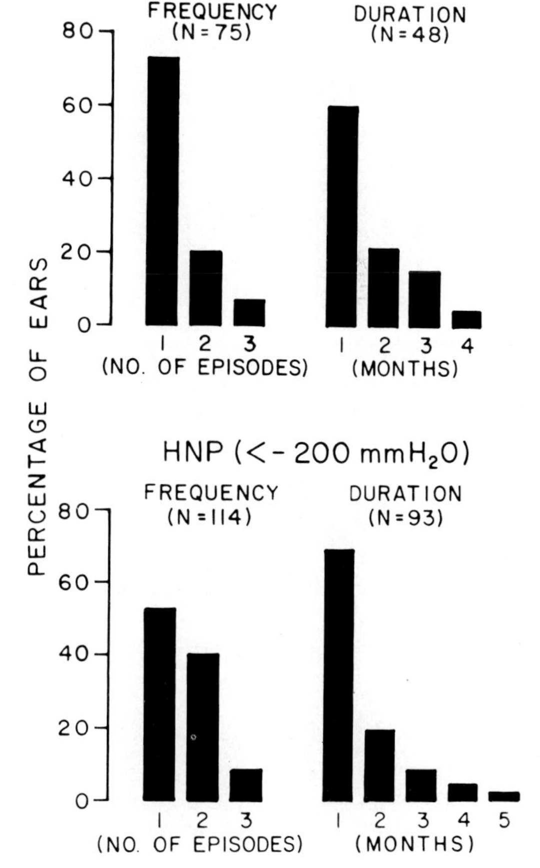

Figure 2 Frequency and duration of otitis media with effusion (OME) and high negative pressure (HNP) during a one-year observation period.

OME or HNP within one month. Of the 48 episodes of OME with known duration, 60 percent resolved in one month and 20 percent resolved in two months. Similarly, 70 percent of the 93 HNP episodes with known duration were resolved within a one-month period.

The seasonal distribution of upper respiratory infections was found to be closely related to the seasonal distribution of OME, and the findings are summarized in Figure 3. One hundred fourteen episodes of URI were documented in 52 children (79 percent) at the time of examination. The highest prevalence of URI and OME was found during the winter months. For example, in February, 32 percent of the children had URI and 24 percent had OME. Furthermore, 32 percent of the ears examined during a URI bout were identified as having OME, whereas only 7 percent of the ears had OME when the children did not have a URI. During the 12-month follow-up, a total of 153 months of effusion were recorded, 72 of which were in children who had concurrent URIs.

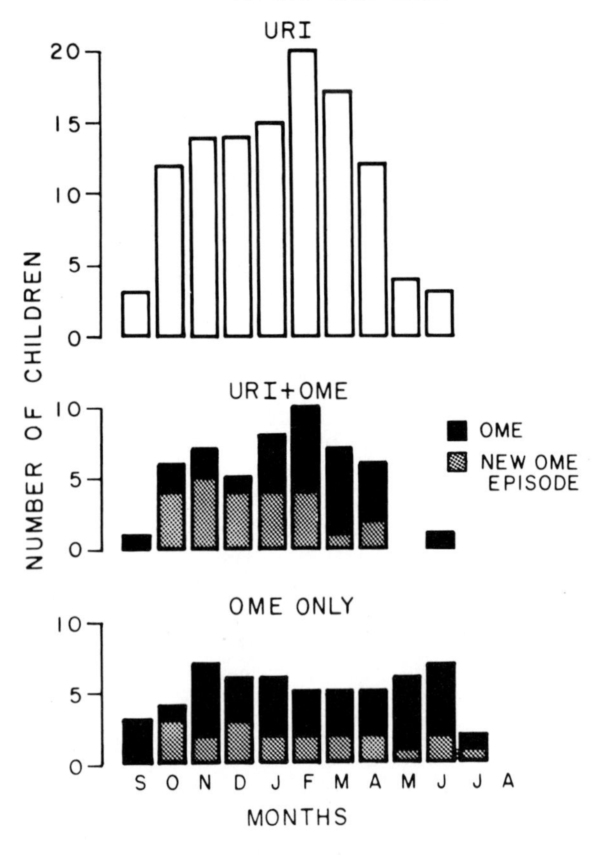

Figure 3 Monthly distribution of upper respiratory infection (URI) and otitis media with effusion (OME) (September 1981 through August 1982).

As a summary and based on the monthly observations for the year, each ear was classified into one of four ME function groups according to the frequency of abnormal ME status. For simplicity, the calculation is based on ears. Except for the 16 ears with persistent effusion that constituted 12 percent of the population and all of which received tympanostomy tubes, three equally distributed groups emerged. The first group comprised 39 ears that were normal at all observations. The second group of 37 ears had only HNP episodes. The third group of 40 ears was characterized by episodes of OME and HNP. About one-half of the ears in this group had only one episode of OME during the entire observation period. These four groups may correspond to a similar set of eustachian tube function types, and the group with tympanostomy tubes may represent the tubal dysfunction type commonly associated with childhood OME.

DISCUSSION

To a large extent our findings are in agreement with other epidemiologic studies of prevalence and incidence of OME and HNP in children. The point prevalence of OME was related to the season of the year, with the highest prevalence during the winter months.[1–3] There was a correlation between OME and URI that previously had been reported.[7,8] The middle ear status fluctuated, with deteriorations and spontaneous recovery.[2,3,7,9] More boys than girls developed the disease,[10] and for both the incidence of OME decreased with age.[7,11]

Few investigations have been concerned with the duration of an OME episode. Lous and Fiellau-Nicholajsen found a mean duration of two to three months in 7-year-old children, with a preponderance of episodes of one month's duration.[3] In our group of children, we found that 60 percent of the OME episodes had resolved in one month or less.

The monthly prevalence reported in the present study was somewhat higher than that reported in previous studies. This difference might be explained by two factors. First, our observations from otoscopy, tympanometry, and acoustic reflex measurements were combined into an algorithm to determine the presence or absence of OME, which provided a more objective method with higher sensitivity than tympanometry alone.[6] Second, the population examined was attending a nursery school, and such children have been shown to be at higher risk for development of OME and a longer course of the disease.[7,12,13] However, the duration of the OME episodes in our children was usually short.

This study differs from the previous epidemiologic studies in two main aspects: the use of the highly accurate diagnostic method to identify OME and the frequent assessment of ear status. Thus, it was possible to document the number of episodes of OME and HNP and the duration of these episodes. Our objective was to determine the prevalence, incidence, and natural history of OME in a group of preschool children and to develop a method that could be applied to a larger number of children in several geographic areas.

REFERENCES

1. Fiellau-Nicholajsen M: Tympanometry in three-year-old children: II. Seasonal influence on tympanometric results in non-selected groups of three year old children. Scand Audiol 8:181, 1979
2. Tos M, Holm-Jensen S, Sørensen CH: Changes in prevalence of secretory otitis from summer to winter in four-year-old children. Am J Otol 2:324 1981
3. Lous J, Fiellau-Nicholajsen M: Epidemiology of middle ear effusion and tubal dysfunction. A one year prospective study comprising monthly tympanometry in 387 non-selected seven-year-old children. Int Ped Otorhinolaryngol 3:303, 1981
4. Bluestone CD, Cantekin EI: Design factors in the characterization and identification of otitis media and certain related conditions. Ann Otol Rhinol Laryngol 88(60):13, 1979
5. Paradise JL, Smith CG, Bluestone CD: Tympanometric detection of middle ear effusion in infants and children. Pediatrics 58:198, 1976
6. Cantekin EI, Bluestone CD, Fria TJ, et al: Identification of otitis media with effusion in children. Ann Otol Rhinol Laryngol 89(68):190, 1980
7. Fiellau-Nicholajsen M.: Tympanometry and secretory otitis media: Observations on diagnosis, epidemiology treatment and prevention in prospective cohort studies of three-year-old children. Acta Otolaryngol Suppl 394: 1983
8. Tom M, Poulsen G, Haucke AB: Screening tympanometry during the first year of life. Acta Otolaryngol 88:388, 1979
9. Tos M, Poulsen G: Tympanometry in 2 year old children. Seasonal influence on frequency of secretory otitis and tubal dysfunction. ORL 41:1, 1979
10. Brooks D: The use of the electroacoustic bridge in the assessment of middle ear function. Int Audiol 8:563, 1969
11. Kessner DM, Know CK, Singer J: Assessment of Medical Care for Children: Contrasts in Health Status, vol 3, Washington DC: Institute of Medicine, National Academy of Sciences, 1974
12. Tos M, Poulsen G, Borch G: Tympanometry in 2 year old children. ORL 40:77, 1978
13. Sørensen CH, Holm-Jensen S, Tos M: Middle ear effusion and risk factors. J Otolaryngol 11:1, 1982

EPIDEMIOLOGY OF ACUTE OTITIS MEDIA IN CHILDREN—A COHORT STUDY IN AN URBAN POPULATION

LEIF INGVARSSON, M.D., KAJ LUNDGREN, M.D., and BERTIL OLOFSSON, Ph.D.

The epidemiology of acute otitis media (AOM) is still inadequately explored.[1–3] Most studies have been carried out in selected groups of children[4–8], and among earlier epidemiologic studies there are very few cohort studies penetrating the relationship between AOM and demographic and socioeconomic factors.[9–11] Prospective investigations in a sufficiently large cohort of unselected children from a well-defined population have been recommended.[12]

Malmö, Sweden, is a well-defined geographic unit with unique conditions for epidemiologic studies. The aim of this investigation was (1) to study the incidence rate of AOM in children in a prospective long-term epidemiologic study, and (2) to analyze the possible influence of different demographic and social factors on the observed incidence of AOM.

MATERIALS AND METHODS

Since 1977 all cases of AOM among children living in Malmö have been registered.[13] In the first year (1977) all children up to 3 years old were registered. In each of the following two years a new age class was introduced. Since 1980 children up to 15 years old have been registered. All children born in 1977 or later are included in a cohort study; these children have been followed from birth until December 1981—the present end point—implying a maximum observation time of 60 months. The cohort study will continue for a ten-year period.

The investigation implies that all children diagnosed as having AOM by a doctor in the city are registered. All doctors who work in acute pediatric medical practice are participating. Episodes of AOM are defined as the presence of reddened and bulging eardrums with or without spontaneous perforation. Information on the patient's name, ten-digit birth number, and date and place of diagnosis is forwarded from the ENT and Pediatrics departments at the General Hospital and from all individual physicians in the city (general practitioners, otologists, pediatricians, and physicians on duty). These reports are completed from official computerized data files containing information about the patient's dwelling in the city, type of housing, and type of day care at the time of diagnosis. All information is computerized and processed in a specially designed statistical program.[14]

Malmö is the leading industrial and commercial center in southern Sweden, with 235,000 inhabitants of whom about 37,000 are children up to 15 years of age. Each age class covers between 2200 and 2700 children. There is only one hospital in the city, Malmö General Hospital.

In Sweden day care centers with 15 to 25 children in each group and family day care homes with three to six children in each group are the main forms of public out-of-home care for children up to 11 years old. In Malmö about 17 percent of all children up to 5 years of age are cared for in day care centers and 14 percent in day care homes, while about 70 percent are cared for at home or by private babysitters.

RESULTS

Incidence Study

The annual incidence rates in children up to 15 years old for 1980 and 1981 are given in Figure 1. The largest number of episodes, 44 to 45 per 100 children at risk, was seen in 1-year-old children, that is, children from 1 year to 2 years of age. In this age group about 30 percent of the children had at least one episode of AOM annually. Above this age the proportion of children with AOM, as well as the number of episodes of AOM, steadily decreased.

Cohort Study

In 1977, 2404 children (1277 boys and 1127 girls) were born in Malmö. At the end of 1981, 542 of the boys and 433 of the girls had been registered for 1254 and 938 episodes of AOM respectively. Forty-four percent of the boys and 47 percent of the girls had only one episode each of AOM during the period. Twenty percent of the boys and 17 percent of the girls had more than four episodes each of AOM, and there was no difference between the sexes in this respect.

The cumulative incidence rate (CIRs) for the first episode of AOM in the boys and girls born in 1977 are illustrated in Figure 2. At the age of 12 months, 20 percent of the boys and 17 percent of the girls had had at least one episode of AOM. At the end of the observation period, 60 months, about 60 percent of the boys and 55 percent of the girls had had at least one episode of AOM. The CIR for boys and girls of comparable ages differed

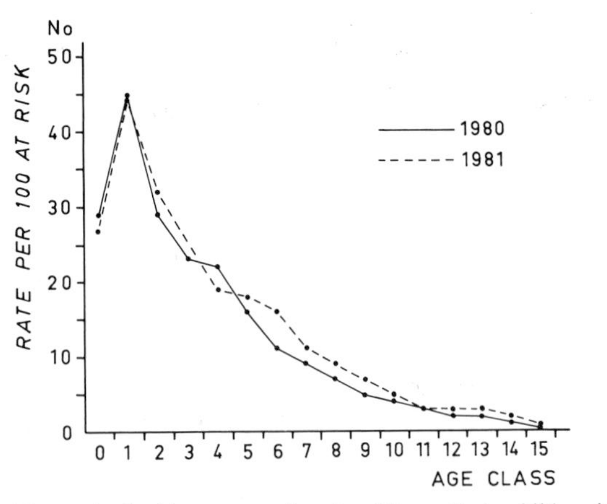

Figure 1 Incidence rate of acute otitis media in children in Malmö.

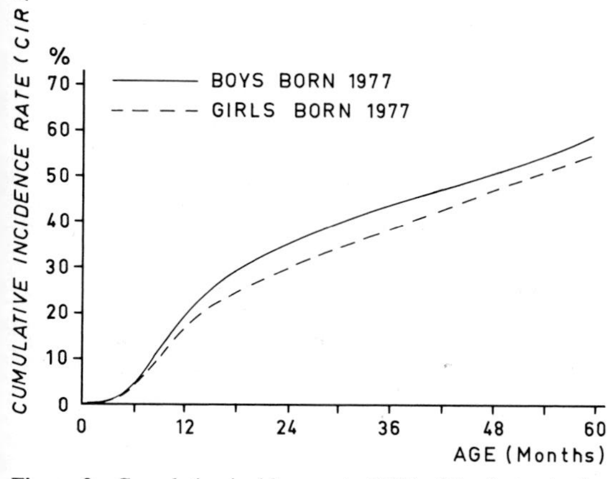

Figure 2 Cumulative incidence rate (CIR) of the first episode of AOM in relation to sex.

significantly ($p < 0.001$). The highest incidence rate (greatest risk of getting AOM) was found in the age interval 6 to 11 months for both boys and girls.

The distribution of the total population of children aged up to 5 years old in Malmö among the different types of day care was 17 percent in day care centers, 14 percent in day care homes, and about 70 percent at home or with private babysitters. The corresponding distribution in children with episodes of AOM at the time of diagnosis is illustrated in Figure 3. Among the children born in 1977 who had occasional (one or two) episodes of AOM, 28 percent of the episodes were diagnosed in children attending day care centers, 17 percent in children in family day care homes, and 55 percent in children cared for at home or by private babysitters. The corresponding distribution

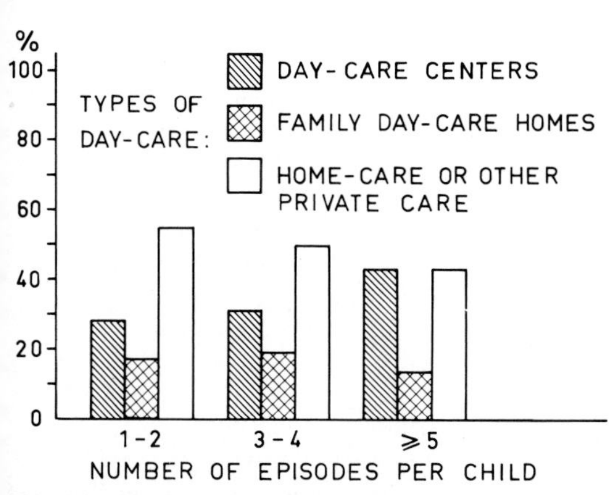

Figure 3 Distribution among different types of day care at the time of diagnosis in the children with AOM born in 1977.

in children with five or more episodes was 43, 14, and 43 percent, respectively, during the same period. The three groups (children with one or two, three or four, and more than five episodes of AOM) differed significantly ($p < 0.001$) in their distribution among the different types of day care.

The registration revealed differences in the incidence rate of AOM among children living in different districts of the city. Three different districts (center of the city, Rosengård, and Oxie) were studied. In the center of the city most families live in older, mainly well maintained apartment houses. Rosengård is a modern crowded tenement house district built in the 1960s and 1970s. Oxie is a modern crowded villa suburb outside Malmö built during the latter part of the seventies. The children born in 1977 who lived in Oxie had the highest CIR. At the end of the observation period of 60 months, about 65 percent of the children had had at least one episode of AOM. The corresponding figures for the children living in Rosengård and in the center of the city were about 55 and 45 percent, respectively. The differences between the districts were significant ($p < 0.001$). The children living in the three districts had the same type of distribution among different types of day care in the districts, and therefore the differences could not be explained by the type of day care.

DISCUSSION

The results in our study showed that the incidence of AOM was greatest in the 1-year-olds. About 30 percent of the children of this age get at least one episode of AOM. The cohort study showed that children aged 6 to 11 months run the greatest risk of getting the first episode of AOM within their first five years of life. The boys had significantly higher CIRs than the girls of corresponding ages. At the age of 5 years about 55 percent of all children have had at least one episode of AOM. The incidence of AOM was greatest among children in day care centers, and these children run a greater risk of getting recurrent AOM than those at home or in family day care homes. The incidence was also found to vary among children living in different districts and in different types of housing.

It has not yet been possible to investigate other factors that probably influence the incidence of AOM in children in the present study. Such factors might be heredity, the degree of immunologic defense, and the importance of breast versus bottle feeding. External factors, such as type and quality of housing, degree of air humidity and ventilation in the apartment, and cigarette smoke inhalation and other air pollution might also be of interest. The next step in our epidemiologic study of AOM in children includes an analytic case-control study, comparing a group of children with recurrent episodes of AOM with an equivalent group of healthy children, in which factors mentioned above will be studied.

This study was supported by grants from the Swedish Medical Research Council (B82-27X-06279-01).

REFERENCES

1. Hinchcliffe R: Epidemiological aspects of otitis media. In Glorig A, Gerwin K (eds): *Otitis Media: Proceedings of the National Conference*. Springfield, IL: Charles C Thomas, 1972, pp 36–43
2. McEldowney D, Kessner DM: Review of the literature. Epidemiology of otitis media. In Glorig A, Gerwin K (eds): *Otitis Media: Proceedings of the National Conference*. Springfield, IL: Charles C Thomas, 1972, pp 11–25
3. Manning P, Avery ME, Ross A: Purulent otitis media: Differences between populations in different environments. Pediatrics 53:135, 1974
4. Lowe JF, Bamforth JS, Pracy R: Acute otitis media. One year in a general practice. Lancet 2:1130, 1963
5. Cambon K, Galbraith JD, Kong G: Middle-ear disease in Indians of the Mount Currie Reservation, British Columbia. Can Med Assoc J 93:1301, 1965
6. Paavolainen M: Incidence, etiology and prognosis of acute purulent otitis media in Helsinki residents of various ages. Acta Otolaryngol (Stockh) Suppl 224:360, 1967
7. Brownlee RC Jr, Deloache WR, Cowan CC Jr, Jackson HP: Otitis media in children. Incidence, treatment, and prognosis in pediatric practice. J Pediatr 75:636, 1969
8. Howie VM, Ploussard JH, Sloyer J: The "otitis-prone" condition. Am J Dis Child 129:676, 1975
9. Reed D, Struve S, Maynard JE: Otitis media and hearing deficiency among Eskimo children: A cohort study. Am J Public Health 57:1657, 1967
10. Teele DW, Klein JO, Rosner BA: Epidemiology of otitis media in children. Ann Otol Rhinol Laryngol 89 (Suppl 68):5, 1980
11. Pukander J: Occurrence of acute otitis media. Department of Clinical Sciences, University of Tampere, Finland. Acta Universitatis Tamperensis, Series A, vol 135, 1982
12. Kudrjavcev T, Schoenberg BS: Otitis media and developmental disability. Epidemiologic considerations. Ann Otol Rhinol Laryngol Suppl 60:88, 1979
13. Ingvarsson L, Lundgren K, Olofsson B, Wall S: Epidemiology of acute otitis media in children. Acta Otolaryngol (Stockh) Suppl 388, 1983
14. Persson T: *New Mathematical Statistics Package*. Department of Mathematical Statistics, Institute of Technology, University of Lund, Lund, Sweden, 1981

EPIDEMIOLOGIC ASPECTS IN CHILDREN WITH RECURRENT ACUTE OTITIS MEDIA

KAJ LUNDGREN, M.D., LEIF INGVARSSON, M.D., and BERTIL OLOFSSON, Ph.D.

Recurrent episodes of acute otitis media (AOM) are very common in children during the first years of life. In many cases the recurrences appear after a relatively short interval. The recurrent nature of AOM has been related to anatomic, pathologic, and immunologic factors and even to the type of therapy.[1] Studies have also shown that early onset of AOM increases the risk of recurrent episodes.[1] But in many cases the underlying causes are not evident. Different approaches, such as adenoidectomy with or without tonsillectomy, antimicrobial prophylaxis, the use of tympanostomy tubes, and liberal use of myringotomy and vaccination, have been recommended to prevent recurrent AOM or at least to decrease the number of episodes.[2] In spite of all treatment regimens recurrent AOM is still a great problem.

Many authors have emphasized the need for epidemiologic data concerning recurrent AOM.[3,4] Most such data are derived from selected populations, and the children have not been followed up for a sufficient length of time. However, the interest in epidemiologic studies has increased considerably during recent years, and a number of studies have been published.[5–9]

In 1977 a prospective longitudinal epidemiologic study of AOM in children began in Malmö, Sweden.[5] The study is intended to continue for at least ten years and this report is a part of that study. The aim is to study children with recurrent episodes of AOM at different ages and the recurrence in relation to sex, type of dwelling in the city, and type of day care.

MATERIALS AND METHODS

The design and method of the epidemiologic study have been described in detail elsewhere.[5] Comparisons of different statistical distributions were made with the *Chi*-square analysis. The material in this report consists of all cases of AOM, otoscopically diagnosed by a doctor, in children born in Malmö in 1977 and still living in Malmö at the end of 1981. Thus, the observation period is a maximum of five years. Episodes of AOM are defined as the presence of reddened and bulging eardrums with or without spontaneous perforation. A new episode of AOM was considered to have occurred if at least ten days had elapsed since the previous episode. In a few cases it is possible that a recurrent episode was an exacerbation or a continuation of a previous episode that had never completely resolved. Every episode of AOM was registered. Children with only one episode were registered only once, while children with more than one episode (2 to 13) were registered in connection with each episode.

RESULTS

In 1977, 2404 children (1277 boys and 1127 girls) were born in Malmö. Of these children 975 had at least one episode of AOM and all together the children had 2192 episodes. There was no sex-related difference among children with AOM in relation to the distribution of boys and girls in the total population. However, boys had significantly more episodes than girls.

The number of episodes of AOM per child is given in Table 1. Of the children with AOM 45 percent had only one episode and 6 percent had more than six episodes. Of these, two children had 11 episodes and one child 13 episodes. There was no difference between boys and girls in the number of episodes per child.

Table 2 shows the age at the first episode of AOM in relation to the number of episodes per child. Children who had their initial episode in the first year of life had many recurrences, in contrast to children who had their first episode after the age of 1 year. The risk of getting recurrent episodes of AOM was significantly higher ($p < 0.001$) in children having their first episode before the age of 1 year. Table 2 also shows that 50 (14 percent) of the children having their first episode of AOM before 1 year of age experienced six or more episodes, while only nine children (1 percent) of those with their initial episode after 1 year of age had six or more episodes. This difference was statistically significant ($p < 0.001$).

The percentage of distribution of the total number of episodes of AOM in different types of day care at the time of diagnosis is shown in Table 3. Children who got only one episode of AOM accounted for 15, 18, and 25 percent of the episodes in the three types of day care. The corresponding figures for children having six or more episodes were 24, 18, and 16 percent. Thus, children attending day care centers run a greater risk of having recurrent episodes of AOM than those cared for at family day care homes or at home. The differences among the different types of day care were significant ($p < 0.001$).

Table 4 shows the percentage of distribution of the number of episodes of AOM in three different districts in Malmö at the time of diagnosis. Children who had only one episode of AOM accounted for 26, 22, and 15 percent of the total number of episodes in the three districts. The cor-

TABLE 1 Number of Episodes of AOM per Child

No. of Episodes per Child	*Boys*		*Girls*		*Total*	
	No.	*%*	*No.*	*%*	*No.*	*%*
1	241	45	204	47	445	45
2–3	197	36	159	37	356	37
4–5	68	13	47	11	115	12
6–13	36	6	23	5	59	6
Total	542	100	433	100	975	100

TABLE 2 Age at First Episode of AOM in Relation to Number of Episodes per Child

No. of Episodes per Child	*Age at First Episode*					*Total*
	0–1	*1–2*	*2–3*	*3–4*	*4–5*	
1	101	109	92	82	61	445
2–3	150	112	49	40	5	356
4–5	60	43	11	1		115
6–13	50	5	4			59
Total	361	269	156	123	66	975

TABLE 3 Percentage Distribution of Number of Episodes of AOM in Different Types of Day Care at Time of Diagnosis

No. of Episodes per Child	*Type of Day Care* Day Care Center (N = 726)	Family Day Care Home (N = 374)	Home Care (N = 1092)
1	15	18	25
2–3	36	38	40
4–5	25	26	19
6–13	24	18	16
Total	100	100	100

responding figures for children having six or more episodes were 8, 24, and 13 percent. The risk of getting six or more episodes of AOM is greater in Rosengård, the apartment house district, than in Oxie, the modern villa suburb district, or in the center of the city, the older apartment house district. The differences among the districts were significant ($p < 0.001$).

DISCUSSION

The information on the sex distribution of AOM varies. In most studies the incidence of AOM has been found to be higher in boys than in girls.[7,9,10] On the other hand, a few studies have shown no sex differences.[11,12] In the present report, in which a birth cohort has been followed for five years, more boys than girls had at least one episode of AOM, but this corresponded to a greater number of boys than girls in the population. However, boys had a significantly greater number of episodes of AOM than girls.

TABLE 4 Percentage of Distribution of Number of Episodes of AOM in Three Districts in Malmö at Time of Diagnosis

No. of Episodes per Child	*District* City (N = 271)	Rosengård (N = 366)	Oxie (N = 191)
1	26	22	15
2–3	47	31	47
4–5	19	23	25
6–13	8	24	13
Total	100	100	100

According to Howie, children having their initial episode of AOM in the first year of life are more prone to get recurrent AOM than those having their first episode after 1 year of age.[1] Children having six or more episodes of AOM before the age of six were termed "otitis prone." In the present study 14 percent of the children having their initial episode before 1 year of age had six or more episodes, compared with 1 percent among children having their first episode after 1 year of age. These results agree closely with those of Howie.

Recent studies in Scandinavia have shown that children cared for in larger groups such as in day care centers have more episodes of AOM and upper respiratory tract infection than those cared for at home.[6,8] The first report of the epidemiologic study of AOM in children in Malmö showed that children attending day care centers had AOM more often than those cared for at home.[5] Children attending family day care homes occupied an intermediate position. In this part of the study with special reference to recurrent AOM it was shown that children with six or more episodes of AOM accounted for a greater portion of the episodes in children attending day care centers than corresponding children cared for at home. Children attending family day care homes occupied an intermediate position.

Studies have shown a higher incidence of AOM in children living in apartments than among those living in houses.[8] The first report of the epidemiologic study of AOM in children in Malmö showed important differences in the incidence rate for the first episode of AOM among children living in different districts in Malmö.[5] Children living in a modern villa suburb had a significantly higher incidence rate than those living in the apartment house district and in the center of the city. In this part of the study it was found that children having six or more episodes of AOM accounted for a greater portion of the episodes among children in the apartment house district than in the modern villa suburb district and in the center of the city.

This report shows that it is not only the age at the time of the initial episode that is important to the number of episodes of AOM. The type of dwelling and the type of day care are also factors associated with an increased risk of recurrent episodes of AOM. It is vital, in different ways and early in life, to identify the "otitis prone" children in order to take appropriate measures. If recurrences of AOM can be prevented or substantially reduced the result will be of great medical and socioeconomic importance to society.

REFERENCES

1. Howie VM, Ploussard JH, Sloyer O: The "otitis-prone" condition. Am J Dis Child 129:676, 1975
2. Paradise JL: Antimicrobial prophylaxis for recurrent acute otitis media. Ann Otol Rhinol Laryngol Suppl 84:53, 1981
3. Kudrjavcev T, Schoenberg BS: Otitis media and developmental disability. Epidemiologic considerations. Ann Otol Rhinol Laryngol Suppl 60:88, 1979
4. Biles RW, Buffler PA, O'Donell AA: Epidemiology of otitis media: A community study. Am J Public Health 70:593, 1980
5. Ingvarsson L, Lundgren K, Olofsson B, Wall S: Epidemiology of acute otitis media in children. Acta Otolaryngol (Stockh) Supp 388:5, 1982
6. Strangert K: Otitis media in young children in different types of day-care. Scand J Infect Dis 9:119, 1977
7. Teele DW, Klein JD, Rosner BA: Epidemiology of otitis media in children. Ann Otol Rhinol Laryngol Suppl 68:5, 1980
8. Vinther B, Elbrønd O, Brahe Pedersen C: Otitis media in childhood. Socio-medical aspects with special reference to day-care and housing conditions. Acta Otolaryngol Suppl 386:121, 1982
9. Pukander J, Luotonen J, Sipilä M, et al: Incidence of acute otitis media. Acta Otolaryngol (Stockh) 93:447, 1982
10. Feingold M, Klein J, Haslam G, et al: Acute otitis media in children. Am J Dis Child 111:361, 1966
11. Medical Research Council (MRC): Acute otitis media in general practice. Lancet 2:510, 1957
12. Lowe JF, Bamforth JS, Pracy R: Acute otitis media. One year in a general practice. Lancet 2:1130, 1963

SOME FACTORS OF POSSIBLE ETIOLOGIC SIGNIFICANCE RELATED TO OTITIS MEDIA WITH EFFUSION

IAN STEWART, M.B., Ch.B., F.R.C.S. (Ed), CORALIE KIRKLAND, Dip.H.Sc., ANNE SIMPSON, M.B., Ch.B., PHIL SILVA, M.A., Ph.D., and SHEILA WILLIAMS, B.Sc.

The Dunedin Multidisciplinary Child Development Study is a comprehensive longitudinal study of 1037 of the 1661 children born at the Queen Mary Hospital, Dunedin, New Zealand, between April 1, 1972, and March 31, 1973. Virtually all births in Dunedin city occur at Queen Mary Hospital. The group of 1037 children studied at age 3 did not differ in terms of birth characteristics from the 624 who could not be studied at age 3.[1] The children studied received a variety of medical, psychological, and educational assessments.

This chapter describes the otologic and audiologic aspects of the study and relates these measurements to factors of possible significance in the origin of otitis media with effusion (OME).

MATERIALS AND METHODS

Otomicroscopy was carried out by a trained examiner whose observations have been shown in an independent study to be in greater than 99 percent agreement with those of the otologist concerned.[2] Immediately following microscopy, impedance tympanometry was carried out "blind" by a trained audiometrist using an Amplaid 702 tympanometer with XY plotter. The same examiner carried out pure-tone audiometry using an Interacoustics Screening Audiometer AS7 in a quiet but not soundproof room.

These studies were made in 962 children at age 5, 855 children at age 7, and 754 at age 9 at the study center. Data were available from elsewhere for many of those children unable to attend the center. Any child in the sample detected as having a significant ear or hearing problem was followed by the otolaryngology service until the problem had resolved. The data are complete up to age 9 for groups 1 and 2 of the "etiologic grouping" (see below), and any missing observations relate to the less severely affected groups.

Examination of the nose, mouth, and neck was made at ages 7 and 9. Posterior rhinoscopy was not performed. At age 9, respiratory function tests (FEV_1) were carried out before and after methacholine challenge. Skinfold thickness was measured by a trained examiner.

The history was obtained by a trained recorder using a questionnaire; it included breast-feeding history (obtained at age 3 years); socioeconomic status and smoking habits of the parents; ENT symptoms, including otalgia, otitis media, aural discharge, nasal obstruction, tonsillitis and hay fever; and lower respiratory symptoms.

RESULTS

On the basis of data available from the study center and the otolaryngology service until the age of 9, the 962 children for whom results were available were divided into 11 groups (Table 1).

For analyzing factors of possible etiologic significance, these groups were combined into six major groups (Table 2).

Analysis of variance was used to test for significant differences among the group means, followed by post hoc comparisons if the significance level was $p < .05$. A significance level of $p < 0.05$ was also used for the post hoc comparisons.

There were no significant differences in socioeconomic status among the groups. There was, however, a slight over-representation of the higher socioeconomic groups in the Dunedin population, but the lower socioeconomic groups had adequate access to medical services.[1]

There was a significant male preponderance in children who had at least one episode of OME (58 percent). This male preponderance was even more marked in those children with persistent bilateral otitis media with effusion, in which the male:female ratio was 2:1.

Based on our data, breast-feeding for a minimum of three months appears to protect significantly against OME (significant at the 0.05 level).

A history of nasal obstruction, a clinical diagnosis of nasal obstruction by the examiner, and increased turbinate size on examination were all significantly related to OME ($p \leq 0.05$). A history of tonsillitis, tonsil size to examination, or the presence of cervical adenitis on examination was not significantly associated with OME.

Despite frequent suggestions that OME may have an allergic basis, there was no significant association between it and a history of wheezing, hay fever, eczema, or bronchitis. On the basis of the respiratory function tests as carried out at the age

TABLE 1 Children Classified According to Severity of Otologic Features (N = 962)

Descriptive Grouping	*No.*	*%*	*Description*
A	13	1.4	Bilateral tubes on more than one occasion
B	40	4.2	Bilateral tubes on one occasion for hearing loss exceeding 25 dB
C	30	3.1	Bilateral tubes on one occasion without hearing loss exceeding 25 dB
D	15	1.6	Bilateral persistent otitis media with effusion, no tubes
E	45	4.7	Bilateral transient otitis media with effusion
F	18	1.9	Unilateral tube
G	8	0.8	Unilateral persistent otitis media with effusion, no tube
H	73	7.6	Unilateral transient otitis media with effusion
I	138	14.3	Never proven otitis media with effusion, scarred tympanic membrane
J	133	13.8	Never proven otitis media with effusion, no scar in tympanic membranes, always bilateral A tympanogram when assessed
K	449	46.7	The remainder (essentially C tympanogram on at least one occasion, never otitis media with effusion or B tympanogram)

TABLE 2 Combined Groups for Analysis of Possible Etiologic Factors (N = 962)

*Descriptive Grouping**	*New Group*	*No.*	*Description*
A, B, C, D	1	98	Persistent bilateral otitis media with effusion, with or without tubes
F, G	2	26	Persistent unilateral otitis media with effusion, with or without tubes
E, H	3	118	Transient unilateral or bilateral otitis media with effusion
I	4	138	Never proven otitis media with effusion, scarred tympanic membrane
K	5	449	Ears showing a C tympanogram on at least one occasion but never otitis media with effusion or a B tympanogram
J	6	133	Never proven otitis media with effusion, no scarred tympanic membranes, always bilateral A tympanogram when assessed

*See Table 1.

of 9, no relationship could be demonstrated between OME and evidence of hyper-reactive airways.

TYMPANOGRAMS BY MONTH, AGES 5-9

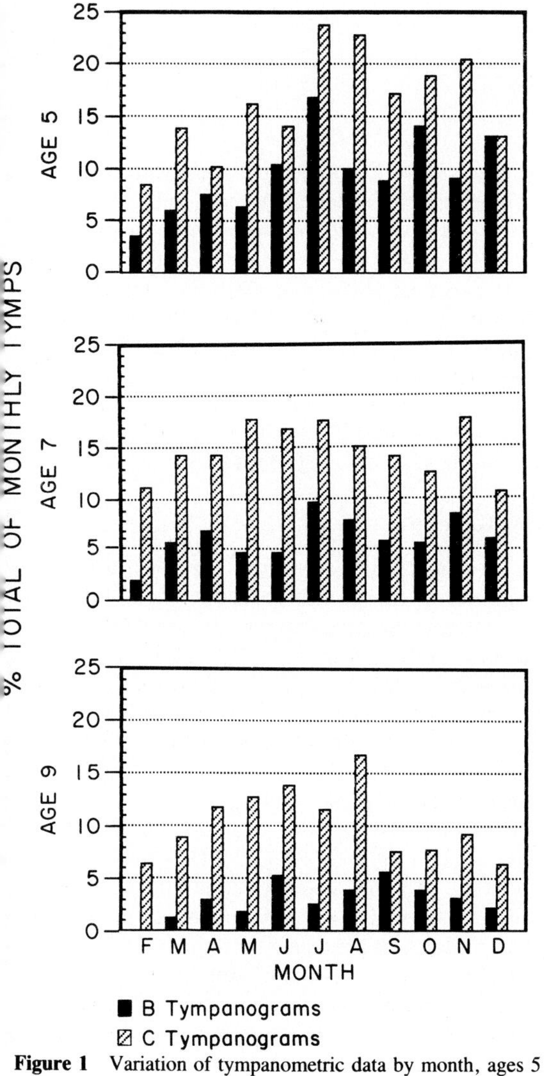

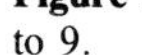

Figure 1 Variation of tympanometric data by month, ages 5 to 9.

Figure 1 shows the variation in prevalence of OME, as defined by tympanometry, between the ages of 5 and 9. It should be noted that type B tympanograms were more prevalent in the winter and spring months and also that the prevalence of type B tympanograms declined between ages 5 and 9. Type C_2 tympanograms (defined as a middle ear pressure more negative than -200 mm H_2O) showed a comparable seasonal and age-related variation in prevalence.

Otitis media with effusion showed no significant relationship to gestational age (pre- or postmaturity) nor was it related to nutritional status as defined by skinfold thickness. It was also not related to parental smoking habits.

Finally, it should be pointed out that no child in the sample developed a spontaneous chronic perforation, although 16 chronic perforations occurred following extrusion of tympanostomy tubes. Eleven of these closed spontaneously and five required surgical treatment. One child developed a cholesteatoma and two developed severe posterosuperior retraction pockets, all of which required surgical reconstruction. All three serious complications occurred in the group of children with refractory OME who required tympanostomy tubes on more than one occasion.

This study was supported by the Medical Research Council of New Zealand, the National Children's Health Research Foundation, the Departments of Education and Health of New Zealand, and the Deafness Research Foundation.

REFERENCES

1. McGee RO, Silva PA, A thousand New Zealand children: Their health and development from birth to seven. Auckland: Medical Research Council of New Zealand, Special Report No. 8, 1982
2. Stewart IA, Jenkin L, Kirkland C, et al: A preliminary evaluation of the use of an automatic impedance tympanometer in the diagnosis of otitis media with effusion in children: A report from the Dunedin Multidisciplinary Health and Development Research Unit. NZ Med J 96:252, 1983

SOME PREDISPOSING FACTORS IN OTITIS MEDIA WITH EFFUSION

PAUL B. VAN CAUWENBERGE, M.D., and PAUL M. KLUYSKENS, M.D., Ph.D.

When we consider the natural history of otitis media with effusion (OME), it is obvious that nearly all children have at least one episode of OME during their first six years of life.[1,2] The majority will recover spontaneously within weeks or months, but a minority will develop chronic OME or chronic otitis with perforation and discharge. Only a few factors predisposing to OME are well documented: age, race,[3,4] season and climate,[5] recurrent upper respiratory tract infections,[2,6] cleft palate,[7] and types of day care.[8] Many authors have demonstrated that the sex of the child is not a determining factor.[5] The possible role of adenoids, allergic processes,[9–12] and antibiotics[2] is still quite controversial.

To determine the influence of some of these and other possible predisposing factors, a prospective epidemiologic study was performed in Belgium on 2069 healthy schoolchildren between 2½ and 6 years of age.

MATERIALS AND METHODS

A complete otolaryngologic examination, including tympanometry, rhinomanometry, and, when possible, audiometry, was performed on 2069 healthy children attending different kindergartens, between May 1979 and January 1980. All children attending these kindergartens were enrolled; there was no selection. A questionnaire comprising 65 questions was completed by the parents, while the teachers were asked to give their opinions concerning some psychosocial characteristics of each child.

Tympanometry screening was performed with the 1722 Grason Stadler middle ear analyzer. The children showing abnormal tympanograms were retested with the 1723 otoadmittance recorder from the same company on the same day and again with the 1722 type three to four weeks later. When discussing the role of some predisposing factors in this chapter, we will make use only of the tympanograms obtained during the first screening.

To determine the seasonal influence on the prevalence of OME, we performed monthly tympanometry in a group of 97 nonselected children in three different schools from October 1979 through June 1980.

RESULTS

Prevalence

At the initial screening we found a flat tympanometric curve with absent stapedial reflex and an otoscopic picture compatible with OME in 12.0 percent of the left (n = 1946) and 11.5 percent of the right (n = 1952) ears. In addition, we recorded a flat curve in another 8.7 percent of left ears and 9.4 percent of right ears, but with a positive stapedial reflex or with an unsatisfactory otoscopic evaluation.

In the left ear a normal middle ear pressure (between −49 and +49 mm H_2O) was recorded in 33.9 percent, a positive middle ear pressure (≥ +50 mm H_2O) in 3.0 percent, a slightly negative middle ear pressure (between −50 and −100 mm H_2O) in 24.3 percent, and a more pronounced negative middle ear pressure (lower than −100 mm H_2O) in 18.1 percent. For the right ear the figures were 33.1 percent, 2.7 percent, 23.1 percent, and 20.2 percent respectively.

Age

The highest number of flat curves was recorded in children between 36 and 48 months of age (Fig. 1). The number of flat curves gradually decreased after the age of 4. These findings correlate with the epidemiologic studies of Tos and Poulsen,[13] Fiellau-Nikolajsen and Lous,[14] Viro-

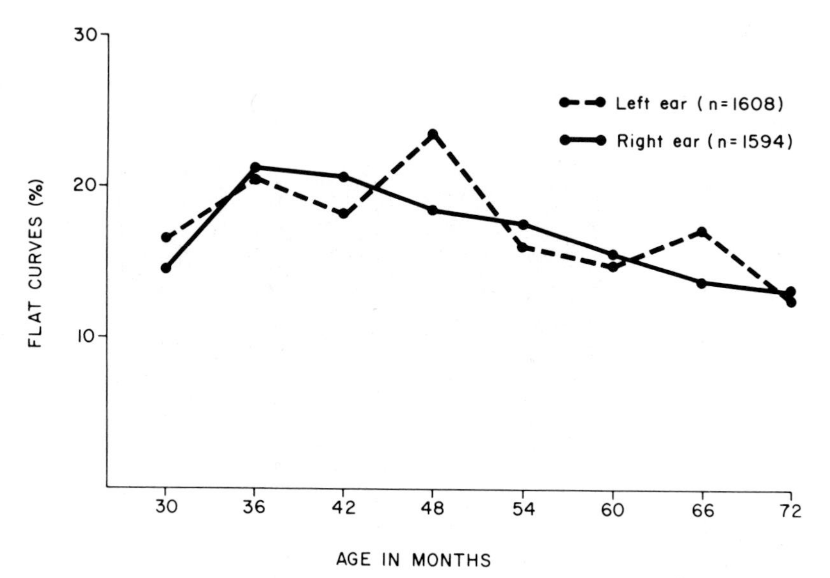

Figure 1 The percentage of flat tympanograms according to age of the child.

lainen and colleagues,[15] and Tos and associates,[16] who all showed the highest prevalence at between 2 and 6 years of age.

Seasonal Influence

Monthly tympanometric screening of 97 children from October 1979 through June 1980 showed that the highest number of flat curves was recorded in December (26.7 percent of the total number of ears), while the initial number in October was 9.2 percent and in November 17.0 percent. During the whole period from January through April the number of flat curves remained high: 20.1 percent in January, 21.9 percent in February, 21.0 percent in March, and 18.6 percent in April. In the late spring the number of flat tympanograms was lower: 15.0 percent in May and 17.0 percent in June.

We also noted that the peak number of flat tympanograms did not occur in the same period in the three schools tested: in two schools it occurred in December and in one school in March, a period in which the number of flat curves was already low in the first two schools. The distance between the schools was not more than 20 km. The occurrence of OME in a kind of epidemic demonstrated that not only climatologic conditions but also concomitant upper respiratory tract infections may influence the middle ear status.

Weight, Length, and Skull Circumference

Little is now known about the influence of birth weight and birth length on the development of OME in childhood. From our data (Fig. 2) it is obvious that children with very low birth weights (under 2.4 kg) are at greater risk for OME than children with higher birth weights ($p < 0.05$). Birth weights above 2.3 kg no longer influenced the percentage of flat tympanograms, although the percentage of completely normal tympanograms increased with increasing birth weight (statistically not significant). Similar findings were made with regard to the degree of prematurity, which was of course directly proportional to the birth weight.

Statistics on skull circumference were similar to those of birth weight: children with skull circumferences below the 2.5 percentile had a significantly higher number of flat tympanograms than the others ($p < 0.05$).

Birth length and present length of the child, and present weight, had a certain influence on the middle ear condition; there was a greater prevalence of OME in children with the lowest weights and lengths, but this was not statistically significant.

Episodes of Acute Otitis Media

The annual number of episodes of acute otitis media has a very definite influence on OME. There

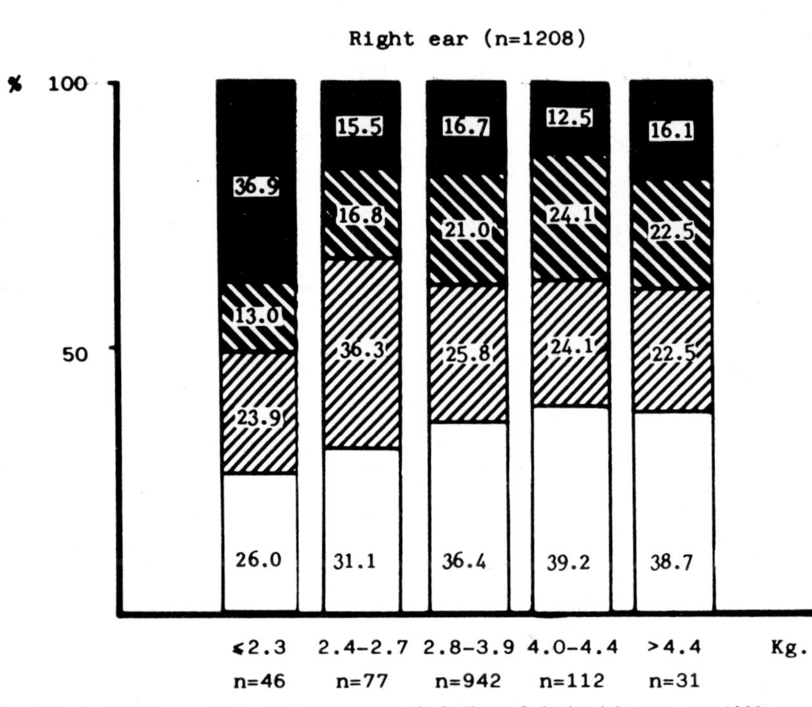

Figure 2 The relationship between birth weight and tympanometric findings. Only the right ears (n = 1208) are considered. There is a statistically significant difference between the findings in children with a birth weight lower than 2.4 kg and those with a higher birth weight ($p < 0.05$). Each bar represents from top to bottom: flat curves, middle ear pressure < -100 mm H_2O, pressure between -50 and -100 mm H_2O, normal middle ear pressure.

is a highly statistically significant difference in the prevalence of OME between children who never had acute otitis, children with one or two annual episodes of acute otitis, and those with three or more ($p < 0.001$).

The lapse of time between the latest episode of acute otitis media and the tympanometric screening also determines the tympanometric findings. If the latest episode occurred within one month before screening, only 44.2 percent of the children had bilateral normal or negative middle ear pressures, while 26.9 percent had unilateral and 20.8 percent bilateral flat curves. The number of bilateral normal or negative pressure curves went up to 50.0 percent when there was a five- to eight-week period between the latest episode of acute otitis and the tympanometric screening, to 53.3 percent when this period was between nine and 28 weeks, and up to 70.1 percent when there was more than 28 weeks between. We found bilateral normal or negative middle ear pressures in 73.2 percent of children who had never had acute otitis media ($p < 0.001$).

Nasal Condition

We found a very close relationship between nasal and middle ear pathologic conditions. A statistical analysis showed (1) the more common colds, the more episodes of acute otitis media ($p < 0.0001$); (2) the more common colds, the higher the risk of a negative middle ear pressure below -100 mm H_2O ($p < 0.05$); (3) children with open-mouth breathing and snoring have a higher risk of pronounced negative middle ear pressure and OME ($p < 0.01$); (4) pathologic nasal secretions and nasal edema predispose to negative middle ear pressures and OME ($p < 0.005$ and < 0.001 respectively); (5) even minor septal deviations have an unfavorable effect on the patency of the eustachian tube ($p < 0.05$).

Cigarette Smoking of the Parents

Our study shows that if parents smoke in the presence of the children this does not influence the development of OME in the children. The children of smoking parents have, however, a higher tendency toward negative middle ear pressure.[17] The only statistically significant difference we found concerned smoking of the mother during pregnancy. If the mother smoked more than 15 cigarettes daily during her pregnancy (whether in the first trimester or the last semester) the child was at higher risk for OME than a child of a nonsmoking mother or one who smoked less ($p = 0.05$).

Consumption of Antibiotics

It is assumed but not proven by numerous authors that the present high incidence of OME is due to the more frequent consumption of antibiotics for all kinds of infections and especially for acute otitis media. OME is explained as a kind of masked otitis media. This hypothesis seems to be contradicted by our findings (Table 1). We could not find any correlation between the antibiotic consumption of the child (expressed in number of episodes of antibiotic treatment) and the prevalence of OME or negative middle ear pressure. Also, when the results were analyzed per age group (6 months), no significant correlation was found between antibiotic consumption and tympanometric findings. Another finding was that the number of normal tympanometric curves increased at the cost of the number of negative middle ear pressures with increasing mean duration of antibiotic treatments ($p = 0.14$, not significant).

TABLE 1 Influence of Antibiotic Treatment on Middle Ear Status

		Tympanograms (%)			
Total Number of Antibiotic Treatments	*n*	*Normal*	*−50 to −100 mm H_2O*	*−100 mm H_2O*	*Flat Curve*
0	248	33.4	31.0	16.5	18.9
1–4	447	36.4	25.7	21.9	15.8
5–10	293	28.3	26.6	24.2	20.8
11–20	64	39.0	28.1	15.6	17.1
> 20	37	29.7	32.4	27.0	10.8
Mean Duration of Antibiotic Treatments					
3 days	34	23.5	29.4	29.4	17.6
3–5 days	322	38.5	27.6	15.3	18.3
6–8 days	304	38.1	21.3	23.0	17.4
9–12 days	76	46.0	26.3	11.8	15.7
> 12 days	15	26.6	26.6	33.3	13.3

n = number of ears tested

Note: There is no significant difference between the different treatment groups ($p = 0.17$ for the number of antibiotic treatments and $p = 0.14$ for the mean duration of antibiotic treatments).

DISCUSSION

From our figures we can conclude that the prevalence of OME in our target group (healthy children between 2½ and 6 years of age living in Belgium) was comparable to that in North America and Scandinavia. The highest prevalence was found at the age of 3 and during the winter. We also confirmed the positive correlation between the number of episodes of upper respiratory tract infections and the risk of OME. In this respect the time lapse between the most recent bout of acute otitis media and the tympanometric screening is very important. It was demonstrated that the condition of the nasal cavity had a definite influence on the middle ear pressure and on the development of OME. Cigarette smoking of the parents was shown to be less important; only if the mother smoked more than 15 cigarettes daily during pregnancy did the child have a higher risk of showing a flat tympanogram. Very low birth weight (< 2.4 kg) and small skull circumference (< 2.5 percentile) are factors predisposing to OME. Contrary to what has been suggested by many, antibiotic consumption did not influence middle ear pressure and development of OME in our series of 2069 children.

This study was supported financially by the Belgian Ministry of Labour and morally by the Ministry of National Education. Technical assistance was provided by Mrs. K. Coenegrachts, Mrs. P. Huijer, Dr. A. Derycke, Dr. S. Vandesande, and Mr. C. Lagrain.

REFERENCES

1. Teele DW, Klein JO, Rosner BA: Epidemiology of otitis media in children. Ann Otol Rhinol Laryngol 89 (Suppl 69):5, 1980
2. Tos M, Poulsen G, Borch J: Etiologic factors in secretory otitis. Arch Otolaryngol 105:582, 1979

3. Griffith TE: Epidemiology of otitis media—an interracial study. Laryngoscope 89:22, 1979
4. Wiet RJ, de Blanc GB, Stewart J, Weider DJ: Natural history of otitis media in the American native. Ann Otol Rhinol Laryngol 89 (Suppl 68):14, 1980
5. Draper WL: Secretory otitis media in children: A study of 540 children. Laryngoscope 77:639, 1967
6. Grote JJ, Kuijpers W: Middle ear effusion and sinusitis. J Laryngol 94:177, 1980
7. Bennett M, Ward RH, Tait CA: Otologic-audiologic study of cleft palate children. Laryngoscope 78:1001, 1968
8. Strangert K: Otitis media in young children in different types of day-care. Scand J Infect Dis 9:119, 1977
9. Lim DJ, Liu YS, Schram J, Birck HG: Immunoglobulin E in chronic middle ear effusions. Ann Otol Rhinol Laryngol 85 (Suppl 25):117, 1976
10. Bluestone CD: Eustachian tube dysfunction and allergy in otitis media. Pediatrics 61:753, 1978
11. Bernstein JM: Immunological reactivity in otitis media with effusion. In *Advances in Allergology and Clinical Immunology*. Oxford: Pergamon Press, 1980, p 139
12. Van Cauwenberge P: Otitis media with effusion. Functional morphology and physiopathology of the structures involved. Acta Otorhinolaryngol Belg 36:5, 1982
13. Tos M, Poulsen G: Screening tympanometry in infants and two-year-old children. Ann Otol Rhinol Laryngol 89 (Suppl 68):217, 1980
14. Fiellau-Nikolajsen M, Lous J: Prospective tympanometry in 3-year-old children. Arch Otolaryngol 105:461, 1979
15. Virolainen E, Puhakka H, Aantaa E, et al: Prevalence of secretory otitis media in seven to eight year old school children. Ann Otol Rhinol Laryngol 89 (Suppl 68):7, 1980
16. Tos M, Holm-Jensen S, Sørensen CH: Changes in prevalence of secretory otitis from summer to winter in four-year-old children. Am J Otol 2:324, 1981
17. Van Cauwenberge P: The influence of passive smoking on the upper respiratory tract mucosa in children. Acta Otol Rhinolaryngol Belg, in press

DETECTION OF ASYMPTOMATIC OTITIS MEDIA IN EARLY INFANCY

COLIN D. MARCHANT, M.D., PAUL A. SHURIN, M.D., MIMI A. TUTIHASI, M.D., VIRGINIA A. TURCZYK, R.N., P.N.A., DIANA E. WASIKOWSKI, R.N., P.N.A., and JOAN C. FEINSTEIN, R.N., P.N.A.

The onset of otitis media in the first year of life is of particular interest because (1) the majority of children with recurrent episodes of otitis media have their first episode before age 1[1,2] and (2) younger children have slower resolution of middle ear effusion following otitis media than do older ones.[3] Accordingly, we performed a prospective study of otitis media in the first year of life to determine the course of otitis media and to identify strategies for detection of otitis media in early infancy.

MATERIALS AND METHODS

Infants were recruited from among normal newborns in nurseries. The only entry criterion was willingness to participate in a prospective study of middle ear disease. They were followed according to an explicit protocol that outlined diagnostic criteria, medical management, and follow-up visits for the first year of life. Regular well-child visits were performed at ages 2 weeks, 2, 4, 6, 9, and 12 months. In addition, infants were examined whenever acute illnesses occurred.

Methods will be presented in detail elsewhere (Marchant CD, et al, 1983, Journal of Pediatrics: In press).

Histories of acute illness were sought at all visits using a standard questionnaire. Pneumatic otoscopy was performed by one of two physicians without knowledge of clinical symptoms or other otoscopic findings. Cerumen was carefully removed from the external auditory canal with a blunt curette before otoscopic examination. The term "middle ear effusion" was used to describe the finding of markedly decreased tympanic membrane mobility or a visible air-fluid level by pneumatic otoscopy. The otoscopists' diagnostic accuracy is supported by substantial agreement among observers and between otoscopy and tympanometry (Kappa, 0.65 to 0.76) in an independent sample.[4]

The otoscopic observations and symptoms were used to define the following conditions. *Acute otitis media* was defined as middle ear effusion with a recent history of fever or irritability. *Asymptomatic otitis media* was defined as middle ear effusion not present at the previous visit and without fever or irritability. *Recurrent otitis media* was defined as three or more episodes of otitis media (acute or asymptomatic). *Chronic otitis media* was defined as middle ear effusion lasting three months or longer.

Acute and asymptomatic otitis media were treated with 14-day courses of antimicrobial therapy. Each child was examined two weeks later and at monthly intervals until the middle ear effusion had resolved. Infants who experienced recurrent otitis media were given prophylactic antimicrobial agents.

RESULTS

Seventy infants (35 males and 35 females) were followed for the first year of life. Forty-four were white and 26 were black. Sixteen (23 percent) had no otitis media and 24 (34 percent) had onset of otitis media after age two months. The first episode of otitis media was acute (symptomatic) in 29 of 54 (54 percent); 25 (46 percent) presented at well-child visits without symptoms of otitis media. Subsequent episodes of otitis media were acute in 65 (69 percent) and asymptomatic in 29 (31 percent). Chronic otitis media, as defined above, occurred in ten infants. The practice of performing otoscopic examinations in asymptomatic infants at well-child visits detected 31 new cases of otitis media in the 70 children: four at 2 weeks of age, nine at 2 months of age, eight at 4 months of age, eight at 6 months of age, and two at 9 months of age. Asymptomatic otitis media at well-child visits accounted for 31 of all 148 (21 percent) cases of otitis media. If well-child examinations had not been performed, the diagnosis in six of ten infants with chronic bilateral otitis media would have been missed.

DISCUSSION

These findings demonstrate that infants with early onset of otitis media are at high risk for chronic otitis media. The results are particularly important in the light of data reported by the Greater Boston Collaborative Otitis Media Study Group.[5] In their large prospective study, time spent with otitis media during the first six months of life was most strongly associated with depressed scores of speech and language function at age 3 years. This suggests that the infants with early onset of otitis media are at high risk for delayed language development.

The second important finding is the high rate of asymptomatic otitis media in early infancy. Since the initial episode is asymptomatic in almost 50 percent of cases, otoscopic examination at well-child visits in the first year of life is essential to determine the full extent and duration of otitis media in infancy. Practitioners will underestimate the duration of otitis media, and the timing of therapy such as tympanostomy tubes will not be optimal. Moreover, epidemiologic studies of risk factors or outcome of otitis media which do not identify otitis media with minimal or absent symptoms may yield misleading estimates of risk.

This work was supported by Biomedical Research Support grant # RR05410 awarded to the Case Western Reserve University School of Medicine and by the Perinatal Clinical Research Center, Cleveland Metropolitan General Hospital, NIH USPHS grant # 5M01-RR00210.

REFERENCES

1. Howie VM, Ploussard JH, Sloyer J: The "otitis prone" condition. Am J Dis Child 129:676, 1975
2. Teele DW, Klein JO, Rosner BA: Epidemiology of otitis media in children. Ann Otol Rhinol Laryngol 89 (Suppl 68):5, 1980
3. Shurin PA, Pelton SI, Donner A, Klein JO: Persistence of middle-ear effusion after acute otitis media in children. N Eng J Med 300:1121, 1979
4. Kramer MS, Feinstein AR: Clinical Biostatistics LIV: The biostatistics of concordance. Clin Pharmacol Ther 29:111, 1981
5. Klein JO, Teele DW, Marros R, et al: Otitis media with effusion during the first three years of life and development of speech and language. In Lim DJ et al (eds): *Otitis Media*. Philadelphia, Toronto: BC Decker Inc, 1984

INCIDENCE OF SECRETORY OTITIS MEDIA AFTER ACUTE INFLAMMATION OF THE MIDDLE EAR CLEFT AND THE UPPER RESPIRATORY TRACT

Y. KANEKO, M.D., T. OKITSU, M.D., M. SAKUMA, M.D., Y. SHIBAHARA, M.D., R. YUASA, M.D., T. TAKASAKA, M.D., and K. KAWAMOTO, M.D.

The purpose of this chapter is to define the primary occurrence and the incidence of secretory otitis media (SOM) in children and to consider the pathogenesis of SOM statistically. The SOM described here was diagnosed based on the findings of an accumulation of fluid in the middle ear without any sign of acute inflammation; therefore, persistent middle ear effusion following acute otitis media (AOM) was considered as a sequela of AOM and was excluded from this study.

Although many factors such as race, economy, environment, sex, various diseases, and so on, have been mentioned as having a relationship to SOM, acute otitis media seems clinically to have the closest one.[1,2]

A total of 347 schoolchildren who had no past histories of SOM or any other ear disease were carefully followed up longitudinally to delineate the cases of SOM. In addition, 238 children (328 ears) suffering from AOM were followed up for several years to investigate the relationship between AOM and SOM.

INCIDENCE OF SOM IN SCHOOLCHILDREN

Materials and Methods

Three hundred forty-seven children who entered the elementary school located in the suburbs of Sendai, Japan, with a population density of 9100 persons per kilometer^2 in 1976, 1978, and 1979 were longitudinally investigated every spring and fall for three to six years to establish the incidence of primary SOM. Pupils were excluded who had SOM before entering school and who had effusion as a sequela of AOM. Children with abnormal findings of the tympanic membrane and B or C type tympanograms were re-examined at a hospital within one to two weeks. Middle ear effusion was confirmed by myringotomy. At each examination the parents were asked to answer questionnaires on AOM and upper respiratory tract infection within the last six months.

Results

The incidence of primary SOM was 0.5 to 4.0 percent in the pupils of the first (6- to 7-year-olds), second (7- to 8-year-olds), and third (8- to 9-year-olds) grades in each of the years examined. A few cases of SOM were picked up in the upper grade pupils; however, they were regarded as recurrence of SOM, not primary SOM. The cases of primary SOM were classified into two groups: with and without histories of AOM. Twelve cases (16.9 percent) of primary SOM were seen among 71 pupils with histories of AOM; 8 cases (6.1 percent) were found in 131 pupils without histories of AOM for a total of 9.9 percent of cases among 202 pupils. The *chi*-square value in these data would be significant at the $p = 0.01$ level.

OCCURRENCE OF SOM AFTER PRIMARY ATTACK OF AOM

Materials and Methods

Three hundred twenty-eight ears of 238 children with AOM were selected in our clinic for our investigation of the clinical course of AOM in the previous five years (1976 to 1980); they had no history of ear disease other than primary AOM. After AOM was cured, they received examinations at least once a month for two years. The patients were divided into four groups according to their age (0–1, 2–3, 4–5, and 6–12 years old) when they first suffered from AOM.

TABLE 1 Incidence of SOM after Primary AOM (Ears)

	Age Group (Years)				
	0–1 (n = 66)	*2–3 (n = 92)*	*4–5 (n = 113)*	*6–12 (n = 57)*	*Total (n = 328)*
1st year	18.2%	6.5%	21.2%	8.7%	14.3%
2nd year	13.6%	14.1%	23.0%	10.5%	16.5%
2 years old	30.3%	17.4%	35.4%*	15.8%	25.9%

*$P < 0.01$

Treatment of AOM

The patients with AOM associated with high fever and severe earache underwent myringotomy and antibiotic therapy. Less severe cases were treated with antibiotics without myringotomy. Almost all the cases were cured within 30 days. The ear was confirmed to be normal by the finding of (1) mobile eardrum by pneumotoscopy, (2) A- or C-type tympanogram, and (3) diminished air-bone gap in audiogram. When these conditions continued for more than one month, the AOM was regarded as cured.

Treatment of SOM

The patients with SOM underwent inflation of the middle ear (politzerization or catheterization) after the nose and throat had been cleaned for the first two weeks. When middle ear effusion was still suspected, even after the treatment of two weeks, suction of the fluid in the middle ear was performed after myringotomy. This procedure was repeated once or twice a month if the middle ear effusion persisted for more than 30 days. Children without effusion for one month were considered to be cured.

Results

Almost all the children with SOM had a history of infection of the upper respiratory tract within the previous two weeks.

Forty-seven (14.3 percent) of the 328 ears with AOM had suffered from SOM within one year after the first attack of AOM. In the second year, a similar incidence of SOM (16.5 percent) was noted. Within two years, 85 cases (25.9 percent) of SOM were found among the 328 ears (Table 1).

Noticeable differences were demonstrated in the incidence of SOM among the age groups. The 0–1 and the 4–5-year-old groups had higher incidences of SOM than the other age groups (Table 1).

About half of the cases of SOM had multiple episodes in every age group except for the 0–1-year-old group, in which only one of 12 cases recurred (Table 2).

Almost all the cases of primary AOM were cured within 30 days, but about half the cases of SOM required more than 30 days to heal.

DISCUSSION

The present study indicated that the primary occurrence of SOM is not found in children older than 9 years. This may be attributed to the fact that the immunoglobulin system of the middle ear matures with age until the ninth year.[3] Accordingly, patients under the age of 9 should be observed carefully for the occurrence of SOM.

Although only 6 percent of SOM cases were schoolchildren without histories of AOM, 17 percent of children with histories of AOM suffered from SOM. This result showed that a history of AOM seems to have a close relationship with SOM.

TABLE 2 Recurrence of SOM in the Next Year (Ears)

	Age Group (Years Old)				
	0–1 (n = 12)	*2–3 (n = 6)*	*4–5 (n = 24)*	*6–12 (n = 5)*	*Total (n = 47)*
Recurrence	1 (8.3%)	3 (50.0%)	11 (41.7%)	2 (40.0%)	17 (34.0%)

According to the immunologic studies mentioned previously, each of the age groups belongs to a different developmental stage of the immunologic system. The children in the 4–5-year-old group have a greater enlargement of adenoids and palatine tonsils and also an immature immunologic system in the middle ear. These situations may cause the highest incidence of SOM following AOM in the 4–5-year-old group.

It is well known that SOM often occurs during or after inflammation of the upper respiratory tract.[1,2,4] Almost all the cases of SOM in this study also had such histories within the previous two weeks.

Although the 0–1 and 4–5-year-old groups showed similar incidences of SOM within the year after the primary attack of AOM, there was a significant difference in the incidence of recurrence in that year. That is, in the 0–1-year-old group, SOM recurred in only one of 12 cases, whereas SOM recurred in half of the 4–5-year-old group in the next year. This difference may be due to the absence of immunologic reaction in the middle ear cavity in the 0–1-year-old group, as suggested by many investigators.[3,5,6] SOM in the 0–1-year group might have a different pathogenesis.

Based on the findings in this study, the important factors for the primary occurrence of SOM seem to include a history of AOM, inflammation of the upper respiratory tract and the immunological immaturity of the middle ear.

Based on our findings in this study and the reports from the immunologic studies, we consider SOM to occur as follows: First, an immunologic memory is induced by acute inflammation in a middle ear cavity that is immunologically immature. The middle ear mucosa becomes immunocompetent owing to the initial inflammation. Then the immunologic response in the immunocompetent middle ear is stimulated by an inflammation of the upper respiratory tract, which can transmit the antigen to the middle ear cavity. This response may cause SOM.

REFERENCES

1. Virolainen E, Puhakka H, Aantaa E, et al: Prevalence of secretory otitis media in seven to eight year old school children. Ann Otol Rhinol Laryngol 89 (Suppl 68):7, 1980
2. Schutte PK, Beales DL, Dalton R: Secretory otitis media—a retrospective general practice survey. J Laryngol Otol 95:17, 1981
3. Liu YS, Lim DJ, Lang RW, Birck HG: Chronic middle ear effusions: Immunochemical and bacteriological investigations. Arch Otolaryngol 101:278, 1975
4. Tos M, Poulsen G, Borch J: Etiologic factors in secretory otitis. Arch Otolaryngol 105:582, 1979
5. Sloyer JL Jr, Howie VM, Ploussard JH, et al: Immune response to acute otitis media in children. Infect Immun 9:1028, 1974
6. Branefors-Helander P, Dahlberg T, Nylén O: Acute otitis media. Acta Otolaryngol 80:399, 1975

NATURAL HISTORY OF SECRETORY OTITIS MEDIA

MIRKO TOS, M.D., SVEN-ERIC STANGERUP, M.D.,
ULRIK KOKS ANDREASSEN, M.D., GERD HVID, M.D.,
JENS THOMSEN, M.D., and SVEND HOLM-JENSEN, M.D.

The course of secretory otitis media varies greatly, with regard to both duration and degree of severity. Between the two extremes—that is, the scarcely recognized single episode of middle ear effusion of about one month's duration and the most protracted or recurrent course, lasting throughout childhood and continuing in the form of adhesive otitis or atelectasis—there are several intermediate stages, from which some patients recover without sequelae whereas others develop eardrum changes of varying character and degree. Any description of an average episode of secretory otitis could not possibly cover all its many facets, nor would a description of the natural history of the most frequently occurring cases of secretory otitis be representative of the disease.

In this study the natural history has been subdivided into several fairly typical forms of secretory otitis, each of which involves a substantial percentage of children. In this way we hope to be able to encompass the many aspects of the disease. The epidemiologic studies of secretory otitis performed during recent years, involving children born in different years who were followed with tympanometry and otoscopy from birth or infancy until school age, enable us to calculate the percentage of children with a certain disease pattern and the number of children who develop sequelae. Although the description of the natural course today can be based on many more data than previously,[1] many aspects of the course of secretory otitis are still unknown.

MATERIALS AND METHODS

The screening series comprised three cohorts of randomized, healthy children who were followed with tympanometry and otomicroscopy through preschool age.

Cohort I

Cohort I consisted of 150 randomized, healthy children[2] born in the maternity ward of the Gentofte Hospital from January through April 1977; they were examined with tympanometry two days after birth. The screening was repeated every three months until the end of the second year of life, and in February 1979, 1980, 1981, 1982, and in 1983 when the children were 6 years old. In all, tympanometry was repeated 13 times. At the trials performed from 1980 through 1983 otomicroscopy was also performed.

Cohort II

Cohort II comprised 278 randomized, healthy children[3–5] born during the first ten days of every month in 1976 in two municipalities of Copenhagen County, which has 120,000 inhabitants. They underwent tympanometry for the first time in November 1977 when they were 2 years old. Tympanometry was repeated every third month until August 1978, and in February 1979, 1980, 1981, 1982, and in 1983 when the children were 7 years old. The last four examinations also included otomicroscopy. A total of nine screenings has been performed in this group.

Cohort III

Cohort III included 373 healthy children[6–8] born during the first ten days of every month in 1975 in two municipalities. They were first seen in Feburary 1979 at the age of 4. Tympanometry was repeated every third month, five times in all, until February 1980, and repeated in February 1981, 1982, and 1983. A total of eight screenings was performed and the children were 8 years old at the last trial. The last four examinations also included otomicroscopy. The natural history has been analyzed on the basis of those children who until 1982 appeared at all trials, that is, 116 ears in cohort I, 254 ears in cohort II, and 444 ears in cohort III. We have previously shown that drop-outs did not influence the composition of the groups.[2,6,7]

RESULTS

Several of the epidemiologic aspects have already been published,[2–8] since each of the annual reevaluations of the cohorts brought new information. Thus, we found that the point prevalence of a type B tympanogram ranged between 10 and 18 percent at the many tympanometries performed when the children were between the ages of 1 and 6 years. After the age of 6 it was 7 percent. Age and seasonal variations thus had an influence on the point prevalence. During the first year of life the period prevalence of type B was 14 percent in cohort I and 44 percent during the first two years. In cohort II the period prevalence during nine months at the age of 2 years was 29 percent, and during 27 months at the age of 2 to 3 years it was 39 percent. In cohort III the period prevalence during one year at the age of 4 was 32 percent.[9]

In addition, it was demonstrated that about 50 percent of the ears changed type between trials, and the rate of spontaneous improvement of type B varied between 40 and 70 percent.

SEVERITY–DURATION CURVE OR TYMPANOMETRIC PROFILE

The alternation of tympanogram types from trial to trial in a series comprising up to 12 examinations can be analyzed only if the tympanometric profile of each ear is graphically presented. This has been done for each ear in all three cohorts, but to render these intelligible is almost impossible, as the number of possible variations in cohort I, with

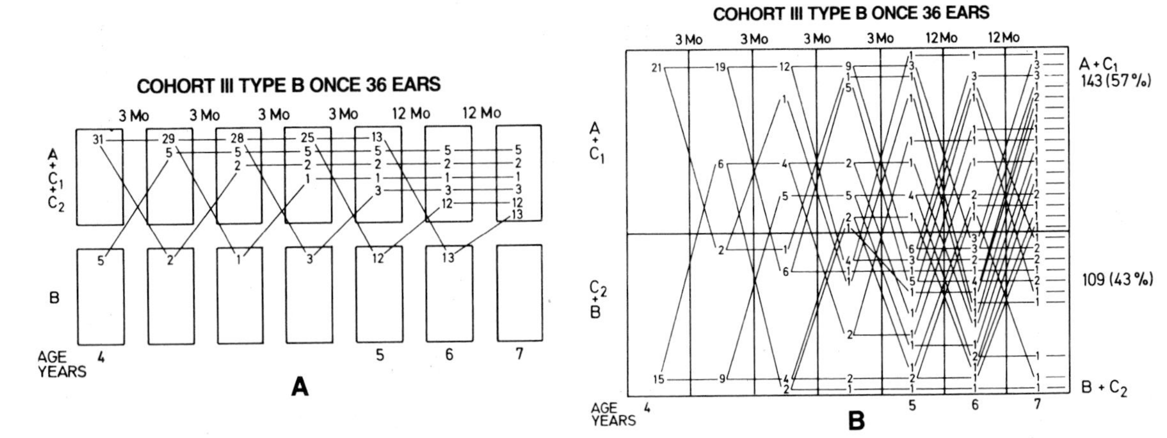

Figure 1 Spontaneous course in untreated ears in cohort III, which have had type B once. Cohort III represents 444 ears from 222 randomized, otherwise healthy children born in 1975. A, Type A, C_1, C_2 as one variable; type B as the other. B, Type A and C_1 as one variable; type B and C_2 as the other.

four types of tympanograms and 12 screenings performed, amounts to 16,777,216 (4^{12}); in cohort II with eight screenings, 65,500 (4^8); and in cohort III with seven screenings, 16,400 (4^7). Simplification to two variables was necessary: Types A, C_1, and C_2 were cumulated into one variable and type B constituted the other (Fig. 1A). The number of variations was thereby reduced to 4,096 (2^{12}), 256 (2^8), and 128 (2^7). However, much information is lost this way, especially the possibility of calculating the duration of type C_2. We know that fluid may be found in up to 50 percent of ears with this type. In an attempt to counter this, types A and C_1 were cumulated into one variable and types B and C_2 into another (Fig. 1B). By comparing the curves of the two figures, the duration and incidence of type C_2 could also be calculated.

The percentage of distribution of ears according to degree of severity and course of disease was obtained by subdividing each cohort into nine subgroups. Some examples are as follows: (1) Ears with type B only once (see Fig. 1); (2) ears with recurrent type B; (3) ears with long-lasting type B, that is, at two successive trials (Fig. 2); and (4) ears with type B for a very long period, that is, at three or more successive trials. Ears that had not had type B, but only type C_2, were likewise subdivided into groups with (1) C_2 at one trial, (2) recurring C_2, (3) long-lasting C_2, and (4) very long lasting C_2. There thus remained ears with types A or C_1 (Table 1).

Each of the nine groups was further subdivided into two groups, one with normal eardrums at the last otomicroscopic examination in

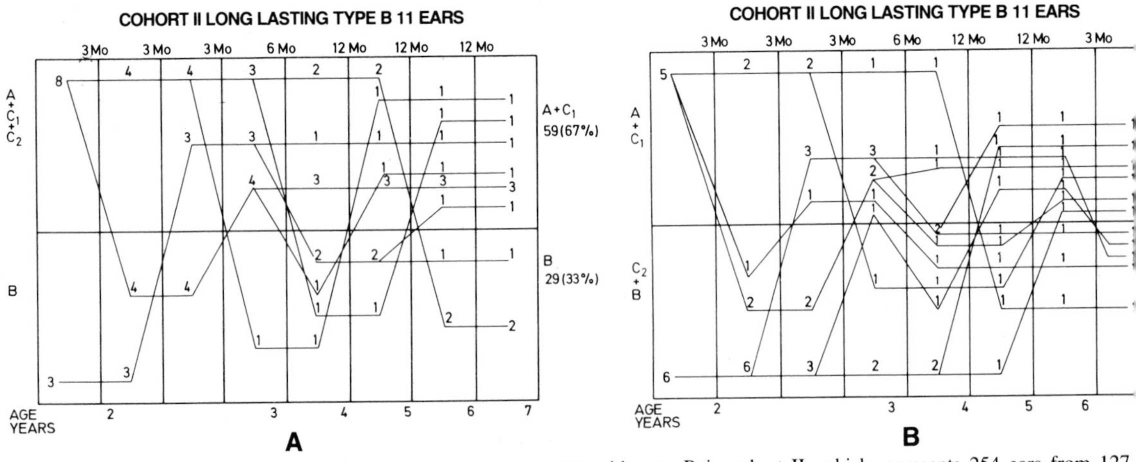

Figure 2 Spontaneous course in untreated, long-lasting cases with type B in cohort II, which represents 254 ears from 127 randomized, otherwise healthy children born in 1976. A and B are the same as in Figure 1.

TABLE 1 Percentage of Distribution According to Degree of Severity of Three Cohorts With and Without Pathologic Changes of the Eardrum

Severity Groups	*Cohort I (116 Ears)* Pathology −	+	All Ears	*Cohort II (254 Ears)* Pathology −	+	All Ears	*Cohort III (444 Ears)* Pathology −	+	All Ears
Always A or C_1	12.9	0.9	13.8	21.7	0.8	22.4	17.8	1.4	19.2
Once C_2	12.1	2.6	14.7	15.0	4.7	19.7	12.2	2.9	15.1
Recurrent C_2	7.8	1.7	9.5	4.3	1.6	5.9	6.3	2.3	8.6
Long-lasting C_2	10.3	0.9	11.2	6.3	1.6	7.9	6.3	4.3	10.6
Very long lasting C_2	3.4	1.7	5.1	2.4	1.2	3.5	4.1	3.4	7.4
Once B	14.7	12.1	26.8	10.2	8.7	18.9	10.1	9.5	19.6
Recurrent B	1.7	0.9	2.6	3.2	3.5	6.7	0.5	2.7	3.2
Long-lasting B	0.9	5.2	6.1	4.3	3.9	8.3	2.5	5.9	8.4
Very long lasting B	4.3	6.3	10.3	2.0	4.7	6.7	1.1	7.0	8.1
Totals	68.1	32.0	100.1	69.4	30.7	100.0	60.9	39.4	100.2

Note: Type A, middle ear pressure = 0 to −99 mm H_2O; C_1, middle ear pressure = −100 to −199 mm H_2O; C_2, middle ear pressure = −200 to −350 mm H_2O; B, flat curve without impedance minimum.

1982 and one with pathologic changes in the eardrum. Each of the 18 groups was then subdivided into a treated and an untreated group. For each cohort 72 drawings were made, 36 based on the principle shown in Figures 1A and 2A, and 36 similar to those in Figures 1B and 2B. Obviously, these 216 drawings cannot be published, but they do allow a thorough and fairly reliable study of the course of secretory otitis. A very short summary is presented in Table 1, but, owing to limitations of space, no distinction has been made between treated and untreated groups.

We have previously shown that at least 80 percent of all children have had at least one episode of secretory otitis before school age.[4] The percentage of distribution according to degree of severity is shown in Table 1 for all ears in the three cohorts. Type B occurred in 46 percent of the ears in cohort I, in 49 percent in cohort II, and in 39 percent in cohort III. At a single screening type B occurred in 27 percent, 19 percent, and 20 percent, respectively. Since the cohorts comprise children at different ages it can be assumed that half of the ears in cohort II and the majority of those in cohort III with type B at a single trial must be recurrent cases. Furthermore, we have calculated that, on an average, ears with a single type B had type C_2 at two other trials. So the apparently short episode of secretory otitis may be of longer duration, and an ear with a single type B may in fact be a case of recurrent type B within the same cohort. Table 1 also shows that 26 to 27 percent of ears in each cohort have had recurrent or long-lasting type C_2, although they did not have type B at any trial. If these ears were screened more frequently or at other times, type B could probably have been demonstrated. A small percentage of the ears had eardrum changes, although they had either had type C_2 once, or else type A or C_1 at all trials (Table 1). These ears have probably had secretory otitis too. In total, secretory otitis occurred in 75 percent of ears in cohort I, in 63 percent in cohort II, and in 70 percent in cohort III. These percentages confirm our earlier calculations that at least 80 percent of preschool children have had at least one episode of secretory otitits and at least 40 percent have had recurrence of the disease. Based on numerous calculations, the following preliminary conclusions may be drawn about the natural history of secretory otitis:

1. Single episodes of one to six months' duration occurred in 15 percent of ears. Only a few ears had serious changes in the eardrum.

2. Short but recurring episodes of one to six months' duration occurred in about 25 percent of ears. The prognosis is good and a relatively small percentage had pathologic findings in this eardrum.

3. Protracted episodes of six to 12 months' duration occurred in 15 percent of ears. The tympanogram type often alternated between B and C_2. Pathologic changes in the eardrum were frequently found in this group.

4. Protracted cases that improved but deteriorated again had an incidence of about 15 percent. Pathology changes were frequently found in the eardrum.

5. Very protracted cases of one to four years' duration had an incidence of 10 percent. Severe eardrum pathologic changes were found in almost all ears.

REFERENCES

1. Sadé J: *Secretory Otitis Media and Its Sequelae*. New York: Churchill Livingston, 1979
2. Tos M, Poulsen G, Hancke AB: Screening tympanometry during the first year of life. Acta Otolaryngol 88:388, 1979
3. Tos M, Poulsen G, Borch J: Tympanometry in two-year-old children. ORL 40:77, 1978
4. Tos M: Frequency of secretory otitis and histology of normal middle ear mucosa. Int J Ped Otorhinolaryngol 1:241, 1979
5. Tos M: Spontaneous improvement of secretory otitis and impedance screening. Arch Otolaryngol 106:345, 1980
6. Tos M, Holm-Jensen S, Sørensen CH, Mogensen C: Changes in point prevalence of secretory otitis in four-year-old children. Arch Otolaryngol 108:4, 1982
7. Tos M, Holm-Jensen S, Stangerup S-E, Sørensen CH: Changes in point prevalence of secretory otitis in preschool children. ORL, in press
8. Tos M, Stangerup S-E, Holm-Jensen S, Sørensen CH: Spontaneous course of secretory otitis and changes of the eardrum. Arch Otolaryngol, in press
9. Tos M: Epidemiology and spontaneous improvement of secretory otitis. Acta Otolaryngol Belg, in press

OTITIS MEDIA IN NEWBORNS: LONG-TERM FOLLOW-UP, BACTERIOLOGIC AND CYTOLOGIC INVESTIGATIONS

G. PESTALOZZA, M.D., C. CIOCE, M.D.,
M. ROMAGNOLI, M.D., F. TACCONE, M.D., L. DE LUCA, M.D.,
M. FACCHINI, D.S., and E. PACIFICO, D.S.

The incidence of otitis media in a normal population of newborn infants is uncertain since different reports[1–7] have been based on different patient populations. There are authors, such as Berman and associates,[3] who have identified effusion in as many as 30 percent of 125 examined infants in a neonatal intensive care unit. Other studies[8] claim that otitis media in newborns is "uncommon." In a previous study performed in our hospital (including both the intensive care unit and the normal nursery) otitis media was identified in 5.76 percent of newborns.[5]

Bacteriologic investigations of otitis media strictly limited to the neonatal period are very rare: most studies include infants up to the fourth month or to 6 weeks of age. According to Klein and Bluestone,[6] a study of children of this age group revealed *Streptococcus pneumoniae* and *Hemophilus influenzae* to be the most frequent bacteria cultured from the middle ear fluid. According to Narcy,[9] *Staphylococcus* spp. (*aureus, epidermidis,* and so on), *H. influenzae* and *Pseudomonas aeruginosa* are the predominant organisms. In both studies, however, enteric bacteria were found more frequently than in older children, whereas the role of coagulase-negative staphylococci is still uncertain.[10]

Histopathologic investigations of the middle ear[11–13] showed early alterations of the epithelial cells lining the entire middle ear following surgically induced otitis media. Owing to uncertain early clinical manifestations, diagnosis of otitis in the newborn is often rather difficult[5,14,15]; tympanometry is of no value at this age.[16] Previous clinical studies[5,7,17–19] point to the extreme variability of incidence and low specificity of symptoms.

MATERIALS AND METHODS

The present study was based on 3072 newborns hospitalized a few days after birth in the years 1977 to 1982. The number of newborns undergoing otoscopy was 970; the number of newborns affected and treated for otitis media was 205.

Newborns were referred from the neonatologist to the otologist because they presented clinical and/or laboratory signs of infection. Clinical features of otitis media in newborns based on otoscopy are described elsewhere.[5]

A retrospective chart review was prepared to collect case histories and clinical data, including (1) diseases of the mother during pregnancy, (2) type of delivery, (3) time interval between ruptured membranes and delivery (more than 6 hours), (4) characteristics of amniotic fluid, (5) causes of hospitalization, and (6) associated illnesses.

With regard to course and treatment of otitis media during hospitalization, the following factors were marked in the chart: (1) date of diagnosis to otitis media (in days from birth); (2) duration of the disease; (3) type of antibiotic treatment; (4) duration of the treatment; (5) number of paracenteses and type of effusion; (6) bacterial etiologic factors (paracentesis and spontaneous otorrhea); (7) cytology; and (8) follow-up, including case history from birth to the date of the visit, otoscopy, and tympanometry. Seventy-two children were studied in the follow-up group. When paracentesis was required, aspiration of middle ear fluid for bacteriologic and cytologic tests was performed as follows without prior anesthesia: the ear canal was cleaned, sterilized with Cetavlon or Betadine, the ear drum was incised, and the end of a PVC suction with a special container (Xomed JUHN TIM-TAP) was introduced. Aspirated materials were sent to the laboratory in two separate sterile containers.

RESULTS

Otitis was unilateral in 159 and bilateral in 46 newborns. Cause of disease and results of treatment refer only to the worst ear, that is, to the ear that had a longer duration of disease or was submitted to paracentesis. Thus, all results refer to 205 ears of 205 newborns.

Physiologic and pathologic conditions of the mother during pregnancy were not significant. Meconium-stained amniotic fluid recurred in 26.3 percent of cases in association with otitis media. This result is significant when compared with an 8.8 percent incidence of this finding in cases reported by Gregory and colleagues[20] in a normal population.

Symptoms and illnesses associated with otitis media are presented in Table 1. This classification

TABLE 1 Otitis Media in Newborns (N = 205)

Symptoms		*Associated Illnesses*	
Irritability, lethargy, cry	48	Severe jaundice	46
Vomiting	23	Dystrophia	24
Seizures	9	Immaturity	22
Hypothermia or fever	6	Postasphyxia syndrome	21
Hepatosplenomegaly	4	Infections*	17
Hypotonia	3	Small for date	10
		Congenital heart disease	7
Total	93	Total	147

*Conjunctivitis, omphalitis, gastroenteritis, urinary tract infection

is not as accurate as we would like; symptoms of otitis media could actually be present in cases of associated illnesses as well. Newborns with "symptoms" include those referred by the neonatologist to the otologist with no other manifest disease. In this group otitis media must be considered responsible for the symptoms causing hospitalization. This was true in 93 cases of 205 (45.4 percent). In Table 1 we can see that the most frequent signs have very low specificity for otitis (prolonged cry, irritability, lethargy, vomiting). Newborns with "associated illnesses" include those who were hospitalized for a particular disease or condition (dystrophia, severe jaundice, immaturity, and so on); otitis media was discovered in the course of otoscopy requested by the neonatologist. This was true in 143 cases (71.7 percent).

There were 132 newborns with serous otitis (64.4 percent); 55 (26.8 percent) underwent paracentesis. Seventy-three newborns (35.6 percent) had purulent discharging otitis at the first visit. The duration of the disease was 9.2 days ± 5.6. We considered those newborns recovered in whom purulent discharge had completely disappeared at the time of the last visit and in whom the eardrum was normal or nearly normal. In Figure 1 duration of antibiotic treatment and the number of paracenteses from the day of the beginning of the disease are shown. Duration of antibiotic treatment was 6.93 days ± 3.4. In most cases we use cephalosporins (50.7 percent) or aminoglycosides (43.4 percent); ampicillin and amoxicillin were rarely used (5.9 percent) on the basis of the neonatologist's experience in the treatment of other bacterial infections of the newborn. A great many newborns (18 percent) underwent paracentesis on the second day of the disease or on the seventh day, that is, when the number of children submit-

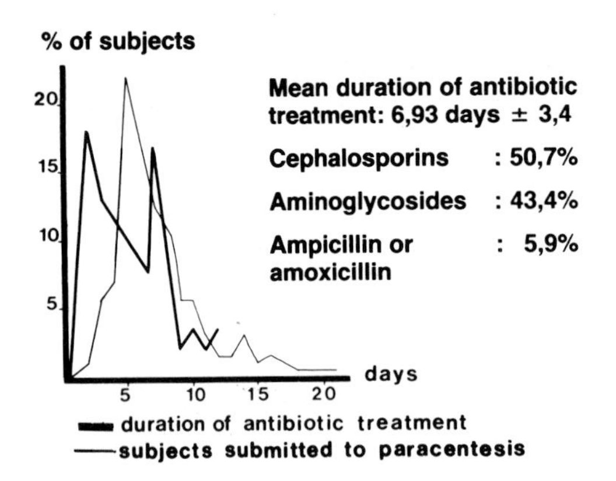

Figure 1 Antibiotic treatment and paracentesis. The paracentesis group curve indicates that some newborns underwent paracentesis on the second day after the beginning of the disease, whereas another group had paracentesis on the seventh day, when antibiotic treatment was stopped in most subjects.

ted to antibiotic treatment decreased. According to our experience this means that if otitis media in newborns does not respond to antibiotic treatment within five or six days, paracentesis should be performed.

Bacteriologic cultures were sterile or showed nonpathogenic bacteria in 57.4 percent of cases. Pathogenic bacteria had the following distribution: *S. aureus,* 10.7 percent; *S. pneumoniae,* 5.3 percent; *H. influenzae,* 6.7 percent; *P. aeruginosa,* 10.7 percent; *Enterobacter,* 4 percent; and *Escherichia coli,* 5.3 percent. We found eight significant cytologic tests out of 16. We found both inflammatory cells (polymorphonuclear neutrophils, macrophages, lymphocytes) and epithelial cells. Some of them were normal, with preserved cilia and sharp eosinophilic terminals; others had some cellular modifications, of inflammatory origin (increased relationships between nucleus and cytoplasm, loss of cilia).

The purpose of the cytologic studies was to define the types of cells commonly seen in middle ear fluid and to establish, whenever possible, the "age" of the lesion based on the type of cellular alterations. It is important to note that modified ciliated cells and numerous inflammatory cells were found in the middle ear fluid of newborns three to five days old. These results are similar to those obtained by Goycoolea and associates[11] in studies on the cat. Observing the early appearance of cellular degeneration, we could argue that middle ear infection probably began before birth as a consequence of early ruptured amniotic membranes, prolonged delivery, and meconium-stained amniotic fluid. Meconium is supposed to be sterile, but it could be contaminated by the fluids of the birth canal as a result of early ruptured membranes.

FOLLOW-UP

We could control only 72 of 205 children born between 1977 and 1982 who suffered from otitis media during the neonatal period; 50 (24.4 percent) came to the hospital for a visit and 22 had only a telephone interview regarding history and frequency of otitis after birth. At the time of the visit 52 percent of the children were less than 2 years of age (the youngest was 10 months), and 48 percent were more than 2 years (the oldest 4½ years). Results are summarized in Figure 2; we can see that infection of the upper airways occurred frequently (35 percent). Twenty-five percent of children had two or more attacks of otitis media (earache with fever for 2 days or more); 4.2 percent had purulent discharge.

At otoscopy eardrums were normal in only 55 percent of the cases; in 15 percent eardrums were severely retracted (major tympanic lesions). Many children (30 percent) had congested eardrums at the time of the visit. In Figure 3 a correlation is illustrated between long-term anatomic–functional results and type of neonatal otitis. On one side children with normal or slightly congested eardrums and type A or C tympanometries were considered, and on the other side children with major tympanic lesions and type B tympanometry were considered. We could argue that the best long-term anatomic and functional results were found in chil-

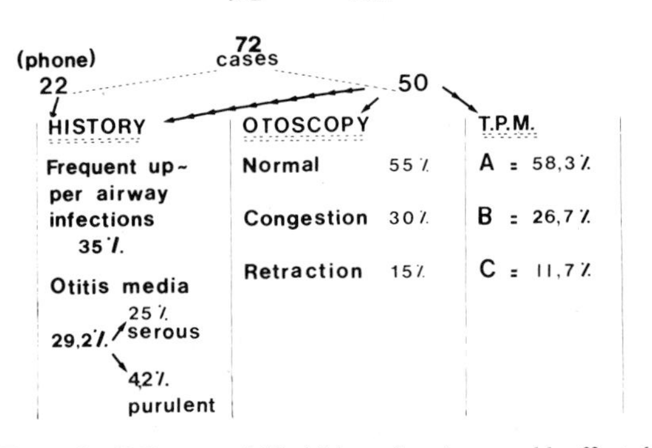

Figure 2 Follow-up of 72 children, 1 to 4 years old, affected by otitis media in the neonatal period.

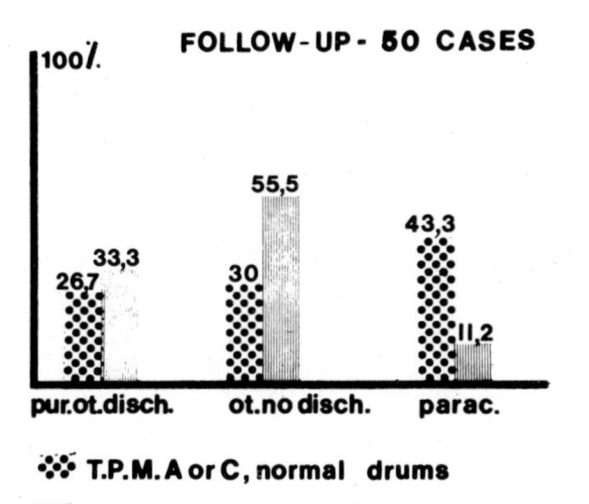

Figure 3 Long-term anatomic and functional results in relation to neonatal otitis. In most cases children who underwent paracentesis at birth presented normal drums and type A tympanograms.

dren whose neonatal otitis was treated by means of paracentesis. Among children who were submitted to antibiotic treatment only (serous otitis, purulent discharging otitis) there was a lower percentage of good results.

CONCLUSIONS

The retrospective study (history, clinical course, bacteriologic and cytologic investigations) of 205 hospitalized newborns allowed us to clarify several epidemiologic aspects of neonatal otitis and to define some useful rules of treatment with the purpose of preventing recurrent otitis in early childhood. We can make the following conclusions:

No significant relationship was found between neonatal otitis and pathologic conditions of the mother during pregnancy.

The incidence of 26.3 percent of cases of meconium-stained amniotic fluid following ruptured amniotic membranes in newborns affected by otitis media is significant.

Signs and symptoms of otitis media are not specific; diagnosis was based chiefly on otoscopy.

Mean duration of the disease (with or without purulent discharge) in 205 newborns who underwent antibiotic treatment was 6.9 days. The most frequently used antibiotics were cephalosporins and aminoglycosides.

Fifty-five children underwent paracentesis, mostly on the second day or after the seventh day of the disease if antibiotics did not lead to recovery.

Bacteriologic studies revealed a high incidence of sterile cultures or cultures that were not pathogens. Among pathogens discovered there was a high relative incidence of enteric bacteria (*Enterobacter, E. coli*) and *Pseudomonas*.

Cytologic examination revealed numerous inflammatory cells and early alterations of ciliated cells of the middle ear in cases of otitis in the third or fourth day of life. It could be argued that otitis started before birth (from infected meconium-stained amniotic fluid?).

Long-term follow-up involved 72 cases (50 underwent otoscopy and tympanometry). In the period between birth and control (from 2 to 4 years), the incidence of pathologic changes of the upper airways was 35 percent. Two or more attacks of otitis media (serous or purulent) occurred in 29.2 percent of children. A recent study on the epidemiology of otitis media in infancy in the United States[8] reports that by 3 years of age approximately two-thirds of children have had at least one episode of acute otitis media and one-third have had three or more episodes. The results obtained from our group of children are within the range of those in this study.

REFERENCES

1. Warren WS, Stool SE: Otitis media in low-birth weight infants J Pediatr 79:740, 1971
2. Jaffe BV, Hurtado F, Hurtado E: Tympanic membrane mobility in the newborn with seven month's follow-up. Laryngoscope 80:36, 1970
3. Berman SA, Balkany TJ, Simmons MA: Otitis media in infants less than 12 weeks of age: Differing bacteriology among in-patients and out-patients. J Pediatr 93:43, 1978
4. de Sa DJ: Infection and amniotic aspiration of middle ear in stillbirths and neonatal death. Arch Dis Child 48:872, 1973
5. Cioce C, Canubi A: L'otite nel neonato. Annali di Laring Otol Rinol Faringol 76:571, 1978
6. Klein JO, Bluestone CD: Acute otitis media. Pediatr Infect Dis 1:66, 1982
7. Shurin PA, Howie VM, Pelton SI, et al: Bacteriology and etiology of otitis media during the first six weeks of life. J Pediatr 92:893, 1978
8. Teele DW, Klein JO, Rosner BA: Epidemiology of otitis media in children. Ann Otol Rhinol Laryngol 89 (Suppl 68):5, 1980
9. Narcy P, Arronio C, Margo JN, et al: Etude bacteriologique de l'otite moyenne aiguë. Ann Otorhinol 99:383, 1982
10. Bernstein JM, Myers D, Kosinsky D, et al: Antibody coated bacteria in otitis media with effusion. Ann Otol Rhinol Laryngol 89 (Suppl 68):104, 1980

11. Goycoolea MM, Paparella MM, Juhn SK, Carpenter AM: Cells involved in the middle ear defense system. Ann Otol Rhinol Laryngol 89 (Suppl 68):121, 1980
12. Sadé J: The biopathology of secretory otitis media. Ann Otol Rhinol Laryngol 83 (Suppl 11):59, 1974
13. Lim DJ: Functional morphology of the lining membrane of the middle ear and Eustachian tube. Ann Otol Rhinol Laryngol 83 (Suppl. 11):5, 1974
14. Klein JO: Microbiology of otitis media. Ann Otol Rhinol Laryngol 89 (Suppl 68):98, 1980
15. McLellan MS, Strong JP, Johnson QR, Dent JH: Otitis media in premature infants: A histopathologic study. J Pediatr 61:53, 1962
16. Pestalozza G, Cusmano C: Evaluation of tympanometry in diagnosis and treatment of otitis media of the newborn and of the infant. Int J Pediatr Otorhinolaryngol 2:73, 1980
17. Tetzlaff TR, Ashworth C, Nelson JD: Otitis media in children less than 12 weeks of age. Pediatrics 59:827, 1977
18. Bland RD: Otitis media in the first six weeks of life. Pediatrics 49:187, 1972
19. Shurin PA, Pelton SI, Klein JO: Otitis media in the newborn infant. Ann Otol Rhinol Laryngol 85 (Suppl 25):216, 1976
20. Gregory GA, Gooding CA, Phibbs H, Tooley WH: Meconium aspiration in infants: A prospective study. J Pediatr 85:848, 1974

PHYSIOLOGY AND PATHOPHYSIOLOGY

STATE OF THE ART: PHYSIOLOGY AND PATHOPHYSIOLOGY OF THE EUSTACHIAN TUBE

ERDEM I. CANTEKIN, Ph.D.

Otitis media is the result of an unfavorable combination of endogenous and exogenous factors that alter the mucous membrane of the middle ear. Eustachian tube (ET) function is probably the single most important entity involved in the endogenous factors. The three known functions of the ET are pressure regulation, protection, and drainage. Drainage is assumed to be responsible for clearance of middle ear secretions and is accomplished by mucociliary transport. Since this function has not been extensively investigated in the past, we have little knowledge of clearance of middle ear secretions through the ET.[1,2] The remaining two functions (pressure regulation and protection) have been more thoroughly studied, and therefore this report will focus on these two functions as they relate to physiology and pathophysiology of the system.

Tasks of pressure regulation and protection are accomplished by active and passive functions of the ET. Mechanics of tubal function related to active and passive functions are illustrated in Figure 1. Tubal opening secondary to inferolateral pull of the tensor veli palatini (TVP) muscle is defined as active function in contradistinction to tubal closing or tubal opening due to a pressure differential between the two ends of the tube, which is defined as passive function. Contractions of the TVP muscle displace the lateral wall with a fixed amount during active opening, and, if there is a pressure differential between nasopharynx and middle ear, there will be a flow of gas through the ET (Fig. 1B). Closing of the tube, after termination of TVP activity, is a passive event due to elastic recoil of surrounding tissue (Fig. 1C). Without TVP activity, the tube may open passively when pressure exceeds the closing forces around the lumen. In this situation the tubal walls would be displaced a variable distance, depending upon the magnitude of pressure (Fig. 1D). Assessment of passive function provides a measure of mechanical properties of the ET, and active function measures reveal information about the efficiency of TVP muscle in actively dilating the tubal lumen.

During the last two decades, numerous laboratory and clinical investigations have been conducted to understand the physiologic function of the ET in patients with intact and nonintact tympanic membranes[3–20] (also see pp. 59, 62). In these studies various methods and techniques were used to define the limits of normal function in subjects without a history of otologic disease. Findings in subjects with various forms of ear disease were then compared with the normal data to establish abnormal function parameters. Existing tubal function evaluation techniques can be classified into four general groups: (1) radiographic, (2) manometric, (3) tympanometric, and (4) sonometric. Of these, the macroflow- or microflow-based manometric techniques have yielded the most discriminating quantitative data on active and passive functions of the ET.

These quantitative manometric data from the previous studies were used to construct conceptual schematic illustrations to exemplify the tubal function types. Figure 2A shows a two-dimensional space relating active and passive functions. The normal limits as well as the gray area of the operational tolerance are depicted by the two concentric semicircles. The symbol convention of the plot is such that the origin represents a perfect active function corresponding to complete equilibration capacity of applied positive or negative pressures. Increasing distance on the ordinate represents diminishing active function. On the abscissa, the normal passive function is defined as the origin.

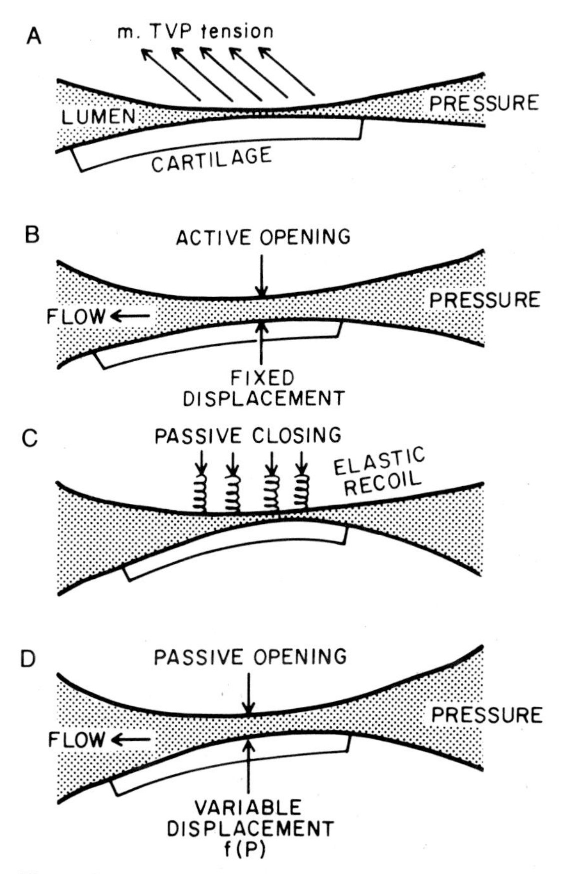

Figure 1 Schematics of eustachian tube mechanics during pressure equilibration; (A) At rest, (B) fixed displacement during active opening by the tensor veli palatini muscle (TVP), (C) passive closing due to the elastic recoil of the surrounding tissue, (D) passive opening of variable dilation as a function of overpressure (f [P]).

Increasing values on this axis represent a shift toward inadequate ventilation. Conversely, decreasing values signify a move toward inadequate protection. Figure 2B depicts three extreme cases of tubal dysfunction to exemplify the utility of this active-passive function space. Total functional obstruction representing the deficiency in the tubal opening mechanism without mechanical abnormalities is shown on the top of the ordinate. Pure mechanical obstruction, such as total blockage of the tube by a tumor, is shown on the extreme right. In this hypothetical case, active function is shown to be normal, assuming that the integrity of the muscle has not been affected. The third example illustrates a tubal dysfunction secondary to inadequate protection, such as a patulous tube, in which the pathophysiologic change stems from closing failure of the tube.

The remaining six frames in Figure 2 illustrate different categories of tubal function derived from the findings of various studies in the literature. Figure 2C depicts improvement in active function by increasing age for children with and without otitis media. Normal children have passive function parameters within normal limits of adults. A recent longitudinal study in children with negative otologic histories demonstrated that, with increasing age, there was an improvement in their active function.[20] In the otitis media group, the maturation process of tubal function is more obscure.[24] However, there is some evidence for active and passive function improvement with advancing age in this group which is supported by indirect evidence of decreased incidence of chronic or recurrent middle ear disease in older children.

The patients with unrepaired cleft palates are generally characterized by high passive function[9] (also see page 59). The effect of surgical repair of the palate in this population is shown in Figure 2D. With conventional palatoplasty, the active function would not be affected, but inadequate ventilation due to high passive function may be corrected.[9,15] It has been suggested that by performing a levator veli palatini sling operation, tightening of the muscle may improve ET function, since both active and passive functions may be altered during the surgical procedure.[21]

Inadequate protection of the middle ear is exemplified by the patulous tube syndrome. The effects of two different procedures to correct this defect are illustrated in Figure 2E. The lower example shows a Teflon injection around the tube in which the closing failure of the tube is corrected by increasing the passive function. The second example is a newly described procedure, transposition of the TVP muscle medial to the hamulus, which is purported also to increase passive function.[22] However, these procedures may compromise the active function, and functional obstruction of the tube may become a postsurgical problem.

In Figure 2F the function space concept is used to show the effect of inflammation secondary to upper respiratory infection.[12,20] The top example shows a subject who has marginal normal tubal function. During inflammation, the change in passive function due to increase in opening and closing pressures would move the subject to an inadequate ventilation zone. This could result in middle ear disease. The lower example represents a subject who has ET function that is within normal limits prior to inflammation. In this case, after changes in the passive function secondary to the inflammation, tubal function would remain within

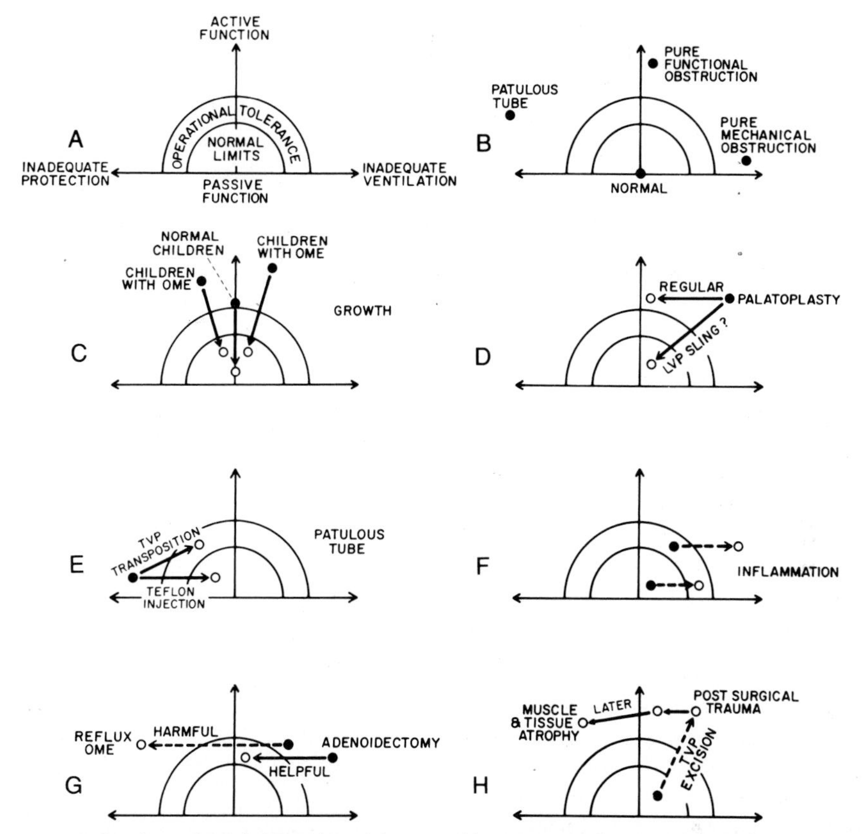

Figure 2 The concept of active and passive function of the eustachian tube as it relates to the specific examples. (A) Limits of normal function and extremes of passive function, such as inadequate protection or ventilation; (B) various tubal function types (normal function, functional obstruction, mechanical obstruction, and patulous tube); (C) effect of growth on tubal function of children with and without otitis media; (D) effect of palatoplasty in cleft palate children; (E) repair of patulous tube; (F) effect of inflammation; (G) tubal function before and after adenoidectomy; (H) effect of tensor veli palatini (TVP) muscle excision in the experimental animal model of otitis media.

operational tolerance of the system, and no ear disease would occur.

The effect of adenoidectomy on tubal function is illustrated in Figure 2G.[8] Preoperatively, the first example is a patient who has high opening and closing pressures, signifying inadequate ventilation due to high passive function. The beneficial effects of the adenoidectomy on this patient would be evidenced by improved tubal function status after surgery. Contrary to this, the second example depicts a patient with almost normal passive function prior to surgery. This patient would not benefit from the surgery, since the postoperative tubal function would be within the inadequate protection zone. This unfavorable change would be the result of adenoid tissue removed, which could reduce the mechanical support of the medial tubal wall. This type of tubal function is generally associated with reflux otitis media.

The final example (Fig. 2H) is the experimental animal model of otitis media secondary to ET dysfunction.[23] In the Rhesus monkey active tubal function was totally abolished following TVP excision. Also there was an increase in opening and closing pressures due to postsurgical trauma, indicating a change in passive function as well. When the trauma decreased, passive function returned to normal presurgical values. However, passive function further decreased months later due to atrophy of muscle and tissue surrounding the tube.

In an effort to understand the differences in ET function of various populations with and without ear disease, the parameters of passive function (forced opening pressure, closing pressure, passive resistance) and active function (equilibration ability of positive or negative middle ear pressure, constriction or dilation during swallowing) were compiled from past studies to establish a qualitative centroid point for each population in the two-dimensional active–passive tubal function space. The resultant spectra of centroids repre-

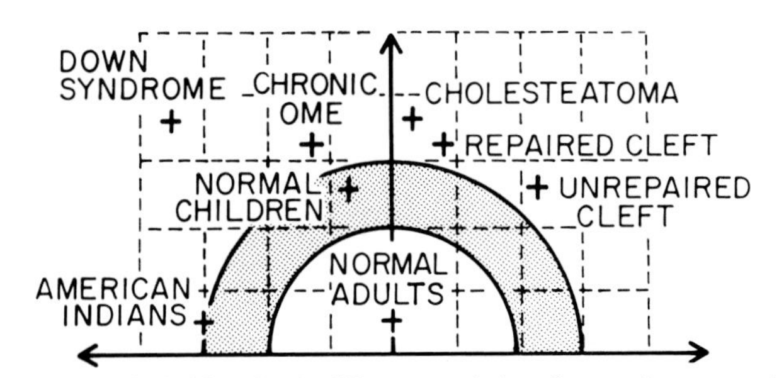

Figure 3 The spectra of tubal function in different populations from various reports in the literature.

senting tubal function types in different populations is depicted in Figure 3. The data from normal children and adults are assumed to represent normal limits.[6,10,13,17,20] Children are shown above adults with respect to their active function; this is to say that their normal function is at the operational limits of the system.[20] Two special populations, American Indians and those with Down's syndrome, represent tubal dysfunction groups whose problem stems from inadequate protection[16] (also see page 62). The difference between them is the finding that the American Indians have almost normal active function, in contrast to the total lack of active function in the Down's syndrome group. Another population, infants with unrepaired cleft palates, have both active and passive function deficiency[9] (also see page 59). The group of cholesteatoma patients presented has normal passive function and abnormal active function, which is contrary to the tubal closing failure or sniff-induced disease hypothesis.[14,19]

Figure 3 should be interpreted with caution, since it is basically a schematic and conceptual display of the relative position of centroids of tubal function distributions of various populations. Furthermore, the centroid determinations were made by rank ordering of different passive and active function parameters rather than by numerical computations. Therefore, this schema is intended to be only qualitative. It is hoped that in the future, a quantitative spectrum of tubal function types can be constructed to reveal the underlying pathophysiologic changes in various tubal dysfunction groups.

Further understanding of this important endogenous factor, ET function, as it relates to the pathogenesis of otitis media will help clinical management of this disease process.

This study was supported in part by grant NS-16337 from the National Institutes of Health.

Most of the ideas and concepts in this manuscript are the result of discussions with my coworkers Charles D. Bluestone and William John Doyle.

REFERENCES

1. Bluestone CD: Eustachian tube obstruction in the infant with cleft palate. Ann Otol Rhinol Laryngol 80(2):1, 1971
2. Nuutineu J, Karja J, Karjalainen P: Measurement of mucociliary function of the eustachian tube. Arch Otolaryngol 109:669, 1983
3. Flisberg K, Ingelstedt S, Ortegren U: On the function of middle ear and eustachian tube. Acta Otolaryngol (Stockh) Suppl 182:1, 1963
4. Flisberg K: Ventilatory studies on the eustachian tube. Acta Otolaryngol (Stockh) Suppl 219:1, 1966
5. Ingelstedt S, Ivarsson A, Jonson B: Mechanics of the human middle ear. Acta Otolaryngol (Stockh) Suppl 228:1, 1967
6. Elner Å, Ingelstedt S, Ivarsson A: The normal function of the eustachian tube—a study of 102 cases. Acta Otolaryngol (Stockh) 72:320, 1971
7. Andreasson L: Kronisk Slemhinneotit. Thesis, Lund University, Malmo, Sweden, 1973
8. Bluestone CD, Cantekin EI, Beery QC: Certain effects of adenoidectomy on eustachian tube ventilatory function. Laryngoscope 85:113, 1975
9. Bluestone CD, Beery QC, Cantekin EI, Paradise JL: Eustachian tube ventilatory function in relation to cleft palate. Ann Otol Rhinol Laryngol 84:333, 1975
10. Cantekin EI, Bluestone CD, Parkin LP: Eustachian tube ventilatory function in children. Ann Otol Rhinol Laryngol 85(25):171, 1976
11. Virtanen H: Eustachian tube sound conduction—sonotubometry, an acoustical method for objective measurement of auditory tubal opening. Thesis, University of Helsinki, Finland, 1977
12. Bluestone CD, Cantekin EI, Beery QC: Effect of inflammation on the ventilatory function of the eustachian tube. Laryngoscope 87:493, 1977
13. Cantekin EI, Saez CA, Bluestone CD, Bern SA: Airflow through the eustachian tube. Ann Otol Rhinol Laryngol 88:603, 1979
14. Magnuson B: Mellanoresjukdom av Retraktionstyp. Thesis, University of Linkoping, Linkoping, Sweden, 1980
15. Doyle WJ, Cantekin EI, Bluestone CD: Eustachian tube function in cleft palate children. Ann Otol Rhinol Laryngol 89(68):34, 1980
16. Beery QC, Doyle WJ, Cantekin EI, Bluestone CD, Wiet

RJ: Eustachian tube function in an American Indian population. Ann Otol Rhinol Laryngol 89(68):28, 1980
17. Groth P: Eustachian tube function in aviation—an experimental study in man. Thesis, Lund University, Malmo, Sweden, 1981
18. Lildholdt T, Cantekin EI, Bluestone CD, Rockette HE: Effect of a topical nasal decongestant on eustachian tube function in children with tympanostomy tubes. Acta Otolaryngol 94:93, 1982
19. Bluestone CD, Casselbrant ML, Cantekin EI. Functional obstruction of the eustachian tube in the pathogenesis of aural cholesteatoma in children. In Proceedings of the Second International Conference on Cholesteatoma and Mastoid Surgery. Amsterdam: Kugler Publications, 1982
20. Bylander A: Eustachian tube function in healthy children—a pressure equilibration study with an adult reference group. Thesis, Lund University, Malmo, Sweden, 1983
21. Honjo I, Harada H, Okazaki N: Significance of levator muscle sling formation in cleft palate surgery: Evaluation by electrical stimulation. Plast Reconstr Surg 65:443, 1980
22. Virtanen H, Palva T: Surgical treatment of patulous eustachian tube. Arch Otolaryngol 108:735, 1982
23. Cantekin EI, Phillips DC, Doyle WJ, Bluestone CD, Kimes KK: Effect of surgical alterations of the tensor veli palatini muscle on eustachian tube function. Ann Otol Rhinol Laryngol 89(68):47, 1980
24. Beery QC, Doyle WJ, Cantekin EI, Bluestone CD: Longitudinal assessment of eustachian tube function in children. Laryngoscope 89:1446, 1979

NEW TECHNIQUES FOR MEASURING EUSTACHIAN TUBE RESPONSES

BENGT MAGNUSON, M.D., and BERNT FALK, M.D.

The classic "ex vacuo" theory states that middle ear effusion is a result of negative pressure caused by resorption of air in the middle ear cavity. It is presumed that when the eustachian tube fails to open at regular intervals the gas enclosed in the middle ear cavity is resorbed, and eustachian tube malfunction is defined in terms of failure of opening. Results of recent studies in patients with chronic ear disease and in patients with middle ear effusion indicate a need to reconsider the part played by the tube in the development of ear disease, and consequently lead to a restatement of the "ex vacuo" theory.

Direct pressure measurements in patients with manifest ear disease, for example, atelectatic ears, adhesive otitis, and retraction cholesteatoma, have shown that negative middle ear pressure is induced instantly by direct evacuation of the middle ear space during the act of sniffing.[1–3] The primary disturbance of the eustachian tube function is thus failure of closing. As a consequence of the locking effect on the tube, the sniff-induced negative pressure remains in the middle ear space for a period of time. The induced negative pressure is usually on the order of 2 to 3 kPa (200 to 300 mm of water), but in exceptional cases the negative pressure may exceed 10 kPa, or 1000 mm water pressure.[1] The middle ear pressure is often reduced in several steps in response to repeated sniffing. Some patients with chronic ear disease are suffering from patulous tube symptoms (autophonia, drumhead flutter, and hyperacusis) and have developed a habitual sniffing behavior to suppress their symptoms.[4] They are thus sniffing constantly, trying to keep their eustachian tubes closed. Some children with recurrent middle ear effusion seem to suffer from the same type of malfunction, but most frequently a disorder denoted "relative closing failure" is found.[3–5] This means that the eustachian tube is seldom, if ever, wide open. However, the tube fails to resist the high negative pressure generated in the nasopharynx during vigorous sniffing, and the middle ear is evacuated of air.[5]

METHODS

In some cases evacuation of the middle ear on sniffing can be seen when the ear is examined under the otomicroscope. The clinical sniff test is performed by having the patient inflate his ear and then sniff sharply.[4] This test is not always reliable, partly because otomicroscopic examination is usually done with the patient lying on the examination table. In the horizontal position the elevated venous pressure causes the tube to close more firmly.

Also, it may be difficult to observe the movements of the tympanic membrane.

Two methods for performing an objective sniff test are available: tympanometry and direct pressure recording. Serial tympanograms taken before and after sniffing can provide a qualitative determination of whether evacuation of the middle ear takes place.[6] In normal ears the indirect determination of the middle ear pressure obtained with tympanometry is also reliable, but in an atelectatic ear with very small middle ear volume and a flaccid tympanic membrane the measured pressure value is often misleading. In such cases the tympanometric method is impaired by a systematic numerical overestimation of the real pressure, and a too high negative pressure is indicated. This depends on the fact that the pressure sweep of the tympanometer forces the retracted tympanic membrane back to the midposition. The middle ear space is thus expanded by the lateral movement of the eardrum and, subsequently, the pressure is changed by the action of the tympanometer.

Ears with middle ear effusion are well suited for direct pressure recording because the use of transmyringeal ventilation tubes is part of the treatment. When a pressure transducer is connected to the ear canal, airtight, the response to sniffing can be recorded. This method leads to a systematic underestimation of the numerical value of the middle ear pressure. The error can be reduced if the volume of the measuring system is minimized. With direct pressure recording the course of pressure change in the middle ear can be followed, and this method is preferred.

Our method for pressure recording is illustrated in Figure 1. Three pressure transducers are mounted on a headpiece and the transducers are connected to the nose and the ear canals by short catheters and made airtight. Pressures in the nose and both ears are recorded simultaneously to an ink-jet recorder. The headpiece also includes a pressurizing system consisting of a glass syringe and a mechanical manometer for display. This equipment is used when forced opening of the tube is performed and for application of test pressures in the pressure equalization tests.

Figure 2 shows a typical pressure curve obtained in a boy with persistent bilateral middle ear effusion. During the test the patient is standing in front of the recorder to achieve a positive feedback. When the patient can see the immediate result of his sniffing or Valsalva blowing on the curves, he becomes interested in what is going on and cooperation is facilitated.

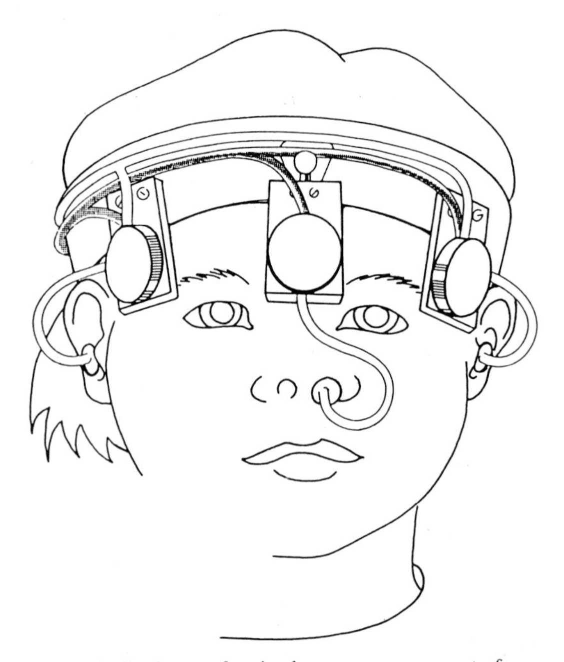

Figure 1 Equipment for simultaneous measurement of pressures in the nose and both ears. Three transducers are mounted as a headpiece with short catheters connected to the nose and ears.

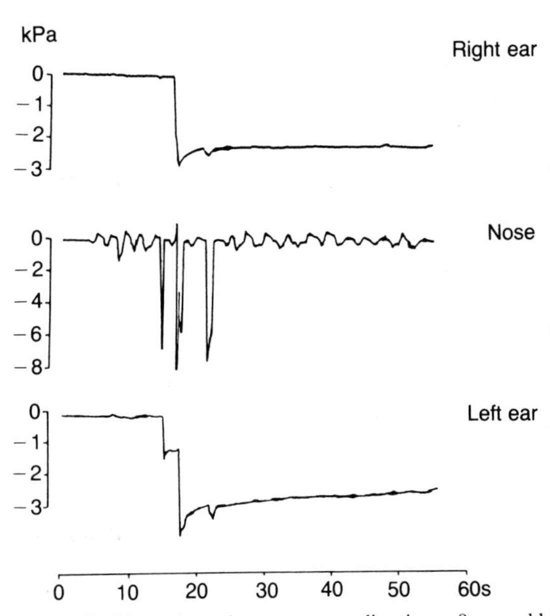

Figure 2 Three-channel pressure recording in an 8-year-old boy. He had persistent bilateral middle ear effusion and was treated with ventilating tubes. The pressure of normal respiration was not transmitted to the ears. However, both of the middle ears were easily evacuated to stable negative intratympanic pressure levels on sniffing. The subject was unable to equalize negative middle ear pressure by swallowing.

Figure 3 shows the internal construction of our pressure measuring unit. A small piezo-resistive pressure transducer (AME type 831, AS Mikkroelektronik, Horten, Norway) is enclosed within a Plexiglas housing, which is also supplied with an integral stopcock mechanism. The lid on top of the housing is pressed airtight against the housing by a spring and is held in place by a center screw. The lower connector is for the measuring catheter, and the connector on top of the lid connects to the pressurizing system. When the lid is turned, the latter connection can be cut off, or, alternatively, the system can be opened to ambient pressure. The volume enclosed in the transducer housing is 0.07 ml and the total volume, including the catheter, is 0.5 ml. The three pressure transducers on the headpiece are connected to a multichannel ink-jet recorder (Mingograf 81 Siemens, Solna, Sweden). It is essential not to use extensive filtering in the amplifying systems to avoid distortion of the pressure curves.

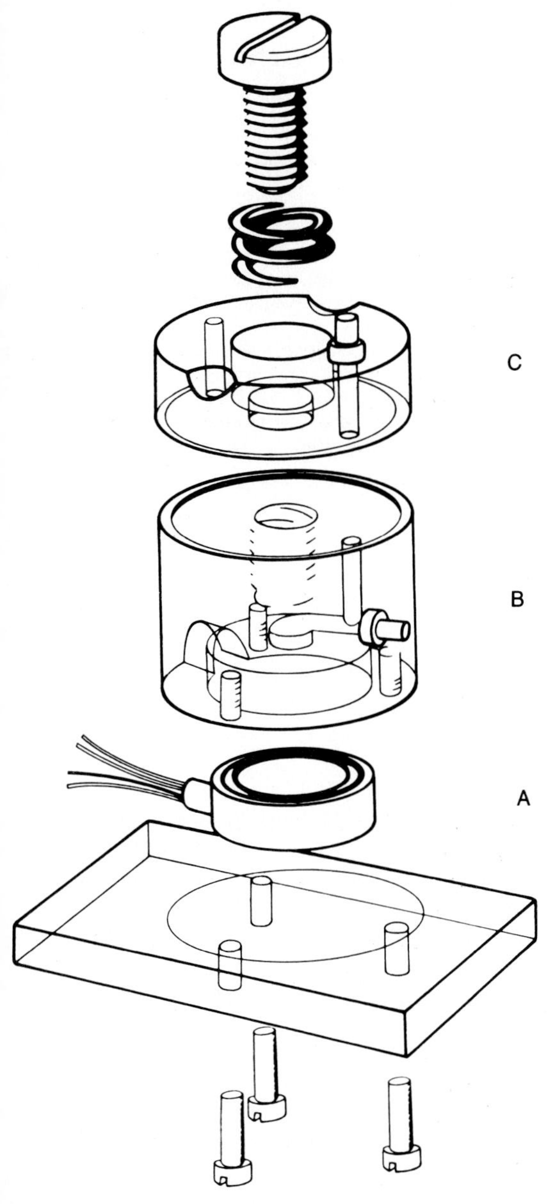

Figure 3 The internal construction of the pressure measuring unit. A, Piezo-resistive pressure transducer. B, Plexiglas housing with connector for the measuring catheter. C, Cover lid serving as a swivel stopcock mechanism, with connector for the pressurizing system.

RESULTS OF MEASUREMENTS

In a group of 100 children, comprising a consecutive series of subjects with persistent middle ear effusion treated with ventilating tubes, we found that 63 percent of ears were evacuated on sniffing. (In all, 156 ears were tested and 98 ears were evacuated.) Seventy-three percent of subjects showed positive evidence of evacuation of one or both ears on sniffing. The range of sniff-induced negative middle ear pressure was 0.6 to 9.4 kPa, with a mean of 2.4 kPa (Falk and Magnuson, unpublished data).

DISCUSSION

Fluid is normally produced by the middle ear mucosa and is transported down the eustachian tube by ciliary activity. Middle ear effusion may be looked upon as the result of imbalance between production and elimination of fluid. Increased production of fluid may be produced by different irritants. One strong irritant, and a very common one, is sniff-induced negative middle ear pressure. Primarily, effusion may be seen not as a disease entity but as a normal reaction in response to negative pressure. The accumulation of fluid may compensate for the negative pressure. In some cases, however, the compensatory effect of effusion may not suffice to prevent the development of manifest structural lesions.

Manifest ear disease encompasses a spectrum of different lesions, ranging from atrophy to severe retraction of the eardrum with formation of local retraction pockets. Ear disease develops differently in different individuals and also shows different characteristics in different communities. It is well known that children in poor communities have a very high incidence of perforated tympanic membranes. In contrast, in developed communities permanent perforations of the eardrum are less common, and middle ear disease is characterized by atrophic changes with retraction of the eardrum. An intermediate lesion is frequently seen: a "perforated retraction" formed by primary retraction and partial adhesion of the retracted tympanic membrane, followed by perforation of an area of the membrane that has not become adherent to underlying structures. The result is a perforated retraction of the eardrum.

CONCLUSIONS

To a great extent pressure equalization is an artificial demand on eustachian tube function connected with modern technology: deep-sea diving, flying, riding express elevators, and so on. The present findings lead to a new a priori statement: The most important physiologic role of the tube is to protect the middle ear from the nasopharyngeal environment with its loud sounds, its bacterial flora, and, most notably, from its extensive pressure variations. In failure of tubal closing the tube is unable to protect the middle ear reliably, and the middle cavity is evacuated by the high negative pressure in the nasopharynx caused, for example, by sniffing. Sniff-induced negative pressure in the middle ear may well be the most common cause of development of middle ear effusion.

REFERENCES

1. Magnuson B: On the orgin of the high negative pressure in the middle ear space. Am J Otolaryngol 2:1, 1981
2. Magnuson B: The atelectatic ear. Int J Ped Otolaryngol 3:25, 1981
3. Falk B: Tubal dysfunction in patients with cleft palate. In Sadé J (ed): Cholesteatoma and Mastoid Surgery. Amsterdam: Kugler Publications, 1982 pp 229-233
4. Magnuson B: Tubal closing failure in retraction type cholesteatoma and adhesive middle ear lesions. Acta Otolaryngol 86:404, 1978
5. Falk B: Sniff-induced negative middle ear pressure: Study of a consecutive series of children with otitis media with effusion. Am J Otolaryngol 3:155, 1982
6. Falk B: Negative middle ear pressure induced by sniffing. J Otolaryngol 10:299, 1981.

SONOTUBOMETRY

TORBEN BRASK, M.D., Ph.D., and TORBEN LILDHOLDT, M.D.

Clinical and experimental investigations have clearly demonstrated that dysfunction of the eustachian tube is a very important factor in the pathogenesis of otitis media, including otitis media with effusion. It is therefore of great importance to have reliable methods for testing the tubal function. If the tympanic membrane is intact the acoustic impedance method is an excellent way of testing tubal function. However, in many severe cases of otitis media the tympanic membrane is not intact. It is thus necessary to use other methods. Until now none of these seemed to be able to give a physiologic measurement of the tubal function.

From a theoretical point of view, sonotubometry might be ideal. The principles of sonotubometry were first described by Politzer in 1869.[1] He observed that a vibrating tuning fork in front of the nostrils could be heard better during swallowing. It was assumed that the tubal opening increased the sound transmission from the nasopharynx to the middle ear. On this principle, Pearlman[2] in 1939 used electric equipment with low frequency test sounds. Since then increasing efforts have been made to use the method in the clinic.[3–10] It is thus remarkable that Virtanen[11] found a discrepancy between results of sonotubometry and of tympanometry in normal adults with common colds. In eight of 12 patients with flat tympanograms good tubal function was found by sonotubometry.

The primary purpose of this study was to compare sonotubometry recordings from normal subjects with those from patients with middle ear effusion and to explain the phenomena influencing the sonotubometry recordings.

METHODS

The principle of sonotubometry is to record changes of sound intensities in the external auditory canal in relation to swallowing when a constant sound source is applied to the ipsilateral nostril.

A Heterodyne analyzer (Brüel and Kjaer type 2010) consisting of a beat frequency oscillator and an analyzer section including a band-pass slave filter was used. This instrument feeds a phone connected to the nostrils by a nasal olive tip. Inside the tip is a tube for recording the sound pressure in the nasal cavity. The subjects were investigated in a sitting position holding the nasal olive tip themselves. The signals from the external auditory canal are picked up by a condenser microphone (Brüel and Kjaer type 4134) and connected to the analyzer section, followed by a filtering through a 3.16 Hz band-pass slave filter. The signals were recorded by a level recorder (Brüel and Kjaer type 2307).

After recording a baseline of the "constant" sound level in the external auditory canal, the subject was asked to swallow a sip of water. The recorded signals had the baseline as reference. The signal-to-noise ratio should be higher than 1.5 (3.5 dB).

Normal subjects were required to have a normal otoscopic examination, normal tympanogram, and hearing better than 20 dB HL. The patients with dysfunction of the eustachian tube all had flat tympanograms. At a subsequent myringotomy it was demonstrated that the middle ear was filled with effusion in all the investigated patients.

RESULTS

According to the theory of sonotubometry, the sound intensity should increase in the external auditory canal when the eustachian tube is opened, and no change of the baseline should appear if the tube remained closed. Nevertheless, three main types of signals were recorded: positive, "biphasic," and negative, as shown in Figure 1. The results in percentages from normal persons and from patients with severe tubal dysfunction are seen in Table 1. No signals could be recorded in from 6 to 43 percent of normal persons, depending on the test frequency. The most unexpected results were that patients with severe tubal dysfunction had signals similar to those in normal subjects in relation to swallowing.

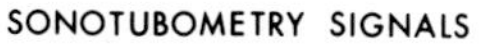

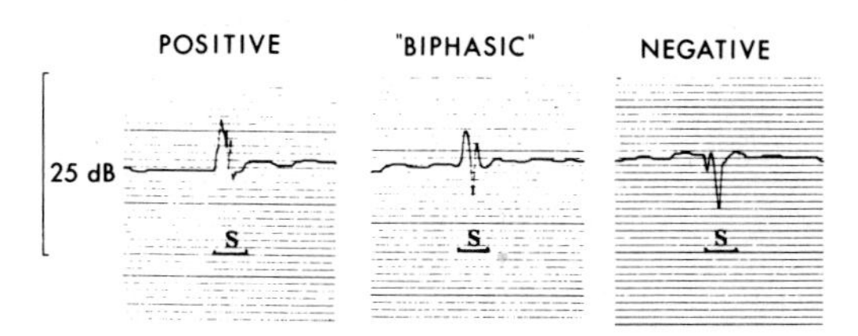

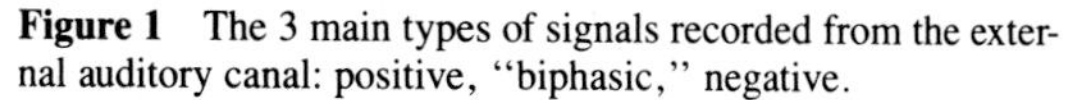
Figure 1 The 3 main types of signals recorded from the external auditory canal: positive, "biphasic," negative.

DISCUSSION

As the signals were sharp slave filtered and most of them were negative or "biphasic," even at 7000 Hz,[7] it seems improbable that they were artifacts due to noise from the swallowing procedure. From a simple acoustic point of view, the sound impedance of the eustachian tube should be least for low frequencies due to the dimensions of the tube. Because spectral analysis of the noise from the swallowing procedure has a content of special frequencies below 5 kHz, it is difficult to preestimate the optimal frequency for testing tubal function. Only empiric investigations can demonstrate the optimal test frequency.

The ideal condition for sonotubometry is a constant sound pressure level of the test tone at the opening of the eustachian tube in the nasopharynx. Because of the results from normal subjects and patients with middle ear effusion, together with the configurations of the signals, it seemed imperative to investigate whether the sound pressure level at the opening of the eustachian tube really remained constant. During the swallowing procedure the soft palate decreases the volume of the space into which the test tone is delivered. From a simple acoustic point of view, this should probably increase the sound pressure level at the opening of the eustachian tube. However, the acoustic conditions in biologic cavities with changing volumes and wall tensions are very complex. The changing of the equivalent acoustic volume in front of the nasal olive tip will also probably load the phone in a complex way. So the whole acoustic system is reacting in a nearly unpredictable way during the swallowing procedure.

To illustrate the variability of the sound pressure level in relation to changing volumes and frequencies, some model experiments were performed by connecting the nasal olive tip in an airtight fashion to a syringe. The piston was hollow

TABLE 1 Sonotubometry Results in Normal Persons and Persons with Severe Tubal Dysfunction

Sonotubometry Signals	*Normal Persons*				*Persons with Tubal Dysfunction*			
	0.5 kHz	*1.0 kHz*	*2.0 kHz*	*7.0 kHz*	*0.5 kHz*	*1.0 kHz*	*2.0 kHz*	*7.0 kHz*
Positive	14	77	11	22	27	18	46	28
"Biphasic"	27	16	46	13	28	18	9	0
Negative	51	51	30	22	36	64	45	45
Total signals	92	94	87	57	91	100	100	73
No signals	8	6	13	43	9	0	0	27

Note: All values are given in percentages.

and filled with rock wool to minimize standing waves and resonance.

It is shown in Figure 2 that at 500 Hz the sound pressure level of the test tone decreases when the volume increases, as could be expected from a simple acoustic point of view. At 2000 Hz the sound pressure level varies in relation to increasing volumes. At 7000 Hz the sound pressure level is nearly constant when the volume is increasing.

The conclusion from these experiments is that the sound pressure level in a cavity in relation to the used sound source depends on both the frequency and the volume in front of the phone.

For recording the conditions in the nasopharynx, a plastic tube was situated near the opening of the eustachian tube. The plastic tube was connected to a steel tube passing through the nasal olive tip. The other end of the steel tube was connected to a microphone. As shown in Figure 3, the recorded sound pressure levels were not constant during swallowing, as sonotubometry requires. The configurations of the sound pressure level in the nasopharynx were similar to those measured in the external auditory canal. By performing simultaneous recordings from the external auditory canal and the nasopharynx, we found a little difference in the configurations of the recorded sound pressure levels. This difference can be explained as a sound filter function of the tissue between the nasopharynx and the external auditory canal and/or effect of the tubal opening.

Our conclusion is that the interpretations of the ear canal signals in the hitherto performed sonotubometry measurements are quite uncertain as regards tubal function. However, by using a compressor controlled test tone intensity and other technical methods it is possible to keep the test tone intensity constant. A constant test tone intensity is thus a prerequisite for future investigations, which finally may demonstrate the clinical value of sonotubometry.

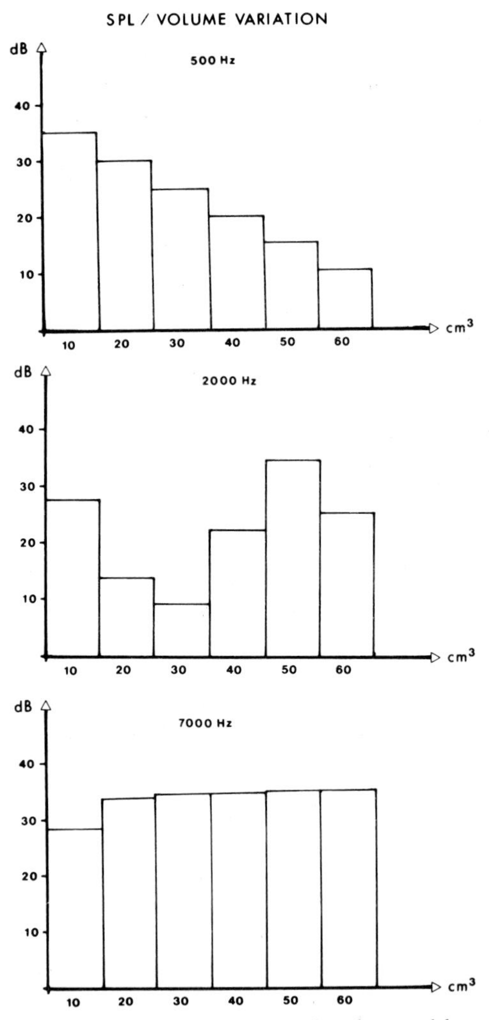

Figure 2 Sound pressure level recordings from model experiments. The recorded sound pressure levels (SPL) depend on both the frequency and the volume in front of the phone.

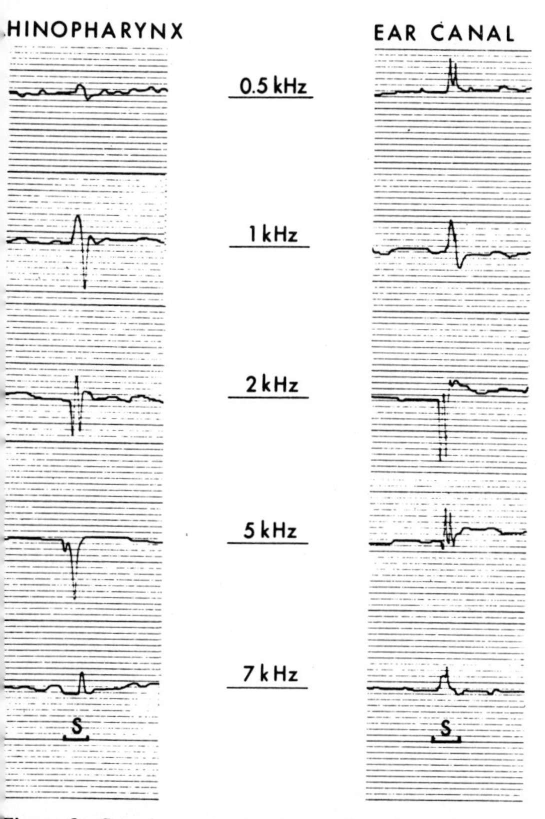

Figure 3 Sound pressure level recordings from the nasopharynx and the external auditory canal at different frequencies. The recordings were not performed simultaneously.

This study was supported by Danish Medical Research Council grant #12-1865, and by the Oticon Fund. The instruments for tympanometry were provided by Danplex-Danamedica, Odense, Denmark.

We are deeply in debt to Stig C. Dalsgaard, M.Sc., of the Research Laboratory for Technical Audiology, Odense University Hospital, for his technical and theoretic expertise.

REFERENCES

1. Politzer A: Physiologie der Tuba Eustachii. In *Lehrbuch der Ohrenheilkunde*. Stuttgart: Verdinand Enke, 1908
2. Pearlman HB: The Eustachian tube: Abnormal patency and normal physiologic state. Arch Otolaryngol 30:212, 1939
3. Elpern BS, et al: Objective measurement of middle ear function: the Eustachian tube. Laryngoscope 74:359, 1964
4. Flach M, Seidel P: Elektroakustische Prüfung der Tubendurchgängigkeit. HNO 15:41, 1967
5. Satoh I, et al: Measurement of Eustachian tube function. Arch Otolaryngol 92:329, 1970
6. Cole RM, et al: Eustachian tube function in cleft lip and palate patients. Arch Otolaryngol 99:337, 1974
7. Virtanen H: Eustachian tube sound conduction. Thesis, Helsinki, Finland, 1977
8. Holmquist J, Olén L: Evaluation of Eustachian tube function. J Otol 94:15, 1980
9. Murti KG, et al: Sonometric evaluation of Eustachian tube function using broadband stimuli. Ann Otol 89 (Suppl 68):178, 1980
10. Lildholdt T, et al: Interpretation of sonotubometry. A critical view of the acoustical measurement of the opening of the Eustachian tube. Acta Otolaryngol, in press
11. Virtanen H, Marttila T: Middle ear pressure and Eustachian tube function. Arch Otolaryngol 108:766, 1982

EUSTACHIAN TUBE FUNCTION IN CHILDREN WITH AND WITHOUT OTOLOGIC HISTORY

ANITA BYLANDER, M.D., ÖRJAN TJERNSTRÖM, M.D.,
ALF IVARSSON, Ph.D., and LEIF INGVARSSON, M.D.

Today it is generally accepted that dysfunction of the eustachian tube is involved in otitis media with effusion (OME)[1]. So far, however, there is no conclusive evidence that the dysfunction is a primary etiologic factor. It might just as well be secondary to an underlying infection. To evaluate the role of the eustachian tube in OME in children it is necessary to study its function not only in children with middle ear disease but also in those who are otologically healthy. To clarify further whether the dysfunction is primary or secondary it seems necessary to study the eustachian tube function at free intervals in the children with recurrent episodes of OME.

MATERIALS AND METHODS

Twenty-five children (ages 5 to 9 years) with histories of secretory otitis media (SOM) and/or recurrent acute otitis media (AOM) and 32 otologically healthy children (ages 5 to 9 years) were selected for the present study. In the latter group there was no history of either airway allergy or obstructing adenoid. Thirteen children with positive histories had long-lasting (more than three months) episodes of SOM, treated with tympanostomies with and without tubes, and 12 had at least six episodes of AOM only. All children, with and without otologic history, were healthy at the time of investigation, that is, had no history of a present or recent upper respiratory tract infection, audiometry within 20 dB, and V-shaped tympanograms. The children with positive histories had all been healthy for at least two months before the investigation.

The equipment and procedures of the different tests of eustachian tube function were identical with those described in detail in previous papers[2–4] and will be only briefly summarized here.

The eustachian tube function was measured using a pressure chamber for static and dynamic pressure changes, with an impedance bridge. The following tests were performed:

1. Middle ear pressure by tympanometry.
2. Active equilibration of static pressure differences across the eardrum after a decrease and an increase in chamber pressure of 1 kPa. Depending on the results of equilibration of applied over- and underpressures by a method of free choice,[1] the subjects were distributed in tubal function groups I through IV according to the method of Elner and associates.[5] Those in groups I and II were considered to have good muscular opening function, since they could equilibrate both over- and underpressures, and those in groups III and IV to have poor function, since either only overpressure (III) or no pressure at all (IV) could be equilibrated.
3. Deflation test in a pressure chamber. The change in chamber pressure required to induce an overpressure in the middle ear forcing the tube open was called the pressure opening level (Pol). The residual overpressure in the middle ear when the tube closed after the pressure opening was called the pressure closing level (Pcl).
4. Inflationary maneuvers. The subject was instructed to perform Valsalva's maneuver and mouth-to-nose inflation. The latter test was performed with a nose olive connected to a catheter held in the mouth. Those who could build up a positive pressure in the middle ear by either maneuver were called responders to inflation.
5. Deflationary maneuvers. The subject was instructed to inspire forcefully with one nostril connected to the pressure transducer, the other open (sniffing) or closed (reversed Valsalva's maneuver). Those who could create a negative pressure in the middle ear by either maneuver were called responders to deflation.

The maximal over- and underpressures in the rhinopharynx during the inflationary and deflationary maneuvers, respectively, were also recorded.

RESULTS

Muscular Opening Function

The muscular opening function was poorer in children with otologic histories than in those without. Sixty-four percent of the children with positive histories could not equilibrate underpressures, compared with 25 percent of the children with negative histories (Table 1). There was no difference in the distribution of tubal function groups (I–IV) between younger and older children with positive histories. In the children with negative histories, however, an age-related difference was seen (Fig. 1). Improvement with age in healthy children was confirmed by retests of the muscular opening function after one and a half years in 31 children, of whom ten also were tested after three years. Ten of 13 children with histories of both recurrent AOM and long-lasting episodes of SOM had poor muscular opening function compared with only six of the 12 who had histories of recurrent AOM only.

Middle Ear Pressure by Tympanometry

The middle ear pressures were significantly more negative in the children with otologic histories than in the other children (Table 2).

TABLE 1 Distribution of Muscular Opening Function in Tubal Function Groups I–IV and of the Response Rate to Inflation and Deflation in 25 Children with a Positive History of Middle Ear Disease and 32 Children with a Negative History

Tubal Function Tests	Positive History No.	Positive History %	Negative History No.	Negative History %
Group I	—	—	14	44
Group II	7	28	9	28
Group III	12	48	5	16
Group IV	4	16	3	9
PT	2	8	1	3
Inflation	15/25	60	24/32	75
Deflation	6/25	24	7/32	21

Note: PT = patulous tube.

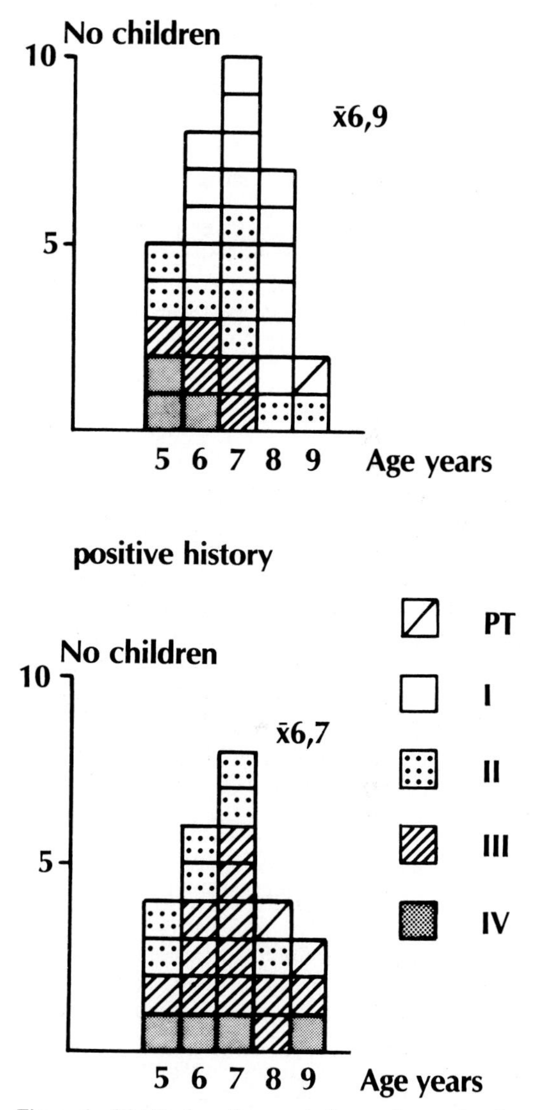

Figure 1 Distribution of age and of muscular opening function in tubal function groups I–IV in 32 children with negative otologic histories and in 25 children with positive histories.

Pressure Opening and Closing Functions by Deflation in a Pressure Chamber

There was no significant difference of Pol and Pcl between the children with and without otologic histories (Table 2). The children with histories of AOM only had significantly lower mean Pcls than

TABLE 2 Pressure Opening Levels (Pol), Pressure Closing Levels (Pcl), and Middle Ear Pressures (Pm) in kPa in Children with Negative and Positive Histories of Middle Ear Disease

	Pol			*Pcl*			*Pm*		
	No	$\bar{x}$	*SD*	*No*	$\bar{x}$	*SD*	*No*	$\bar{x}$	*SD*
Negative history	31	3.98	1.30	31	1.33	0.75	32	−0.24	0.35
Positive history	25	3.00	1.33	25	1.22	0.74	25	−0.72	0.74

those who had histories of long-lasting episodes of SOM.

Inflationary and Deflationary Maneuvers

There was no difference in the response rate to inflation and deflation in the two groups of children (Table 1). The response rate to inflation was related to the magnitude of applied overpressure in the rhinopharnyx during the maneuvers. The response rate to deflation was related not only to the magnitude of applied rhinopharyngeal underpressure, but also to low Pol and Pcl. All children with negative histories who responded to deflation belonged to tubal function group I except one, who had a patulous tube. In the other group two were in group II, two were in group III, and two had patulous tubes.

DISCUSSION

It is claimed that the muscular opening function of the eustachian tube is poor and remains poor in the majority of children with OME for up to several months.[6–11] The studies suggest that eustachian tube dysfunction is involved in the pathogenesis of OME but they cannot answer whether the dysfunction is a primary factor or secondary to the disease.

In a previous study we demonstrated that otologically healthy children had a higher frequency of poor muscular opening function of the eustachian tube than healthy adults, suggesting a primary hypofunction that improves with age.[1] The present study shows that the muscular opening function of the eustachian tube is even poorer in children with positive histories of middle ear disease measured when they are well than in those who are otologically healthy. This is also reflected in the greater number of negative middle ear pressures in the group with positive histories of OME. The results provide further evidence that there is a primary muscular opening hypofunction of the tube that may be an underlying etiologic factor in the development of OME. In the children in this study the poor muscular opening function is, however, sufficient to maintain adequate middle ear pressure under normal conditions. However, they constitute a risk group, since other etiologic or pathogenic factors may aggravate the hypofunction or contribute in other ways to the development and maintenance of OME.[12]

REFERENCES

1. Bluestone CD, Klein JO: Otitis media with effusion, atelectasis, and eustachian tube dysfunction. In Pediatric Otolaryngology, Bluestone CD, Stool SE (eds): W.B. Saunders Company, Philadelphia, pp 356–512, 1983.
2. Bylander A, Ivarsson A, Tjernström Ö: Eustachian tube function in normal children and adults. Acta Otolaryngol (Stockh) 92:481, 1981
3. Bylander A, Tjernström Ö, Ivarsson A: Pressure opening and closing functions of the Eustachian tube in children and adults with normal ears. Acta Otolaryngol (Stockh) 95:55, 1983
4. Bylander A, Tjernström Ö, Ivarsson A: Pressure opening and closing functions of the Eustachian tube by inflation and deflation in children and adults with normal ears. Acta Otolaryngol (Stockh), 96:255, 1983
5. Elner Å, Ingelstedt S, Ivarsson A: The normal function of the Eustachian tube. A study of 102 cases. Acta Otolaryngol (Stockh) 72:320, 1971
6. Silverstein H, Miller GF, Lindeman RC: Eustachian tube dysfunction as a cause for chronic secretory otitis in children. (Correction by pressure-equalization). Laryngoscope 76:259, 1966
7. Renvall U, Holmquist J: Eustachian tube function in secretory otitis media. Scand Audiol 3:87, 1974
8. Briggs DR, Applebaum EL, Noffsinger D: Eustachian tube function in children. J Otolaryngol 5:12, 1976
9. Neel HG, Keating LW, McDonald TJ: Ventilation in secretory otitis media. Effects on middle ear volume and Eustachian tube function. Arch Otolaryngol 103:228, 1977
10. Poulsen G, Tos M: Tubal function in chronic secretory otitis media in children. ORL 39:57, 1977
11. Beery QC, Doyle WJ, Cantekin EI, Bluestone CD: Longitudinal assessment of Eustachian tube function in children. Larynogoscope 89:1446, 1979
12. Tos M, Poulsen G, Borch J: Etiologic factors in secretory otitis. Arch Otolaryngol 105:582, 1979

EUSTACHIAN TUBE FUNCTION IN CHILDREN WITH UNREPAIRED CLEFT PALATES

WILLIAM J. DOYLE, Ph.D., JAMES S. REILLY, MD., SYLVAN E. STOOL, M.D., and ERDEM I. CANTEKIN, Ph.D.

Children with cleft palate are considered to be at risk for the development of otitis media with effusion (OME), with an incidence approaching 100 percent.[1,2] Clinical and experimental studies have supported the contention that compromised eustachian tube (ET) function underlies the pathogenesis of the disease in this population. Specifically, these studies in infants and children with both repaired and unrepaired cleft palates have documented a retrograde obstruction to fluid flow, a limited ability to equilibrate applied positive middle ear pressures, and an inability to equilibrate applied negative middle ear pressures.[3,4] This deficient function was termed functional ET obstruction by Bluestone and associates.[3] A more recent study of children with repaired palatal clefts used an expanded test protocol that included the forced-response test.[5] The results confirmed those of the earlier studies and documented that in the majority of patients the ET constricted with swallowing. However, with few exceptions these studies have been conducted on patients with patent tympanostomy tubes inserted because of unresolved or repeated bouts of OME. Assuming that those children with the worst ET function are those who also develop the most severe and protracted course of OME, the limitation of a testing procedure that requires a patent tympanostomy tube biases the test results toward poorer function. It has become the practice at the Cleft Palate Center of the University of Pittsburgh to insert tympanostomy tubes in all children before surgery. These children provide an ideal sample population from which to draw unbiased conclusions concerning the function of the ET in the general cleft palate population. The present study reports the results of these tests.

MATERIALS AND METHODS

Thirty-one patients with unrepaired palatal clefts, 17 males and 14 females, were enrolled in the study at approximately 6 months of age. Eleven children had bilateral complete palatal clefts, eight had unilateral complete palatal clefts, and 12 had clefts of the soft palate only. All children had had bilateral tympanostomy tubes inserted by 6 months of age and were tested bestween 6 and 18 months. ET function tests were conducted on 47 ears of these patients. Twenty-seven ears were tested once, 16 twice, two three times, and two four times, for a total of 73 tests.

Each test session included two testing protocols: the inflation-deflation and forced-response tests. The procedures and equipment used have been described in detail previously.[6] In general, an attempt was made to define the parameters of the forced-response test for three flow rates: 12, 24 and 48 cc/min. Because of the young age of these children, the tests could not be completed in a number of cases because of the child's irritability. However, for all tests included in this study results for at least one flow rate, usually 12 cc/min., were recorded.

The results of the inflation-deflation tests were compared with those reported for adults and children without cleft palates who had traumatic perforations and otherwise negative otologic histories (hereafter called the normal group)[6] and with those reported for a group of children with repaired cleft palates and a history of chronic OME,[5] referred to as the repaired cleft group. The results of the forced-response test are compared with those of the repaired cleft palate group and with those of a second normal group reported by Cantekin and associates.[7]

RESULTS

The study population is a rather heterogeneous group that is bounded by a number of parameters including age, sex, type of cleft, and number of tests per year. While these parameters may influence the distribution of test variables, the various individual cells contained too few observations to allow for meaningful tests of parametric influence. Consequently, in this preliminary review, all tests are considered to be independent observations and of equal weight.

Of the 73 tests performed, the passive opening pressure in seven tests was greater than 1000 mm H_2O. Because of the discomfort experienced at this rather great middle ear pressure, application of pressure was discontinued at this point and the test results were omitted from the calculation of the descriptive statistics.

The inflation-deflation test assesses the ability to reduce applied positive and negative middle ear pressures. Of the 53 tests in which these functions were evaluated, 19 (35.9 percent) evidenced an ability to reduce applied positive middle ear pressure although none showed an ability to reduce negative middle ear pressure. These results compare favorably with those reported for the repaired cleft palate population, of whom 33 percent showed an ability to reduce applied positive and 11 percent evidenced an ability to reduce applied negative middle ear pressures. In the group of normals previously studied, 97 percent were able to equilibrate applied positive and 42 percent were able to equilibrate applied negative middle ear pressures. Thus, both cleft palate groups showed deficient function when compared with these normals.

Figure 1 shows the comparison of the three groups with respect to the opening and closing pressures. The average opening pressure of 385 ± 161 mm H_2O recorded for the cleft palate infants in the present study was greater than the mean opening pressure of 337 mm H_2O reported for the repaired cleft palate group or the mean opening pressure of 330 mm H_2O reported for the normals. However, the mean closing pressure for the unrepaired and repaired cleft palate groups were essentially identical, being 143 ± 94 and 147 ± 70.4, respectively. These closing pressures were greater than those reported for the normal population (110 mm H_2O).

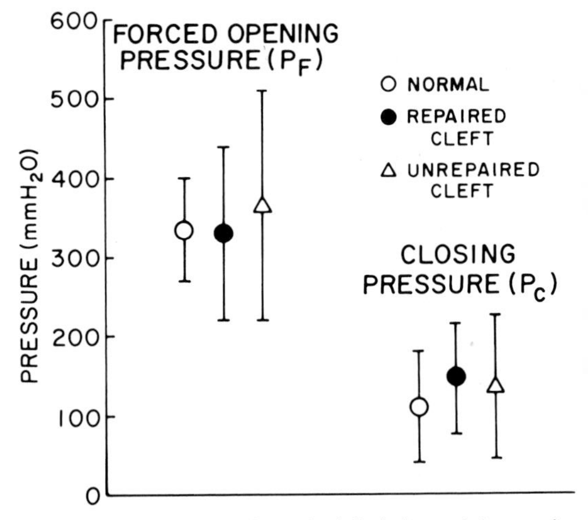

Figure 1 The means and standard deviations of the opening pressure (P_F) and closing pressure (P_C) for the children with unrepaired cleft palates and the two comparison groups.

During the forced-response test, two parameters of eustachian tube function were recorded at each of three flow rates. These were the passive and active tubal resistances. Figure 2 shows a comparison of the mean passive tubal resistance as a function of flow rate for the normals and the repaired and unrepaired cleft palate groups. This parameter was essentially identical in the normals

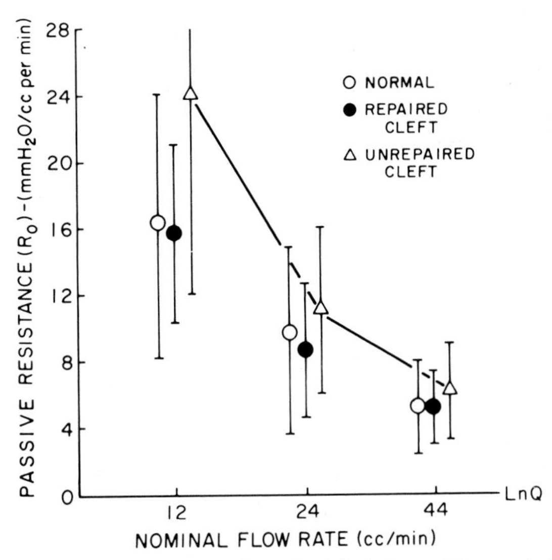

Figure 2 The means and standard deviations of the passive tubal resistance as a function of flow rate for the children with unrepaired cleft palates and the two comparison groups.

and the repaired cleft palate group. The mean values of passive tubal resistance in the unrepaired cleft palate group were 23.6, 11.0, and 6.1 for flow rates of 12, 24, and 48 cc/min, respectively. The corresponding mean values for the repaired cleft palate children were 15.5, 8.7, and 5.3. Thus, the unrepaired cleft palate children in the present study had a higher passive tubal resistance than either repaired cleft palate children or normals.

By convention, active tubal resistance is defined for tests in which the passive resistance is greater than the active resistance, a condition that is satisfied when a predilated tube dilates further with swallowing. The distribution of tests for the three groups with respect to this condition is shown in Figure 3 for the three constant flow rates. The percentage of tests characterized by dilation decreased with increasing flow rate for both the repaired and unrepaired cleft palate groups. Furthermore, this trend was most pronounced in the children with unrepaired palatal clefts. At a flow rate of 12 cc/min, dilation was observed in 100 percent of the tests on normals. However, only 23 percent of the repaired cleft palate tests evidenced

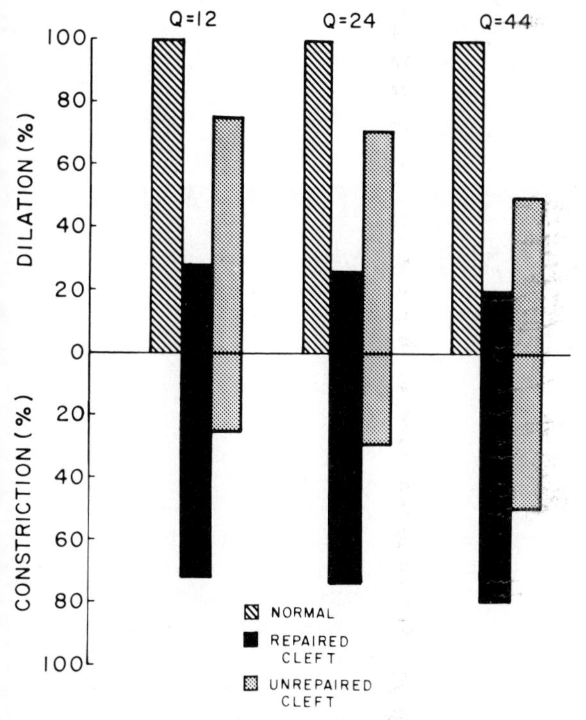

Figure 3 A comparison of the percentage of tests evidencing tubal dilation and constriction at each of the three flow rates for the children with unrepaired cleft palate and the two comparison groups.

dilation. Significantly, 75.4 percent of the tests reported in the present study showed tubal dilation with swallowing, an improvement over the repaired cleft palate population. For these tests the mean active resistances recorded were 5.8, 3.7, and 3.2 for flow rates of 12, 24, and 48 cc/min, respectively.

The resistance ratio (Ro/Ra) is a normalized measurement of tubal dilation efficiency, with higher valued ratios corresponding to more efficient tubal systems. The mean values of the ratio for the normals were 9.7, 5.0, and 4.0, and for the 75.4 percent of tests in the present study in which active resistance could be defined the corresponding values were 7.2 ± 5.9, 4.6 ± 3.3, and 3.1 ± 2.2. While slightly less than the normal means, they do indicate a relatively efficient mechanism of active tubal dilation.

A relationship between active function variables and passive function variables has been suggested. To investigate this possibility, the mean opening and closing pressures for two subgroups of the data set were computed. Subgroup I consisted of those patients capable of reducing applied positive pressure, indicative of better tubal dilation. Subgroup II consisted of the 24.6 percent of the patients evidencing tubal constriction with swallowing. For subgroup I the mean opening and closing pressures were 302 ± 105 and 136 ± 70, respectively. Mean values in subgroup II were 378 ± 154 and 155 ± 124. Thus it appears that, on the average, lower opening and closing pressures were associated with better active tubal function.

DISCUSSION

In an early report on ET ventilatory function, Bluestone and coworkers reported that children with unrepaired cleft palates had a higher forced opening pressure and poorer active dilating function than children with repaired cleft palates.[4] A control group of children with traumatic perforations had lower opening pressures and better dilating function than either cleft group.[6] Our results are consistent with those findings. Furthermore, in the present study the ET closing pressure in the children with unrepaired palatal clefts was shown to be greater than that of normal children. It is interesting that the subgroup of children with unrepaired cleft palates capable of reducing applied middle ear pressure had lower mean opening and closing pressures than did the subgroup of children whose ET constricted with swallowing. This supports a relationship between the active and passive functions of the tube as postulated by Bylander.[8]

In the present study, approximately 75 percent of the tests showed tubal dilation during the forced response test, in contrast to 23 percent of the children with repaired cleft palates studied previously. An explanation for this difference may lie with the bounding parameters of the two study populations. All of the children with repaired cleft palates tested had had tympanostomy tubes inserted because of long histories of OME, whereas the children in the present study had tympanostomy tubes inserted without knowledge of the course of an OME. Since in a significant proportion of children with cleft palates OME resolves following repair of the palate, the population described here is composed of two subpopulations, one that will continue to have OME following palate repair and a second that will not. Assuming ET dysfunction underlies the development of OME, it is reasonable to suggest that the majority of those children capable of tubal dilation represent the second subpopulation. Continued follow-up of these children will allow for testing this interesting hypothesis.

This study was supported in part by a grant from the National Institutes of Health DE-O1969.

REFERENCES

1. Stool SE, Randall P: Unexpected ear disease in infants with cleft palate. Cleft Palate J 4:99, 1967
2. Paradise JL, Bluestone CD, Felder H: The universality of otitis media in fifty infants with cleft palate. Pediatrics 44:35, 1969
3. Bluestone CD, Wittel RB, Paradise JL: Roentgenographic evaluation of the eustachian tube function in infants with cleft and normal palates. Cleft Palate J 9:93, 1972
4. Bluestone CD, Berry QC, Cantekin EI, Paradise JL: Eustachian tube ventilatory function in relation to cleft palate. Ann Otol Rhinol Laryngol 84:333, 1975
5. Doyle WJ, Cantekin EI, Bluestone CD: Eustachian tube function in cleft palate children. Ann Otol Rhinol Laryngol 89(Suppl 68):34, 1980
6. Cantekin ET, Bluestone CD, Parkin LP: Eustachian tube ventilatory function in children. Ann Otol Rhinol Laryngol 85(Suppl 25):171, 1976
7. Cantekin ET, Saez CH, Bluestone CD, Been S: Airflow through the eustachian tube. Ann Otol Rhinol Laryngol 88:603, 1979
8. Bylander A: Comparison of eustachian tube function in children and adults with normal middle ears. Ann Otol Rhinol Laryngol 89(68):34, 1980

EUSTACHIAN TUBE FUNCTION IN INFANTS AND CHILDREN WITH DOWN'S SYNDROME

BENJAMIN LeM. WHITE, M.D., WILLIAM J. DOYLE, Ph.D., and CHARLES D. BLUESTONE, M.D.

It has become increasingly apparent that individuals with Down's syndrome frequently have decreased auditory sensitivity levels. Beginning in 1968, several investigators have reported hearing loss in from 42 percent to 77 percent of the Down's population.[1–5] Most of the hearing problems were reported to be conductive in nature.

Eustachian tube (ET) dysfunction is thought by many to be the primary etiologic factor in otitis media with effusion (OME) in children. Jahn and Becker suggested that hearing loss in Down's syndrome is usually secondary to a middle ear effusion (MEE) brought on by ET dysfunction.[6] Several investigators have presented strong evidence that other populations at risk for the development of OME are characterized by a dysfunction of the ET,[7–9] which Bluestone and Beery have defined as functional ET obstruction.[10] No data have been reported on the ET function in the Down's syndrome population. Therefore, the present study was designed to evaluate the function of the ET in patients with Down's syndrome in order to determine whether dysfunction is present and, if so, the characteristics of that dysfunction.

MATERIALS AND METHODS

The subjects were 14 children with Down's syndrome. There were seven males and seven females ranging in age from 8 months to 17 years 8 months, with a mean age of 9 years 11 months. All children had functioning tympanostomy tubes that had been inserted because of chronic OME. Of the 14 subjects, eight were tested bilaterally and six unilaterally, yielding a total of 22 ears tested.

Two different protocols were followed in the testing procedures: inflation-deflation testing and forced-response testing. The procedure and testing equipment used in this study have been described in detail previously.[11] The results of these tests were compared with those previously reported for four different populations. A description of all five groups is provided in Table 1.

RESULTS

Twenty-two ears were evaluated by the inflation-deflation test. Of these only four (18 percent) were able to reduce positive ME pressure, while only one (5 percent) was able to reduce negative ME pressure by swallowing. The remainder were unable to actively reduce applied ME pressures by swallowing. These results are similar to those reported for children with cleft palates (33 percent and 11 percent) and significantly different from the other groups: group I, 97 percent and 41 percent, group II, 70 percent and 30 percent; and group III, 79 percent and 7 percent.

The mean opening pressure recorded for the Down's syndrome population in this study was 326 ± 151 mm H_2O and the mean closing pressure was 66 ± 36 mm H_2O. These values and those previously reported for the four comparison groups are shown in Figure 1. With the single exception of the American Indians, all mean values of opening pressure were remarkably similar. The American Indians had a lower opening pressure (245 ± 100 mm H_2O) when compared with the other groups. The mean closing pressure of the ET in patients with Down's syndrome of 66 mm H_2O was much lower than that of the other groups. In contrast, the mean closing pressure of 145 ± 70 mm H_2O reported for the children with cleft palates was much higher than that of the other groups.

Passive tubal resistance was determined at each of three flow rates: 12, 24, and 48 cc/min. For the children with Down's syndrome the mean passive resistances recorded for these flow rates were 13.0 ± 4.6, 6.8 ± 2.2, and 4.0 ± 0.8, respectively. Figure 2 shows a comparison between these values and those recorded for the other four populations. For group III these values were available only for a rate of 24 cc/min. The mean passive resistance for patients with Down's syndrome was consistently lower than the mean for normals and approaches the mean reported for the American In-

TABLE 1 Sample Size, Text Abbreviation, Source of Data, and Population Characteristics for the Five Comparison Groups

Group	*Abr*	*N*	*Ref*	*Characteristics*
I	NL	29	Cantekin et al, 1976	Children and adults with traumatic perforations of the TM and otherwise negative otologic histories
		6*	Cantekin et al, 1979	
II	AI	23	Beery et al[8]	Children and adult American Indians with chronic tympanic membrane perforations secondary to otitis media
III	CO	137	Cantekin et al, 1976	Children without cleft palate or Down's syndrome who had tympanostomy tubes inserted because of chronic otitis media with effusion
		40†	Lildholdt et al[13]	
IV	CP	55	Doyle et al[9]	Children with repaired palatal clefts and tympanostomy tubes inserted because of chronic otitis media with effusion
V	DS	22	Present study	Children with Down's syndrome and tympanostomy tubes inserted because of chronic otitis media with effusion

Key: Abr, text abbreviation; N, sample size; Ref, source of data; NL, normal; AI, American Indian; CO, chronic otitis; CP, cleft palate; DS, Down's syndrome

*Source for Passive Resistance values

†Source for Opening Pressures, Closing Pressures and Passive Resistance

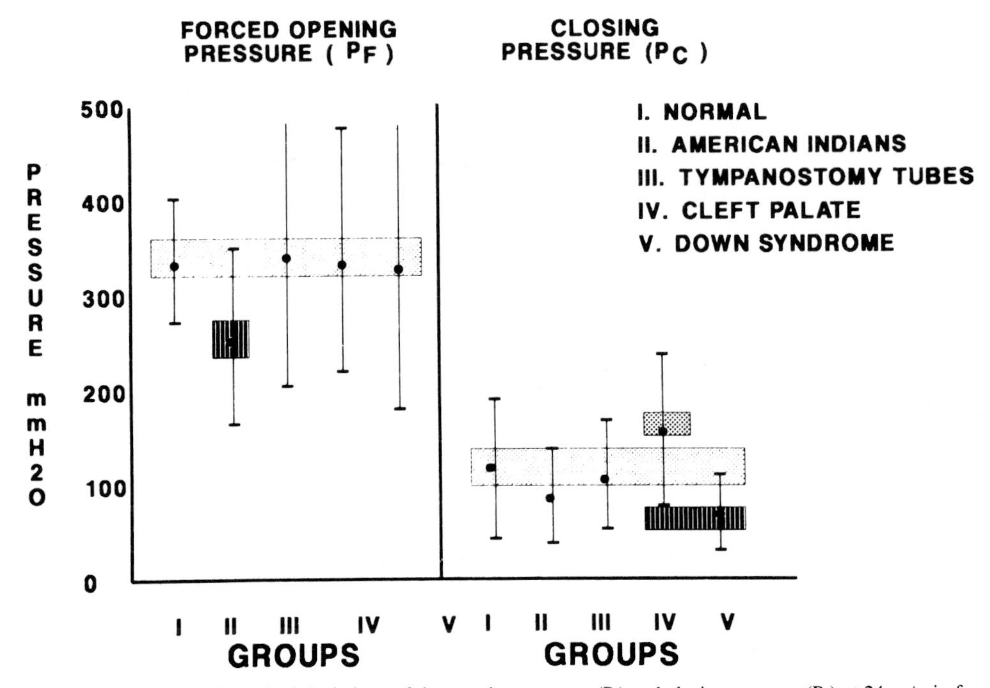

Figure 1 The mean values and standard deviations of the opening pressure (P_f) and closing pressure (P_c) at 24 cc/min for each of the five groups in Table 1.

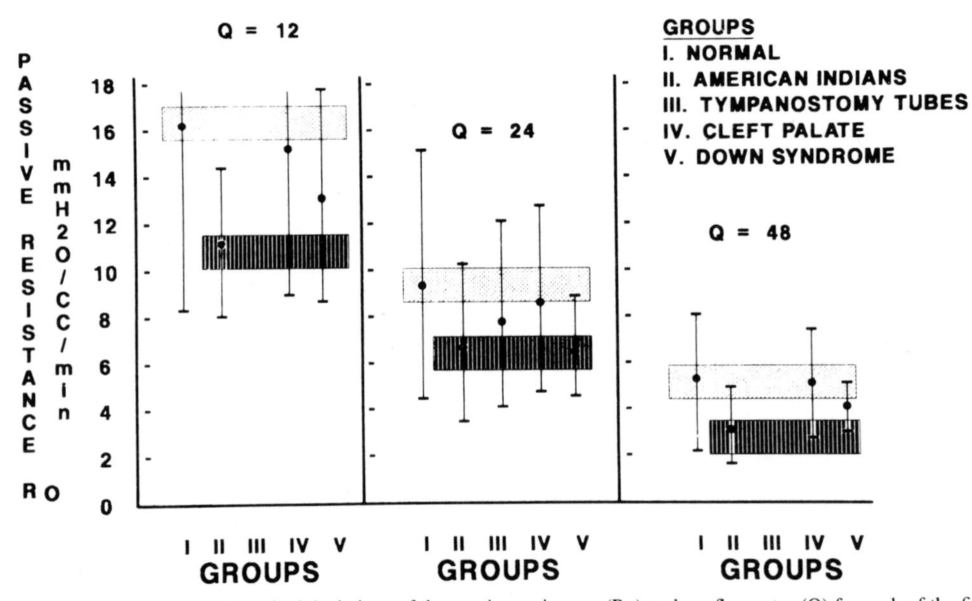

Figure 2 The mean values and standard deviations of the passive resistance (Ro) at three flow rates (Q) for each of the five groups in Table 1

dians. Patients with cleft palates had mean values similar to those of the normals. The mean values of resistance for children with chronic OME fall between those for children with cleft palates and those for children with Down's syndrome.

The active tubal resistance is determined by dividing the steady state pressure by the maximum flow during a swallow. In the normal condition this value is always less than the passive tubal resistance recorded at a given flow rate. For the patients with Down's syndrome studied, this relationship was true of only three ears tested. In one additional ear the active resistance was equal to the passive resistance, which indicated that there was no change in either pressure or flow during swallowing. For this ear, the tensor veli palatini (TVP) muscle was ineffective in dilating the ET. For the remaining 18 ears the active resistance was greater than the passive resistance, a condition that results from tubal constriction with swallowing.

DISCUSSION

It has been recognized that children with craniofacial abnormalities, and those with Down's syndrome in particular, have a high prevalence of conductive hearing loss and MEE.[12] The role of ET dysfunction in the pathogenesis of MEE has been outlined by Bluestone and Beery[10] as well as by other investigators.[8–9] The present study showed a dysfunction of the ET in children with Down's syndrome characterized by a low passive tubal resistance, a low closing pressure, constriction of the ET on swallowing, and inability of most of these children to equilibrate positive or negative ME pressure.

Previous studies of other populations considered to be at risk for OME have investigated ET function. Doyle and coworkers showed that 67 percent of children with cleft palates could not reduce positive middle ear pressure and 89 percent could not equilibrate negative middle ear pressure.[9] This compares well with the values of 82 percent (18/22) and 95 percent (21/22) reported in the present study. They further reported that 73 percent of the tests evidence ET constriction, compared with 71 percent in the present study, and suggested that the inability of the TVP muscle to dilate the ET actively during swallowing was the major factor responsible for the pathogenesis of OME in children with cleft palates.

Beery and coworkers found an abnormally low passive tubal resistance and a possible impairment of the protective function of the ET in the White Mountain Apache Indians of Arizona, which they postulated as being responsible for the high incidence of otitis media in this population.[8] This lowered resistance is similar to our consistent finding of low passive tubal resistance in children with Down's syndrome.

Thus, patients with Down's syndrome may represent a unique population group doubly at risk for OME because of two functional abnormalities of the ET. First, the ET does not dilate and the middle ear is therefore subject to high negative pressures and MEE. Second, because of the low resistance, unwanted secretions from the nasopharynx can more easily gain access to the ME space, resulting in middle ear infection.

These factors suggest that children with Down's syndrome are at high risk for OME and, consequently, hearing loss. Because developmental problems resulting from hearing loss may be magnified in the already mentally and physically handicapped child, aggressive treatment of even the seemingly minor problem at an early age may provide considerable improvement in the quality of life of the handicapped child.

This study was supported in part by grant #NS16337 from the National Institutes of Health.

REFERENCES

1. Fulton RT, Lloyd LL: Hearing impairment in a population of children with Down's syndrome. Am J Ment Defic 73:298, 1968
2. Brooks DN, Wooley H, Kanjilal GC: Hearing loss and middle ear disorders in patients with Down's syndrome (mongolism). J. Ment Defic Res 16:21, 1972
3. Schwartz DM, Schwartz RH: Acoustic impedance and otoscopic findings in young children with Down's syndrome. Arch Otolaryngol 104:652, 1978
4. Downs MP. Identification of children at risk for middle ear effusion problems. Ann Otol Rhinol Laryngol 89(68):168, 1980
5. Balkany TJ, Downs MP, Jafek BW, Krayjcek MJ: Hearing loss in Down's syndrome. Clin Pediatr 18(2):116, 1979
6. Jahn AF, Becker A: Ear disease in adults with Down's syndrome. Otolaryngol Head Neck Surg 90:184, 1982 (Abstr)
7. Bluestone CD, Wittel RA, Paradise JL: Roentgenographic evaluation of the eustachian tube function in infants with cleft and normal palates. Cleft Palate J 9:93, 1972
8. Beery QC, Doyle WJ, Cantekin EI, et al: Eustachian tube function in an American Indian population. Ann Otol Rhinol Laryngol 89(68):28, 1980
9. Doyle WJ, Cantekin EI, Bluestone CD: Eustachian tube function in cleft palate children. Ann Otol Rhinol Laryngol 89(68):34, 1980

10. Bluestone CD, Beery QC: Concepts in the pathogenesis of middle ear effusion. Ann Otol Rhinol Laryngol 85(25):182, 1976
11. Cantekin EI, Saez CA, Bluestone CD, Bern S.A: Airflow through the eustachian tube. Ann Otol Rhinol Laryngol 88:603, 1979
12. Cantekin EI, Bluestone CD, Parkin LP: Eustachian tube ventilatory function in children. Ann Otol Rhinol Laryngol 85(25):171, 1976
13. Lildholdt T, Cantekin EI, Bluestone CD, Rockette HE: Effect of a topical nasal decongestant on eustachian tube function in children with tympanostomy tubes. Acta Otolaryngol 94:93, 1982

FLUID CLEARANCE OF THE EUSTACHIAN TUBE

TSUNEKI NOZOE, M.D., NOBUHIRO OKAZAKI, M.D.,
YOKO KODA, M.D., NOBUO AYANI, M.D.,
and TADAMI KUMAZAWA, M.D.

Recent studies on the eustachian tube have shown that the tensor veli palatini muscle is the most important muscle in tubal function. It has been demonstrated by experiments with an open tympanum that contraction and relaxation of the tensor results in a pumplike function of the tube that milks fluids out of the tympanum.

The aim of the present study was to examine the detailed mechanism of this function in a closed tympanum, which more closely approximates the normal physiological state than an open tympanum.

MATERIALS AND METHODS

Experiment One

Fluid clearance from a closed tympanum, both upon electrical stimulation of the tensor veli palatini muscle and upon swallowing, was examined.

Ten cats were used. Under general anesthesia with ketamine hydrochloride, saline solution or radiopaque medium (80 percent Iodamide meglumine) was gently instilled into the tympanum through a Teflon tube inserted through the tympanic bulla in an airtight manner. Then the tympanic cavity was adjusted to atmospheric pressure and closed by a three-way stopcock connected to the Teflon tube. Electrical stimulation of the tensor muscle was performed using a palatal approach.[1] A bipolar hooked electrode was directly inserted into the belly of the tensor muscle, which was stimulated with a 0.4-second duration, 3V amplitude, and 100 Hz square wave pulse. Swallowing was induced by mechanical stimlation of the pharynx under light anesthesia. Expulsion of fluid was observed through an operating microscope or endoscope at the pharyngeal orifice of the tube and recorded on cinefilm.

Experiment Two

Change of pressure in a closed tympanum was measured during fluid clearance by both tensor stimulation and swallowing.

In 15 cats, fluid was instilled into the tympanum in the manner described above. A manometric system was connected to the tympanum through a Teflon tube and a stopcock. The change of intratympanic pressure was recorded simultaneously with signals of tensor stimulation or EMG of the tensor upon swallowing.[2]

Experiment Three

In human beings, a change of middle ear pressure was measured during fluid clearance by swallowing.

Ten adults with dry perforation of the tympanic membrane were examined. After the application of the inflation-deflation test to assess their tubal function, fluids were instilled into the middle ear through a perforation of the drum. Then a manometric system was connected to an inflatable ear cuff sealed in the external auditory canal, and subjects were induced to swallow repeatedly.

RESULTS

Experiment One

Fluid in a closed tympanum was expelled to the pharynx by both tensor stimulation and swallowing. At the pharyngeal orifice of the tube, periodic outflow of fluid was observed (Fig. 1). During tensor stimulation and swallowing we observed the opening of the orifice, but there was no expulsion of fluid. However, fluids were pushed out to the pharynx simultaneously with closure of the orifice upon cessation of the stimulation or completion of swallowing. The amount of fluid expelled gradually diminished in quantity with each tubal closure and finally disappeared. When the stopcock was opened and ambient pressure restored, expulsion of fluid with each tubal closure resumed.

Experiment Two

Intratympanic pressure dropped stepwise simultaneously with tensor stimulation and swallowing to produce negative pressure in a closed tympanum. The relationship between electrical stimulation of the tensor muscle and change of intratympanic pressure is shown in Figure 2. Tympanic pressure, which was first equal to ambient, dropped simultaneously with the onset of tensor stimulation and remained negative even after cessation of the stimulation. Repeated stimulation of the tensor muscle resulted in an increase in negative pressure, and the drop in pressure with each stimulation gradually became smaller and finally disappeared. However, a change of tympanic pressure in this manner would resume after the release of negative pressure and the adjustment of tympanic pressure to ambient. Also, during swallowing tympanic pressure changed in the same manner.

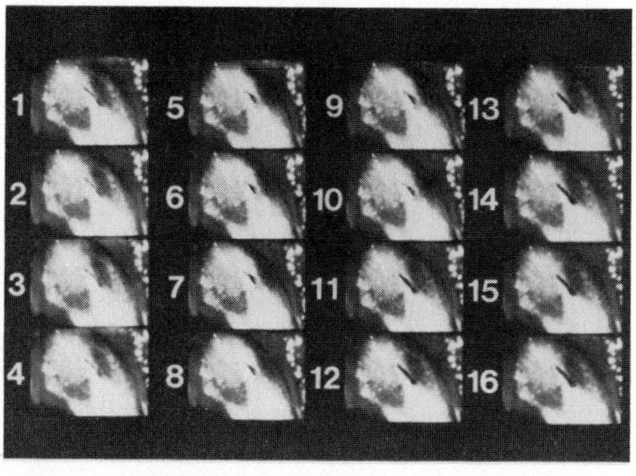

Figure 1 Cinephotographs showing sequence of expulsion of middle ear fluid from the pharyngeal orifice.

Experiment Three

In five of ten subjects, relatively good tubal function was revealed by the inflation-deflation test. That is, lower than 450 mm H_2O opening pressure, lower than 50 mm H_2O residual positive pressures, and residual negative pressures of nearly 0 mm H_2O were found. In these subjects with good tubal function, a drop in middle ear pressure was detected simultaneously with swallowing. On the other hand, no change in middle ear pressure occurred in subjects who appeared to have poor tubal function.

DISCUSSION

From previous studies on fluid flow through the eustachian tube, several concepts related to clearance function of the tube have been proposed. It has often been reported that the tube rapidly clears the tympanum of fluids[3,4] and swallowing accelerates it.[5] Recently, it has been revealed that the eustachian tube has a pumplike activity that actually milks fluids out of the tympanum.[2] That is, fluids in the tympanum are sucked in and accumulated in the tube by dilation of the tube upon tensor contraction, and fluids in the tube are forced to flow out to the pharynx by tubal closure upon tensor relaxation. Because of the mechanical aspects of the middle ear system, however, fluid clearance out of a tympanum with an intact tympanic membrane may be affected by negative pressure that develops in the tympanum.[6]

In the present study, experiment one was conducted to examine fluid clearance from a closed tympanum. Concurrent expulsion of fluid with

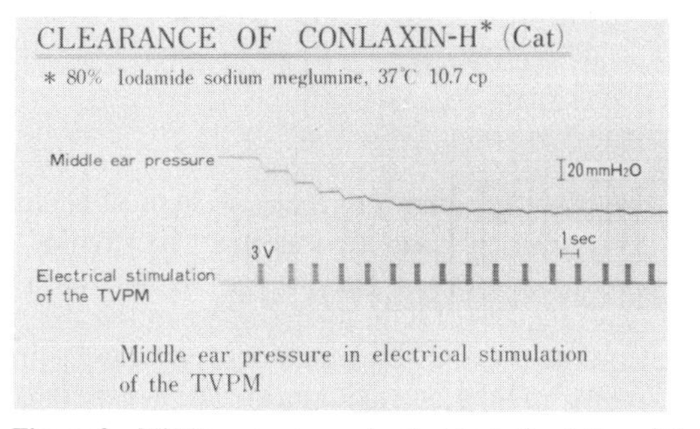

Figure 2 Middle ear pressure in electrical stimulation of the tensor veli palatini muscle (TVPM).

tubal closure means that the pumplike function of the tube works similarly in a closed and an open tympanum. However, it appears that any change of tympanic pressure must be induced by fluid clearance in a closed tympanum, since fluid outflow decreased and disappeared with each tubal closure and was restored by a procedure of adjusting tympanic pressure to ambient.

The second and third experiments demonstrated that intratympanic pressure, which was adjusted to ambient, dropped with each expulsion of fluid and a negative pressure was produced in the tympanum. A sudden drop of tympanic pressure at the instant of tensor stimulation or swallowing is attributed to tubal dilation,[2,7] and the remaining negative pressure after tubal closure is the result of a decrease in fluid volume in the closed tympanum. Relative negative pressure that develops in the tympanum is considered to obstruct the tube functionally, since the pressure drop upon tubal dilation gradually became smaller and finally disappeared. The functional obstruction is further confirmed with the characteristic change of pressure, which is always reproducible with the release of negative pressure in the tympanum. Thus, progressively restrained tubal dilation results in inhibition of fluid clearance, and the pumplike function of the tube is completely abolished by the collapse of the tube.

In summary, fluids in a closed tympanum are rapidly expelled by both tubal opening and closure. When the tympanum is not adequately ventilated, negative pressure is gradually produced in the tympanum. This negative pressure inhibits tubal opening and finally stops fluid clearance by the tube. Therefore, we conclude that ventilation of the tympanum is essential to the pumplike clearance function of the eustachian tube in a closed tympanum.

REFERENCES

1. Honjo I: Experimental study of the eustachian tube function with regard to its related muscles. Acta Otolaryngol 87:84, 1979
2. Honjo I: Experimental study of the pumping function of the eustachian tube. Acta Otolaryngol 91:85, 1981
3. Compere WE Jr: Tympanic cavity clearance studies. Trans Am Acad Ophthalmol Otolaryngol 62:444, 1958
4. Compere WE Jr: The radiologic evaluation of eustachian tube function. Arch Otolaryngol 71:386, 1960
5. Rogers RL: The evaluation of eustachian tubal function by fluorescent dye studies. Laryngoscope 72:456, 1962
6. Bluestone CD: Concepts on the pathogenesis of middle ear effusions. Ann Otol Rhinol Laryngol 85 (Suppl 25): 182, 1976
7. Flisberg K: Ventilatory studies on the eustachian tube. Acta Otolaryngol (Stockh) Suppl 291:44, 1966

MASS SPECTROMETRIC ANALYSIS OF GAS COMPOSITION IN THE GUINEA PIG MIDDLE EAR–MASTOID SYSTEM

JACOB SEGAL, M.D., ERVIN OSTFELD, M.D., M.Sc., JEHUDAH YINON, Ph.D., ALEXANDER SILBERBERG, Ph.D., and JACOB SADÉ, M.D.

On the grounds of their mechanical behavior, the gas-filled body cavities may be divided into two categories: collapsible (as in the lung) and noncollapsible (as in the middle ear and the paranasal sinuses). The contact between the gas in the cavity and the outside atmosphere is generally restricted, although in most cases, in a normally functioning system, periodic contact at least is maintained. In the case of the middle ear this is done through the eustachian tube, which is normally closed but opens periodically for brief intervals that serve to equalize pressure and permit a partial exchange of the gas content of the cavity, thereby maintaining the gas ambiance with respect to both mean pressure and composition.[1]

Very few and incomplete data are available

on the composition of middle ear gas (MEG)[2-5] because many of the associated fundamental difficulties, biologic and technologic, have not yet found their solution. Matsumura in 1955 was the first to determine the MEG composition,[6] but his gasometric method of analysis was not sensitive enough to give adequate indications and he failed to detect the CO_2. More reliable results were reported by Riu and associates in 1966, who, examining the MEG composition by a gas chromatographic method, found the following composition: N_2, 85 percent; O_2, 9.5 percent; and CO_2, 5.5 percent;[7] by Morgenstern and associates, who examined the partial pressure by microelectrodes introduced into guinea pigs' bullae and found 10.9 percent oxygen;[8] and by Sadé and Weisman, who examined the CO_2 content of normal human MEG obtained after direct aspiration by a pH blood analysis and found a mean of 2.66 percent.[9] Ostfeld and colleagues, in air ventilated dogs (gas chromatographic analysis) found: N_2, 83.2 percent ($\pm$ 5.0); O_2, 12.1 percent ($\pm$ 2.2), and CO_2, 4.7 percent ($\pm$ 0.7)[10]—but it is very likely that the results could have been influenced by a state of artificially induced hyperventilation.

In all of these experiments, the problem of contamination of the gas sample by the atmosphere was not entirely resolved. Moreover, the volume of the gas sample withdrawn was far in excess of the physiologic order of magnitude. These considerations explain the scatter in the results and raise serious questions about their reliability. This was clearly also the feeling of Cantekin and associates, who concluded that the composition of the middle ear gas has not yet been definitively determined.[11] Elner calculated that during each act of swallowing—that is, eustachian tube opening—1 μl of air enters the middle ear.[4] Thus, a sampling amount of 1 μl or less could be regarded as physiologic.

We believe that the best way to perform the gas analysis of such small samples is by mass spectrometry (MS) and that the quadrupole system fits our requirements. In a pilot study gas analysis was performed on a VG micromass Q4 quadrupole gas analyzer. We scanned the mass range of 26 to 46 atomic mass units.

The reproducibility of the mass spectrometric gas analysis was demonstrated by a relatively low coefficient of variability of the peaks found by the use of samples of standard gas mixtures (Table 1).

The sensitivity of detection of all middle ear gas components, namely, CO_2, O_2, and N_2, was less than 1 μl.

In the present study the normal middle ear mastoid integral gas composition was determined in healthy guinea pigs by mass spectrometric analysis.

TABLE 1 Reproducibility of Mass Spectrometric Analysis of N_2, O_2, and CO_2 As Found by the Height of Peaks of Ten Microsamples (1 μl) of a Standard Gas Mixture

Gas	*Mean Height of Peak*	*Standard Deviation*	*Coefficient of Variability (%)*
N_2	88.64	0,35	0,39
O_2	10,15	0,308	3,03
CO_2	1,2	0,08	6,6

MATERIALS AND METHODS

The experiments were carried out on healthy adult guinea pigs under general anesthesia induced by Ketamine and Rompun. The animals were allowed to breathe air spontaneously.

For the experiments, a trepanation hole of approximately 3 to 4 mm in diameter was made surgically in the mastoid bulla of each animal. The trepanation hole was closed by a biocompatible material (a septum of Silastic, 2 mm thickness) and sealed by histoacryl. Using the seal as septum, one can sample the middle ear gas from outside for analysis. The samples for MEG analysis were taken 24 to 36 hours following the surgical preparative procedure.

Gas samples of 1 μl were aspirated into a gastight syringe (Hamilton–Model 7100) through the Silastic septum.

Mass Spectrometer

The sensitivity of the VG micromass Q4 gas analyzer was increased by incorporating an electron multiplier detector (Galileo Channeltron type) which increased the overall sensitivity of the mass analyser by a factor of 10^4.

A special inlet system was devised, enabling direct injection of samples with the gastight syringe through a septum into the ion source. In this way we prevented the sample dilution as in the conventional inlet system. This method of sample injection increased the detection sensitivity but extensively shortened the effective life of the sample in the ion source (3 to 6 seconds) before being pumped out. Therefore, ion measurement at the detector had to be done quickly, which was accom-

TABLE 2 The Relative Guinea Pig Middle Ear–Mastoid Space Gas Composition (30 Microsamples)

Gas	Mass	Relative Concentration (%)	Standard Deviation
N_2	28	80.8	2.1
O_2	32	11.7	1.2
CO_2	44	7.5	1.0

plished by connecting a memory oscilloscope to the detector and measuring the peaks obtained from the fast mass scan.

RESULTS AND COMMENT

The middle ear mastoid space gas composition determined by mass spectrometric analysis in 30 microsamples of 1 μl each is shown in Table 2.

The purpose of the present study was to develop a reliable method of gas analysis in microsamples of the order of 1 μl. The quadrupole mass spectrometer proved a reliable tool of analysis of gasses with masses between 2 and 60. The spectrum of gasses in the middle ear ($N_2 = 28$, $O_2 = 32$, and $CO_2 = 44$) fitted the quadrupole scan range.

The high sensitivity of the mass spectrometric analysis was demonstrated by the ability to perform scanning of all the middle ear gas components in a microsample of only 1 μl. This low volume of gas sample permits multiple sampling of the middle ear gas content without altering intratympanic pressure.

As in previous studies, the findings of this study indicate that the relative oxygen concentration in the middle ear even under physiologic conditions is lower than in the surrounding environment. The CO_2 content of the MEG was surprisingly high, and it can be suggested that this high CO_2 level may reflect an active production by the mucociliary epithelium.

REFERENCES

1. Sadé, J: Eustachian tube function. In Sadé J ed: Secretory Otitis Media and Its Sequelae. London: Churchill Livingston 1979, pp 212–253
2. Drettner B: The oxygen tension in transudate of the middle ear. Acta Otolaryngol 79:396, 1975
3. Elner Å: Normal gas exchange in the human middle ear. Ann Otol Rhinol Laryngol Suppl 25:161, 1976
4. Elner Å: Quantitative studies of gas absorption from the normal middle ear. Acta Otolaryngol 83:25, 1977
5. Ostfeld E, Crispin M, Blonder J, Szeinberg A: Micromethod for determination of middle ear gas composition. Ann Otol Rhinol Laryngol 88:562, 1979
6. Matsumura H: Studies on the composition of air in the tympanic cavity. Acta Otolaryngol 61:220, 1955
7. Riu R, Flottes J, Bouche J, et al: *La Physiologie de la Trompe d'Eustache,* Paris: Librarie Arnette, 1966
8. Morgenstern C: Oxygen supply of middle ear mucosa under normal conditions and after eustachian tube occlusion. Ann Otol Rhinol Laryngol 89 (Suppl 68): 76, 1980
9. Sadé J, Weisman Z: The phenotypic expression of middle ear mucosa. In *First International Cholesteatoma Conference*, Birmingham, AL: Aesculapius Publishing Co, 1977, p 52
10. Ostfeld E, Blonder J, Crispin M, et al: The middle ear gas composition in air ventilated dogs. Acta Otolaryngol 89:105, 1980
11. Cantekin EI, Doyle WS, Phillips DC, et al: Gas absorption in the middle ear. Ann Otol Rhinol Laryngol 89 (Suppl 68):71, 1980

ANATOMY AND PATHOLOGY

ANATOMY, MORPHOLOGY, CELL BIOLOGY, AND PATHOLOGY OF THE TUBOTYMPANUM

DAVID J. LIM, M.D.

Many significant contributions to our knowledge of the tubotympanum have been made during the four years since the Second International Symposium on Recent Advances in Otitis Media with Effusion in 1979. Because of the numerous publications during this period, including review articles,[1] this review will be selective rather than exhaustive, and many worthy papers cannot be cited.

In the area of comparative anatomy, descriptions of the tubotympanum in the rhesus monkey, rat, cat, gerbil and hamster have been published during this period,[2,3] and these studies have contributed to the development of several new animal models for otitis media. These models were used to correlate physiologic data and anatomy, which has helped to better our understanding of tubal and mucosal physiology. Anatomic descriptions of the tubotympanum have been reported for the human fetus and neonates,[4,5] for change with age,[6] in the cleft palate population,[7–9] and for normal surface morphology in humans.[10] Morphologic variations of tubal cartilage in otitis-free subjects have also been reported.[11] This information is critically needed for defining the anatomic basis of otitis proneness.

The introduction of computer-assisted image analysis systems has led to attempts to reconstruct various substructures of the tubotympanum, using serial sections for light microscopy.[12] The image storage capability allows investigators to quantitate various anatomic structures and also allows electronic resectioning of the reconstructed structures to provide different sectional views.

Descriptive morphology of the round window membrane has been reported for both humans and animals.[13,14] Furthermore, by use of various tracers in normal animals and in animals with inflamed middle ears, the permeability of the round window membrane has been established.[15,16] Using macromolecules, Saijo and Kimura[17] demonstrated that horseradish peroxidase (HRP) introduced into the middle ear is found in the endolymphatic sac within 48 hours after its injection, which suggests that the round window membrane allows HRP to pass through the round window to the perilymph, and the tracers are then taken in by the endolymphatic sac. HRP was not found in the endolymphatic sac after the endolymphatic duct had been obliterated. These observations have a profound implication in that toxic substances introduced into the middle ear may have access to the inner ear, causing inner ear pathologic changes.

Considerable progress has also been made in quantitating the cellular responses in normal and pathologic specimens by the use of a water-soluble plastic embedding medium (methyl methacrylate), which can be thin-sectioned (1 to 5 μm). These thin sections will greatly improve the resolution of light microscopic observation over that of conventionally thick-sectioned material, which is cut at 20 μm thickness. Using methyl methacrylate embedding, Kuijpers and van der Beek[18] and Okazaki and colleagues[19] investigated experimental middle ear pathologic changes. In addition, by using a digitizer interfaced with a computer, the quantitative analysis of cell responses in these thin sections is readily obtained and stored for statistical analysis. Using this method, Okazaki and colleagues[19] demonstrated distinctly different cellular responses in the middle ear induced by *Hemophilus influenzae* type b and nontypable *H. influenzae* (biotype II) in chinchillas. The striking difference was that *H. influenzae* type b caused a strong initial polymorphonuclear leukocyte response, whereas biotype II caused a strong initial macrophage response and a late lymphocyte response about ten days after middle ear inoculation. Quantitative histology is critical for comparing various experimental pathologic changes and for defining the temporal sequences of cell responses in experimental animal models.[18,20,21]

Using the digitizing technique, Webster[22] demonstrated for the first time the critical period that significantly affects the development of neurons in the brain stem auditory nuclei by experimentally induced conductive hearing loss.

Another significant contribution is the use of immunocytochemistry for the demonstration of antileukoprotease,[23] cyclooxygenase (prostaglandin),[24] and collagenase,[25] as well as secretory immunoglobulins and enzymes, which were reported earlier, in the middle ear tissues. Takasaka and associates[26] reported localizing immune complex in the interciliary surfaces and in the endothelial cells of blood capillaries, suggesting that immune complex may affect both mucociliary system and capillaries in this animal model, leading to serous effusions.

Another significant contribution that used enzyme cytochemistry and immunocytochemistry is the characterization of the autonomic innervation of the tubotympanum. The presence of adrenergic and cholinergic fibers has been well established.[27-30] The adrenergic fibers were found in the lamina propria of the pharyngeal mucosa and the cartilage portion of the tubotympanum. Adrenergic fibers were found innervating the blood vessels and tubal glands. Electron microscopic cytochemistry[29] demonstrated that there are two types of nerve terminals in the eustachian tube mucosa, one type innervating the area along the blood vessel walls and the other running independently of the blood vessels. Some nerve terminals were observed close to the myoepithelial cells of the tubal gland. Recent immunocytochemical studies[29,30] demonstrated the presence of peptidergic innervation. This includes vasoactive intestinal peptide (VIP) and gastrin-releasing peptide. In these two major neuropeptides, Uddman and colleagues[30] reported the presence of neuropeptide Y, substance P, and enkephalin. The VIP-ergic nerve is thought to derive from the pterygopalatine ganglion, whereas neuropeptide Y derives from the superior cervical ganglion. The proposed functions of autonomic innervation are blood flow, which regulates oxygen supply; blood volume regulation, which affects tubal patency or resistance; and regulation of secretory activity, tubal muscles, and sensory feedback from the tympanum.

Another important contribution in the pathology of otitis media is the further investigation of the relationship between otitis media and inner ear pathologic changes. Paparella and his associates suggested that patients with chronic otitis media appear to have a greater incidence of high-tone hearing loss[31] and endolymphatic hydrops.[32] It is postulated that these disorders are mediated by toxic substances passed from the middle ear through the permeable round window membrane. Walby and colleagues[33] studied temporal bones of patients who had suffered from otitis media and found depressed bone conduction in these patients, but suggested that the changes in sound transmission mechanics might be responsible for the depression of bone conduction. Animal experiments combining electrophysiologic with histologic methods demonstrated that otitis media may adversely affect the cochlea, particularly the basal turn.[34] If otitis media adversely affects the inner ear, it could lead to serious consequences for hearing conservation in children, since it remains one of the most common childhood infectious diseases.

Another interesting concept proposed is that of "silent otitis media," which is characterized by histologic evidence of otitis media without clinical manifestations,[35] but this remains controversial.

In summary, quantitative morphology has in recent years provided statistical analysis of various pathologic changes. The improvement of immunocytochemistry has helped us to identify and localize antigens and antibodies, neurotransmitters and enzymes. The use of tracer techniques has allowed us to investigate the macromolecular transport mechanism in the middle ear. These areas will play a vital role in future research. In their future studies, more investigators should attempt to combine other methods with anatomy and cell biology techniques, such as physiology, biochemistry, microbiology, and immunology.

This work was supported in part by grant # NS 08854 from NINCDS/NIH.

REFERENCES

1. Van Cauwenberge P: Otitis media with effusion: Functional morphology and physiopathology of the structures involved. Acta Otorhinolaryngol Belg 36:5, 1982
2. Daniel HL, Fulghum RS, Brian JE, Barret KA: Comparative anatomy of eustachian tube and middle ear cavity in animal models for otitis media. Ann Otol Rhinol Laryngol 91:82, 1982
3. Saad M, Doyle WJ, Gest TR: The morphology of the mid-

dle ear in the rhesus monkey. Acta Anat 112:117, 1982
4. Akaan-Penttila E: Middle ear mucosa in newborn infants. Acta Otolaryngol 93:251, 1980
5. Spector GJ, Ge X-X: Development of the hypotympanum in the human fetus and neonate. Ann Otol Rhinol Laryngol 90 (Suppl 88), 1981
6. Tomoda K, Morii S, Yamashita T, Kumazawa T: Histologic characteristics of human eustachian tubal muscles with regard to their functions and the effect of aging. Ann Otol Rhinol Laryngol, 1984, in press
7. Lathan RA, Long RE, Lathan EA: Cleft palate velopharyngeal musculature in a five month old infant: A three dimensional reconstruction. Cleft Palate J 17:1, 1980
8. Doyle WJ, Kitajiri M, Sando I: The anatomy of the auditory tube and paratubal musculature in a one month cleft palate infant. Cleft Palate J, 20:218–226, 1984
9. Kitajiri N, Sando I, Hashida T, et al: Histopathologic study of otitis media in cleft palate and in high arched palate infants. In Lim DJ et al (eds): *Otitis Media*. Philadelphia, Toronto: BC Decker Inc, 1984
10. Hiraide F, Inouye T: The fine surface view of the human adult eustachian tube. J Laryngol Otol 97:149, 1982
11. Rood SR, Doyle WJ: An extreme morphologic variation of the auditory tube cartilage. Cleft Palate J 18:693, 1981
12. Todhunter JS, Siegel MI, Doyle WJ: Computer generated eustachian tube shape analysis: A preliminary report. In Lim DJ (eds): *Otitis Media*. Philadelphia, Toronto: BC Decker Inc, 1984
13. Schachern PA, Paparella MM, Duvall AJ: The normal chinchilla round window membrane. Arch Otolaryngol 108:550, 1982
14. Schachern PA, Paparella MM, Duvall AJ, Shea D: The chinchilla and human round window membrane: a preliminary electron microscopic study. In *Abstracts of the Sixth Midwinter Research Meeting, Association for Research in Otolaryngology*, 1982, p 45
15. Goycoolea MV, Paparella MM, Goldberg B, Carpenter A-M: Permeability of the round window membrane in otitis media. Arch Otolaryngol 106:430, 1980
16. Goycoolea MV, Paparella MM, Goldberg B, et al: Permeability of the middle ear to staphylococcal pyrogenic exotoxin in otitis media. Int J Pediatr Otorhinolaryngol 1:301, 1980
17. Saijo S, Kimura RS: Distribution of horseradish peroxidase in the inner ear after injection into the middle ear cavity. In *Abstracts of the Research Forum, AAO-HNS/ARO*, 1981
18. Kuijpers W, van der Beek JNH: Experimental occlusion of the eustachian tube: The role of short- and long-term infection and its sequelae. In Lim DJ et al (eds): *Otitis Media*. Philadelphia, Toronto: BC Decker Inc, 1984
19. Okazaki N, DeMaria TF, Briggs BR, et al: Cytological and histological study of experimental otitis media with effusion induced by *H. influenzae*. In Lim DJ et al (eds): *Otitis Media*. Philadelphia, Toronto: BC Decker Inc, 1984
20. Tos M, Wiederhold M, Larsen P: Experimental long-term tubal occlusion in cats: A quantitative histopathological model to study the normalization of the middle ear mucosa. In Lim DJ et al (eds): *Otitis Media*. Philadelphia, Toronto: BC Decker Inc, 1984
21. van der Beek JNH, Kuijpers W: The short- and long-term effects of tubal occlusion in a germfree animal model. In Lim DJ et al (eds): *Otitis Media*. Philadelphia, Toronto: BC Decker Inc, 1984
22. Webster DB: Conductive loss affects auditory neuronal soma size only during a sensitive postnatal period. In Lim DJ et al (eds): *Otitis Media*. Philadelphia, Toronto: BC Decker Inc, 1984
23. Carlsson B, Ohlsson K: Localization of antileukoprotease in middle ear mucosa. Acta Otolaryngol 95:111, 1983
24. Jung TTK, Shea D, Giebink GS, et al: Comparative histopathology of animal models of otitis media in chinchillas. In Lim DJ et al (eds): *Otitis Media*. Philadelphia, Toronto: BC Decker Inc, 1984
25. Gantz BJ, Maynard J, Bumsted RM, et al: Bone resorption in chronic otitis media. Ann Otol Rhinol Laryngol 88:693, 1979
26. Takasaka T, Kaku Y, Shibahara Y, et al: Experimental otitis media with effusion: An immunoelectron microscopic study. In Lim DJ et al (eds): *Otitis Media*. Philadelphia, Toronto: BC Decker Inc, 1984
27. Uddman R, Alumets J, Densert O, et al: Innervation of feline eustachian tube. Ann Otol Rhinol Laryngol 88:557, 1979
28. Yamashita T, Amano H, Kumazawa T, et al: Adrenergic innervation in the eustachian tube of guinea pigs. Arch Otorhinolaryngol 225:279, 1979
29. Amano H, Yamashita T, Kitajiri M, et al: Adrenergic innervation in the eustachian tube of guinea pigs: Histochemical and electron microscopic observations. In Lim DJ et al (eds): *Otitis Media*. Philadelphia, Toronto: BC Decker Inc, 1984
30. Uddman R, Kitajiri M, Sundler F: Autonomic innervation of the tubotympanum. In Lim DJ et al (eds): *Otitis Media*. Philadelphia, Toronto: BC Decker Inc, 1984
31. Paparella MM, Oda M, Hiraide F, Brady D: Pathology of sensorineural hearing loss in otitis media. Ann Otol Rhinol Laryngol 81:632, 1972
32. Paparella MM, Goycoolea MV, Meyerhoff WL, Shea D: Endolymphatic hydrops and otitis media. Laryngoscope 89:43, 1979
33. Walby AP, Barrera A, Schuknecht HF: Cochlear pathology in chronic suppurative otitis media. Ann Otol Rhinol Laryngol 92 (Suppl 103), 1983
34. Morizono T, Giebink GS, Sikora MA, et al: Sensorineural hearing loss in an animal model of purulent otitis media. In Lim DJ et al (eds): *Otitis Media*. Philadelphia, Toronto: BC Decker Inc, 1984
35. Paparella MM, Mancini F, Shea D, et al: Silent otitis media. In Lim DJ et al (eds): : *Otitis Media*. Philadelphia, Toronto: BC Decker Inc, 1984

N.B.: The book listed here as *Otitis Media* is an abbreviation of the title of this work, *Recent Advances in Otitis Media with Effusion*.

ADRENERGIC INNERVATION IN THE EUSTACHIAN TUBE OF THE GUINEA PIG: HISTOCHEMICAL AND ELECTRON MICROSCOPIC OBSERVATIONS

H. AMANO, M.D., T. YAMASHITA, M.D., M. KITAJIRI, M.D.,
T. KUMAZAWA, M.D., C. TANAKA, M.D., and Y. IBATA, M.D.

The eustachian tube plays an important role in the pathogenesis of otitis media with effusion; however, its mechanism has not yet been elucidated completely.

The patency of the tube is affected by vasoconstriction, vasodilation, or secretion of the tubal glands. There is good clinical evidence to suggest that the autonomic nervous system influences eustachian tube function. The patency of the tube is affected by the blocking of the superior cervical ganglion, and it is controlled by the blood flow through the autonomic nervous system.[1]

Although autonomic innervation of the nose[2] and the inner ear[3,4] has been thoroughly studied by several investigators, knowledge of the distribution of the adrenergic nerve fiber in the eustachian tube which is part of the autonomic innervation is scanty. Only recently has demonstration of the adrenergic innervation of the eustachian tube using Falck-Hillarp's histochemical method[5] been reported by Uddman[6] and by us[7] on the light microscopic level.

Recently available special staining techniques were helpful in specifically identifying the fibers containing biogenic amines and in distinguishing them from other nerve terminals on the ultrastructural level.[8,9] The reliability of this method is also increased by pretreatment with a false transmitter, such as 5-hydroxydopamine (5-OHDA), and the adrenergic innervation of the tube using this method has been reported recently.[10]

In this study we have attempted to demonstrate the adrenergic fibers in the tube by the glyoxylic acid method using stretch preparation[11] and the Falck-Hillarp method using frozen sections. In addition, an electron microscopic method was used to detect the exact adrenergic terminals.

MATERIALS AND METHODS

Fluorescent Microscopic Study

We used guinea pigs weighing about 300 gm, and pentobarbital was used as an anesthetic. For fluorescent microscopic investigation, all animals received, while under anesthesia, an intracardiac perfusion with 400 to 600 ml/kg of 2 percent glyoxylic acid solution with phosphate buffer. The temporal bone was removed and the tube was carefully dissected out in the glyoxylic acid solution. Then the tubal cartilage was removed and the dissected tubal mucous membrane was stretched on a slide glass and heated. For the study of detailed adrenergic innervation in the tube, tubes obtained in the same way were frozen quickly, freeze dried, and treated with paraformaldehyde according to the Falck-Hillarp method. After the whole-mount specimens were embedded in paraffin, they were sectioned and observed under a Zeiss fluorescent microscope.

One group of animals received surgical sympathectomy by removal of the superior cervical ganglion. One week after the sympathectomy, the tubes were obtained and examined as described above.

Electron Microscopic Study

Guinea pigs weighing about 300 gm were anesthetized and 200 to 250 mg/kg of 5-OHDA was injected into the carotid artery of each. Three hours after injection, they underwent general perfusion with a solution of 2.5 percent glutaraldehyde and 2 percent paraformaldehyde buffered with phosphate at pH 7.2. The temporal bone was removed and put in the same fixative. The tissues from the entire eustachian tube were immediately excised and sectioned into 1 mm sections. These sections were immersed again in renewed fixative for another hour. After being washed with phosphate buffer, the blocks were dehydrated through a graded series of alcohol and embedded in Spurr medium. Ultrathin sections of the tube were stained with uranyl acetate and lead citrate and examined under a JEM-100B electron microscope.

RESULTS

Fluorescent Microscopic Studies

The adrenergic nerve fibers reveal a distinct

green fluorescence when treated with glyoxylic acid owing to the preservation of catecholamines with acid. These nerve fibers are characterized by varicose thickening and by the fact that they run as individual fibers, in parallel curved rows.

In the stretch preparation of the tube, fluorescent adrenergic nerves were observed throughout the tubal mucosa. The nerve fibers were most abundant in the pharyngeal area, sparser in the middle, and even more sparse near the tympanic orifice. They were seen to be arranged essentially longitudinally in all specimens. In the pharyngeal area, the adrenergic plexus forms a loose network of varicose fibers.

Much detailed localization of adrenergic nerves was observed using the freeze-dried sections and the Falck-Hillarp method. Scattered adrenergic fibers were seen in the lamina propria of the pharyngeal area. The lamina propria in the middle part and near the tympanic orifice is much thinner, and only a few fibers were seen in several specimens.

Most of the arteries that reach the tube arise from the external carotid artery, and many arteries or arterioles run through the connective tissue of the lamina propria and the tubal glands. Numerous adrenergic nerve fibers were observed surrounding those blood vessels.

In the coronal section, the fibers were seen forming a network close to the vessel's wall. Numerous fibers were observed just around the perivascular layer of a relatively large artery in the connective tissue not far from the tubal epithelium, and a few of the fibers branched out in the connective tissue.

Adrenergic nerve fiber was also seen in the interacinal spaces of the tubal glands. A few of the fibers were observed arising from the plexus of the vessels that supply the tubal glands and running along the bottom of the acinus. No nerve fiber was seen running through the basal layer of the acinus.

The specimens from both the stretch preparation and the Falck-Hillarp method after the sympathectomy showed a remarkable decrease of the adrenergic nerve fibers.

Electron Microscopic Studies

Small, dense-cored granular vesicles were seen in the adrenergic nerve terminals. The appearance of high electron density in these vesicles is attributed to the fact that 5-OHDA is taken up into the amine-containing vesicles.

The epithelial layer had no adrenergic terminals. In the lamina propria of the eustachian tubal mucosa, two types of adrenergic nerve terminals were observed. One innervated the area along the blood vessel wall and the other ran quite independent of the blood vessel. Some of the nerve terminals were observed close to the myoepithelial cells of the tubal gland, but most of the nerve terminals were found in the vicinity of the blood vessel close to the tubal gland. No clear adrenergic innervation was detected in the intra-acinal region. The adrenergic nerve terminals were also observed in the tubal muscle. Most of the adrenergic nerve fibers terminated close to the artery that supplies the tubal muscle. On the other hand, a few nerve terminals were observed as free endings in the space close to the tubal muscle and cartilage.

Most of the adrenergic nerve terminals around the arteries were located just beneath the smooth muscle layer, but some terminated as free endings lying close to the endothelial cells of the arteries.

CONCLUSIONS

Our findings give a morphologic conception about the adrenergic innervation and its regulatory mechanism in the function of the eustachian tube. The studies of sympathectomy suggest that the adrenergic nerve arises from the superior cervical ganglion and reaches the tube along the vessels.

Abundant adrenergic nerve fibers were seen in the pharyngeal area. In the freeze-dried sections and electron microscopic studies, the adrenergic nerve fibers and their terminals were observed in the lamina propria, tubal gland, and especially around the vessels. Some of those fibers were also observed running independent of the vessel.

The patency of the eustachian tube is changed easily by blood pressure.[1,12] The adrenergic nerve seems to affect tubal patency through the control of vasoconstriction. It can also be speculated that secretory activity of the tubal gland is affected by the adrenergic nervous system. Although it is highly speculative, the adrenergic nerve fiber just beneath the epithelium may control a mucociliary system in the pharyngeal area.

The secretions of the tubal gland and mucociliary system are suspected to be controlled by both the adrenergic nervous system and the cholinergic nervous system. Also, the existence of the peptidergic nerve has been reported. It can be suggested that, in association with cholinergic and peptidergic nerves, the adrenergic nervous system might play an important role in the function of the eustachian tube.

REFERENCES

1. Nathanson SE, Jackson RT: Vidian nerve and the eustachian tube. Ann Otol 85:83, 1976
2. Densert O: Adrenergic innervation in the rabbit cochlea. Acta Otolaryngol 78:345, 1974
3. Spoendlin H, Lichtensteiger W: The sympathetic nerve supply to the inner ear. Arch Klin Exp Ohrres Nasen Kehlk-heilk 189:346, 1967
4. Terayama Y, Holz E, Beck C: Adrenergic innervation of the cochlea. Ann Otol 75:69, 1966
5. Falck B, Hillarp N-Å, Thieme G, Torp A: Fluorescence of catecholamines and related compounds condensed with formaldehyde. J Histochem 10:348, 1962
6. Uddman R, Alumets J, Densert O, et al: Innervation of the feline eustachian tube. Ann Otol Rhinol Laryngol 88:557, 1979
7. Yamashita T, Amano H, Kumazawa T, et al: Adrenergic innervation in the eustachian tube of the guinea pigs. Arch Otorhinolaryngol 225:279, 1979
8. Richardson KC: Electron microscopic identification of autonomic endings. Nature 210:756, 1966
9. Tranzer JP, Thoenen H: Electron microscopic localization of 5-hydroxydopamine (3,4,5-trihydroxy-phenyl-ethylamine), a new "false" sympathetic transmitter. Experientia 23:743, 1967
10. Kitajiri M, Yamashita T, Shinomiya M, Ibata Y: Electron-microscopical observation of adrenergic innervation in guinea pig Eustachian tube. Arch Otorhinolaryngol 228:123, 1980
11. Axelsson S, Björklund A, Falck B, et al: Glyoxylic acid condensation: A new fluorescence method for the histochemical demonstration of biogenic monoamines. Acta Physiol Scand 87:57, 1973
12. Jackson RT: Pharmacological mechanisms in the eustachian tube. Ann Otol 80:313, 1971

AUTONOMIC INNERVATION OF THE TUBOTYMPANUM

ROLF UDDMAN, M.D., MASANORI KITAJIRI, M.D., and FRANK SUNDLER, M.D.

In contrast to the rich literature on the autonomic innervation of the nasal mucosa and lower respiratory tract, there are relatively few reports on the autonomic nervous supply to the tubotympanic region. Nevertheless, early histologic studies, using methylene blue or gold chloride staining, have revealed numerous nerve fibers in, for example, the tympanic membrane, some of which enter from the middle ear.[1]

With development of new histochemical techniques it became possible to differentiate between two types of nerve fibers; those containing noradrenalin and those giving a positive acetylcholinesterase staining. Studies using the acetylcholinesterase method of Koelle[2] and the Falck-Hillarp method for the demonstration of noradrenalin[3] revealed a rich supply of nerve fibers around the eustachian tube and in the middle ear mucosa.[4–6] Both types of nerves were distributed around small blood vessels, around seromucous glands, and in the subepithelial layer. Such studies supported the classic subdivision of the autonomic nervous system into adrenergic and cholinergic components.

The rapid progress in immunology and immunocytochemistry during the last decade has resulted in the localization of a number of peptides in neurons. Among such peptides are vasoactive intestinal peptide (VIP), substance P (SP), gastrin-releasing peptide (GRP), enkephalin and neuropeptide Y (NPY). Some of these peptides were first detected in the brain and subsequently found to exist also in peripheral nerves, particularly in the gut. Conversely, other peptides were first detected in the gut and later found to exist also in the brain.

The studies have led to the view that the autonomic nervous system is composed not only of adrenergic and cholinergic components but also of a variety of peptidergic neurons. There are, however, recent data indicating that peripheral adrenergic and cholinergic neurons may also contain peptides. This chapter summarizes available data on the occurrence and distribution of peptide-containing neurons in the tubotympanic region.

MATERIALS AND METHODS

Middle ear mucosa and specimens from the eustachian tube were taken from adult guinea pigs and cats. The specimens from the eustachian tube were immersed in ice-cold fixative solution (4 percent formaldehyde in 0.1M sodium phosphate) for 12 hours. They were rinsed in a Tyrode's solution containing 10 percent sucrose at 4°C for 48 hours, frozen on dry ice, and sectioned in a cryostat at −20°C. The specimens from the middle ear mucosa were stretched on chrome-alun subbed slides as whole mounts and fixed in a buffered solution of formaldehyde and picric acid. They were

TABLE 1 Details of the Antisera

Antigen	*Code*	*Raised Against*	*Working Dilution*	*Source*
Vasoactive intestinal peptide	7852	Unconjugated porcine VIP	1:160	Milab, Malmö, Sweden
Substance P	SP-8	Protein-conjugated bovine substance P	1:40	P. C. Emson, Cambridge, England
Leu-enkephalin	leu-enk	Protein-conjugated leu-enkephalin	1:80	K. J. Chang, Burroughs Wellcome Research Laboratory, Research Triangle Park, North Carolina, USA
Gastrin releasing peptide	R-6902	Protein-conjugated porcine GRP	1:640	N. Yanaihara, Shizuoka, Japan
Avian pancreatic polypeptide	APP 123	Unconjugated chicken PP	1:360	J. R. Kimmel, Kansas City, Kansas, USA
Neuropeptide Y	NPYY	Unconjugated porcine NPY	1:400	P. C. Emson, Cambridge, England

then dehydrated, cleared in xylene, and hydrated in a series of ethanol solutions. The cryostate sections and the whole mounts were processed for the immunocytochemical demonstration of the various peptides using the indirect immunofluorescence methods of Coons and associates.[7] Details of the antisera are given in Table 1. The site of the antigen–antibody reaction was revealed by fluorescein isothiocyanate-labeled goat-antirabbit IgG in dilution 1:20. Specimens and whole mounts incubated with antiserum inactivated by the addition of excess antigen were used as controls.

RESULTS AND COMMENTS

In the tubotympanun numerous fibers containing VIP were seen around the eustachian tube and in the middle ear mucosa. The fibers surrounded small blood vessels and seromucous glands. In addition, VIP fibers were seen in the subepithelial layer of the eustachian tube. Previous studies have revealed a rich supply of VIP-containing nerve fibers in the upper respiratory tract, most of which originate in the pterygopalatine ganglion.[8] VIP has a wide range of biologic effects, including dilatation of blood vessels, relaxation of smooth muscle, and stimulation of secretion from several exocrine and endocrine glands.

A moderate supply of SP fibers was seen in the tubotympanic area. In the wall of the eustachian tube the fibers were distributed around small blood vessels, in the subepithelial layer, and sometimes within the epithelium. In the middle ear mucosa SP fibers formed a wide-meshed network, often in close association with small blood vessels. SP evokes dilatation of blood vessels, an effect that can be blocked by SP antagonists.[9] Capsaicin is a drug with neurotoxic effects, and systemic treatment with capsaicin causes depletion of SP in primary sensory afferents. Since most SP fibers in the epithelium and around blood vessels disappear upon administration of capsaicin, it has been suggested that these SP fibers mediate sensory information.[10]

Recently, GRP was isolated from porcine gastric mucosa. The carboxy terminal portion of GRP is almost identical in amino acid sequence with bombesin, isolated from amphibian skin. GRP also shows some structural similarity with substance P in that they share the carboxy terminal 2 amino acids. Radioimmunologic and immunocytochemical findings have demonstrated the occurrence of GRP fibers in the mammalian brain and gut.[11] In the tubotympanic region a moderate supply of GRP fibers was seen distributed around small blood vessels. In the middle ear mucosa, however, GRP fibers without obvious relation to blood vessels could be found.

Enkephalin is a neuropeptide with a high affinity for opiate receptors which has been demonstrated immunocytochemically in both the central and peripheral nervous system.[12] The distribution pattern of peripheral enkephalin neurons suggests that this peptide also serves functions other than those involving modulation of pain transmission. In our study a scarce supply of enkephalin fibers was seen in the middle ear mucosa. Little information is available to explain the role enkephalin may play in this tissue.

Pancreatic polypeptide (PP) is a 36-amino-acid hormone candidate produced by a population of endocrine cells in the pancreas and gastrointestinal tract. With antisera raised against the avian variety of pancreatic polypeptide (APP) it has been possible to demonstrate immunoreactive PP in neuronal elements in both the central and peripheral nervous systems. Previous studies have revealed a rich supply of APP-immunoreactive nerve fibers in the tubotympanic area.[13] Since the neurons could not be demonstrated by all antibodies against APP, nor were they demonstrated by antibodies raised against mammalian PP, it appeared likely that they demonstrated a PP-like peptide rather than PP itself. A likely candidate for this peptide is NPY, recently isolated from brain by Tatemoto and colleagues[14] and found to resemble PP in the amino acid sequence. In the tubotympanic region NPY-immunoreactive fibers were abundant. The fibers were located close to small blood vessels, arteries having a very rich supply and veins a scarce supply. Sequential staining with antisera to APP and NPY revealed that the immunostained nerves are identical. It therefore appears likely that the previously demonstrated neuronal PP-like peptide in fact represents NPY. The superior cervical ganglia contain numerous NPY-immunoreactive nerve cell bodies, and on extirpation of these ganglia the NPY fibers to the tubotympanic area disappear. Thus, it is conceivable that the NPY fibers constitute a population of adrenergic neurons.

In conclusion, the eustachian tube and the middle ear mucosa harbor numerous cholinergic and adrenergic nerve fibers. In addition, there are nerve fibers containing peptides such as VIP, SP, GRP, enkephalin, and NPY. Generally, the peptide-containing fibers are distributed around small blood vessels, seromucous glands, and in the subepithelial layer. Occasionally, SP fibers can be seen within the epithelium. The distribution of the peptide-containing nerve fibers suggests a role for neuropeptides in the local control of blood flow and seromucous secretion. In addition, some fibers, notably those containing SP, may participate in sensory transmission.

REFERENCES

1. Wilson JG: The nerves and nerve-endings in the membrana tympani. J Comp Neurol 17:459, 1907
2. Koelle GB: Cytological distributions and physiological functions of cholinesterases. In Koelle GB (ed): *Handbook of Experimental Pharmacology*. Berlin: Springer Verlag 1963, p 187
3. Björklund A, Falck B, Owman C: Fluorescence microscopic and microspectrofluorometric techniques for the cellular localization and characterization of biogenic amines. In Berson SA (ed): *Methods of Investigative and Diagnostic Endocrinology*, Vol 1: Rall JE, Kopin IJ (eds): *The Thyroid and Biogenic Amines*. Amsterdam, North-Holland Publishing Company, 1972 pp 318–368
4. Ishii T, Kaga K: Autonomic nervous system of the cat middle ear mucosa. Ann Otol Rhinol Laryngol 85 (Suppl 25): 51, 1976
5. Uddman R, Alumets J, Densert O et al: Innervation of the feline Eustachian tube. Ann Otol 88:557, 1979
6. Yamashita T, Amano H, Kumazawa T, et al: Adrenergic innervation in the Eustachian tube. Arch Otorhinolaryngol 225: 279, 1979
7. Coons AH, Leduc EH, Conolly JM: Studies on antibody production. I. A method for the histochemical demonstration of specific antibody and its application to a study of the hyperimmune rabbit. J Exp Med 102:49, 1955
8. Uddman R, Malm L, Sundler F: The origin of vasoactive intestinal polypeptide (VIP) nerves in the feline nasal mucosa. Acta Otolaryngol 89:152, 1980
9. Edvinson L, McCulloch J, Rosell S, Uddman R: Antagonism by (D-Pro^{2}, D-Trp^{7,9})–substance P of the cerebrovascular dilatation induced by substance P. Acta Physiol Scand 116:411, 1982
10. Furness JB, Papka RE, Della NG, et al: Substance P-like immunoreactivity in nerves associated with the vascular system of guinea pigs. Neuroscience 7:447, 1982
11. Yanaihara N, Yanaihara C, Mochizuki T, et al: Immunoreactive GRP. Peptides 2 (Suppl 2): 185, 1981
12. Elde R, Hökfelt T, Johansson O, Terenius L: Immunohistochemical studies using antibodies to leucine-enkephalin: Initial observations on the nervous system of the rat. Neuroscience 1:349, 1976
13. Uddman R, Håkanson R, Sundler F: Immunoreactive avian pancreatic polypeptide occurs in nerves of the mammalian nasal mucosa and Eustachian tube. ORL 42:242, 1980
14. Tatemoto K, Carlquist M, Mutt V: Neuropeptide Y—a novel brain peptide with structural similarities to peptide YY and pancreatic polypeptide. Nature 296:659, 1982

SILENT OTITIS MEDIA

MICHAEL M. PAPARELLA, M.D., TIMOTHY T.K. JUNG, M.D., Ph.D., FERNANDO MANCINI, M.D., DON SHEA, M.A., and SUDHIR P. AGARWAL, M.D.

INTRODUCTION

In assessing various pathogenic factors in otitis media, it is important to consider the clinically silent (undetected or undetectable) existence of pathologic findings in the mucoperiosteal membrane, which upon stimulation may become clinically active. Otitis media can, in certain cases, occur along a continuum. As animal and human studies demonstrate, various forms of otitis media with effusion (OME) can, over time, lead to other active infectious forms and ultimately to chronic otitis media (COM) characterized by granulation tissue, including cholesterol granuloma and cholesteatoma.[1-8] OME usually resolves with treatment.

On the other hand, otitis media can become clinically inactive (burned out or noninfectious) and can result in sequelae of hearing loss, both conductive and sensorineural, atelectasis, tympanosclerosis, and a variety of pathologic changes in the middle ear that may or may not be associated with a hearing loss, including perforation of the tympanic membrane, atrophic tympanic membrane/healed perforation or retraction pockets, ossicular discontinuity or fixation, adhesions and scar tissue, osteolysis and osteogenesis, and a thick, granular mucoperiosteum.[9] Because of the widespread use of antibiotics, the mucoperiosteum may undergo partial resolution but remain diseased and be masked or silent with an apparently normal ear and tympanic membrane. This is comparable to "masked" mastoiditis, which because of antibiotic coverage may also escape clinical detection,[10,11] and to chronic inactive maxillary sinusitis, in which radiograms demonstrate thick mucosa.

In certain infants and young children, mesenchyme can persist in the middle ear after birth. The possible relationship of unresolved mesenchyme and otitis media in children will be discussed from a review of the literature and from temporal bone studies in our laboratory. Unresolved mesenchyme can also mimic otitis media and may produce false-positive tympanometric findings in infants. We will expand our temporal bone study of silent otitis media to include all forms of otitis media, with emphasis on clinical correlation. Finally, individual cases will be selected to demonstrate the syndrome of silent otitis media.

ROLE OF MESENCHYME

Much discussion has arisen as to the time of disappearance of the mesenchyme in the middle ear, which indeed presents numerous paradoxes. Typically, mesenchymal cells are transient elements awaiting differentiation; however, many authorities maintain that cells of this "embryonic" type persist in the adult.[12] Wolff reported the distinct absence of mesenchyme in specimens from humans older than 13 months.[13] Keibel and Mall stated that areolar tissue (mesenchyme) disappeared only after birth, the tympanic cavity at that time almost or completely lacking a lumen.[14] More recently, Guggenheim and colleagues reported that the resorption process begins in the third fetal month and should ideally be completed by the eighth month.[15] In actuality, traces of this tissue may be present up to the fourth or fifth year, and a few children retain even larger amounts until the onset of puberty when, under the influence of hormones, any mesenchymal remnants tend to differentiate into adult fibrous tissue. This is substantiated by Buch and Jorgenson, who believe that from the middle of fetal life the mesenchyme seems to start its regression, which presumably may take place at a highly varied rate.[16] The point of agreement among most investigators is that there is a fairly regular reduction of embryonic connective tissue with increasing maturity under normal circumstances.

The question now arises as to what is the behavior of mesenchyme under abnormal circumstances, such as in the presence of otitis media. Aschoff considered, as early as 1897, that mucosal changes predispose to infection, which presumably would inhibit the mesenchymal regression.[17] Meyer believed that prenatal otitis and otitis during infancy were purulent, but that owing to differences in the tendency to organization their manifestations differed.[18] Singer attributed the mesenchymal metamorphosis to decreasing viscosity and dissolution and absorption as well as normal growth, but he also considered exogenous actions, such as inflammation, to influence the reactive properties of mesenchyme.[19] Wolff reported that infection and mesenchyme in the middle ear had a mutually unfavorable effect upon each other, infection stimulating differentiation of mesenchyme into scar tissue, and mesenchyme interfering with effectiveness of myringotomy.[13]

The unfavorable effect of unresorbed mesenchyme on the course of otitis media through interference with drainage of exudate was further emphasized by Guggenheim in his study of temporal bones from children dying of complications of ear infections.[20] There was a striking incidence of large masses of tympanal mesenchyme infiltrated with inflammatory cells, with walled-off pockets of pus throughout the tympanic cavity. Wilson stressed the special anatomic factors applying to the eustachian tube in fetuses and newborns and considered the entrance of amniotic fluid and infection to be of great importance.[21] Guggenheim and associates suggested that the deleterious effects of unresorbed mesenchyme upon the course of otitis media are more subtle and difficult to detect in this antibiotic age than formerly, and one would hardly be in a position to consider an unfavorable course of events as diagnostic of the persistence of mesenchyme.[15] Buch and Jorgenson reported that infections play no major role in the fate of the mesenchymal tissue in newborn infants,[16] while this influence no doubt increases later and, as emphasized by Wittmaack,[22] presumably affects formation of the cavity apart from the tympanic cavity proper.

All of this leads to intriguing questions regarding the role and association of mesenchyme in the pathogenesis of otitis in infants. Are genetic factors related to mesenchymal absorption, as Guggenheim and Buch and Jorgenson argue,[15,16] or are there other factors, such as endocrinopathy or metabolic disturbance[15] or ventilatory function of the eustachian tube, or is mesenchymal regression induced by invasion of epithelium from the foregut?[22]

In a recent study, the hypothesis was put forth that the presence of clinically undetectable silent otitis media in neonates and infants might help explain why certain children are prone to otitis media.[24] One hundred eleven temporal bones harvested from neonates and infants were studied and histologic analysis demonstrated normal findings in some, while significant numbers of others showed all forms of otitis media, including acute purulent (POM), COM, serous (SOM), mucoid (MOM) and overlap of types. A meaningful outcome of this study was the finding of a marked degree of unresolved mesenchyme in the group with clinically manifest otitis media and in the group with silent otitis media as compared with a control group. Most of these infants died in intensive care units, which might explain the high incidence of pathologic factors found. Unresolved mesenchyme has also been seen in Hurler's syndrome in the temporal bones of three patients 2 to 6 years of age[25] and in a 17-year-old.[26] Tympanometric findings in premature infants show an abnormal middle ear function compatible with persistent mesenchymal tissue as contrasted with normal findings in full-term infants.[27]

SURGICAL FINDINGS

Other evidence for the existence of "silent otitis media" or silent sequelae from otitis media can be found at surgery. Exploratory tympanotomy for otherwise undiagnosable conductive losses of 35 dB or greater (250 cases) revealed silent otitis media or sequelae of otitis media to be the most common finding.[28] In 118 cases with evidence of OM, the main findings were a thick, granular mucosa with adhesive changes, ossicular fixation and discontinuity, and granulation tissue. Often more than one feature or sequela of otitis media was found in one ear, such as ossicular fixation associated with fluid and an atrophic tympanic membrane.

Clinically, in some cases it appears that "silent otitis media" can cause insidious changes in the inner ear behind an intact tympanic membrane in the absence of active otitis media. Rarely, this can lead to sensorineural hearing loss, presumably due to invasion of the round window.[29] Meniere's syndrome can develop after otitis media in certain patients. Typically, active otitis media early in life is followed by inactive (silent) otitis media and, years later, full-blown Meniere's syndrome can occur.[30] Occasionally, evidence of thickened, granular mucoperiosteum is found within a sclerotic mastoid of these patients as in a subclinical form of masked mastoiditis. The classic description of the first case of Meniere's disorder by Hallpike and Cairns in 1938 was associated with extensive pathologic findings of chronic otitis media.[31] Reduced development of periaqueductal cells of the vestibular aqueduct and endolymphatic sac, hypodevelopment of Trautmann's triangle, and anterior displacement of the lateral sinus in patients with Meniere's disorder have been discussed by several authors in association with hypocellularity of the mastoid and a possible relationship to subclinical otitis media during childhood.[32,34] Endolymphatic hydrops has also been seen in association with experimentally induced otitis media in animals.[35,38]

TEMPORAL BONE STUDIES IN HUMANS

In a previous study of neonates and infants, all forms of otitis media in patients with an intact tympanic membrane were seen, including POM, SOM, MOM, and COM, with overlap of types.[24] These children had serious systemic diseases and it is likely that otitis media, especially the acute forms, occurred in some as part of their terminal illness, thus explaining the absence of clinical diagnosis. This explains some, perhaps, but not all, of the positive findings. It can be safely assumed

TABLE 1 Silent Otitis Media

	No. of Cases	Average Age	Temporal Bones	Perforations of TM (%)	Positive History of Otitis Media: No. of Cases	Temporal Bones	Temporal Bones with Silent Otitis Media
COM	112	50	163	36 (22.1)	37	51	112
POM	60	40	79	5 (6.3)	5	7	72
SPOM	66	45	94	2 (2.1)	5	7	87
SOM	15	52	21	1 (4.8)	3	3	18
MOM	5	4	9	— (0)	—	—	9

that otitis media was not clinically detected or *detectable* in most of these infants with positive histologic evidence.

Chronic otitis media is generally described in association with a perforated tympanic membrane. A review of clinical records and temporal bone findings was undertaken on 90 patients with histologic findings of COM. Of particular interest was the low incidence of associated perforations of tympanic membrane (19.5 percent). Furthermore, only 24 patients had symptoms or findings of otologic disease recorded in their charts.[39]

This study represents an expansion of the study noted above. Eleven hundred thirty human temporal bones were reviewed for histopathologic findings of otitis media, and 366 temporal bones (32 percent) were found to have evidence of otitis media. Based on these findings, the otitis media was classified as COM, POM, SPOM (seropurulent), MOM, or SOM. Clinical records were carefully reviewed for positive history or findings of otitis media, and absence or presence of perforation of tympanic membrane was noted. The findings are summarized in Table 1.

Silent (undetected or undetectable) otitis media was diagnosed in 208 cases (298 temporal bones). Perforation of the tympanic membranes was seen in 12 percent of cases, ranging from none in the group with MOM to 22 percent in the group with COM.

In reviewing the histopathology of 366 bones with otitis media, we also noted the presence of unresolved mesenchyme in the middle ear cleft. In 70 temporal bones (20 percent), mesenchyme was present in mild (22 cases), moderate (30 cases), and marked (18 cases) amounts (Table 2). All but two patients having unresolved mesenchyme in the middle ear were below age 2. One was a 6-year-old male and the other an 18-year-old male.

CLINICAL EXAMPLES

The best examples of silent otitis media are those in which pathologic changes of the mucoperiosteum coexist with normal otologic and audiologic findings. In certain patients, in whom temporal bone studies confirmed pathologic evidence of silent otitis media, audiometric data revealed sensorineural hearing losses in the absence of conductive losses or positive tympanometric studies, presumably unrelated to middle ear pathologic findings (Fig. 1). Examples of temporal bone pathologic findings in cases of silent otitis media are seen in Figure 2.

DISCUSSION

From this study of temporal bones and a review of the literature, we have presented evidence that otitis media can exist in a subclinical state that we term "silent otitis media." This entity may have certain features in common with "adhesive

TABLE 2 Unresolved Middle Ear Mesenchyme

	Number of Temporal Bones	Total (%)	Mild (%)	Moderate (%)	Marked (%)
COM	163	15 (9.2)	3 (4.7)	4 (2.4)	8 (4.9)
POM	79	26 (32.9)	10 (12.6)	11 (13.9)	5 (6.3)
SPOM	94	19 (20.2)	5 (5.3)	11 (11.7)	3 (3.1)
SOM	21	3 (14.2)	1 (4.7)	2 (9.5)	0 (0)
MOM	9	7 (77.7)	3 (33.3)	2 (22.2)	2 (22.2)

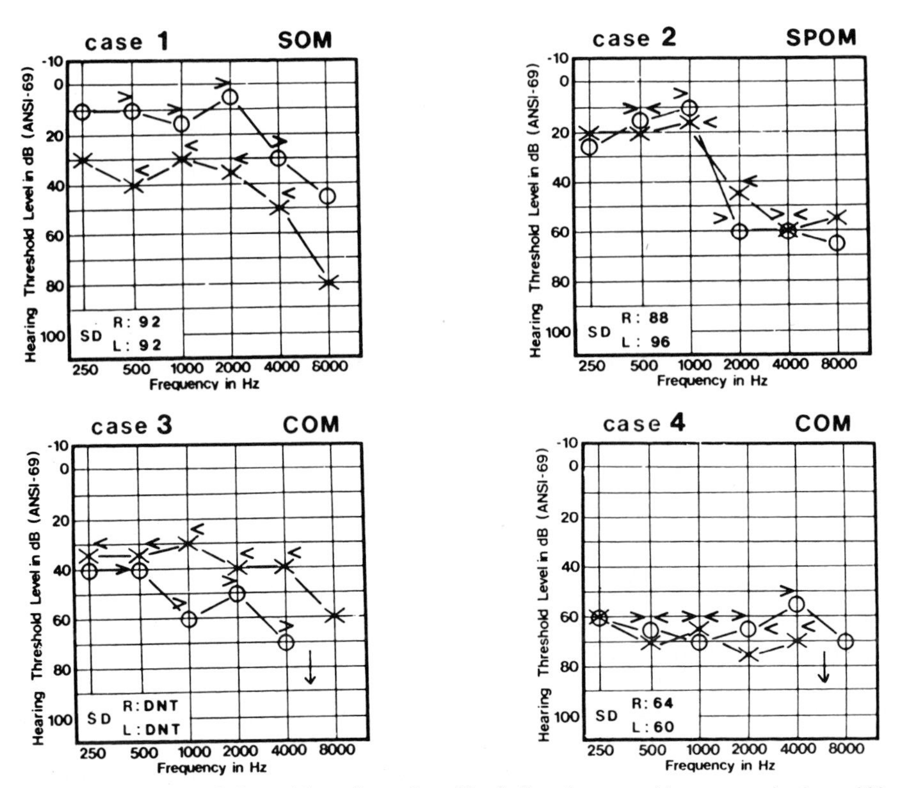

Figure 1 In these four examples of silent otitis media confirmed by findings in temporal bones, examinations within days or a few months before death demonstrated sensorineural hearing losses. Conductive losses and positive tympanometric findings were not demonstrated. It is still possible that acute otitis media could have developed subsequent to testing in Cases 3 and 4 (COM).

Case 1: age 45, examined nine days before death; cause of death, multiple myeloma. Case 2: age 52, examination 20 days before death, cause of death, chronic heart failure. Case 3: age 28, treated with kanamycin on several occasions. Case 4: age 52, had hearing loss "all her life," with a positive family history.

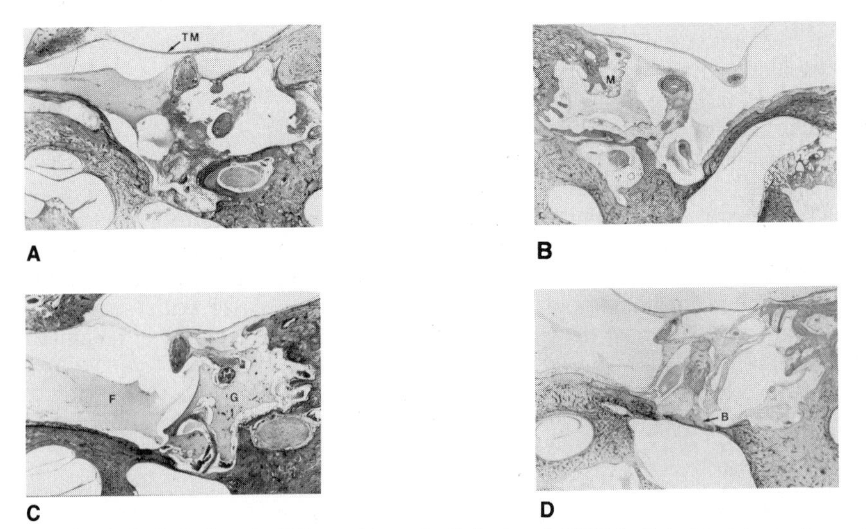

Figure 2 Examples of pathologic findings in "silent otitis media." A, Age 6 (SPOM): Note intact tympanic membrane (TM); clinical record negative. (Approximately x10 magnification.) B, Age 2 (MPOM): No history of ear problems; note unresolved mesenchyme (M). (Approximately x10 magnification.) C, Age 70 (COM): No history or findings of ear problems; note granulation tissue surrounding stapes (G) and fluid (F); tympanic membrane intact. (Approximately x10 magnification.) D, Age 3½ (COM): Fibrous granulation tissue destroying stapes; new bone formation on stapes footplate (B). (Approximately x10 magnification.)

otitis media'' as described, but differs clinically. Adhesive otitis presents with a conductive loss and may be confused with otosclerosis.[10] Unresolved mesenchyme in certain infants and young children may be associated with OM or silent otitis media and may mimic OM on tympanometric testing. Temporal bone studies in infants, older children, and adults demonstrate a surprisingly high incidence of pathologic findings of OM in the presence of an intact tympanic membrane, associated with undetected or undetectable OM by history or findings as noted on the clinical record. Further evidence comes from surgical findings of OM through exploratory tympanotomy and in certain patients who appear to develop sensorineural hearing loss in latent Meniere's syndrome from subclinical otomastoiditis.

Silent otitis media can refer to clinically undetected forms of OM but it especially refers to clinically undetectable OM. It seems likely that the negative clinical records of our cases with positive findings in the temporal bones include more undetected than undetectable cases. Our classification ''undetected OM'' includes many children with OME or adults with OM in whom the diagnosis of OM is overlooked or missed. The assumption is made that with a proper history and examination, including otoscopy and audiometry (tympanometry), a correct diagnosis of OM can be made. This, however, is not always the case.

As temporal bone studies[24,39] and exploratory tympanotomy findings[28] indicate, often more than one pathologic lesion will coexist, so it is possible to diagnose one and not the other. For example, in children the emphasis in diagnosis and treatment is on the fluid in OME. The fluid is removed by myringotomy and a ventilation tube is inserted. In some children, an associated ossicular disruption or fixation can lead to a continued conductive hearing loss after the fluid is removed. In other children, the hearing may return to normal or close to normal; however, a granular, thickened mucoperiosteum (silent otitis media) may continue indefinitely.

Our concept of the pathogenesis of silent otitis media or a subclinical form of otitis media is based on otitis media occurring along a continuum. The various forms of OME can evolve one into another; thus, POM can become SOM or MOM, or SOM can become MOM. It is unlikely that MOM can convert to a pure form of SOM. Most children have OME resulting from activity both in epithelial (secretory) and in subepithelial (transudative) spaces, and have seromucinous otitis media. With proper treatment in the majority of children, OME resolves to a normal state. In some children, OME can persist in a chronic state and over time (years) may lead to chronic otitis media characterized by the intractable presence of tissue, including cholesteatoma, granulation tissue, and cholesterol granuloma. In other patients, clinically active and infectious OM can become ''silent,'' leading to sequelae of otitis media, including hearing losses, tympanosclerosis, atelectasis, changes in tympanic membrane, ossicular changes, and so on.

From the above, we see that active OME can lead to active COM or inactive OM characterized by various sequelae of OM. In another subset of patients, OME (after treatment) undergoes apparent resolution with loss of fluid from the middle ear and a normal or intact tympanic membrane. In these patients, clinically inactive pathologic changes in the mucoperiosteum, including both epithelial and subepithelial components, can persist. Insidious sequelae in the middle ear and inner ear (for example, hearing loss) can occur and otologic findings can be obscured. Upon stimulation, due to extrinsic or intrinsic causes, otitis media can again become clinically active. When assessing factors in the pathogenesis of OM, the prior existence of a pathologic mucoperiosteum should be considered. It is to this entity of subclinical otitis media that we apply the term ''silent otitis media.''

This study was supported by grant #NS-14538 from NIH.

REFERENCES

1. Main TS, Shimada T, Lim DJ: Experimental cholesterol granuloma. Arch Otolaryngol 91:356, 1970
2. Paparella MM, Hiraide F, Juhn SK, Kaneko Y: Cellular events involved in middle ear fluid production. Ann Otol Rhinol Laryngol 79:766, 1970
3. Juhn SK, Paparella MM, Kim CS, et al: Pathogenesis of otitis media. Ann Otol Rhinol Laryngol 86:481, 1977
4. Goycoolea MV, Paparella MM, Carpenter AM, Juhn SK: A longitudinal study of cellular changes in experimental otitis media. Otolaryngol Head Neck Surg 87:685, 1979
5. Paparella MM, Schachern PA, Shea D: Genesis of granulation tissue. In: *Cholesteatoma and Mastoid Surgery*, Sadé J (ed). Amsterdam: Kugler Publications, 1982
6. Paparella MM, Lim DJ: Pathogenesis and pathology of the ''idiopathic blue ear drum.'' Arch Otolaryngol 85:35, 1967
7. Palva T, Kokko E: Middle ear effusions—complications of disease and treatment. J Otolaryngol 5:459, 1976
8. Tos M: Upon the relationship between secretory otitis in childhood and chronic otitis and its sequelae in adults. J Laryngol Otol 95:1011, 1981

9. Paparella MM, Schachern PA: Complications and sequelae of otitis media with effusion—state of knowledge. In Lim DJ et al (eds): *Otitis Media*. Philadelphia, Toronto: BC Decker, Inc, 1984
10. Mawson SR, Ludman H: *Diseases of the Ear: A Textbook of Otology*, 4th ed. Chicago: Year Book Medical Publishers, Inc, 1979
11. Holt RG, Gates GA: Masked mastoiditis. Presented at the Southern Section of the 1983 Triological Meetings. Laryngoscope, to be released
12. Arey LB: *Human Histology: A Textbook in Outline Form*, 1st ed. Philadelphia: WB Saunders Co, 1957
13. Wolff D: Significant anatomic features of the auditory mechanism with special reference to the late fetus. Ann Otol Rhinol Laryngol 42;136, 1933; 43:193, 1934
14. Keibel F, Mall FP (eds): *Manual of Human Embryology*, 2nd ed. Philadelphia: JB Lippincott Co, 1910-1912
15. Guggenheim P, Clements L, Schlesinger A: The significance and fate of the mesenchyme of the middle ear. Laryngoscope 66:2, 1956
16. Buch NH, Jorgenson MB: Embryonic connective tissue in the tympanic cavity of the fetus and newborn. Acta Otolaryngol 58:111, 1964
17. Aschoff L: Die Otitis Media Neonatorum. Ein Beitrag zur Entwicklungsgeschichte der Paukenhohle. A Offrenheilk 31:295, 1897
18. Meyer M: Über die Konstitution und Mettelohrs Schleimhaut. Z Ohrenheilk 29:106, 1931
19. Singer L: Über Entzündliche Erkrankungen des Mittelohres und der Pneumatischen Hohlaume des Schlafenbeines. Z Ohrenheilk 32:110, 1933
20. Guggenheim LK: Therapy of deafess: Report of cases. Part II. Laryngoscope 50:503, 1943
21. Wilson TG: The surgical anatomy of ear, nose and throat in the newborn. J Laryngol 69:229, 1955
22. Wittmaack K: Über die normale und die pathologische Pneumatisation des Schlafenbeines. Jena: G. Fisher, 1918
23. Von Wreden R: Die Otitis Media Neonatorum vom anatomischpathologischen Standpunkte. Berlin: CH Norging, 1868, p 12
24. Paparella MM, Shea D, Meyerhoff WL, Goycoolea MV: Silent otitis media. Laryngoscope 90:1089, 1980
25. Schachern PA, Shea D, Paparella MM: Mucopolysaccharidosis I-H (Hurler's syndrome) and human temporal bone histopathology. Ann Otol Rhinol Laryngol, in press.
26. Hayes E, Babin R, Platz C: The otologic manifestations of mucopolysaccharidoses. Am J Otol 2:65, 1980
27. Fouad H, El-Hoshy Zoheir, Seous I, et al: Tympanometry in premature and newborn infants. Med J Cairo Univ 50:231, 1982
28. Paparella MM, Koutroupas S: Exploratory tympanotomy revisited. Laryngoscope 92:531, 1982
29. Paparella MM, Oda M, Hiraide F, Brady D: Pathology of sensorineural hearing loss in otitis media. Ann Otol Rhinol Laryngol 81:632, 1972
30. Paparella MM, de Sousa LCA, Mancini F: Meniere's syndrome and otitis media. Laryngoscope 93:1408, 1983.
31. Hallpike CS, Cairns H: Observations on the pathology of Meniere's syndrome. J Laryngol 53:625, 1938
32. Paparella MMP, Griebie MS: Trautmann's triangle and Meniere's disease. Am J Otol, in press
33. Arslan M: On the etiology of Meniere's disease. Boll Mal Orec Gola Naso 15:121, 1972
34. Stahle J, Wilbrand H: The vestibular aqueduct in patients with Meniere's disease. Acta Otolaryngol 78:36, 1974
35. Wittmaack K: Die Ortho und Pathologie des Labyrinthes. Stuttgart: Georg Thieme, 1956
36. Kimura RS: Experimental production of endolymphatic hydrops. Otolaryngol Clin North Am 1:457, 1968
37. Kimura RS: Animal models of endolymphatic hydrops. Am J Otol 3:447, 1982
38. Meyerhoff WL, Shea DA, Giebink GS: Experimental pneumococcal otitis media: A histopathologic study. Otolaryngol Head Neck Surg 88:606, 1980
39. Meyerhoff WL, Kim CS, Paparella MM: Pathology of chronic otitis media. Ann Otol Rhinol Laryngol 87:749, 1978

EXPERIMENTAL OTITIS MEDIA WITH EFFUSION INDUCED BY NONVIABLE *HEMOPHILUS INFLUENZAE*: CYTOLOGIC AND HISTOLOGIC STUDY

NOBUHIRO OKAZAKI, M.D., THOMAS F. DeMARIA, Ph.D., BRUCE R. BRIGGS, and DAVID J. LIM, M.D.

The etiology of otitis media with effusion (OME) has not been conclusively established. Bacteria have been implicated in the pathogenesis of OME,[1,2] but their exact role in its production has not been determined.

The gram-negative bacterium *Hemophilus in*

fluenzae ranks as the primary pathogen in cases of OME, and serous effusions are associated predominantly with this organism.[3] Our laboratory recently reported that formalin-killed *H. influenzae* induces sterile OME in chinchillas,[4] which suggests that certain dead bacteria or bacterial components trapped in the middle ear can initiate inflammation and middle ear effusion (MEE). The purpose of the present study was to investigate and quantitate the morphologic changes in the middle ear after injection with nonviable *H. influenzae* and to compare the pathologic changes induced by type b with those induced by nontypable (biotype II) *H. influenzae*.

MATERIAL AND METHODS

Animals

A total of 29 healthy chinchillas (360 to 290 gm) were used.

Injection of PBS and Nonviable Bacteria

Both the type b and nontypable (serologically not typable but belonging to biotype II) isolates were originally isolated from cases of otitis media. The bacteria were cultured and inactivated, and inoculum was prepared for injection as previously described.[4]

Morphologic Study

The effusions were collected under general anesthesia, and the temporal bones were fixed immediately following decapitation in cacodylate-buffered 2.5 percent glutaraldehyde, pH 7.2 to 7.4, for 24 hours. They were further dissected and decalcified with 0.1 M EDTA in 2 percent glutaraldehyde for three to six weeks. EDTA solutions were changed every one to three days. Tissues from selected areas—the inferior bulla, eustachian tube orifice (tympanum side), and superior bulla—were routinely used for light microscopy. For light microscopy, the specimens were embedded in glycol methacrylate (JB-4, Polysciences, Warrington, PA), and 5-μ sections were made using glass knives and stained with H & E. For electron microscopy the specimens were postfixed with 0.11 M *s*-collidine buffered 1.33 percent osmium tetroxide for 1 hour and embedded in epoxy resin. One-micron sections were made for phase contrast microscopy, and thin sections were made for transmission electron microscopy.

For the quantitative study, macrophages, polymorphonuclear neutrophils (PMNs), and lymphocytes were counted in ten randomly selected unit areas in each section. Each area was traced with a drawing tube attached to a light microscope, and the response was digitized to quantitate cell densities. Capillary areas were also traced to quantitate the extent of vascular engorgement.

Statistics

The two-tailed Student's *t* test was used to determine the statistical significance of the pathologic findings quantitated.

RESULTS

Three features were examined as an index of the inflammatory responses: the thickness of the middle ear connective tissue, the percentage of capillary area in the sections, and the cell density in the connective tissue. Data were collected for up to 14 days after injection with formalin-killed *H. influenzae* type b, nontypable, or PBS.

The thickness of the connective tissue and submucosa was significantly higher ($p \leq 0.05$) in the animals after injection with killed *H. influenzae* type b at each sample time when compared with PBS control values. The same significant increase ($p \leq 0.05$) over control values was observed in chinchillas injected with the nontypable (biotype II) isolate of *H. influenzae*. There was no significant difference in the increased thickness caused by each isolate. The thickness of the connective tissue increased steadily to a maximum of 41 μm by day 4 in animals injected with type b. The response to the nontypable (biotype II) isolate was more rapid since the values exhibited a twofold increase within 24 hours that persisted through almost the entire duration of the experiment.

When the percentage of capillary area was measured to assess the degree of capillary engorgement after injection with killed *H. influenzae,* the maximum capillary engorgement occurred at day 2, and the percentage of capillary area was significantly higher ($p \leq 0.05$) in animals injected with *H. influenzae* type b than in the control animals. This significant increase persisted through, but was no longer evident after, the fourth day of the experiment. The percentage of capillary area was also significantly higher ($p \leq 0.05$) in animals injected with the killed

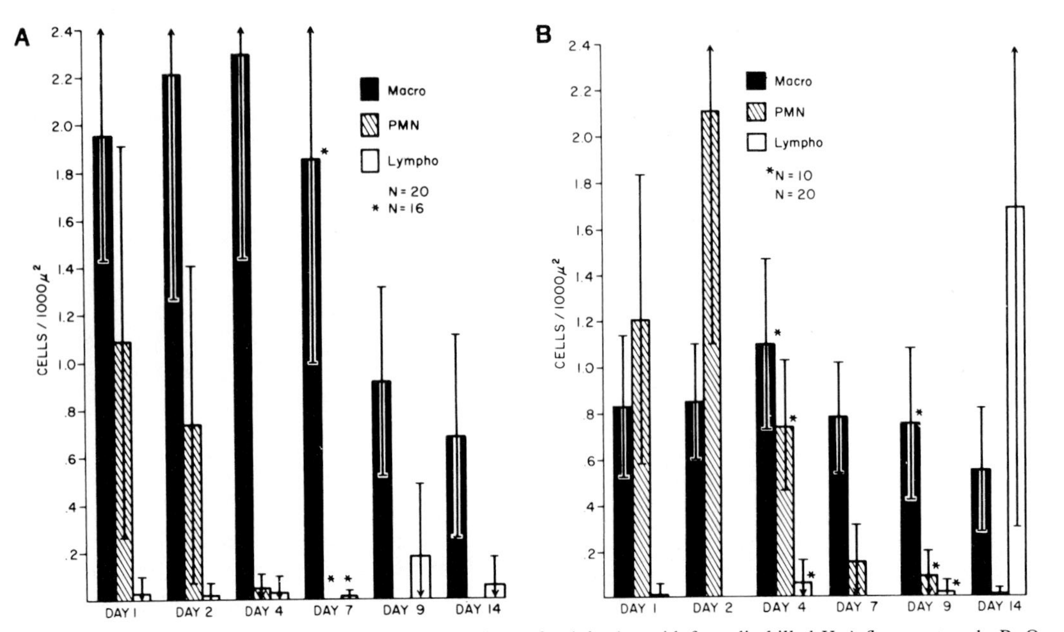

Figure 1 A, Quantitative cellular response in connective tissue after injection with formalin-killed *H. influenzae* type b. B, Quantitative cellular response in connective tissue after injection with formalin-killed, serologically nontypable *H. influenzae* (biotype II).

nontypable (biotype II) isolate, and this significantly increased level of dilated capillaries persisted to the seventh day of the experiment.

The cellular density in the connective tissue was examined after injection of both isolates of *H. influenzae* and PBS (Fig. 1). The number of macrophages per 1000 μm^2 gradually increased in the middle ear submucosa of animals injected with type b (Fig. 1A) and the nontypable (biotype II) isolate (Fig. 1B). In both instances the PMN levels per 1000 μm^2 peaked by day 2 and rapidly declined by four days after injection with either type. A significant increase ($p \leq 0.05$) in the number of lymphocytes per 1000 μm^2 was evident in both experimental groups. The increase in lymphocytes was most dramatic by day 14 in animals injected with the nontypable (biotype II) isolate. The cell counts in the control sections were all significantly lower than in both experimental groups.

There were also striking differences in the cellular responses in the submucosal connective tissue between the experimental groups, although both groups showed the same biphasic response observed in the cytocentrifuge preparations of MEEs after injection with type b or the nontypable (biotype II) isolate of *H. influenzae*.[4]

The PMN response was most dramatic in the type b group at days 1 through 2 after injection (Fig. 1A), whereas the macrophage response was most dramatic in the nontypable (biotype II) group from day 1 through day 4 (Fig. 1B).

The lumens of capillaries contained PMNs, and hyperemia and bleeding were found in the connective tissue in both groups at days 1 and 2. The osteoclasts were found in both groups in the early stage of inflammation.

At days 4 through 9 capillary dilatation, bleeding and tissue edema persisted. There were some macrophages and a few PMNs in the connective tissue. The capillary lumens contained many lymphocytes and monocytes. The connective tissue was noticeably thicker. Evidence of bone remodeling was found during this period, characterized by numerous osteoblasts at the endosteal margin. The lumen of the eustachian tube contained macrophages and PMNs, but the tubal mucosa had no marked change.

At day 14 in the type b group, new bone formation and bleeding were still evident in the connective tissue, but the connective tissue was as thin as in the controls, largely due to ossification of the thickened connective tissue. In contrast, in the nontypable group, connective tissue was still thick and had considerable lymphocyte and plasma cell infiltration. At day 28 the connective tissue returned to normal and new bone formation was complete.

Half the experimental animals (8 of 12 in the nontypable [biotype II] group and 5 of 12 in the type b group) had histologic evidence of adhesive otitis media characterized by threadlike abnormal epithelial growth with fibrotic bands in the bullae and the promontory area (Fig. 2). The most dramatic example is seen in a day 4 animal from the type b group. Often the original mucosal epithelium and the proliferative epithelium formed a pocket containing MME (Fig. 3). Numerous macrophages were found in these trapped effusions.

DISCUSSION

The histologic evidence from these experiments indicates that formalin-killed *H. influenzae* induces severe inflammatory changes in the middle ear comparable to the pathologic changes observed in biopsy specimens from cases of human OME.[5] Our earlier report[4] describing the induction of OME by formalin-killed *H. influenzae* suggested that the endotoxin on the surface of these bacteria is probably responsible for the inflammation and fluid accumulation in the middle ear. The more rapid and persistent capillary dilation and connective tissue thickening induced by the killed nontypable (biotype II) *H. influenzae* in this study supports this concept. Serologically nontypable *H. influenzae* do not contain a polyribophosphate capsule which partially masks endotoxin on the surface of the encapsulated (serologically typable) strains. Therefore, more endotoxin is likely to be

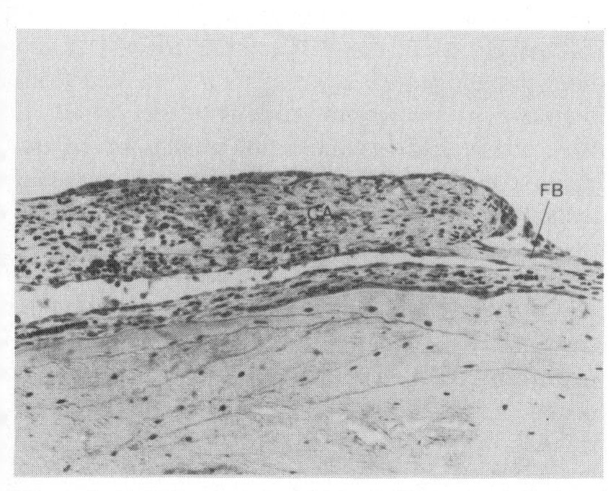

Figure 2 A LM photomicrograph of EDTA-decalcified and JB-4 embedded chinchilla bulla showing extensive proliferation of connective tissue with a fibrotic band (FB) 14 days after injection of *H. influenzae* (biotype II). CA, capillary (X160 magnification).

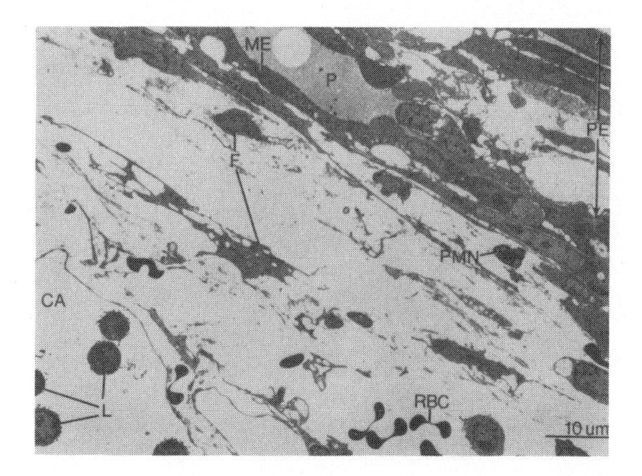

Figure 3 A TEM photomicrograph of mucosa of a chinchilla middle ear showing extensive epithelial growth (proliferation) (PE) forming a pocket (P) containing effusions. A large number of lymphocytes (L) are found in the dilated capillary vessel (CA). Numerous red blood cells (RBC) and some inflammatory cells are evident in the connective tissue 4 days after injection with *H. influenzae* type b. PMN, polymorphonuclear leukocytes; F, fibrocyte; ME, middle ear epithelium.

in direct contact with the middle ear epithelial surfaces after injection with the nontypable *H. influenzae*.

Bernstein and colleagues[6] reported, and our own data also indicate,[7] detectable levels of endotoxin in the MEEs from OME patients. Recently our laboratory was successful in inducing serous MEEs in animals injected with endotoxin, suggesting a possible role of endotoxin from nonviable *H. influenzae* in the pathogenesis of OME.

The pathogenesis of chronic adhesive otitis media is not well established.[8] The current study shows marked mucosal proliferation in nearly half the experimental animals injected with either type b or the nontypable formalin-killed *H. influenzae*. The threadlike abnormal epithelial growths with fibrotic bands and pockets containing MEE strikingly resemble the histologic description of adhesive otitis media.[9,10] The availability of the killed *H. influenzae* model provides the first opportunity to study this disease.

In conclusion, the results of this study indicate that nonviable bacteria (*H. influenzae*) can induce inflammatory response in the middle ear tissue with middle ear effusion in large amounts in the absence of tubal occlusion, and can also produce pathologic findings similar to those of human adhesive otitis media.

This study was supported in part by grants from NINCDS/NIH (NS08854) and The Deafness Research Foundation.

REFERENCES

1. Senturia BH, Gessert DF, Carr DC, Baumann ES: Studies concerned with tubotympanitis. Ann Otol Rhinol Laryngol 67:440, 1958
2. Liu YS, Lim DJ, Lang RW, Birck HG: Chronic middle ear effusions: Immunochemical and bacteriological investigations. Arch Otolaryngol 101:278, 1975
3. Giebink GS, Mills EL, Huff JS, Edelman CK, et al: The microbiology of serous and mucoid otitis media. Pediatr Pediau 63:915, 1979
4. DeMaria TF, Briggs BR, Lim DJ, Okazaki N: Experimental otitis media with effusion following middle ear inoculation of nonviable *H. influenzae*. Ann Otol Rhinol Laryngol, 93:52, 1984
5. Lim DJ, Birck H: Ultrastructural pathology of the middle ear mucosa in serous otitis media. Ann Otol Rhinol Laryngol 80:838, 1971
6. Bernstein JM, Praino, MD, Neter E: Detection of endotoxin in ear specimens from patients with chronic otitis media by means of the limulus amebocyte lysate test. Can J Microbiol 26:546, 1980
7. DeMaria TF Prior TB, Briggs BR, et al: Endotoxin in middle ear effusions from patients with chronic OME. In Lim DJ et al (eds): *Otitis Media*. Philadelphia, Toronto: BC Decker Inc, 1984
8. Siirala U: Otitis media adhesiva. Arch Otolaryngol 80:287, 1964
9. Ojala L: Pathogenesis and histopathology of chronic adhesive otitis. Arch Otolaryngol 57:378, 1953
10. Lim DJ: Aural sequelae of persistent middle ear effusion. Pediatr Infec Dis 1 (Suppl 5):S125, 1982

EXPERIMENTAL OTITIS MEDIA WITH EFFUSION: AN IMMUNOELECTRON MICROSCOPIC STUDY

T. TAKASAKA, M.D., Y. KAKU, M.D., Y. SHIBAHARA, M.D., K. HOZAWA, M.D., M. TAKEYAMA, M.D., Y. KANEKO, M.D., and K. KAWAMOTO, M.D.

Although several investigators[1-4] have reported the presence of immune complex (IC) in human middle ear effusions, definite morphologic evidence of IC-induced otitis media with effusion (OME) is still insufficient. The recent study by Mravec and associates[5] is the only available publication concerning experimental acute inflammation induced by injection of soluble IC into the bullae of chinchillas.

The purpose of this study is to further clarify morphologic evidence of the detailed immune responses of the tubotympanum using IC prepared by mixing horseradish peroxidase (HRP) with anti-HRP animal serum.

MATERIALS AND METHODS

HRP (Sigma type VI) was chosen as an antigen. To obtain anti-HRP serum, five guinea pigs and chinchillas were immunized by repeated injections of HRP emulsions. Two milliliters of HRP (1.0 mg) emulsions were prepared by mixing 1.0 ml of HRP saline solution with 1.0 ml of complete adjuvant (Freund). In the guinea pigs, immunizations were repeated once a week for three weeks to obtain sufficient anti-HRP titer, whereas, in chinchillas immunizations for seven or eight weeks were necessary. Titers of immunized sera were estimated by both 24-hour passive cutaneous anaphylaxis and a double immunodiffusion method. Soluble HRP–anti-HRP ICs were formed at ten times the antigen excess and then separated from free antigens and serum proteins by gel filtration. After removal of insoluble precipitates by centrifugation at 100,000 g for 30 minutes, a supernatant containing soluble complexes was applied to the top of the gel bed of Sepharose CL-6B. Elution was performed at 4°C by 0.02M Tris buffer solution, pH 8.0, containing 0.5M NaCl. Five partially confluent peaks of soluble ICs were obtained. The mixture of the first and second peaks (high molecular weight IC) and the mixture of the other peaks (low molecular weight IC) were injected into the bullae of 10 albino guinea pigs and 13 adult chinchillas under general anesthesia (ketamine hydrochloride, 20 mg/kg).

Tympanometry was performed on the chinchillas before and after the injections of ICs. The animals were killed for histologic examinations at

6, 12, and 24 hours. The control animals were given HRP solutions alone. Immediately after decapitation, both bullae were dissected and examined macroscopically. The middle ear mucosa and the eustachian tube mucosa were fixed en bloc by 2.5 percent glutaraldehyde in 0.1M phosphate buffer for 2 to 3 hours and transferred to the buffer solution for washing. Benzidine reaction in Graham-Karnovsky's medium was performed for 10 to 15 minutes at room temperature. After postosmification, the specimens were dehydrated by graded ethanol and embedded in the epoxy resin. The thin sections were made by Sorvall MT-5000 Ultratome (DuPont Co., Newtown, Connecticut) and examined under JEM 100C and 1000 electron microscopes (JEOL, Tokyo).

RESULTS

Six-Hour Animals

The gross appearance of the middle ear mucosa was slightly hyperemic, but effusions were not distinctly seen in the bullae. Light microscopic observation clearly demonstrated that numerous red blood cells were disperse in the subepithelial connective tissue, and in some dilated capillary lumens numerous red blood cells were stagnated. The IC precipitates were occasionally visible on the epithelial surface, and some of them were already taken up into the cytoplasm of the epithelial cells. The same fine granules of IC were also found in the capillary endothelium, but migration of the granulocytes was not remarkable in this group.

Twelve-Hour Animals

Edema of the mucous membrane became obvious, and clear serous effusions were consistently present in the bullae. Light and electron microscopic examination of the middle ear mucosa revealed that electron-dense IC-positive cells, most of which were nonciliated, were widely dispersed in the epithelium. Many inflammatory cells, such as polymorphonuclear leukocytes (PMN) and monocytes, were observed in the capillary lumen, and active migration of these cells to the extravascular spaces was also observed. The macrophages were engulfing numerous electron-dense IC granules in the cytoplasm. PMN attachment to the basal lamina was also encountered, and some PMN often migrated into the intercellular spaces of the epithelium through disrupted basal lamina (Fig. 1). Numerous fragments of degenerated cells from the middle ear cavity were observed in the eustachian tubal lumen. These stagnated masses were present from the tympanic orifice to the site near the pharyngeal opening and found only in the tubal lumen supported by cartilage (Fig. 2). The heavy deposits of electron-dense IC were also seen

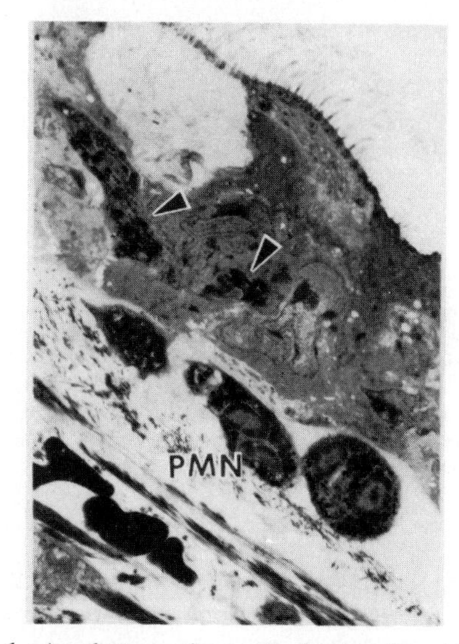

Figure 1 An electron micrograph showing the middle ear mucosa of the 12-hour guinea pigs. Three polymorphonuclear leukocytes (PMNs) are attached to the basal lamina. Some others (arrow heads) have already migrated into the intercellular space of the epithelium. (X1500 magnification)

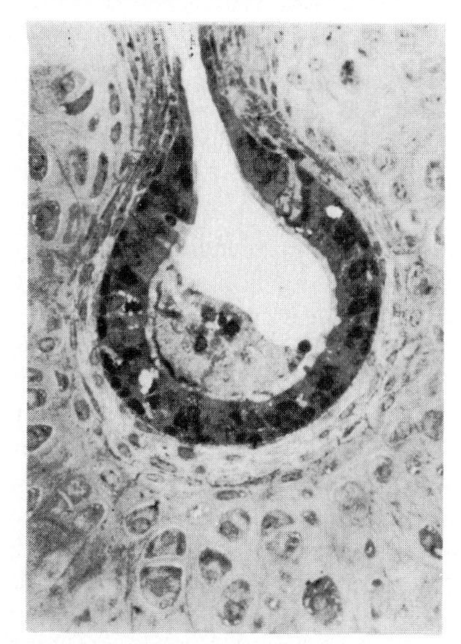

Figure 2 A light micrograph showing the eustachian tube supported by the cartilage. Almost half of the luminal space is occupied by a stagnated mass composed of the degenerated cells and the deposits of immune complexes. (X300 magnification)

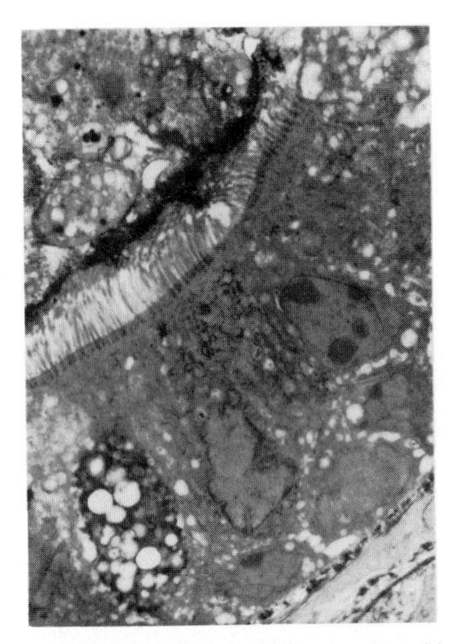

Figure 3 An electron micrograph showing the epithelial cells of a guinea pig's eustachian tube. Electron-dense precipitates of the immune complexes are visible on the surface of the ciliary bundles. (X1500 magnification)

here, and the tips of the numerous cilia of the eustachian tubal mucosa were completely surrounded by these IC deposits (Fig. 3). Electron-dense IC granules were also seen in the epithelial cells of the eustachian tube, but these were less numerous than those in the tympanic mucosa. These characteristic structures in the tube were found in both guinea pigs and chinchillas and were seen most obviously in this 12-hour group.

Twenty-four Hour Group

The most striking reactions were seen in this group. The mucous membrane markedly thickened and bullae contained a considerable amount of effusions. The dilated capillary lumens were filled with numerous granulocytes, many of which migrated toward the mucosal surface. The effusions became mucoid in nature, containing numerous inflammatory cells of various sizes and shapes. Electron-dense IC granules were observed even in the deep capillary walls. The macrophages were accumulated below the thick layer of the IC deposits and showed quite active phagocytotic activities.

In the eustachian tube, effusions with inflammatory cells were observed, but heavy precipitations of IC deposits were not conspicuous in these experiments.

DISCUSSIONS

Since Veltri and Sprinkle[6] first mentioned that one of the etiologic factors of chronic OME might be IC-mediated local immune responses in the middle ear, several investigators[1–3] have supported this possibility and confirmed the presence of IC in the effusions from OME patients. Recently, Mravec and colleagues[5] reported that they could induce experimental OME by IC injections into chinchilla bullae. They observed typical Arthus-type acute reactions of the tympanic mucosa in chinchillas, but it seems possible that these responses were nonspecific for the chinchillas, since the IC was prepared by mixing rabbit serum with goat–antirabbit serum.

To avoid this possibility, we selected HRP as an antigen in the present experimental study and obtained specific ICs for the animals by mixing HRP with anti-HRP serum of the same species. To obtain anti-HRP serum from each animal, HRP immunization was performed. Although the guinea pig immunizations were completed within a month, those of chinchillas took longer to obtain sufficient anti-HRP titers. These results seem to indicate that the animals react differently to HRP immunizations, or that HRP emulsions injected into chinchillas were more rapidly metabolized than those in guinea pigs, as suggested by Hook[7] in 1973. However, it was quite interesting that the acute inflammations induced by specific HRP–anti-HRP IC were not remarkably different between these two groups of animals.

In both guinea pigs and chinchillas, the mild reactions observed in the 6-hour group became more conspicuous in the 12-hour group and even greater in the 24-hour group, which manifested considerable amounts of effusion in the bullae. Numerous inflammatory cells migrated into the subepithelial layer, and many PMNs were attached to the basal lamina in both groups of animals. Actual disruptions of the basal lamina and degenerated epithelial cells as well as increased permeabilities of the capillaries were also observed in the present materials.

These pathologic findings seem to indicate the typical sequence of Arthus-type acute inflammations, but further explanation is hardly possible unless ICs are identifiable under electron microscopy. In this study, however, the definite locations of the IC deposits were visualized by immunohistochemical procedures. As is well known, HRP possesses very high antigenicity as a protein and also an ability to oxidize benzidine, which can be identified as an electron-dense granule. This study revealed that IC deposits were widely dispersed throughout the mucosa, and several electron-dense IC granules often accumulated in the cytoplasm of the fibrocytes and capillary endothelium. Many macrophages phagocytosed these IC granules, and PMN also showed positive chemotaxis toward the IC deposits.

One of the most striking findings of this study was the possibility of mucociliary dysfunction caused by thick depositions of IC precipitates. As morphologic evidence of this possibility, we often observed numerous stagnated masses of the degenerated cell organellae in the tubal lumen, and most of the cilia around these stagnated masses were completely fixed by a considerable amount of IC precipitates. This morphologic evidence may suggest that the concentrations of the glycoprotein component in the mucus can be altered by these abundant precipitates. Sadé and associates[8] previously noted that certain rheologic properties of mucus are required to maintain adequate clearance activities of the mucociliary transport system, and these rheologic requirements are satisfied only by macromolecular systems that are very weak cross-linking gels.

According to the present immunoelectron microscopic observations, it may be considered that the ICs injected into the bullae were transported to the eustachian tube by mucociliary clearance activity, but the IC precipitates damaged the mucosal surface, changing the chemical component of the mucus in the tube, and then retarded the normal beating rate of the cilia. If this is the case, the transport rate of the tube may be remarkably disturbed, resulting in a net accumulation of IC-induced middle ear effusions. To confirm this possibility, it is necessary to develop other animal models in which further sequential evidence of IC-induced OME can be observed.

REFERENCES

1. Maxim PE, Veltri RW, Sprinkle PM, Pusateri RJ: Chronic serous otitis media: An immune complex disease. ORL 84:234, 1977
2. Palva T, Hayry P, Raunio V, Ylikoski J: Immunologic aspects of otitis media. Acta Otolaryngol 89:177, 1980
3. Laurell A-B, Nilsson N-1, Prellner K: Immune complexes and complement in serous and mucoid otitis media. Acta Otolaryngol 90:290, 1980
4. Bernstein JM, Brentjens J, Vladutiu A: Are immune complexes a factor in the pathogenesis of otitis media with effusion? Am J Otolaryngol 3:20, 1982
5. Mravec J, Lewis PM, Lim DJ: Experimental otitis media with effusion: An immune-complex-mediated response. ORL 86:258, 1978
6. Veltri, RW, Sprinkle PM: Secretory otitis media: An immune complex disease. Ann Otol Rhinol Laryngol 85:135, 1976
7. Hook RR: Humoral immune response of the adult chinchilla. Lab Anim Sci 23:837, 1973
8. Sadé J, Meyer FA, King M, Silberberg A: Clearance of middle ear effusions by mucociliary system. Acta Otolaryngol 79:277, 1975

COMPARATIVE HISTOPATHOLOGY OF ANIMAL MODELS OF OTITIS MEDIA IN CHINCHILLAS: A TEMPORAL BONE STUDY

TIMOTHY T. K. JUNG, M.D., Ph.D., DONALD SHEA, M.A., G. SCOTT GIEBINK, M.D., and S. K. JUHN, M.D.

Animal models of otitis media have been developed using various animals, such as guinea pigs, monkeys,[1] cats,[2] rats,[3] and gerbils.[4] Chinchillas *(Chinchilla laniger)* were used to develop pneumococcal purulent otitis media (POM) by direct inoculation[5] or by nasal inoculation and middle ear deflation,[6] and serous otitis media (SOM) by eustachian tube obstruction (ETO).[7] The histopathology of chinchilla POM and SOM has been described.[8,9]

We have developed three additional chinchilla otitis media models by injecting prostaglandin E_2 (PGE_2) or arachidonic acid into the bullae of animals with eustachian tube obstruction and by combining SOM and POM.

The purpose of this chapter is to report the comparative histopathology of seven different models of experimentally induced otitis media in chinchillas, including three new models.

MATERIALS AND METHODS

The seven otitis media models studied and the intervals from the experiment to sacrifice are listed in Table 1. One hundred sixteen ears were studied.

The temporal bones were removed, fixed in buffered 10 percent formalin, decalcified with 5 percent trichloroacetic acid, dehydrated in a graded series of alcohol, embedded in celloidin, and sectioned at a thickness of 20 μ. Every tenth section was stained with hematoxylin and eosin.

Temporal bones were studied and the presence of effusion, leukocyte infiltration, granulation tissue, osteoneogenesis, hyperemia, edema, metaplasia, and hemorrhage was recorded.

The method of nasal inoculation for models 1 and 2 was the same as previously reported.[6,9,12]

POM by direct inoculation (model 3) was induced by injecting live type 7F *Streptococcus pneumoniae* into the dorsal portion of the bullae as described previously.[8]

TABLE 1 Animal Models, Interval to Sacrifice and Number of Ears

Model	*Interval from Experiment to Sacrifice*	*No. of Ears*
1	7 days; 1 month	16
2	7 days; 1, 2 months	16
3	3, 7 days; 1, 3 months	28
4	3, 7 days	6
5	3, 7 days	6
6	3, 7 days; 1, 6 months	31
7	7 days; 1, 3, 6 months; 1 year	13
Total		116

Description of Models:
1. POM by nasal inoculation and middle ear deflation
2. POM by nasal inoculation plus influenza virus
3. POM by direct inoculation
4. ETO + PGE_2
5. ETO + AA
6. ETO
7. ETO + direct inoculation (SOM + POM)

SOM + PGE_2 (Model 4)

Under anesthesia induced by intramuscular ketamine hydrochloride (10 mg/kg) a midline incision was made in the soft palate, and eustachian tubes were obstructed with small pieces of soft silicone sponge. Three to seven days following ETO serial daily injections of 50 μg PGE_2 in Hank's balanced salt solution (HBSS) were given for three and seven days.

SOM and AA (Model 5)

After ETO as described above, serial daily injections of 100 μg arachidonic acid (AA) in HBSS were given for three and seven days.

ETO (Model 6)

After ETO as described above, animals were kept for different periods of time.

ETO + Direct Inoculation (Model 7)

Seven days following ETO, direct inoculation was made through dorsal bullae as described for model 3.

RESULTS

Some degree of inflammation was manifested in all seven models of otitis media. The findings for each model are shown in Table 2.

Hyperemia, edema, PMN infiltration, and hemorrhage are associated with acute inflammation. Chronic inflammation is associated with osteoneogenesis, metaplasia of mucosa, mononuclear leukocyte infiltration, and granulation tissues.

Hyperemia and Edema

Most hyperemia was observed in the ETO model, followed by the ETO + AA and the three POM models; the least was seen in ETO + PGE_2 model. The most edema was seen in the ETO + AA model, followed by ETO, ETO + PGE_2, the POM by direct inoculation, POM by nasal inoculation plus influenza virus, POM by nasal inoculation with deflation, and ETO + direct inoculation.

Hemorrhage

Mucosal hemorrhage was seen most often in the ETO + AA model followed by ETO + PGE

TABLE 2 Temporal Bone Histopathology

Middle Ear Space Pathologic Findings (% of Ears Studied)

Model	*Effusion*	*Leukocytes**		*Granulation Tissue*	*Osteoneogenesis*	*Hemorrhage*
		PMN	*Mono*			
1	43	43	43	31	19	19
2	38	31	38	31	13	25
3	89	61	64	68	36	54
4	17	17	17	33	0	83
5	50	50	50	17	0	66
6	81	26	90	23	65	19
7	85	69	85	77	77	49

Middle Ear Mucosa Pathologic Findings (% of Ears Studied)

Model	*Hyperemia*	*Edema*	*Leukocytes**		*Metaplasia*	*Focal Hemorrhage*
			PMN	*Mono*		
1	13	19	44	44	13	6
2	13	38	44	44	6	31
3	13	50	57	57	14	39
4	0	50	33	33	0	66
5	50	83	67	50	0	83
6	80	78	35	90	23	52
7	8	8	54	46	76	31

*PMN = polymorphonuclear; Mono = mononuclear

and the least in POM by nasal inoculation. Middle ear space hemorrhage was found most often in ETO + PGE_2 model and least often in ETO alone and POM by nasal inoculation.

Cellular Infiltration

Polymorphonuclear leukocyte (PMN) infiltration was most severe in the POM by direct inoculation model and least severe in ETO model. Mononuclear leukocyte infiltration was seen most frequently in the ETO model and the least in ETO + PGE_2.

Metaplasia

"Metaplasia," meaning transformation of normal cuboidal epithelium of middle ear mucosa into pseudostratified columnar epithelium with many goblet cells, was observed most frequently in the ETO + direct inoculation model followed by ETO alone.

Effusion

The three models with the highest rate of effusion were ETO, ETO + direct inoculation, and POM by direct inoculation.

Granulation Tissue

ETO + direct inoculation model showed the most diffuse granulation tissue, followed by POM by direct inoculation and ETO alone.

Osteoneogenesis

Osteoneogenesis was seen the most in the ETO + direct inoculation model, followed by ETO alone and POM by direct inoculation.

Typical mucoperiosteal changes of seven chinchilla otitis media models are shown in Figures 1–3.

Changes associated with acute inflammation, such as hyperemia, edema, hemorrhage, and diffuse infiltration of PMNs, were identified in the ears of those animals killed at short intervals after the experiment. Changes associated with chronic inflammation, such as mononuclear leukocyte infiltration, osteoneogenesis, metaplasia, and granulation tissues, were more frequently identified in ears of the animals kept longer periods of time after the experiment.

Cholesterol granuloma was seen in three of 31 ears (9.7 percent) of the ETO model and three of 13 ears (23 percent) of the ETO + direct inoculation model.

Figure 1 Mucoperiosteal changes of chinchilla purulent otitis media models seven days after inoculation. A, POM by nasal inoculation and middle ear (ME) deflation (model 1): Moderate hyperemia and edema of subepithelial space (SES) and pus in the ME space (X150 magnification). B, POM by nasal inoculation and influenza virus (model 2): Mild edema of SES and thin serous fluid in the ME (X150 magnification). C, POM by direct inoculation (model 3): Hyperemia, edema, and PMN infiltration of mucosa and pus in the ME space (X150 magnification).

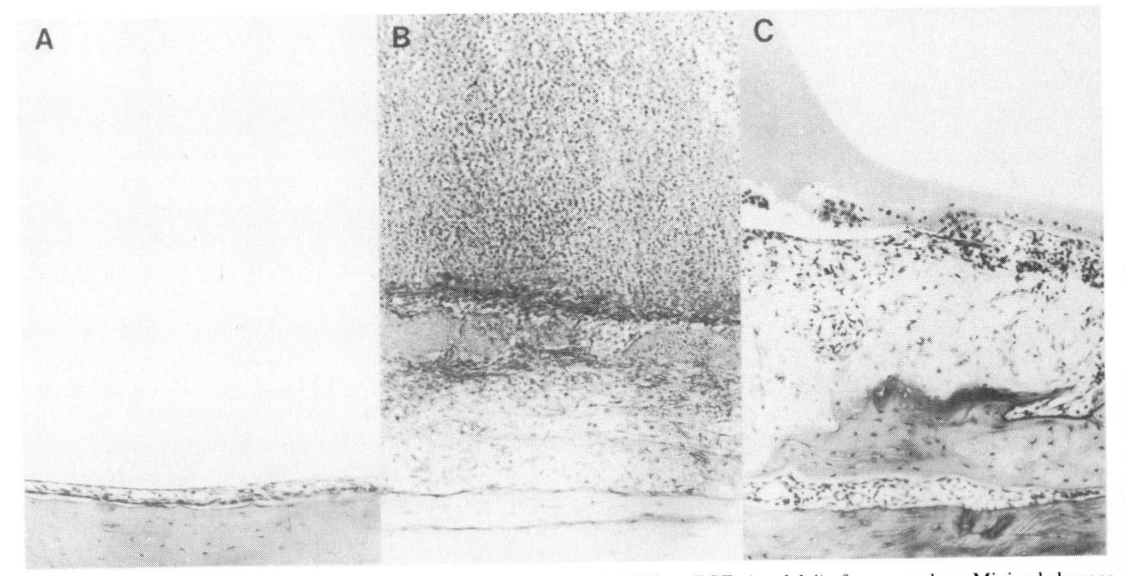

Figure 2 Mucoperiosteal changes of chinchilla otitis media models. A, ETO + PGE_2 (model 4) after seven days: Minimal changes of mucoperiosteum (X150 magnification). B, ETO + AA (model 5) after seven days: Extensive hyperemia and edema of SES with cellular infiltration and thick fluid with many PMNs in the ME. ''Metaplasia'' of mucosa is another prominent feature of this model (X150 magnification). C, ETO (model 6) after one month: Osteoneogenesis and granulation tissue with serous fluid in the ME (X150 magnification).

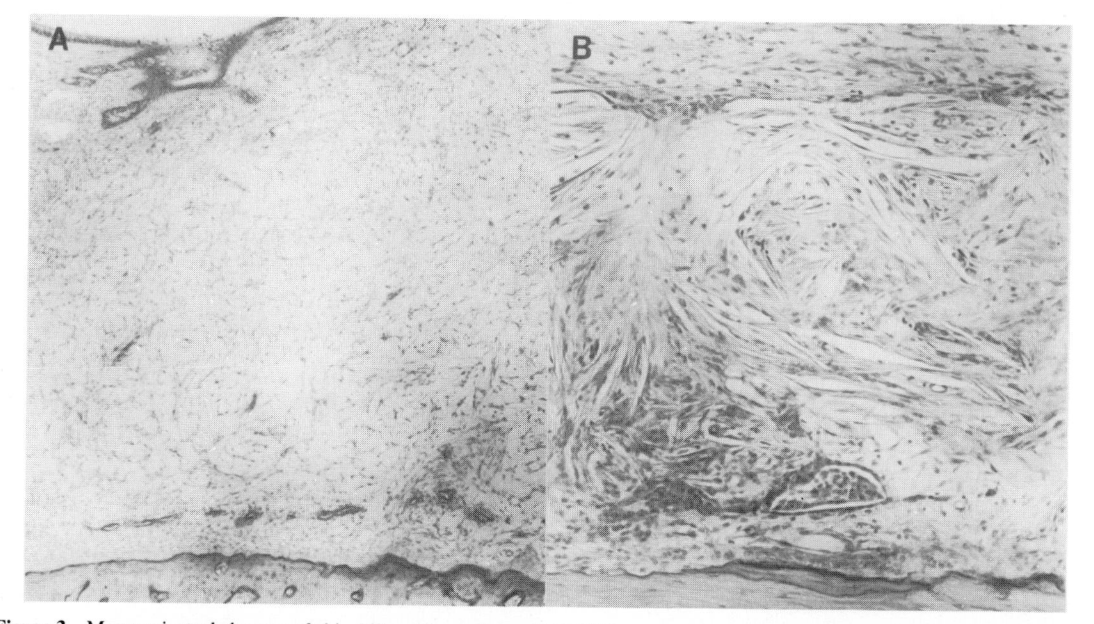

Figure 3 Mucoperiosteal changes of chinchilla otitis media model 7, ETO + direct inoculation (SOM + POM) after three months. A, Osteoneogenesis and granulation tissue with fibrocystic changes (X70 magnification). B, Cholesterol granuloma and granulation tissue (X70 magnification).

DISCUSSION

The pathogenesis of otitis media involves complex interactions of many factors. Perhaps the two most important factors are bacterial infection and eustachian tube dysfunction. Animal models of otitis media provide an opportunity to isolate and control these factors. The chinchilla models of otitis media presented in this study were designed to evaluate these factors singularly and in combination.

Among the three models of POM, the direct inoculation method produced the most consistent severe POM with a high rate of effusion, granulation tissue, and osteoneogenesis. POM by nasal inoculation with middle ear deflation or with influenza virus produced milder POM, which may be more analogous to an ordinary case of human POM.

When the ETO + PGE_2 model was compared with ETO + AA, the latter showed much more severe inflammation. This may be explained by the fact that arachidonic acid is converted to lipooxygenase products (including leukotrienes) as well as cyclooxygenase products (PGs, thromboxanes, prostacyclins), as shown by the AA metabolite studies in chinchillas.[10] It is well known that one of the AA metabolites by the middle ear mucosa, 15-hydroxyeicosatetraenoic acid, is chemotactic to PMNs.[11] It can be postulated from this observation that lipooxygenase products of AA in otitis media can cause inflammation as well as, or perhaps more than, prostaglandins.

Long-term SOM (more than one month) caused by ETO shows features of chronic otitis media, such as cholesterol granuloma, granulation tissue, osteoneogenesis, and mucosal metaplasia. The model of ETO plus direct inoculation (SOM + POM) produced by far the most characteristics of chronic otitis media, with widespread cholesterol granuloma, diffuse granulation tissue, extensive osteoneogenesis, and mucosal metaplasia.

In order of decreasing severity, the most severe acute inflammation was seen in the short-term POM by direct inoculation model, followed by ETO + AA, POM by nasal inoculation and influenza virus, POM by nasal inoculation with deflation, ETO + direct inoculation, ETO + PGE_2, and ETO. In order of decreasing severity, chronic inflammation was most prominent in the ETO + direct inoculation model, followed by ETO, POM by direct inoculation, ETO + AA, ETO + PGE_2, POM by nasal inoculation with influenza virus, and POM by nasal inoculation.

It should be noted that the intervals from the experiment to the sacrifice and the number of ears in each model are not constant. Thus, caution should be exercised in the interpretation of the data. If intervals to sacrifice and the number of ears are kept constant, the results could be somewhat different.

In conclusion, the chinchilla is an excellent animal for otitis media experiments. We found that the most consistent POM model was produced by direct transbullar inoculation. The ETO + AA model showed much more inflammation than the ETO + PGE_2 model, indicating the importance of lipooxygenase products for inducing inflammation in otitis media. ETO + direct inoculation (SOM + POM combination model) seems to be an excellent animal model for chronic otitis media, duplicating the human condition best.

This study was supported by NIH NINCDS grant #NS-14538.

The authors wish to acknowledge the assistance of Sherry Lamey for microphotography and JoAnn Knox for typing the manuscript.

REFERENCES

1. Paparella MM, Hiraide F, Juhn SK, Kaneko Y: Cellular events involved in middle ear fluid production. Ann Otol Rhinol Laryngol 79:766, 1970
2. Goycoolea MV, Paparella MM, Carpenter AM, Juhn SK: A longitudinal study of cellular changes in experimental otitis media. Otolaryngol Head Neck Surg 87:687, 1979
3. Daniel HJ, Carmine FH, Cook RA: Otitis media in two strains of laboratory rats. J Aud Res 11:276, 1971
4. Daniel HJ, Fulghum RS, Brinn JE, Barrett KA: Comparative anatomy of eustachian tube and middle ear cavity in animal models for otitis media. Ann Otol Rhinol Laryngol 91:82, 1982
5. Giebink GS, Payne EE, Mills EL, et al: Experimental otitis media due to *Streptococcus pneumoniae*: Immunopathologic response in chinchilla. J Infect Dis 134:595, 1976
6. Giebink GS, Berzins IK, Schiffman G, Quie PG: Experimental otitis media in chinchillas following nasal colonization with type 7F *Streptococcus pneumoniae*: Prevention after vaccination with pneumococcal capsular polysaccharide. J Infect Dis 140:716, 1979
7. Juhn SK, Paparella MM, Kim CS, et al: Pathogenesis of otitis media. Ann Otol Rhinol Laryngol 86:481, 1977
8. Meyerhoff WL, Shea DA, Giebink GS: Experimental pneumococcal otitis media: A histopathologic study. Otolaryngol Head Neck Surg 88:606, 1980
9. Meyerhoff WL, Giebink GS, Shea DA: Pneumococcal otitis media following middle ear deflation. Ann Otol Rhinol Laryngol 90:72, 1981
10. Jung TTK, Juhn SK, Gerrard JM: Identification of prostaglandins and other arachidonic acid metabolites in experimental otitis media. Prostaglandins Leukotrienes Med 8:249, 1982
11. Goetzl EJ, Sun EF: Generation of unique monohydroxyeicosatetraenoic acids from arachidonic acid by human neutrophils. J Exp Med 150:406, 1979
12. Giebink GS, Berzins IK, Marker SC, Schiffman G: Experimental otitis media following nasal inoculation of *Streptococcus pneumoniae* and influenza A virus in the chinchilla. Infect Immun 30:445, 1980

HISTOPATHOLOGY OF OTITIS MEDIA IN INFANTS WITH CLEFT AND HIGH ARCHED PALATES

MASANORI KITAJIRI, M.D., ISAMU SANDO, M.D., D.M.S., YOSHIE HASHIDA, M.D., and WILLIAM J. DOYLE, Ph.D.

It is well known that children with cleft palates have a high incidence of otitis media with effusion (OME)[1] It has also been well documented that the eustachian tube plays an important etiologic role in otitis media in patients with cleft palates. However, although many investigations[1–6] have focused on the anatomy and pathophysiology of the eustachian tube of patients with cleft palates, to our knowledge no histopathologic studies have described the incidence or extent of pathologic conditions of the middle ear and the eustachian tube in these patients. The study reported here was undertaken to define the relationship between the occurrence of OME and eustachian tube pathologic findings in infants with cleft palates. For comparison, a similar study was performed in infants with high arched palates, a less severe pathologic condition involving the palate and one that has never been investigated with respect to otitis media.

MATERIALS AND METHODS

Twenty temporal bones were studied from 19 infants, aged 45 mintues to 12 months, with cleft palates or high arched palates. Of 20 temporal bones, 12 bones were from infants with complete cleft palates, 4 were from infants with incomplete clefts of the palate, and 4 were from infants with high arched palates.

The temporal bones were removed at autopsy and fixed in 10 percent formalin. Seventeen of the 20 bones were removed using the standard procedure and the remaining 3 specimens were removed in accordance with a procedure described previously,[7] designed to include the entire eustachian tube in the specimen. After decalcification and dehydration, the specimens were embedded in celloidin. The 17 bones that had been removed by trephination were sectioned horizontally, and the remaining 3 bones were sectioned vertically, at 20 μm. Every tenth horizontal section and every twentieth vertical section was stained with hematoxylin-eosin and mounted on a clean glass slide. PAS (periodic acid-Schiff)[8] and Mayer's mucicarmine[9] stains for glycogen and mucin were used for some selected sections. Each stained section was studied under a light microscope to identify any effusion that might be present. Pathologic conditions of the epithelium and subepithelum in the promontory, midpart of the bony portion of the eustachian tube, and tympanic part of the cartilaginous portion of the eustachian tube were identified.

RESULTS

The more general histopathologic findings of the present study are summarized in Table 1 for each specimen studied. The 20 specimens were divided into 3 groups for study. Group I consisted of 12 temporal bones from infants with complete cleft palates. Groups II and III consisted of 4 specimens each from infants with incomplete cleft palates and high arched palates, respectively. Of the 12 specimens from infants with complete cleft palates, OME was present in 11. Most of these effusions were classified as purulent, with one serous and one mucoid effusion. The remaining specimen in this group was from an infant 45 minutes old who had a middle ear effusion that contained amniotic fluid with desquamated epithelial cells. Three of the four bones in Group II had OME and one had otitis media without effusion. In contrast to the type of effusion observed in Group I specimens, all effusions in Group II were serous. Of the four specimens in Group III, two had a middle ear effusion without evidence of inflammation and two had an otitis media with effusion. One of the specimens with a middle ear effusion had a mucoid effusion and the remaining three middle ears had serous effusions.

Epithelial cell types in three areas are presented in Table 1. Flat or cuboidal epithelium, the normal condition, was noted to cover the promontory in 13 of the 20 temporal bones. However, the epithelium of the middle ears of four infants with complete cleft palates, two infants with incomplete cleft palates, and one infant with a high arched palate consisted of ciliated columnar cells, which are not normally found in this area. Pseudostratified ciliated columnar epithelium was observed to line the bony portion of the eustachian tube in 16 of the 20 cases and the cartilaginous portion of the eustachian tube in 13 of the 14 bones in which this portion of the tube was present. This is generally normal epithelium in these areas. In three cases with complete cleft palates and one case with a high arched palate, pseudostratified cuboidal epithelium lined the bony portion of the tube. Similarly, this epithelial type characterized the cartilaginous eustachian tube of one infant with complete cleft palate.

Table 1 catalogues the degree of inflammation of the subepithelium in the three areas studied. Inflammation of the subepithelium in the middle ear was observed in 17 of 20 bones and in the bony portion of the eustachian tube in 15 of 20 bones. However, inflammation of the cartilaginous portion of the eustachian tube was observed in only 6 of 14 bones in which this portion was available for study. Inflammation appeared to be most severe in the middle ear and least severe in the cartilaginous portion of the eustachian tube. This finding is exemplified by Figure 1, which shows a low-power overview of the area of concern (Fig. 1A) and high-powered views of the subepithelium in the three areas of a representative case (Figs. 1B, C, D), an infant 6 weeks old with a complete cleft palate. The same degree of inflammation was observed in four temporal bones that contained serous or mucoid middle ear effusions. When inflammation was present in the cartilaginous portion of the eustachian tube it appeared to be more extensive in the medial part.

Table 2 summarizes the severity of otitis media with respect to the three groups studied.

TABLE 1 Pathologic Conditions of the Middle Ear and the Eustachian Tube in 20 Bones from Infants with Cleft Palates or High Arched Palates

					Middle Ear		*Bony ET*		*Cart. ET*	
	Case No.	*Age*	*ME Condition*	*Type Effusion*	*Ep. +*	*Sub Ep.*	*Ep. +*	*Sub Ep.*	*Ep. +*	*Sub Ep.*
Group I	1	45 min	MEE	AF	N	–	N	–	N	–
	2*	3 d	OME	P	N	+	N	+	N	±
	3	4 d	OME	P	N	+ + +	A	+	A	–
	4	5 d	OME	P	N	+ +	A	+	N	+
	5	6 d	OME	P	N	+	N	+	N	–
	6*	10 d	OME	P	N	+	N	–	N	±
	7	10 d	OME	P	A	+ +	A	+	N	–
	8	13 d	OME	S	N	+ +	N	+	X	X
	9*	1 m	OME	P	N	+ + +	N	+ + +	N	+
	10	6 w	OME	P	A	+ + +	N	+ +	N	±
	11	6 w	OME	M	A	+ + +	N	+	N	+
	12	5 m	OME	P	A	+ + +	N	+ + +	N	+
Group II	13	5 d	OMoE	–	N	+	N	–	X	X
	14	11 d	OME	S	N	+	N	+	N	–
	15	16 d	OME	S	A	+ +	N	+	N	+
	16	12 m	OME	S	A	+ + +	N	+ + +	N	+ +
Group III	17	10 d	MEE	S	N	–	N	–	X	X
	18	4 m	MEE	M	N	–	A	–	X	X
	19	4 m	OME	S	A	+	N	+	X	X
	20	4 m	OME	S	N	+	N	+	X	X

+ Normal and Pathological Findings of the Epithelia

	ME	*Bony ET*	*Cart. ET*
N:	Flat or cuboidal	Pseudostratified ciliated Columnar	Pseudostratified ciliated Columnar
A:	Pseudostratified columnar	Pseudostratified cuboidal	Pseudostratified cuboidal

*Vertical sections

Key: X, Not available for study
- –, No effusion or no inflammation
- ±, Slight
- +, Mild
- + +, Moderate
- + + +, Severe
- A, Abnormal
- AF, Amniotic fluid
- Cart., Cartilaginous
- d, Days
- Ep., Epithelium
- ET, Eustachian tube
- M, Mucoid
- m, Months
- ME, Middle ear
- MEE, Middle ear effusion
- min, minutes
- N, Normal
- OME, Otitis media with effusion
- OMoE, Otitis media without effusion
- P, Purulent
- S, Serous
- w, weeks

Otitis media was more severe in infants with cleft palates than in infants with high arched palates and most pronounced in infants with complete cleft palates. Furthermore, purulent effusion was retained only in the middle ears of infants with complete cleft palates (Table 1). Subepithelial inflammation of the bony portion of the eustachian tube was greater in infants with cleft palates than in infants with high arched palates.

Inflammation of the middle ear and the bony portion of the eustachian tube appeared to be more pronounced in infants over 1 month old than in infants under 1 month old. This tendency was observed particularly in infants with complete cleft palates. Interesting additional comments on this subject may be made with reference to Cases 3 and 4. Marked inflammatory changes (purulent effusion, polyp formation, and fibrosis) in the middle ears were present in these 4- and 5-day-old infants with complete cleft palates.

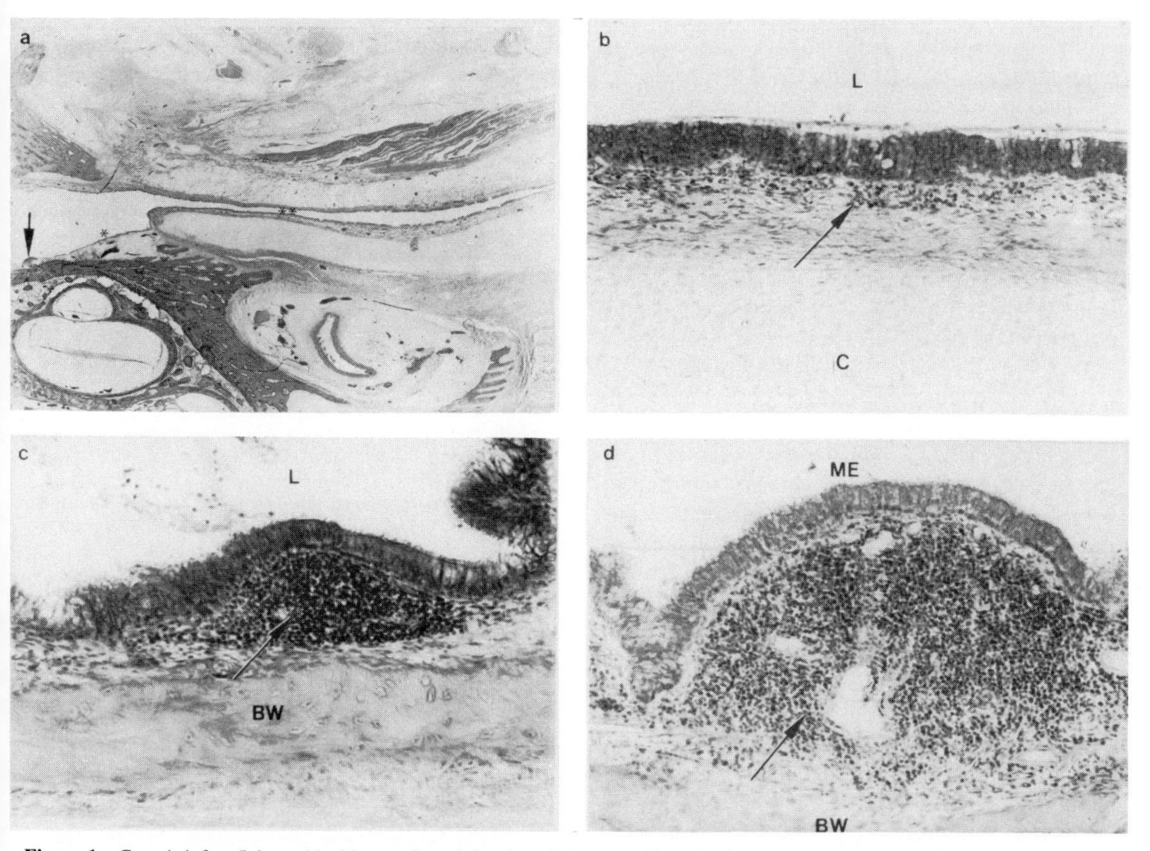

Figure 1 Case 4, infant 5 days old with complete cleft palate, left ear. A, There is a moderate subepithelial inflammatory round cell infiltration (arrow) in the middle ear, whereas very slight inflammation is noted in bot5 bony(*) and cartilaginous(**) portions of the eustachian tube. (H&E stain, X12.5 magnification)

B, Case 10, infant 6 weeks old with complete cleft palate, left ear. A small amount of round cell infiltration (arrow) is present in the subepithelium of the cartilaginous portion of the eustachian tube. C, tubal cartilage, L, tubal lumen. (H&E stain, X275 magnification)

C, Same case as B. Moderate round cell infiltration (arrow) is seen in the subepithelium of the bony portion of the eustachian tube. It is more pronounced than in the cartilaginous portion. BW, bony wall of the internal carotid artery, L, tubal lumen. (H&E stain, X275 magnification)

D, Same case as B. More severe round cell infiltration (arrow) than in the eustachian tube portions is seen in the subepithelium of the promontory. Subepithelial layer is thick, edematous, and polypoid, and epithelial cells showed metaplasia to pseudostratified ciliated columnar cells. BW, bony wall of the promontory; ME, middle ear space. (H&E stain, X275 magnification)

DISCUSSION

In 1967, Stool and Randall reported an unexpectedly high incidence of otitis media in infants with clefts of the palate.[10] Paradise and coworkers[11] reported a 100 percent incidence of OME in infants with cleft palates. The results of the present study showed OME to be present in 94 percent of the middle ears of the cleft palate patients examined. Furthermore, since 11 of the 16 specimens were from infants less than 1 month old, it is suggested that the pathologic process was initiated at an extremely young age. This point is emphasized by the marked inflammatory changes in the middle ear of two infants aged 4 and 5 days with complete

TABLE 2 Severity of Otitis Media in Cleft Palate Infants and High Arched Palate Infants

	Severity of Otitis Media				
	Severe	*Moderate*	*Mild*	*Normal*	
Condition	*N*	*N*	*N*	*N*	*Total*
Complete CP	5	3	3	1*	12
Incomplete CP	1	1	2	0	4
HAP	0	0	2	2	4
Total	6	4	7	3	20

*Newborn (45 minutes old)
Key: CP, Cleft palate
HAP, High arched palate
N, Number of specimens

cleft palates (Cases 3 and 4). These cases raise the interesting possibility that they are the result of a chronic intrauterine inflammation.

Also of interest is the finding of effusion in four middle ears of four infants with high arched palates. We are unaware of any previous studies establishing a relationship between OME and infants with high arched palates. At present we would recommend that such infants be considered tentatively "at risk" for OME and suggest that this possible relationship be explored in the clinical setting.

In a histologic study of temporal bones with OME Zechner[12] reported that eustachian tube inflammation precedes middle ear mucosal metaplasia. Specific intraluminal changes reported included thickened, edematous mucosal folds; increased goblet cell populations; and an intrusive tubal tonsil. The findings of the study reported here showed that inflammation was most severe in the middle ear and least pronounced in the cartilaginous portion of the eustachian tube. Luminal intrusion of subepithelial lymphoid tissue was not observed in the eustachian tube, and epithelial metaplasia was generally confined to the middle ear. The results of the present study fail to support an intrinsic obstruction of the eustachian tube.

The specific pathologic changes secondary to otitis media observed in the present study were similar to those described by Tos[13] and by Ishii and colleagues.[14] For the middle ear, these included an extensive thickening of the subepithelium associated with vascular dilation and transudation, round cell infiltration, and fibrotic proliferation; a metaplasia of the epithelium to pseudostratified ciliated columnar epithelium; mucosal thickening; and an increase in goblet cell numbers. Although gland-like structures were observed, the existence of true secretory glands could not be demonstrated. The degree of these pathologic changes decreased from the middle ear to the nasopharynx, with the cartilaginous portion of the eustachian tube only rarely being affected. In addition, the inflammation of the middle ear and the eustachian tube was more pronounced in infants over 1 month old than in infants less than 1 month old with complete cleft palate. Otitis media and subepithelial inflammation of the bony portion of the eustachian tube appeared to be more pronounced in infants with cleft palates than in infants with high arched palates, and most pronounced in infants with complete palatal clefts.

This study was supported by Research Grants P01 16337-03 and 5 R01 NS 13787-07 from the National Institute of Neurological and Communicative Diseases and Stroke, National Institutes of Health.

REFERENCES

1. Bluestone CD: Eustachian tube obstruction in the infant with cleft palate. Ann Otol Rhinol Laryngol 80 (Suppl 2):1, 1971
2. Ross MA: Functional anatomy of the tensor palatini—its relevance in cleft palate surgery. Arch Otolaryngol 93:1, 1971
3. Dickson DR: Anatomy of the normal and cleft palate eustachian tube. Ann Otol Rhinol Laryngol 85 (Suppl 25):25, 1976
4. Dickson WM, Dickson DR, Rood SR: Anatomy of the eustachian tube and related structures in age-matched human fetuses with and without cleft palate. Trans Am Acad Ophthalmol Otolaryngol 82:159, 1976
5. Bluestone CD, Wittel RA, Paradise JL: Roentgenographic evaluation of eustachian tube function in infants with cleft palate and normal palates—with special reference to occurrence of otitis media. Cleft Palate J 9:93, 1972
6. Bluestone CD, Paradise JL, Beery QC, et al: Certain effect of cleft palate repair on eustachian tube function. Cleft Palate J 9:183, 1972
7. Rood SR, Doyle WJ: An extreme morphologic variation of the auditory tube cartilage: A case report. Cleft Palate J 18:293, 1983
8. McManus JFA: Histological and histochemical uses of periodic acid. Stain Technology 23:99, 1948
9. Preece A: *A Manual for Histologic Technicians,* 3rd Ed. Boston: Little, Brown and Company, 1972, pp 357–359
10. Stool SE, Randall P: Unexpected ear disease in infants with cleft palate. Cleft Palate J 4:99, 1967
11. Paradise JL, Bluestone CD, Felder H: The universality of otitis media in fifty infants with cleft palate. Pediatrics 44:35, 1969
12. Zechner G: Auditory tube and middle ear mucosa in non-purulent otitis media. Ann Otol Rhinol Laryngol 89 (Suppl 68):87, 1980
13. Tos M: Pathogenesis and pathology of chronic secretory otitis media. Ann Otol Rhinol Laryngol 89 (Suppl 68):91, 1980
14. Ishii T, Toriyama M, Suzuki J: Histopathological study of otitis media with effusion. Ann Otol Rhinol Laryngol 89 (Suppl 68):83, 1980

COMPUTER-GENERATED EUSTACHIAN TUBE SHAPE ANALYSIS

JOHN S. TODHUNTER, Ph.D., MICHAEL I. SIEGEL, Ph.D., and WILLIAM J. DOYLE, Ph.D.

It is clear from both epidemiologic studies and private practice surveys that otitis media with effusion (OME) is an age-related pathologic condition. Specifically, the onset of the disease occurs early in postnatal life and decreases in frequency and severity as adolescence approaches. However, general morbidity in the form of speech, language, and educational disabilities consequent to impaired audition may continue throughout the life of the affected individual. Therefore, total management of the disease requires an understanding of the underlying variables responsible for its pathogenesis.

Both clinical and experimental studies evidence a functional obstruction of the eustachian tube (ET) to be causal in the pathogenesis of middle ear disease. Underlying this form of ET dysfunction is the anatomy of the tubal dilating system and specifically the morphology and relations of the cranial base, ET proper, and paratubal musculature. Although a few studies have suggested ontogenetic changes in the morphology of this system to account for the age-related changes in the prevalence of OME, the data have remained cursory and the conclusions extremely speculative.

The objective of this research is to examine the changes in the relations and morphology of the ET, paratubal musculature, and cranial base in a series of 100 extended temporal bone specimens collected at autopsy from persons aged 2 months postconception through adulthood. To date, approximately 30 specimens have been collected, and 12 have completed the processing schedule. In keeping with the objective of this study, a number of representative specimens in each age group are to be reconstructed in three dimensions to allow for more complex analysis of shape and spatial relations. The potential information available from the application of these techniques is enormous. These techniques will allow for resectioning in more favorable planes, isolation of structures and relations of particular interest, and the determination of structural volumes and vectorial relations.

METHODS

During the past 2 years the method for studying anatomic structures through the use of computerized histologic preparations of the nasal capsule has been developed and refined.[1,2] Computerized techniques for reconstruction of three-dimensional structures from a collection of cross-sections have centered in the area of computed tomography[3] and in the past have relied on relatively small data sets. The typical reconstruction program consists of four stages: data acquisition and preprocessing, image alignment, reconstruction, and presentation. The first step involves conversion of analog image data (e.g., photographs or slides) into quantitated form (Fig. 1).

Owing to variations in films, differences in specimen staining, and other environmental effects, preprocessing of digitized images is performed to normalize gray level distribution, enhance contrast, and/or reduce noise. High contrast, low noise, and intersectional gray-level-similar sections simplify later analysis and processing greatly and allow better interpretation during presentation.

During photography or digitization, adjacent slides may be rotated or translated with respect to another. Registration of sections into the correct orientation presents a difficult and often time consuming process. Two general methods are common. The first uses a measure of dissimilarity between areas of the sections under various rotations and shifts.[4,5] A second approach, amenable to both human interaction and automatic procedures, relies on locating special marking positions related to natural or implanted objects within the images. Marks may be selected by a technician or automatically (if marks can be recognized by some algorithm). Points defined by the marks are then matched, and relative rotation and translation may be approximated.[6,7]

In cases where selected marks correspond to

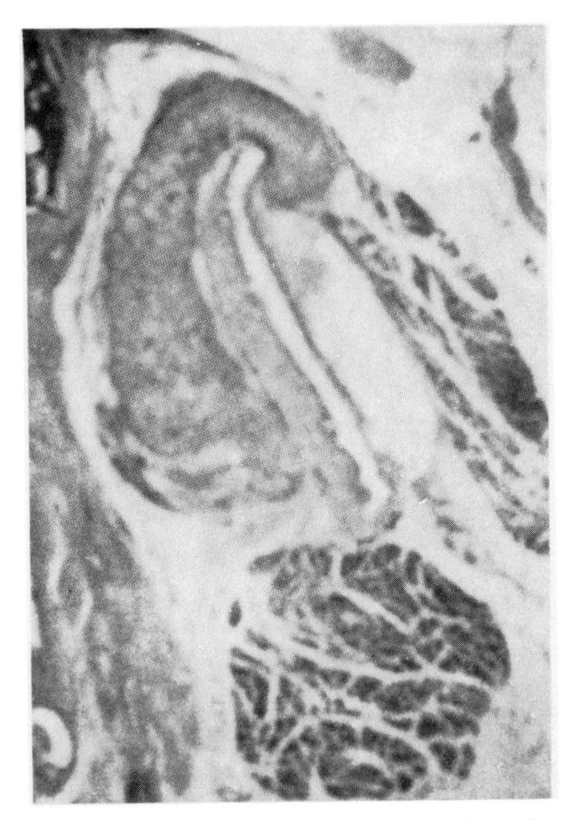

Figure 1 Digitized slide, temporal bone specimen.

natural structures, exact alignment is improbable because of normal variations present in the specimen. Our studies have indicated that excellent alignment is possible using only four marks and relatively coarse point selection. In our studies, marks are selected by human interaction with an approximate 1 percent error in mark selection.

DISCUSSION

After registration, digitized serial sections represent a sampled version of the original continuous data. Reconstruction techniques attempt to recover data lost through sampling. The Nyquist-Shannon sampling theorem gives a limit on the sampling interval so that exact reconstruction is possible. When sampling is too coarse, approximate reconstructions are made, with some expected error.

Three-dimensional reconstruction may be accomplished simply by interpolating gray levels between adjacent sections (e.g., by linear approximation). Alternatively, application of a low-pass filter or, better, a frame recursive filter may be used to recover data.[8] These methods are highly effective in generating oblique sections from the original data so that views from differing angles may be analyzed.

Some interesting problems arise since certain structures within the specimen are transparent. The lumen of the ET is vacant (air-filled) so that for a display of a three-dimensional "block" of reconstructed data, a see-through effect should be generated. Interpolative schemes are highly effective, especially when combined with cutting planes or surfaces so that areas of interest may be exposed for viewing. Drawbacks of these methods are the large amount of data manipulation required, although fast methods have been developed by the investigators.[9] Further, measurements of structural features are not immediately available.

To obtain structural features and to speed reconstruction views, sectional images may be segmented so that individual objects are isolated. From the boundaries of isolated objects or other regional representations,[10] surfaces of the objects may be approximated. Methods for this include simple stacking,[11] optimal triangular tiling,[12] and functional approximation by spline or Bernstein polynomials.[13] These methods have a distinct advantage both in speed of display formation (by standard computer graphics methods) and in determining volume, surface area, center of gravity, and axis of symmetry.

The most difficult aspect of structural representation and reconstruction is the automatic identification of desired objects. To this end, many methods are available;[14] however, ET samples contain a wide variety of object types, such as homogeneous regions (e.g., lumen), textured regions (e.g., muscle), and blending regions (e.g., cartilage). Moreover, many objects split into several parts or merge into one, so that identification of whole structures is somewhat complicated (Fig. 2).

Our present system uses several methods that require a user to supply a starting point and a threshold for a gray level measurement. From this point, regions are determined by finding the outside boundary of the object by a tracking technique. Weakness in edge strength often results in erroneous boundaries; hence, we have developed a program with enough intelligence to remove most of these effects. Finally, detected boundaries are

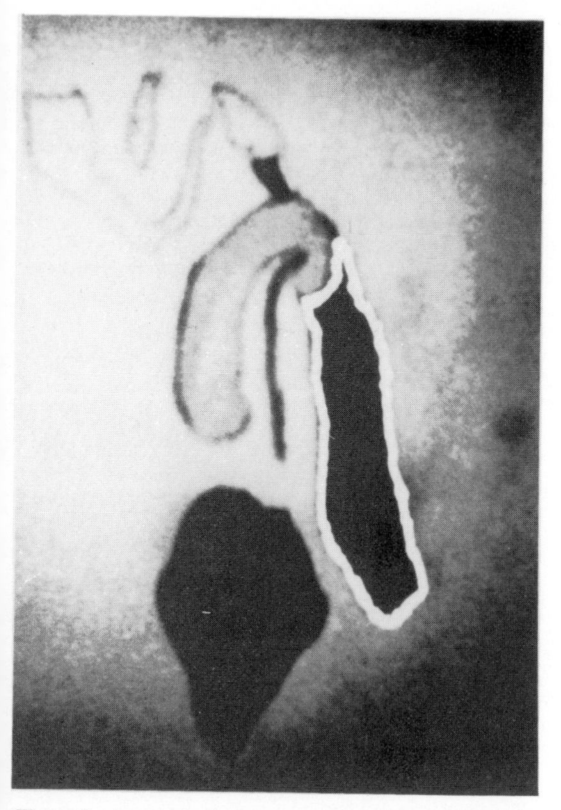

Figure 2 Automatically traced structure of tensor veli palatini (TVP).

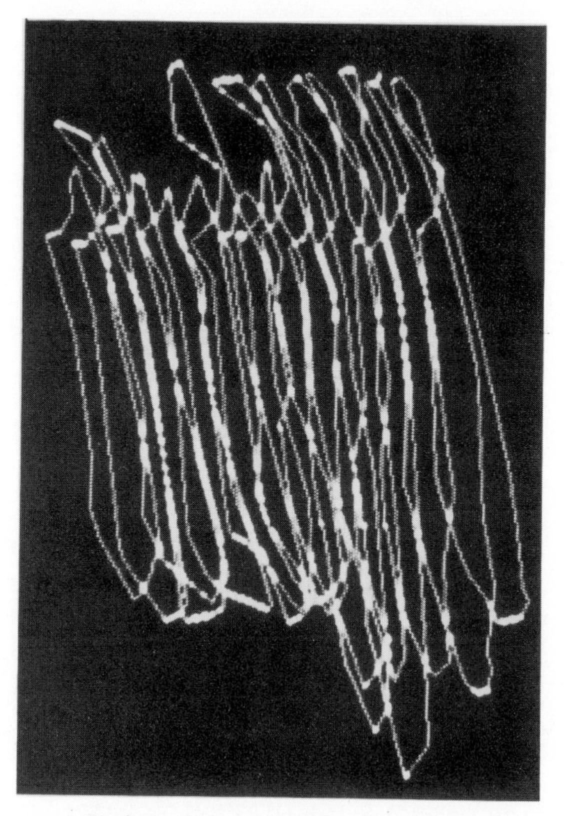

Figure 3 Stacked TVP images (rotated 40°).

approximated by polygons with adjustable accuracy, which are then fed to display processors (Fig. 3).

At present, we are attempting to improve automated segmentation procedures that do not process certain structures successfully. These structures are sectioned perpendicular to the axis of the muscle, which then appears as a large collection of small proto-regions. Also, cartilage blending into other objects has not yet been resolved. Finally, some objects change radically over short distances so that automatic recognition misses portions of the object. Quantitative study of the structures of the eustachian tube–middle ear complex will be based on the reconstructions. Dimensions will be calculated directly, so that exact areas, volumes, and surface shapes can be compared. Since the actual images are stored as digitized information these calculations are easily obtained. Isolated enlarged representations of the middle ear structures will also be studied. The correlation of these relationships with age changes in the face will be related to hypotheses concerning the development of middle ear disease.

REFERENCES

1. Siegel MI, Todhunter JS: Image recognition and reconstruction of cleft palate histological preparations: a new approach. Cleft Palate J 16:4, 381–384, 1979
2. Todhunter JS, Siegel MI, Li CC. Three dimensional reconstruction of histological preparations from cleft palate fetal material. Proceedings of the 14th Hawaii International Conference on System Sciences, pp 409–414, 1981
3. Eden M. The best is yet to come. The Sciences, 18:17, 1978
4. Chow TR, Hsia TC. New results in image alignment. Proc. JACC, 2, 1978
5. Silverman LM, Powell S. Modeling of two-dimensional covariance functions with application to image restoration, IEEE Trans Aut Control AC–19:8, 1974
6. Faugeras O, Price K. Semantic description of aerial images using stochastic labelling. IEEE Trans. PAMI–3:633, 1981

7. Todhunter J. Least-squares point registration. Tech. report TM8201, pattern recognition lab, 1982, University of Pittsburgh
8. Chang SSL. Digital linear processor theory and optimum multidimensional data estimation. IEEE Trans. AC–24:190, 1979
9. Todhunter J. Fast image reconstruction and rotation. Tech. report TM8301, pattern recognition lab, 1983, University of Pittsburgh
10. Merril R. Representation of contours and regions for efficient computer search. CACM–16:69, 1973
11. Rhodes M, Glenn W, Klinger A. Three-dimensional structure isolation using parallel image planes. Proceedings 4th International Conference on Pattern Recognition, 1978, Kyoto
12. Cook N, et al. Three-dimensional reconstruction from serial sections for medical applications, Proceedings of the 14th Hawaii International Conference on System Sciences, 1981
13. Lane J, Riesenfeld R. A theoretical development for the computer generation and display of piece-wise polynomial surfaces. IEEE Trans PAMI–2:35, 1980
14. Fu KS. Special issue on pattern recognition and image processing. Proc. IEEE. 67:3, 1979

MICROBIOLOGY

STATE OF THE ART: MICROBIOLOGY OF ACUTE OTITIS MEDIA WITH EFFUSION

JOHN D. NELSON, M.D.

Streptococcus pneumoniae and *Hemophilus influenzae* remain the undisputed major pathogens of acute otitis media with effusion (AOME) in the United States and most of the rest of the world. For example, in our current study in Dallas, between February 1982 and April 1983, 50 percent of 169 middle ear effusion (MEE) specimens from 125 children contained *S. pneumoniae* and 26 percent contained *H. influenzae* (Odio, C., Nelson, JD, unpublished data). Although a 1983 study from Japan reported an incidence of 19 percent *Staphylococcus aureus* isolations from MEE in AOME,[1] in many other studies during the past decade *S. aureus* has rarely been found.

This status report focuses on new developments and controversial areas of the microbiology of AOME.

BRANHAMELLA CATARRHALIS

The possible pathogenicity of *B. catarrhalis*, like that of *Staphylococcus epidermidis*, has long been debatable, but evidence is accumulating that it is a true pathogen in the middle ear, and it is possible that its prevalence is increasing. Reports in early 1983 from Cleveland[2] and from Pittsburgh[3] of *B. catarrhalis* isolation rates of 27 percent and 22 percent, respectively, support the concept of increasing prevalence. In more than half the cases in those two reports, *B. catarrhalis* was isolated in pure culture. On the other hand, in our current study in Dallas we encountered the organism in only ten patients (8 percent), and in six cases it coexisted with *S. pneumoniae* or *H. influenzae*. Almost 80 percent of *B. catarrhalis* strains elaborate beta-lactamase.[2,3] Leinonen and colleagues in Finland demonstrated IgA antibody to *B. catarrhalis* in 42 percent of MEE specimens and found a significant rise in serum IgG antibodies in 53 percent of children whose MEE specimens had *B. catarrhalis*.[4]

CHLAMYDIA TRACHOMATIS

The first hint that *C. trachomatis* could cause AOME came from studies of experimental eye infection in adults; 11 of 17 volunteers developed otitis.[5] Among 41 babies with chlamydial pneumonia 59 percent had otitis and three of 11 MEE cultures contained *C. trachomatis*.[6] In three subsequent studies summarized by Chang and associates *C. trachomatis* was isolated rarely from MEE.[1] However, most patients were over 1 year old. No systematic study of infants under 6 months old, the peak period for chlamydial infection, has been reported.

ANAEROBIC BACTERIA

Anaerobic bacteria were isolated frequently from MEEs of children with AOME in a study in which the auditory canal was not disinfected before tympanocentesis.[8] However, when the same investigator used disinfection of the canal, anaerobes were isolated from only three (11 percent) of 28 cases, and cultures of the canal after disinfection were positive for anaerobes in two cases.[9] Anaerobes have generally been disregarded as pathogens in AOME. However, in the guinea pig model of otitis media one of three anaerobic genera tested was found to be virulent.[10]

MYCOPLASMAS AND BULLOUS MYRINGITIS

In a thoroughly documented review, Roberts laid to rest two misconceptions: First, that bullous myringitis is a distinct entity, and second, that mycoplasmas are causative.[11] Bullous myringitis is merely one manifestation of AOME caused by the usual bacterial pathogens. Mycoplasmas play no role in the condition.

RESPIRATORY VIRUSES

Respiratory viral infections are important in the epidemiology of AOME, as documented by the 14-year longitudinal study in North Carolina,[12] but their role in direct pathogenesis is less clear. Klein and Teele reviewed the literature in 1976 and uncovered 663 cases in which MEE specimens were cultured for viruses.[13] Twenty-nine (4.4 percent) were positive and respiratory syncytial virus (RSV) accounted for 22 isolations. In a recent study, RSV antigen was detected by the ELISA method in ten (19 percent) of 53 MEE specimens collected at a time when RSV infection was prevalent in the community.[14] Whether RSV is a coincidental inhabitant of the middle ear or whether it invades mucosal cells has not been established.

CONCLUSIONS

Evidence for the pathogenicity of *B. catarrhalis* is becoming increasingly persuasive, and in two locales there appears to be a real increase in its prevalence. Because the majority of strains elaborate beta-lactamase, this would have important implications for therapy. *C. trachomatis* needs to be evaluated in the appropriate age group of patients, but there are hints that it might be an important pathogen in AOME of early infancy. A direct role for pathogenicity of anaerobic bacteria, mycoplasmas, and viruses has not been convincingly demonstrated.

REFERENCES

1. Fujita K, Iseki K, Yoshioka H, et al: Bacteriology of acute otitis media in Japanese children. Am J Dis Child 137:152, 1983
2. Shurin PA, Marchant CD, Kim CH, et al: Emergence of beta-lactamase-producing strains of *Branhamella catarrhalis* as important agents of acute otitis media. Pediatr Infect Dis 2:34, 1983
3. Kovatch AL, Wald ER, Michaels RH: β-Lactamase-producing *Branhamella catarrhalis* causing otitis media in children. J Pediatr 102:261, 1983
4. Leinonen M, Luotonen J, Herva E, et al: Preliminary serologic evidence for a pathogenic role of *Branhamella catarrhalis*. J Infect Dis 144:570, 1981
5. Dawson D, Wood TR, Rose L, et al: Experimental inclusion conjunctivitis in man. III. Keratitis and other complications. Arch Ophthalmol 78:341, 1967
6. Tipple MA, Beem MO, Saxon EM: Clinical characteristics of the afebrile pneumonia associated with *Chlamydia trachomatis* infection in infants less than 6 months of age. Pediatrics 63:192, 1979
7. Chang MJ, Rodriguez WJ, Mohla C: *Chlamydia trachomatis* in otitis media in children. Pediatr Infect Dis 1:95, 1982
8. Brook I, Anthony BF, Finegold SM: Aerobic and anaerobic bacteriology of acute otitis media in children. J Pediatr 92:13, 1978
9. Brook I, Schwartz R: Anaerobic bacteria in acute otitis media. Acta Otolaryngol 91:111, 1981
10. Thore M, Burman LG, Hohn SE: *Streptococcus pneumoniae* and three species of anaerobic bacteria in experimental otitis media in guinea pigs. J Infect Dis 145:822, 1982
11. Roberts DB: The etiology of bullous myringitis and the role of mycoplasmas in ear disease: A review. Pediatrics 65:761, 1980
12. Henderson FW, Collier AM, Sanyal MA, et al: A longitudinal study of respiratory viruses and bacteria in the etiology of acute otitis media with effusion. N Eng J Med 306:1377, 1982
13. Klein JO, Teele DW: Isolation of viruses and mycoplasmas from middle ear effusions: A review. An Otol Rhinol Laryngol 85 (Suppl 5) 140, 1976
14. Klein BS, Dollete FR, Yolken RH: The role of respiratory syncytial virus and other viral pathogens in acute otitis media. J Pediatr 101:16, 1982

THE PATHOGENESIS OF EXPERIMENTAL PNEUMOCOCCAL OTITIS MEDIA DURING RESPIRATORY VIRUS INFECTION IN CHINCHILLAS

G. SCOTT GIEBINK, M.D., and PETER F. WRIGHT, M.D.

Clinical experience suggests that viral upper respiratory infection precedes episodes of acute otitis media in children. Recently, Henderson and associates[1] have demonstrated that certain respiratory viruses, particularly respiratory syncytial virus, adenovirus, influenza, and parainfluenza viruses, are strongly associated with the development of acute otitis media. Others[2,3] have demonstrated that virus species and even strains within a species differ in their association with otitis media. To explore the association between upper respiratory viral infection and otitis media, and to further explore the factors important in the pathogenesis of otitis media, we developed an animal model of pneumococcal otitis media using influenza A virus.[4] This model was based on an earlier observation that gentle mechanical deflation of the middle ear in chinchillas harboring pneumococci in their nasopharynx led to the rapid onset of pneumococcal otitis media with effusion (OME).[5] We reasoned that respiratory viruses that caused negative middle ear pressure might also lead to pneumococcal otitis media.

MATERIALS AND METHODS

Four influenza A virus strains were selected for this study. The prototype strain, A/NWS/33 (ATCC VR-219), is an influenza A virus isolated in Great Britain during an influenza epidemic in 1933 which has undergone multiple laboratory passages since then. For comparison, two wild-type influenza viruses, A/Alaska/6/77 (H3N2) and A/Hong Kong/123/77 (H1N1), obtained during recent influenza outbreaks were selected. In addition, an attenuated, cold-adapted strain (CR29), which is the A/Alaska/6/77 strain further attenuated by recombination with influenza A/Ann Arbor/6/60,[6] was used. This cold-adapted vaccine strain has been shown to cause little or no inflammatory change in the nasopharynx of ferrets. Type 7F *Streptococcus pneumoniae* was used as the bacterial challenge strain in these experiments.

RESULTS

Intranasal inoculation of approximately 10^6 plaque-forming units of each virus consistently caused infection in chinchillas, characterized by a pattern of nasopharyngeal virus shedding for a period of five to seven days after inoculation and by a rise in serum hemagglutinin inhibiting antibody two to three weeks after inoculation.

Tympanometry and otoscopy were performed on virus-infected chinchillas before and at intervals after inoculation. Over 75 percent of chinchillas infected with the A/NWS, A/Alaska, and A/Hong Kong strains developed eustachian tube dysfunction with negative middle ear pressure (Table 1). Middle ear pressure decreased between days 3 and 7 after virus inoculation, especially in chinchillas previously inoculated with the A/Alaska and A/NWS strains. Although most animals infected with the A/Hong Kong strain developed negative middle ear pressure, this finding was not consistent from day to day, and the average middle ear pressure in these animals did not drop nearly as low as the pressure observed in the A/Alaska and A/NWS groups. Significantly fewer animals infected with the CR29 vaccine strain developed negative middle ear pressure.

Tympanic membrane inflammation was seen in 90 percent of A/Alaska-infected animals; in 33 and 35 percent of A/NWS- and A/Hong Kong-infected animals, respectively; and in only 6 percent of the CR29-infected animals.

Chinchillas were sacrificed three to four weeks after inoculation. Only two animals had middle ear effusion present at that time, and both effusions yielded influenza virus on culture. The

TABLE 1 Tympanometry and Otoscopy During Experimental Influenza A Virus Infection

Influenza Strain	*No. of Animals*	*% of Ears Developing:* Negative ME Pressure	TM Inflammation	ME Effusion	*Mortality Rate*
A/NWS/33	32	79	33	0.1	25%*
A/Alaska/77	10	100	90	0	0
A/Hong Kong/77	11	77	36	5	0
CR29	9	28	6	0	0

*Cause of death: Anesthetic (1), *Staphylococcus pneumoniae* (1), killed by cagemate (1), unknown (5)

influenza-related mortality rate was 25 percent in A/NWS-infected animals. It seems likely that the increased mortality rate in this group may have been due to enhanced virulence resulting from serial passage of the strain in chinchillas. None of the animals infected with the other three strains of virus died.

Polymorphonuclear leukocytes (PMNLs) were obtained from the peripheral blood of chinchillas before and at intervals after virus infection, and the chemiluminescence response of these cells was measured as they phagocytized zymosan.[7] Chemiluminescence reflects the ability of PMNLs to kill bacteria by their oxidative mechanisms. Between six and seven days after virus inoculation, animals infected with the A/NWS and A/Alaska

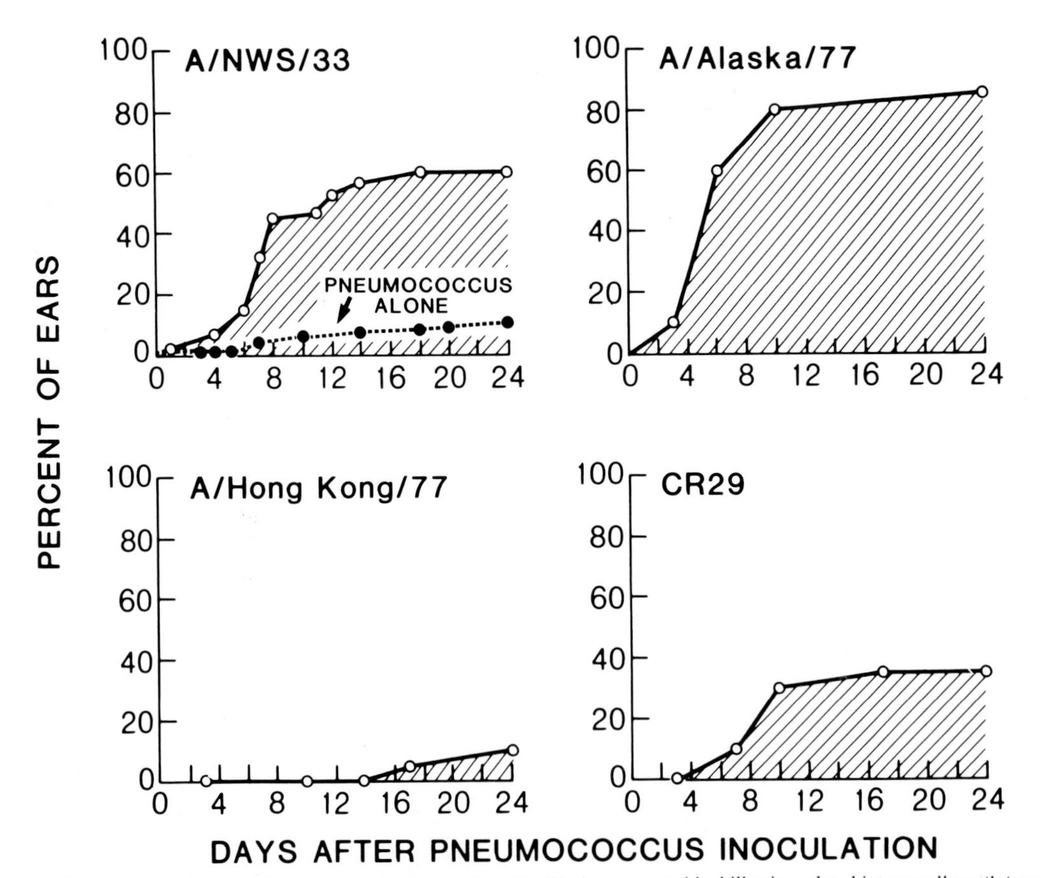

Figure 1 Cumulative incidence of pneumococcal otitis media with effusion among chinchillas inoculated intranasally with type 7F *S. pneumoniae* and influenza A/NWS/33 (upper left), influenza A/Alaska/6/77 (upper right), influenza A/Hong Kong/123/77 (lower left), influenza CR29 (lower right), and with pneumococcus plus saline (nonvirus-infected control, upper left).

strains had a significant decrease in their PMNL chemiluminescence response. A conventional PMN bactericidal assay confirmed the impaired function of these PMNLs.[7]

Four groups of chinchillas were infected with different influenza A strains and were challenged with pneumococcus by intranasal inoculation of 10^5 colony-forming units of type 7F *S. pneumoniae* three to four days after virus inoculation. The highest incidence of pneumococcal OME occurred in animals infected with the A/Alaska strain (85 percent); a somewhat lower incidence was observed in animals infected with the A/NWS strain (60 percent), and a still lower incidence was seen in animals infected with the CR29 vaccine strain (35 percent). The lowest incidence of pneumococcal OME in animals infected with the A/Hong Kong strain (10 percent) did not differ significantly from the incidence of pneumococcal OME in nonvirus-infected control animals inoculated only with pneumococcus (15 percent) (Fig. 1).

Nasal washings were obtained at intervals after intranasal inoculation of pneumococcus to quantitate the number of pneumococci present and to determine the effect of influenza virus infection on pneumococci colonizing the nasopharynx. Animals infected with the A/Alaska influenza strain had significantly higher concentrations of pneumococci in their nasal washings 3, 10, and 17 days after virus inoculation than the nonvirus-infected control group. Animals infected with the attenuated CR29 strain had significantly higher concentrations of pneumococci only on day 3, and A/Hong Kong-infected animals had concentrations of pneumococci similar to control animals. Therefore, the same virus strains that caused negative middle ear pressure, PMNL dysfunction, and pneumococcal otitis also delayed clearance of pneumococci from the nasopharynx.

A preliminary examination of eustachian tube histopathology during experimental influenza infection has been conducted to study the mechanism

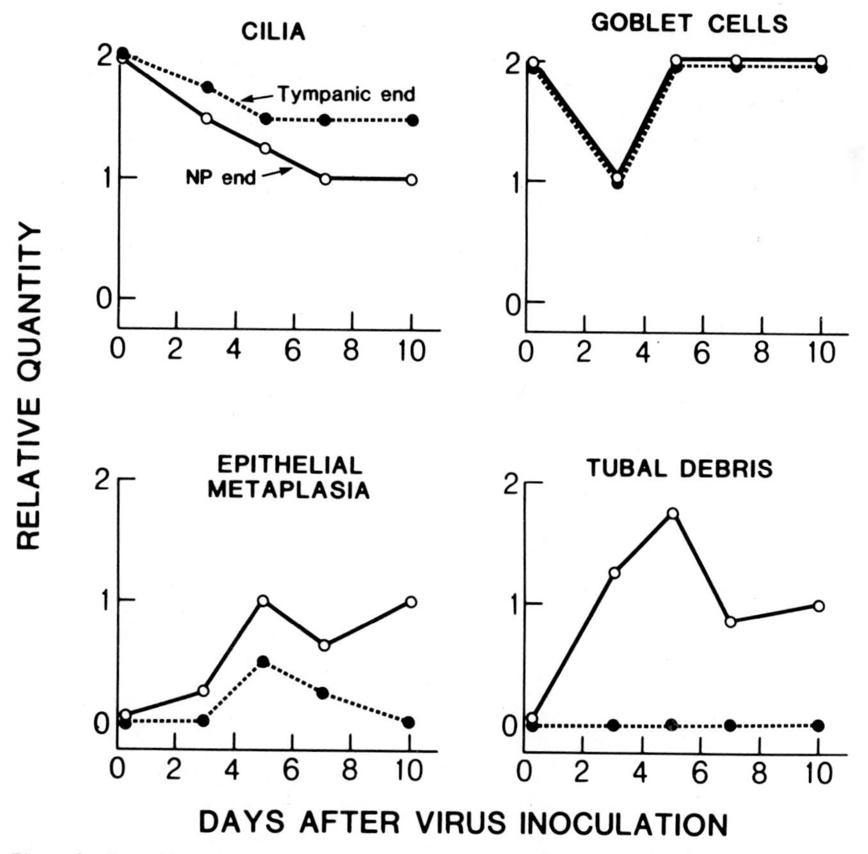

Figure 2 Eustachian tube histopathology in chinchillas during influenza A/Alaska/6/77 infection.

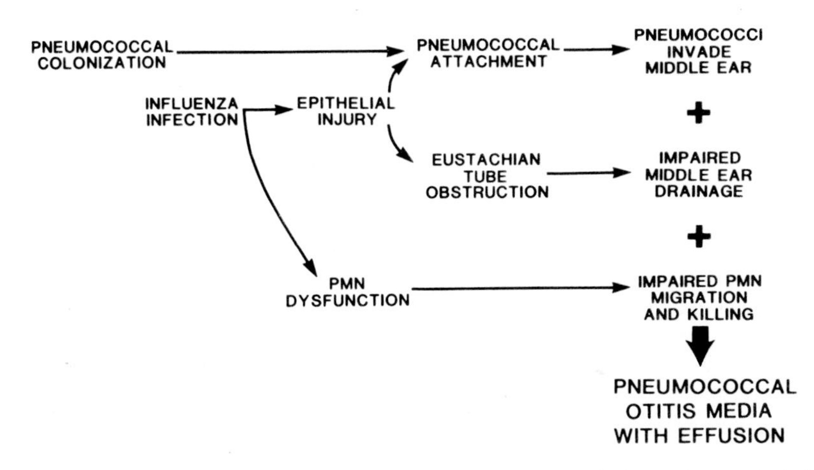

Figure 3 Proposed mechanisms of experimental pneumococcal otitis media with effusion pathogenesis during influenza virus infection.

of eustachian tube dysfunction and impaired pneumococcal clearance. This experiment was performed by sacrificing two chinchillas each on days 3, 5, 7, and 10 after intranasal inoculation of influenza A/Alaska/6/77 virus. Loss of cilia, particularly in the nasopharyngeal end of the tube, was apparent at 3 days, and cilia continued to decline through day 10 (Fig. 2). Epithelial metaplasia with increasing pseudostratification of cells increased through day 10, and goblet cells loss was noted on day 3. A considerable increase in cellular and mucinous tubal debris was noted in the nasopharyngeal end of the tube during the first ten days of virus infection. This debris may have contributed to the tubal dysfunction demonstrated by tympanometry.

CONCLUSIONS

These observations are consistent with the schema of otitis media pathogenesis depicted in Figure 3. Certain influenza virus strains cause epithelial injury and PMNL dysfunction. Epithelial injury might permit increased attachmens of pneumococci to mucosal cells and the larger concentrations of bacteria found in nasal washings. Increased mucosal attachment might permit pneumococci to gain access to the middle ear by a mechanism that is not understood. Since middle ear drainage is impaired by tubal obstruction, and PMNL chemotactic and bactericidal function is impaired, the milieu is perfect for pneumococci to multiply in the middle ear space, causing inflammation and effusion.

This hypothesis is consistent with clinical observations in humans but must be further investigated in the animal model with other respiratory viruses, including strains that do not cause systemic PMN dysfunction, in order to determine the relative importance of bacterial attachment, tubal drainage, and PMN function in the pathogenesis of pneumococcal OME.

This study was supported in part by grant AI-17160 and contract AI-02645 from the National Institute of Allergy and Infectious Diseases, and grant NS-14538 from the National Institute of Neurological and Communicative Disorders and Stroke.

REFERENCES

1. Henderson FW, Collier AM, Sanyal MA, et al: A longitudinal study of respiratory viruses and bacteria in the etiology of acute otitis media with effusion. N Engl J Med 306:1377, 1982
2. Paisley JW, Bruhn FW, Laurer BA: Type A2 influenza viral infections in children. Am J Dis Child 132:34, 1978
3. Wright PF, Thompson J, Karzon DT: Differing virulence of H1N1 and H3N2 influenza strains. Am J Epidemiol 112:814, 1980
4. Giebink GS, Berzins IK, Marker SC, et al: Experimental otitis media after nasal inoculation of *Streptococcus pneumoniae* and influenza A virus in chinchillas. Infec Immun 30:445, 1980
5. Giebink GS, Berzins IK, Schiffman G, Quie PG: Experimental otitis media in chinchillas following nasal colonization with type 7F *Streptococcus pneumoniae*: Prevention after vaccination with pneumococcal capsular polysaccharide. J Infect Dis 140:716, 1979

6. Davenport FM, Hennessey AV, Maassab HF, et al: Pilot studies on recombinant cold-adapted live type 1 and B influenza virus vaccines. J Infect Dis 136:17, 1977

7. Abramson JS, Giebink GS, Mills EL, Quie PG: Polymorphonuclear leukocyte dysfunction during influenza virus infection in chinchillas. J Infect Dis 143:836, 1981

CLINICAL PROFILE OF CHILDREN WITH ACUTE OTITIS MEDIA CAUSED BY *BRANHAMELLA CATARRHALIS*

ANTHONY L. KOVATCH, M.D., ELLEN R. WALD, M.D., RICHARD H. MICHAELS, M.D., MARK M. BLATTER, M.D., KEITH S. REISINGER, M.D., and FREDERICK P. WUCHER, M.D.

Although many case reports associating *Branhamella catarrhalis* with serious systemic infections in adults and children have appeared in the medical literature,[1] the bacterium is still considered by most physicians to be a harmless commensal of the upper respiratory tract.[2] The importance of this organism as a pathogen in acute otitis media was established in 1967 by Coffey and associates,[3] who isolated *B. catarrhalis* in pure culture from the middle ear exudate of 8 percent of 698 symptomatic children with acute otitis. These early investigators considered *B. catarrhalis* a pathogen with little virulence, causing ear infection remarkable for its minimal morbidity and exceptionally low frequency of complications.

Recent clinical investigations[4,5] on acute otitis media have noted frequencies of *B. catarrhalis* higher than the 5 to 8 percent observed in previous series.[3,6,7] The organism was cultured from the middle ear effusions of 22 percent of 146 children studied at our institution; 76 percent of the isolates produced beta-lactamase and were resistant to ampicillin.[4] Shurin and colleagues[5] recognized a significant increase, from 6.4 to 26.5 percent, in the frequency of *B. catarrhalis* cultured from children 6 weeks to 24 months of age with acute otitis studied over consecutive two-year periods; again, the majority of the isolates (77 percent) were beta-lactamase-positive. It is unknown whether the apparent increase in prevalence of *B. catarrhalis* in middle ear disease and the ability to produce beta-lactamase have been accompanied by changes in its clinical characteristics. We therefore sought to compare the presentation and outcome of acute otitis media caused by *B. catarrhalis* with that caused by the other major otic pathogens.

MATERIALS AND METHODS

We reviewed retrospectively the charts of 214 children with acute symptomatic otitis media with effusion (OME) who had been studied in the private office of three pediatricians (all validated otoscopists) in suburban Pittsburgh. Otoscopic criteria for the diagnosis consisted of erythema or white opacification of the tympanic membrane accompanied by varying degrees of bulging and impairment of mobility; the presence of an effusion was corroborated by abnormal tympanograms. The children ranged from 6 months to 13 years of age and were all Caucasian and middle to upper middle class. None had received antibiotic therapy for the present infection before tympanocentesis. The three practitioners were blinded in that they were unaware of the results of middle ear effusion cultures while the patients were being evaluated.

The children examined had been enrolled in one of two consecutive therapeutic studies. The first was an open trial evaluating the efficacy and safety of bacampicillin, which was conducted from August 1980 to November 1980; the 94 patients in this study furnished data on clinical presentation. The second was a randomized, double-blind trial comparing bacampicillin and amoxicillin, which was conducted from August 1981 to May 1982. The 120 patients in this study were followed for one month after antibiotic treatment and therefore supplied data on the short-term outcome of the children, as well as on clinical presentation.

The patients were classified bacteriologically into three groups—*B. catarrhalis, Streptococcus pneumoniae,* and *Hemophilus influenzae*—depending on which pathogen was isolated in pure culture from the middle ear effusion of one or both infected ears. A fourth group consisted of those children whose middle ear cultures were sterile. Although the external auditory canal was cleansed with 70 percent alcohol for 1 minute before each middle ear aspiration was performed, *Staphylococcus epidermidis* was occasionally isolated from pre-entry culture of this area. When it was cultured from both middle ear effusion and external auditory canal, *S. epidermidis* was dismissed as a contaminant. Cases in which the middle ear cultures grew infrequent or doubtful pathogens or combinations of two or more pathogens were excluded from analysis.

Data on the following features were recorded: age, sex, laterality of infection, duration of symptoms (fever or otalgia) before presentation, and the number of ear infections diagnosed in the past year. The oral temperature (or equivalent) recorded at the time of examination or recorded by parents at home before antipyretic therapy was noted. The presence of otalgia was recorded; if the child was too young to report this symptom, irritability was used as an equivalent. Otalgia or irritability was graded as severe if it kept the patient awake and screaming for at least three hours during the night. The presence of symptoms of upper respiratory infection, namely rhinorrhea or cough, was noted. The quality of the effusion obtained by tympanocentesis was characterized on gross inspection as purulent, mucoid, or serous.

All children were examined by otoscope and tympanogram for the presence of a middle ear effusion at the completion of a ten-day course of antibiotic therapy (day 10 of the study) and again one month later (day 42 of the study). Treatment failure was defined as persistence of fever, otalgia, or irritability beyond 48 hours after the start of antibiotic therapy. A recurrence was defined as the development of symptoms and tympanoscopic and tympanometric findings of acute otitis media within one month after documented resolution of the original episode.

Differences among subgroups were statistically analyzed using chi-square with Yates correction, the Fisher exact test, or Student's t-test.

RESULTS

A total of 177 children were assigned to one of the four bacteriologic groups. The clinical characteristics of these children are shown in Table 1. The mean age of the children in the *B. catarrhalis* group (1.8 years) was significantly lower than the mean ages of those in the other three groups ($p < 0.005$). The majority (58 percent) of children in the *B. catarrhalis* group were in the 1- to 3-year age bracket, and a significantly smaller percentage of the children (12.5 percent) were older than 3 years, as compared with the other groups ($p < 0.005$). There were no significant differences in sex, laterality, duration of symptoms less than 24 hours, or the tendency to have repeated ear infections.

A comparison of presenting symptoms is shown in Table 2. There were no differences be-

TABLE 1 Clinical Characteristics of 177 Children with Acute Symptomatic Otitis Media According to Bacteriologic Group

Bacteriologic Group (No.)	*Mean Age (yrs)*	*Older Than 3 Years (%)*	*Male (%)*	*Bilateral (%)*	*Symptoms ≤ 24 hrs (%)*	*> 1 Ear Infection in Past Year (%)*
B. catarrhalis (24)	1.8*	12.5*	62.5	45.8	66.7	20.8
S. pneumoniae (66)	3.3	50.0	56.1	30.3	65.2	31.8
H. influenzae (39)	3.5	51.3	53.8	43.6	41.0	23.1
No pathogen (48)	4.1	54.2	58.3	25.0	47.9	39.6

*$p < 0.005$

TABLE 2 Clinical Presentation of 177 Children According to Bacteriologic Group

Bacteriologic Group (No.)	*Average Temp (°C)*	*Fever > 38.5°C (%)*	*Otalgia† (%)*	*Severe Otalgia† (%)*	*URI (%)*
B. catarrhalis (24)	38.1	12.5	87.5	37.5	91.7
S. pneumoniae (66)	38.2	24.2*	92.4	47.0*	80.3
H. influenzae (39)	37.9	5.1*	79.5	25.6*	87.2
No pathogen (48)	38.2	16.7	91.7	33.3	72.9

*p < 0.05
† Or irritability

tween the *B. catarrhalis* group and the other groups in the average height of fever, the frequency of high fever (≥ 38.5°C), the frequency or severity of otalgia or irritability, or in the frequency of upper respiratory infection symptoms. However, the children in the *S. pneumoniae* group had a significantly greater likelihood of having high fever or severe otalgia than the children in the *H. influenzae* group ($p < 0.05$).

The distribution of purulent (28.6 percent), mucoid (60.7 percent), and serous (10.7 percent) effusions among the children with *B. catarrhalis* otitis media was similar to that of the other groups.

Some features of clinical outcome are shown in Table 3 for 99 children treated with either bacampicillin or amoxicillin; although not shown, there was no difference in outcome between the treatment arms. A significantly lower percentage of children in the "no pathogen" group had middle ear effusion detected on day 10 of the study than in the *B. catarrhalis* group ($p < 0.01$); no differences were observed on day 42 of the study. The frequencies of unsatisfactory outcome—either treatment failure or recurrence—were almost identical among the four groups. The one treatment failure and the four recurrences in the *B. catarrhalis* group all had beta-lactamase–producing strains of the organism isolated from the original middle ear effusion culture. In contrast, all ten recurrences in the *H. influenzae* group had beta-lactamase-negative strains originally isolated. Repeat tympanocentesis was not routinely performed at the time of the recurrences.

DISCUSSION

Several studies attempting to correlate clinical and bacteriologic observations on children with acute otitis media were reported in the late 1960s. After analyzing 585 cases of otitis, Howie and associates[6] concluded that pneumococcal otitis media was more likely than *H. influenzae* otitis media to be associated with severe pain and high fever. Coffey and associates[8] described a population of children with *B. catarrhalis* (then *Neisseria catarrhalis)* "exudative" otitis media; none was acutely sick or febrile, and presenting symptoms referable to the ears were rare. Most of the children were brought to the office because of simple "colds." These authors found the median age of children from whom *B. catarrhalis* was cultured from the middle ear exudate (1 year) to be lower than the median age of those from whom *S. pneumoniae* (1 5/12 years) or *H. influenzae* (also 1 5/12 years) was cultured.

We confirm this early observation that *B. catarrhalis* tends to cause middle ear disease in

TABLE 3 Clinical Outcome for 99 Children According to Bacteriologic Group

Bacteriologic Group (No.)	*Effusion (%)*		*Unsatisfactory Outcome*		
	Day 10	*Day 42*	*Treatment Failure*	*Recurrence*	*Total (%)*
B. catarrhalis (13)	79.6*	20.0	1	4	5 (38.5)
S. pneumoniae (37)	52.8	22.6	1	12	13 (35.1)
H. influenzae (26)	61.5	22.2	0	10	10 (38.5)
No pathogen (23)	39.1*	18.2	0	6	6 (26.1)

*p < 0.01

younger children relative to *S. pneumoniae* or *H. influenzae*. This predilection of *B. catarrhalis* for the younger child has also been noted in acute maxillary sinusitis.[9]

Otherwise, our data indicate that acute symptomatic otitis media caused by *B. catarrhalis* is indistinguishable on clinical grounds from that associated with *S. pneumoniae, H. influenzae,* or a sterile middle ear fluid and may not be a milder disease, as previously thought. Although an association with unsatisfactory outcome has been suggested,[4] the true clinical significance of beta-lactamase production by *B. catarrhalis* as it affects response to antimicrobial therapy is not yet established. Patients with serious systemic illnesses caused by beta-lactamase-producing strains of the organism have responded to penicillin therapy alone in spite of demonstrated resistance.[1] *In vivo* studies in an animal model or in human subjects are necessary to clarify this issue in regard to treatment recommendations for acute otitis media.

This study was supported in part by NIH Grant NS-16337 and Pfizer, Inc.

REFERENCES

1. Doern GV, Miller MJ, and Winn RE: *Branhamella (Neisseria) catarrhalis* systemic disease in humans. Arch Intern Med 141:1690, 1981
2. Jawetz E, Melnick JL, Adelberg EA: *Review of Medical Microbiology*, 15th ed. Los Altos, CA: Lange Medical Publications, 1982, p 205
3. Coffey JD Jr, Martin AD, Booth HN: *Neisseria catarrhalis* in exudate otitis media. Arch Otolaryngol 86:403, 1967
4. Kovatch AL, Wald ER, Michaels RH: β-lactamase-producing *Branhamella catarrhalis* causing otitis media in children. J Pediatr 102:261, 1983
5. Shurin PA, Marchant CD, Kim CH, et al: Emergence of beta-lactamase-producing strains of *Branhamella catarrhalis* as important agents of acute otitis media. Pediatr Infect Dis 2:34, 1983
6. Howie VM, Ploussard JH, Lester RL: Otitis media: A clinical and bacteriological correlation. Pediatrics 45:29, 1970
7. Mandel EM, Bluestone CD, Cantekin EI, et al: Comparison of cefaclor and amoxicillin for acute otitis media with effusion. Ann Otol Rhinol Laryngol 90:48, 1981
8. Coffey JD Jr, Booth HN, Martin AD: Otitis media in the practice of pediatrics. Pediatrics 38:25, 1966
9. Wald ER, Milmoe GJ, Bowen AD, et al: Acute maxillary sinusitis in children. N Engl J Med 304:749, 1981

THE CLINICAL SIGNIFICANCE OF COAGULASE-NEGATIVE STAPHYLOCOCCI IN OTITIS MEDIA WITH EFFUSION

JOEL M. BERNSTEIN, M.D., Ph.D., DIANE DRYJA, and ERWIN NETER, M.D.

The coagulase-negative staphylococci historically have been regarded as saprophytes with little, if any, clinical significance. In persons with decreased resistance to infection these microorganisms can cause opportunistic infections involving the blood,[1] the urinary tract,[2] the meninges,[3] the peritoneum,[4] the joints,[5] and wounds.[6] Coagulase-negative staphylococci comprise several different species, and it is conceivable that species differ in pathogenic potential. Although it has been fairly well established that this organism can cause acute otitis media,[7] its role in chronic otitis media with effusion is not resolved. We have previously reported that under certain conditions coagulase-negative staphylococci are not necessarily contaminants from the external canal, but might play a role in the pathogenesis of otitis media with effusion.[8] Our observations on only some middle ear effusions have suggested that most coagulase-negative staphylococci are coated with IgA antibody[9] and have different biochemical characteristics and antibiograms from strains isolated from the external canal of the same patients.

The present study was undertaken to speciate coagulase-negative staphylococci found in middle ear effusions, on the outer eardrums, postaural skin, tonsils, and adenoids of patients with recurrent otitis media with effusion. Our purpose was to determine whether particular species were more likely to be associated with specific types of effusion and to assess the usefulness of species identification in establishing their clinical significance.

MATERIALS AND METHODS

Study Design

A total of 100 patients with chronic otitis media with effusion were studied, including 64 males and 36 females whose ages ranged from 12 months to 15 years. There were 27 serous, 13 purulent, 27 seromucinous, and 23 mucoid effusions. Ten myringotomy taps were dry.

On receipt in the bacteriology laboratory, specimens were cultured on 5 percent sheep blood, phenylethyl alcohol blood agar (PEA), chocolate and Endo agar, and in brain-heart infusion broth. When sufficient material was available, direct smears were made and methylene blue or Gram stains were performed. The blood, PEA, and chocolate agar plates were incubated at 36°C in air with 2 to 5 percent CO_2. All organisms were identified by conventional means, and, when indicated, antibiograms were performed using the Kirby-Bauer disc diffusion method. All staphylococcus isolates were tested for novobiocin susceptibility and coagulase production. To identify species further, the API Staph-Ident strip was used, which includes the following biochemical tests: phosphatase production, urea utilization, beta-glucosidase production, mannose utilization, mannitol utilization, trehalose utilization, salicin utilization, beta-glucuronidase production, arginine utilization, and beta-galactosidase production. The manufacturer's recommended procedures for inoculation, incubation, and reading of the strips were followed. Organisms were identified with the aid of the charts supplied by the manufacturer. API's computer service was used in cases in which the biotype number was not listed on the differential chart.

A search for more than one organism was undertaken whenever the nature of the colonies from an effusion suggested that more than one organism was present. When only one species was identified on colony growth, the presence of another species could not be rigidly excluded.

RESULTS

Coagulase-negative staphylococci were the most common isolates found in the middle ear effusion. As shown in Table 1, they were present less often in purulent specimens than in other types of effusions. A total of 39 strains were recovered from 100 patients. To exclude the possibility of contamination of the middle ear effusion it was important to determine how frequently coagulase-negative staphylococci were present in the effusion but not on the tympanic membrane or the postauricular skin. As summarized in Table 2, the isolates found in the middle ear were different from those in the tympanic membrane and postauricular skin in 19 patients (50 percent). Furthermore, when considering only the difference between the eardrum and the middle ear, 24 of 39 strains (60 percent) belonged to this group.

Nine different species of coagulase-negative staphylococci were isolated from the middle ear (Table 3). The most common type was *Staphylococcus epidermidis,* recovered from 22 cases. In addition, 24 other isolates included *S. hominis* in six cases, *S. simulans* in three cases, *Staphylococcus hemolyticus* in one case, and *S. cohnii* in one case. Thus, over 50 percent of the isolates reported from the middle ear were species other than *S. epidermidis.* The antibiograms are also summarized in Table 3. Almost half of the isolates (21 of 46) were resistant to penicillin and ampicillin.

TABLE 1 Bacterial Isolates in 100 Cases of Recurrent Otitis Media with Effusion

Fluid Type	*No.*	*Coag-Neg*	*S. aureus*	*S. pneumoniae*	*H. influenzae*	*α Strep*	*β Strep*
Serous	27	12	2	1	1	0	0
Seromucinous	27	17*	2	3	1	4	0
Mucoid	23	15*	1	1	2	0	2
Purulent	13	1	0	3	2	1	1
Dry tap	10	0	1	0	0	1	0
Total	100	45	6	8	6	6	3

*More than one species of Coagulase Negative staphylococci recovered

TABLE 2 Total Number of Middle Ear Aspirates (100)

		With Coagulase-Negative Staphylococci (39)			
Type of Effusion	*No.*	*Different Than Ear Drum and Postaural Skin*	*Different Than Ear Drum*	*Same as Ear Drum*	*Without Coagulase-Negative Staphylococci (61)*
Serous	27	7	7	4	16
Seromucinous	27	7	9	3	15
Mucoid	23	4	7	5	11
Purulent	13	0	0	1	12
Dry tap	10	0	0	0	10
Total	100	18	23	13	64*

*Some middle aspirates had more than one organism

Since colonization of adenoidal tissue could conceivably be a source of middle ear infection, coagulase-negative staphylococci from these two sources were compared. Coagulase-negative staphylococci were found in the adenoidal tissue in 16 cases. The species isolated from the middle ear was identical to that found in the adenoid in eight cases.

DISCUSSION

Coagulase-negative staphylococci are normal inhabitants of the skin, throat, mouth, external auditory canals, conjunctivae, vagina, and urethra.[10] Contamination of bacteriologic cultures with *S. epidermidis* is common and results in difficulty in differentiation between true infection and contamination based on cultures. Suggestive evidence of the possible pathogenic role of coagulase-negative staphylococci can be obtained if middle ear aspirates yield the same microorganism on repeated examination of patients with clinical infection or if the middle ear isolates represent species different from those isolated from possible contaminating areas. Our data indicate that 50 percent of coagulase-negative staphylococci isolated from the middle ear are different from those recovered from both the tympanic membrane and the postaural skin. Furthermore, over 50 percent of the coagulase-negative staphylococci isolated from the middle ear represent species other than *S. epidermidis*. The results of our study are in agreement with the findings of Sipila and associates[11] and others,[12,13] who have reported that the most common bacterial species isolated in chronic otitis media with effusion was *S. epidermidis*.

There are several possible explanations for the isolation of this microorganism from middle ear effusions. It may be a constituent of the normal ear flora. However, in ten subjects with dry taps, coagulase-negative staphylococci were not found

TABLE 3 Classification of Coagulase-Negative Staphylococci in 100 Cases of Recurrent Otitis Media with Effusion

Fluid Type	*No.*	*No. of Staphylococcus Isolates*	*S. epidermidis*	*S. hominis*	*S. warnerii*	*S. capitis*	*S. simulans*	*S. hemolyticus*	*S. hyicus*	*S. intermedius*	*S. cohnii*
Serous	27	12	6 [1] (2)	3 [3] (3)	0	2 [2] (0)	1 [1] (0)	0	0	0	0
Seromucinous	27	17*	8 [2] (3)	1 [1] (1)	5 [3] (1)	1 [1] (1)	1 [1] (1)	1 [0] (1)	0	0	0
Mucoid	23	15*	8 [2] (4)	1 [1] (0)	0	1 [1] (0)	1 [0] (1)	1 [1] (1)	1 [1] (0)	1 [1] (0)	1 [1] (1)
Purulent	13	1	0	1 [0] (1)	0	0	0	0	0	0	0
Dry tap	10	0	0	0	0	0	0	0	0	0	0
Total	100	45	22 [5] (9)	6 [5] (5)	5 [3] (1)	4 [4] (1)	3 [2] (2)	2 [1] (2)	1 [1] (0)	1 [1] (0)	1 [1] (1)

* More than one species of coagulase negative staphylococci recovered
( ) Denotes resistance to penicillin and ampicillin
[ ] Denotes number of coagulase negative staphylococci in middle ear drum

in any fluid obtained from middle ear irrigation. A second possibility is that coagulase-negative staphylococci might have ascended from the nasopharynx into the middle ear. This is a reasonable explanation, because in 16 of the 39 cases coagulase-negative staphylococci were present in the nasopharynx as well, and furthermore, in eight cases (50 percent of this group) the species was identical to that found in the middle ear. A third possibility for the recovery of coagulase-negative staphylococci from the middle ear is that the organism is a contaminant from the ear canal. This could account for 50 percent of our cases. Fourth, it is conceivable that microorganisms from the external canal might penetrate an inflamed eardrum, just as *Pseudomonas aeruginosa* can penetrate severely burned skin.

In conclusion, the frequent occurrence of coagulase-negative staphylococci in the middle ear and the frequent isolation of species other than *S. epidermidis* suggest that routine speciation of coagulase-negative staphylococci could aid in establishing the clinical significance of these isolates. This is particularly so in the case of *S. hominis,* since more than 80 percent of strains of that species are resistant to penicillin and ampicillin.

REFERENCES

1. Munson DP, Thompson TR, Johnson DE: Coagulase-negative staphylococcal septicemia: Experience in a newborn intensive care unit. Pediat 101:602, 1982
2. Wallmark G, Arremark I, Telander B: Staphylococcus saprophyticus: A frequent cause of acute urinary tract infections among female outpatients. J Infect Dis 138:791, 1978
3. Holt RJ: The colonization of ventriculo-atrial shunts by coagulase-negative staphylococci. In Finland M (ed): *Bacterial Infections: Changes in Their Causative Agents, Trends, and Possible Basis.* Bayer-Symposium III. Berlin: Springer-Verlag, pp 81–87, 1981
4. Popovich RP, Moncrief JW, Nolph AJ, et al: Continuous ambulatory peritoneal dialysis. Ann Intern Med 88:449, 1978
5. Patterson FP, Brown CS: The McKee-Farrar total hip replacement. Preliminary results and complications of 368 operations performed in five general hospitals. J Bone Joint Surg 54:257,
6. Morse SI: Staphylococci. In Braude A (ed): *Medical Microbiology and Infectious Diseases.* Philadelphia: WB Saunders Co, 1981, pp 275–281
7. Feigin RD, Shackelford PG, Campbell TO, et al: Assessment of the role of staphylococcus epidermidis as a cause of otitis media. Pediatrics 52:569, 1973
8. Bernstein JM, Dryja D, Neter E: The role of coagulase-negative staphylococci in chronic otitis media with effusion. Otolaryngol Head Neck Surg 90:837, 1982
9. Bernstein JM, Nisengard R, Wisher K, et al: Antibody coated bacteria in otitis media with effusion. Ann Otol Rhinol Laryngol 89(Suppl 68):104, 1980
10. Feigin RD, Shearer WT: Opportunistic infection in children. III. In the normal host. Pediatrics 87:852, 1975
11. Sipila P, Jokipii MM, Jokipii L, Karma P: Bacteria in the middle ear and ear canal of patients with secretory otitis media and with non-inflammed ears. Acta Otolaryngol 92:123, 1981
12. Riding KH, Bluestone CD, Michaels RH, et al: Microbiology of recurrent and chronic otitis media with effusion. J Pediat 93:739, 1978
13. Healy BG, Teele DW: The microbiology of chronic middle ear effusions in children. Laryngoscope 87:1472, 1977

BIOTYPES OF SEROLOGICALLY NONTYPABLE *HEMOPHILUS INFLUENZAE* ISOLATED FROM THE MIDDLE EAR AND PHARYNX OF PATIENTS WITH OTITIS MEDIA WITH EFFUSION

THOMAS F. DeMARIA, Ph.D., DAVID J. LIM, M.D., LEONA W. AYERS, M.D., JEAN BARNISHAN, M.S., and HERBERT G. BIRCK, M.D.

Hemophilus influenzae is the most common bacterial pathogen associated with chronic otitis media with effusion (OME), accounting for 25 percent of the total bacterial isolates.[1] Approximately 95 percent of the *H. influenzae* isolates from cases of OME are unencapsulated and not typable with antisera specific for the six recognized capsular serotypes.[2] Because of this, the majority of the *H. influenzae* involved in OME have not yet been investigated in depth either clinically or experimentally.

Biotyping, a classification system based on various biologic characteristics, was devised by Kilian to assist in the identification and classification of this anonymous group of organisms.[3] The purpose of the present study was to define the biochemical behavior of the serologically nontypable *H. influenzae* isolated from the middle ear effusions (MEEs) and pharynxes of patients with OME according to the established biotyping system for *H. influenzae*.[3] In addition, the antibiotic susceptibility profiles and beta-lactamase production were evaluated in middle ear and pharyngeal isolates of *H. influenzae*.

MATERIALS AND METHODS

Specimens

MEEs and pharyngeal samples were obtained from patients undergoing routine myringotomy and tube insertion for chronic OME at the Children's Hospital, Columbus, Ohio. The patients' ages ranged from 3 months to 11 years. Thirty MEE isolates of serologically nontypable *H. influenzae* and the paired pharyngeal isolates were analyzed at the Clinical Microbiology Laboratory at the Ohio State University Hospitals. For this study, only specimens that exhibited growth of *H. influenzae* in both the MEE and the pharynx were included. Two cases in which only the MEE was culture-positive for *H. influenzae* were excluded from the data analysis.

Bacteria Culture and Isolation

All specimens were cultured for bacteria on sheep's blood and chocolate agar using procedures described previously.[4] Presumptive *H. influenzae* isolates were identified by their typical colonial morphologic features on chocolate agar. Definitive identification was determined by their growth requirements for NAD and hemin on brain-heart infusion agar. Nontypable *H. influenzae* were defined as organisms that failed to agglutinate with commercial, type-specific rabbit antisera prepared against types a through f (Difco, Detroit, MI).

TABLE 1 Condensed Identification Schema of *H. influenzae* Biotypes

Biotype	*Indole*	*Urease*	*Ornithine Decarboxylase*
I	+	+	+
II	+	+	−
III	−	+	−
IV	−	+	+
V	+	−	+
VI	+	−	−

Biotype Analysis

Although a total of 25 different biochemical tests were performed on each isolate, biotypes were assigned by assessing indole, urease, and ornithine decarboxylase in assays modified from those described by Kilian[2,3] by the OSU Clinical Microbiology Laboratory (Table 1).[5] Antibiotic susceptibility patterns were determined to complement biotyping using a battery of 16 antibiotics in supplemented microtube plates (Dynatech Laboratories, Alexandria, VA). Beta-lactamase production was determined for each isolate by the acidometric Beta Test (Malcom Laboratory Supply, Cleveland, OH) and by the chromogenic cephalosporins method (PADAC Calbiochem-Behring, La Jolla, CA).

RESULTS

Fifty-three percent of the middle ear isolates examined belonged to biotype II (Table 2). All *H. influenzae* strains cultured from the pharynxes of these patients were also biotype II. Twenty-three percent of the middle ear *H. influenzae* isolates were designated as biotype III. The remaining isolates were biotype I (10 percent), biotype V (6 percent), or biotype VI (6 percent) (Table 2). No biotype IV isolates were observed in this study. With one exception, the pharyngeal biotypes were identical to the corresponding middle ear isolates.

The incidence of beta-lactamase production was 17 percent, and the results for the middle ear isolates matched those observed for the paired pharyngeal isolates.

The minimum inhibitory concentrations of the antibiotic susceptibility profiles for the paired specimens were the same. The variance of the minimum inhibitory concentration was limited to a single serial twofold dilution, which is not considered a significant difference.[6]

TABLE 2 Biotypes of Nontypable *H. influenzae* from Paired Middle Ear and Pharyngeal Isolates

Biotype	*Paired Isolates*	*Percentage*
I	3	10
II	16	53
III	7	23
IV	0	0
V	2	6
VI	2	6

DISCUSSION

Recent data indicate that the nonencapsulated *H. influenzae* are antigenically diverse and that the development of a serologic classification system for these organisms is not possible at this time.[7] The outer membrane profiles of this organism are also too variable to provide the framework for a classification system.[7] At present, biotyping is the only available framework for the classification of this group of organisms.

The present data indicate that biotype II and III unencapsulated isolates account for 76 percent of the *H. influenzae* isolated from cases of chronic OME. Type II organisms were the predominant biotype, with an overall incidence of 53 percent. No biotype IV organisms were observed in this study, which is compatible with other epidemiologic data that indicate this is a rare biotype with a predilection for colonizing the female genital tract.[8]

The frequencies of the different biotypes among our ear isolates from OME patients are similar to those previously reported in cases of acute otitis media.[7] These findings are compatible with the concept that acute suppurative otitis media and chronic OME are related.

The results from the present study indicate that, with only one exception, the biotype, antibiotic susceptibilities, and beta-lactamase production were identical for the organisms isolated from the paired middle ear and pharyngeal specimens, and that the isolates are probably the same organism. These findings suggest that the natural portal of entry for pathogens into the middle ear is most likely via the eustachian tube from the pharynx, as has been suggested previously.[1] In this regard, it is interesting to note that even at the time of surgery the pharynxes of the patients from whom *H. influenzae* were isolated from the MEEs were also colonized with *H. influenzae*. Even though most species of *Hemophilus* are considered normal inhabitants of the upper respiratory tract,[2] it seems plausible that the chronicity of their condition may be related to the persistent colonization of the pharynx with particular biotypes of *H. influenzae*.

The results of the present study indicate that nonencapsulated *H. influenzae,* biotype II, is the predominant group isolated from the MEEs of patients with OME. The reason biotype II organisms were isolated most often is not known, but this organism is also the predominant biotype of unencapsulated *H. influenzae* isolated from the blood of patients with bacteremia or from the cerebrospinal fluid.[7]

Using *H. influenzae,* biotype II, in the chinchilla model we have sucessfully induced OME that appears to mimic certain types of clinical OME in children.[9] Further study is needed to better understand the clinical course of *H. influenzae* otitis media. According to our data, future experimental studies of OME should focus on this clinically important biotype.

This study was supported in part by grants from NINCDS/NIH (NS08854) and The Deafness Research Foundation.

REFERENCES

1. Lim DJ, DeMaria TF: Panel discussion: Pathogenesis of otitis media. Bacteriology and immunology. Laryngoscope 92:278, 1982
2. Liu YS, Lim DJ, Lang RW, Birck HG: Chronic middle ear effusions: Immunochemical and bacteriological investigation. Arch Otolaryngol 101:278, 1975
3. Kilian M: *Hemophilus.* In Lennette EH, Balows A, Hausler WJ Jr, Truant JP (eds): *Manual of Clinical Microbiology,* 3rd ed. Washington, DC: American Society for Microbiology, 1982 p 330–336
4. Kilian M: A taxonomic study of the genus *Hemophilus,* with the proposal of a new species. J Gen Microbiol 93:9, 1976
5. Bushing W, Svirbely JR, Ayer LW: Evaluation of the Anaerobe-Tek system for identification of anaerobic bacteria. J Clin Microbiol 17:824, 1983
6. Thorsberry C: Methods for dilution in antimicrobial susceptibility tests for bacteria that grow aerobically. National Committee for Clinical Laboratory Standards 3:34, 1983
7. Barenkamp SJ, Munson RS, Jr, Granoff DM: Outer membrane protein and biotype analysis of pathogenic nontypable *H. influenzae.* Infect Immun 36:535, 1982
8. Wallace RJ, Musher DM, Septimus EJ, et al: *Hemophilus influenzae* infections in adults: Characterization of strains by serotypes, biotypes, and β-lactamase production. J Infect Dis 144:101, 1981
9. DeMaria TF, Briggs BR, Okazaki N, Lim DJ: Experimental otitis media with effusion following middle ear inoculation of nonviable *H. influenzae.* Ann Otol Rhinol Laryngol, 93:52, 1984

PNEUMOCOCCI AND THEIR CAPSULAR POLYSACCHARIDE ANTIGENS IN MIDDLE EAR EFFUSION IN ACUTE OTITIS MEDIA

E. HERVA, M.D., V.-M. HÄIVÄ, M.D., M. KOSKELA, M.Sci., M. LEINONEN, M.D., P. GRÖNROOS, M.D., M. SIPILÄ, M.D., P. KARMA, M.D., and P.H. MÄKELÄ, M.D.

Streptococcus pneumoniae is the most common cause of acute otitis media (AOM) in children.[1,2] In a recent study[3] we showed that *S. pneumoniae* could be isolated from the middle ear fluid (MEF) of 40 percent of patients who had AOM and were younger than 7 years of age. In addition, pneumococcal capsular polysaccharide antigen was detected in the MEF in approximately 30 percent of such patients whose MEF cultures were negative or grew other bacteria than pneumococci. Altogether, evidence of involvement of *S. pneumoniae* was obtained in two-thirds of the children who had AOM. Pneumococcal capsular polysaccharide antigen detection, in addition to conventional culture methods, appeared to yield vital information about the role of *S. pneumoniae* in acute otitis media.

We have now applied both these methods to study a larger and more homogeneous group of children who all were less than 2½ years of age and had acute otitis media, most of them for the first time in their lives. The purpose was to test the earlier conclusions and to extend our experience with the use of pneumococcal antigen detection to children with possibly less advanced otitis than in the earlier study. The data reported here confirm the earlier finding of the usefulness of antigen detection methods, but also suggest that antigen-positive, culture-negative MEF is more often encountered in recurrences of AOM, whereas the first attack of pneumococcal AOM in a child is likely to be both culture and antigen positive.

MATERIALS AND METHODS

The patients in the study were drawn from among the participants in the second Finnish otitis vaccination study described in this volume (see page 256). The children selected for this study lived in Tampere and belonged to the control group, who received the control vaccine (saline) at the age of 7 to 9 months and had an attack of acute otitis media with effusion (AOM) after that. Only the first postvaccination attack of AOM in each child was included. Of the 480 children fulfilling these criteria, 336 (70 percent) had not experienced AOM before. All the children in this study were between 8 months and 2½ years old.

The criteria of AOM and tympanocentesis as well as of collection of MEF and its bacteriologic examination were as previously described.[3,4,5] Pneumococcal polysaccharide antigens were detected and identified by counterimmunoelectrophoresis (screening) and latex agglutination (type/group specificity) methods as previously described.[5] The positive reactions were confirmed after holding the sample for 5 minutes in a boiling water bath. After this treatment the reactions of each sample were specific for one or sometimes two serologic types/groups. The bacteriologic cultures and the antigen determinations were performed without our knowing the results of the other.

The findings are presented as previously by defining each attack of AOM according to the main pathogen (in order *S. pneumoniae, Streptococcus pyogenes, Hemophilus influenzae, Branhamella catarrhalis,* other bacteria) found in the MEF drawn from either ear.

RESULTS

S. pneumoniae was found by culture from the MEF in 158 (33 percent) of the 480 patients. *H. influenzae* was the main pathogen in 63 (13 percent) and *B. catarrhalis* in 35 (7 percent) of the patients. Other bacteria only (most often staphylococci and diphtheroids) were present in 94 (20 per-

TABLE 1 Bacterial Culture Findings and Pneumococcal Capsular Polysaccharide Antigen in the Middle Ear Fluid in Children with Acute Otitis Media

Culture	*No. of Patients (%)*	*Patients with Pneumococcal Antigen (%)*
S. pneumoniae	158 (33)	74
H. influenzae	63 (13)	5
B. catarrhalis	35 (7)	9
Other bacteria	94 (20)	10
Negative	130 (27)	9
Total	480 (100)	30

cent) of the patients, whereas all cultures were negative in 130 patients (27 percent) (Table 1).

Of the 158 patients who had AOM caused by *S. pneumoniae,* pneumococcal antigen was detected in the MEF in 117 (74 percent). In all but three cases this was in accord with the culture result. Pneumococcal antigen was also found in the MEF of 25 (8 percent) of the 322 patients whose MEF cultures did not grow pneumococci. Altogether, *S. pneumoniae* was found by antigen detection methods in 142 (30 percent) of the 480 patients (Table 1). Taking into account the 74 percent sensitivity of the method noted above, this figure indicates that 40 percent (192 patients) of all cases were caused by pneumococci. Culture alone detected 158 (83 percent), and both methods together detected 183 (95 percent) of these cases (Table 2).

The sensitivity of the antigen detection was examined separately for the most common types/groups of *S. pneumoniae* (Table 3). The sensitivity was good—70 to 90 percent—for groups 6, 14, 15, and 19, whereas group 23 antigen was detected in only 38 percent of the culture-positive samples. Types 6A and 6B seemed to be detected at differing efficiencies—85 and 61 percent, respectively. Among the *S. pneumoniae* serotypes/groups detected by culture, group 19 (A and F) composed 24 percent; group 6 (A and B), 26 percent; and group 23, 19 percent. However, if *S. pneumoniae* had been sought for by antigen detection alone, the percentage of group 19 would have been higher (34 percent) and that of type 23 lower (9 percent) in accordance with the different sensitivity of the antigen detection method for the different serotypes.

TABLE 2 Comparison of Bacterial Culture and Antigen Determination Methods in the Detection of *S. pneumoniae* in Patients with Acute Otitis Media

S. pneumoniae in MEF Culture	*Pneumococcal Capsular Antigen in MEF*		
	Positive	*Negative*	*Total*
Positive	117	41	158
Negative	25	297	322
Total	142	338	480

CONCLUSIONS

In this study of children 8 months to 2½ years of age with acute otitis media, *S. pneumoniae* was found in 33 percent by culture and in 38 percent by culture and/or antigen detection methods (or in 40 percent if the sensitivity [74 percent] of the antigen detection is taken into account). These percentages are considerably lower than those seen in our earlier study,[3] in which the respective figures were 40 and 57 percent. As reasons for the difference we have considered the following four possibilities.

(1) Method. The methods of sampling, transport, and storage of MEF, of bacterial culture, and of antigen detection were very similar in both studies.[3,5] A possible methodologic difference is noticed in the efficiency of antigen detection in those MEF samples from which pneumococci were isolated by culture—67 percent in the present study, 88 percent in the previous one. The difference was especially marked for the group 23 antigen—38 percent in the present study, 73 percent in the previous one. This kind of difference would easily arise from slight differences in the serum batches used. However, it alone is insufficient to explain the overall difference between the studies.

TABLE 3 Serotype/Group-Specific Detection of Pneumococcal Capsular Polysaccharide Antigens in Middle Ear Fluid Samples Growing *S. pneumoniae*

Type/Group	*No. of Samples*	*Antigen Positive*	
		No.	*%*
6A	20	17	85
6B	31	19	61
14	16	11	69
15	13	10	77
19A	13	12	92
19F	34	31	91
23	37	14	38
All types/groups	196	137	67

(2) Age of the Patients. The patients in the present study were younger (less than 2½ years old) than those (6 months to 6 years) in the previous study.[3] However, the occurrence *S. pneumoniae* detected by culture was similar throughout the age range studied,[3] and the same was true for the pneumococcal antigen (Luotonen, J. and Leinonen, M., 1981, unpublished data).

(3) Otitis History. In the present study, 70 percent of the attacks of AOM occurred in children without previous attacks, whereas in the earlier study[3] only 20 percent of the children were studied during their first attack of AOM and over 50 percent had had several previous attacks. It seems possible that this is an important difference. It also seems possible that the local immune response could prevent the growth of the pneumococcus[8] during a subsequent attack while the antigen could still be detectable for a short time.

(4) Epidemiology. Since the two studies were performed in different years and in different locations, the occurrence of *S. pneumoniae* and/or its individual serotypes/groups might be different. Indeed, a smaller percentage of the pneumococci in the present study were of type 3, and a larger fraction were of groups 6 and 23. Even though this does not readily explain the observed difference, it is possible that the epidemiologic situation had some influence on the occurrence of *S. pneumoniae* in AOM and especially on its demonstration by antigen detection methods.

Altogether, the present study can be considered to reflect the bacteriology of AOM in young children having their first otitis attack. It also suggests that in this kind of material the AOM may be less often (up to 40 percent) caused by pneumococci than in children who have experienced several previous attacks (up to 67 percent when calculated in a similar manner).

Finally, our experience with pneumococcal capsular polysaccharide antigen detection indicates that this method can be used as an adjunct to bacteriologic cultures to study the role of *S. pneumoniae* in otitis media in the same manner in which it has been used in the diagnosis of pneumococcal pneumonia.[9,10] Antigen detection alone may be useful in circumstances in which culture facilities are not available to evaluate the occurrence of *S. pneumoniae* and the role of its separate serotypes/groups—as the etiologic agent in acute otitis media.

We thank Tarja Kaijalainen for expert technical assistance, and Merck Sharp & Dohme Research Laboratories (West Point, PA) for a grant to support the study.

REFERENCES

1. Klein JO: The epidemiology of pneumococcal disease in infants and children. Rev. Infect Dis 3:246, 1981
2. Luotonen J: Studies on the bacteriology of acute otitis media. Ph.D. thesis, The University of Oulu, Oulu, Finland, 1982
3. Luotonen J, Herva E, Karma P, et al: The bacteriology of acute otitis media in children with special reference to *Streptococcus pneumoniae* as studied by bacteriological and antigen detection methods. Scand J Infect Dis 177, 1981
4. Mäkelä PH, Sibakov M, Herva E, et al: Pneumococcal vaccine and otitis media. Lancet ii:547, 1980
5. Leinonen M; Detection of pneumococcal capsular polysaccharide antigens by latex agglutination, counterimmunoelectrophoresis, and radio immunoassay in middle ear exudates in acute otitis media. J Clin Microbiol 11:135, 1980
6. Ogra PL, Bernstein JM, Yurchak AM, et al: Characteristics of secretory immune system in human middle ear: Implications in otitis media. J. Immunol 112:488, 1974
7. Lewis DM, Schram JL, Birck HG, Lim DJ: Antibody activity in otitis media with effusion. Ann Otol 88:392, 1979
8. Sloyer JL Jr, Howie VM, Ploussard JH, et al: Immune response to acute otitis media: Association between middle ear fluid antibody and the clearing of clinical infection. J Clin Microbiol 4:306, 1976
9. Tebbutt GM, Coleman DJ: Evaluation of some methods for the laboratory examination of sputum. J Clin Pathol 31:724, 1978
10. Kalin M, Lindberg AA, Olausson E-H: Diagnosis of pneumococcal pneumonia by coagglutination and counterimmunoelectrophoresis of sputum samples. Eur J Clin Microbiol 1:91, 1982

ENDOTOXIN IN MIDDLE EAR EFFUSIONS FROM PATIENTS WITH CHRONIC OTITIS MEDIA WITH EFFUSION

THOMAS F. DeMARIA, Ph.D., RICHARD B. PRIOR, Ph.D., BRUCE R. BRIGGS, DAVID J. LIM, M.D., and HERBERT G. BIRCK, M.D.

Hemophilus influenzae is considered the most common pathogenic organism associated with chronic otitis media with effusion (OME).[1] Our earlier study[2] indicated that when killed *H. influenzae* organisms were injected into the tympanum they induced clear, amber-colored middle ear effusions (MEEs), and that endotoxin purified from these bacteria also induced middle ear effusion. It was hypothesized that endotoxin on the surface of these gram-negative bacteria might be responsible for the inflammation and fluid accumulation in the middle ear.[2] Endotoxins are lipopolysaccharide complexes present on the outer surface of most gram-negative bacteria.[3] Endotoxin retains its potency after the death of the microbe and is released into the extracellular environment in an active form. The present study was undertaken to determine the possible role of endotoxin in chronic OME by measuring endotoxin levels in human MEEs from children with chronic OME.

MATERIALS AND METHODS

Patient Samples

The study group was composed of 89 patients, aged 6 months to 13 years, who underwent tympanostomy tube placement because of persistent middle ear effusion. MEEs were collected, processed for Gram stain, and cultured for bacteria according to the protocols previously described.[4]

Limulus Lysate Assay for Endotoxin. A total of 89 MEEs was used for this study. The samples were divided into four groups: culture-positive (*H. influenzae* or *Streptococcus pneumoniae*) and culture-negative but Gram-stain-positive or -negative MEEs. The specimens were stored at −80°C before assay for endotoxin, and all the MEEs were assayed within six months. The concentration of endotoxin in the MEEs was determined by the microdilution amebocyte lysate test.[5] The limulus amebocyte lysate used for these studies was obtained from a commercial source (Pyrogent, Mallinckrodt Inc, St. Louis, MO) and a single lot, 2AV, was used throughout. That lot of lysate had a sensitivity of 0.05 ng/ml ref. standard EC2. The microdilution procedure was performed as previously described.[5]

Because of the limited volume of the effusions, aliquots were removed and intitially diluted 1 to 5 (vol/vol) with pyrogen-free saline so that each titration could be performed in duplicate. All the reagents used throughout the test procedure were pyrogen-free materials. Preliminary control experiments were conducted to rule out exogenous endotoxin contamination by assaying for endotoxin in sterile, pyrogen-free water, which was aspirated through the surgical collection devices. In separate experiments selected MEEs were boiled for 10 minutes at 100°C and assayed to ensure that the substrate being measured was actually endotoxin, which is heat stable, and not some other proteolytic substance that might be present in the MEEs. This served to rule out false-positive results. MEEs were also assayed with the addition of Pyrosperse (Mallinckrodt, Inc, St. Louis, MO), a polyionic dispersing agent, to rule out the presence of endotoxin-masking components. Similarly, specific amounts of *Escherichia coli* endotoxin were added to assay wells and monitored to indicate that there were no substances in the MEEs which interfered with the sensitivity of the assay.

Statistical Analysis. The two-tailed Student's t test was used to detect significant differences in endotoxin concentration.

RESULTS

Seventy-one of the 89 MEEs (80 percent) exhibited endotoxin activity, ranging from 0.5 ng/ml to more than 512 ng/ml. With one exception, significant levels of endotoxin were present in MEEs from which *H. influenzae* were cultured. The mean titer of *H. influenzae*-positive MEEs was 157 ng/ml (Table 1). MEEs that contained culturable *S. pneumoniae* contained a mean of 21.8 ng/ml of endotoxin per milliliter, approximately sevenfold less than that measured in MEEs from which *H. influenzae* were cultured ($p < .05$).

Endotoxin was present in 67 percent of the culture-negative MEEs (Table 2). In effusions that did not contain viable bacteria but demonstrated any bacteria by the Gram stain, the mean endotoxin concentration was 3.3 ng/ml. MEEs that did not contain bacteria either by culture or Gram stain had a mean concentration of 12.9 ng/ml. The fourfold difference in the endotoxin concentration between these two samples was not satistically significant ($p > .05$). However, the concentration of endotoxin in both sets of culture-negative MEEs was significantly lower than the levels of endotoxin in the MEEs that grew either *H. influenzae* or *S. pneumoniae* ($p < 0.05$).

Control experiments indicated that the endotoxin titers did not change after boiling, meaning that the substrate being measured was actually endotoxin. The addition of Pyrosperse to the assay system did not increase the titers, which discounts the presence of endotoxin-masking components in the MEEs. The addition of known concentrations of *E. coli* endotoxin and reassaying revealed that there were no substances in the MEEs that interfered with the specificity of the assay.

TABLE 1 Endotoxin (ng/ml) in Culture-Positive Human MEE*

Bacteria Isolated	No. Specimens	Endotoxin (ng/ml) Mean (±S.D.)	Range
Hemophilus influenzae	20	157 (±190)	0–512
Streptococcus pneumoniae	20	21.8 (±29.5)	0–128

*Mallinkrodt Pyrogent ref. standard 50 pg EC_2 used throughout; mean ±1 sd

TABLE 2 Endotoxin (ng/ml) in Culture-Negative Human MEE*

Gram Stain Results	No. Specimens	Endotoxin (ng/ml) Mean (±S.D.)	Range
Positive	25	3.3 (±5.2)	0–16
Negative	24	12.9 (±31)	0–128

*Mallinkrodt Pyrogent ref. standard 50 pg EC_2 used throughout; mean ±1 sd

DISCUSSION

Bacterial endotoxin is an extremely biologically active material and a potent inducer of inflammation and modulator of the immune response. Endotoxin is capable of interaction with complement and components of the clotting system. Endotoxin has been shown to effect the release of various vasoactive amines and other mediators of inflammation by direct interaction with macrophages, polymorphonuclear leukocytes, and other cell types.[3] It can therefore be postulated that endotoxin is responsible for the persistence of the effusions even long after the gram-negative bacteria are no longer viable, if they are trapped in the middle ear.

That endotoxin is present in the highest concentration in effusions containing viable *H. influenzae* is expected, since this organism is gram-negative and contains endotoxin on its surface. However, it is surprising to find that the effusions that grew *S. pneumoniae*, a gram-positive bacterium that does not contain endotoxin, do contain a substantial level of endotoxin. There may be several explanations for these findings. It is well documented that the bacterial species may change during the course of treatment of otitis media,[6] and it is possible that gram-negative bacteria (for example, *H. influenzae, Neisseria* sp., or *Pseudomonas* sp.) had originally been present in the MEEs but were no longer viable at the time of culture.

The levels of endotoxin in the culture-negative MEEs were the same regardless of whether or not bacteria were detectable by the Gram stain procedure. We were puzzled by the presence of endotoxin in those effusions that were culture-negative and Gram stain negative. One possible explanation could be that gram-negative, endotoxin-containing bacteria, once present in the middle ear, became fragmented by antibiotic therapy or by proteolytic enzymes, releasing endotoxin.

Furthermore, the significance of our findings is enhanced by the fact that as little as 0.1 ng of purified endotoxin per milliliter, well below the lower level of endotoxin found in the human MEEs, was capable of inducing inflammation and middle ear effusion in the chinchilla model.[2] Endotoxin remaining in the middle ear might play an important role in the pathogenesis of OME by sustaining the inflammatory response after the acute primary infection has cleared. Our earlier study[7] showed that over 80 percent of the MEEs demonstrated bacteria by Gram stain, while only 47 percent yielded viable bacteria on culture. The frequency and concentration of endotoxin observed in the culture-negative human MEEs in this study lends credence to this hypothesis.

Our data indicate that 67 percent of the sterile MEEs contain endotoxin, which is in contrast to the findings of Bernstein and colleagues.[8] In their study only 7 percent (1 of 14) of the sterile MEEs were positive by the limulus assay. Although this discrepancy cannot be fully explained, three factors must be considered: (1) Their study was qualitative and did not include titration of the endotoxin; (2) two different patient populations were used in the studies; and (3) different commercially available sources of limulus lysate were used, which may have resulted in different sensitivities.

In summary, our data indicate that endotoxin is present in a high percentage of human MEEs, including those that are culture negative, and contributes to the pathogenesis of OME.

This study was supported in part by a grant from The Deafness Research Foundation.

REFERENCES

1. Lim DJ, DeMaria TF: Panel discussion: Pathogenesis of otitis media. Bacteriology and immunology. Laryngoscope 92:278, 1982
2. DeMaria TF, Briggs BR, Okazaki N, Lim DJ: Experimental otitis media with effusion following middle ear inoculation of nonviable *H. influenzae*. Ann Otol Rhinol Laryngol, 93:52, 1984
3. Morrison DC, Ulevitch RJ: The effects of bacterial endotoxin on host mediation systems. Am J Pathol 93:427, 1978
4. Liu YS, Lang RW, Lim DJ, Birck HG: Microorganisms in chronic otitis media with effusion. Ann Otol Rhinol Laryngol 85 (Suppl 25):245, 1976
5. Prior RB, Spagna VA: Adaptation of a microdilution procedure to the limulus lysate assay for endotoxin. J Clin Microbiol 10:394, 1979
6. Howie VM, Ploussard JH: Bacterial etiology and antimicrobial treatment of exudative otitis media: Relation of antibiotic therapy to relapse. South Med J 64:233, 1971
7. Liu YS, Lim DJ, Lang RW, Birck HG: Chronic middle ear effusions: Immunochemical and bacteriological investigation. Arch Otolaryngol 101:278, 1975
8. Bernstein JM, Praino MD, Neter E: Detection of endotoxin in ear specimens from patients with chronic otitis media by means of the limulus amebocyte lysate test. Can J Microbiol 26:645, 1980

CONTRIBUTIONS OF BACTERIA AND POLYMORPHONUCLEAR LEUKOCYTES TO MIDDLE EAR INFLAMMATION IN CHRONIC OTITIS MEDIA WITH EFFUSION

G. SCOTT GIEBINK, M.D., BARBARA A. CARLSON, M.D., SETH V. HETHERINGTON, M.D., MARGARET K. HOSTETTER, M.D., CHAP T. LE, M.D., and S. K. JUHN, M.D.

Children with acute otitis media often have persistent middle ear effusion for weeks after the acute event, and 5 to 10 percent of these children develop otitis media with effusion (OME) lasting 12 weeks or longer.[1,2] Etiologic and pathogenetic factors that result in chronic OME are poorly understood. In an earlier study of 729 children with chronic OME, we reported that 35 percent of the 892 middle ear effusions yielded bacteria on culture, and bacteria were seen on Gram-stained specimens of 17 percent of the 294 sterile effusions.[3] Bacteria cultured from effusions included type b and nontype b *Hemophilus influenzae, Streptococcus pneumoniae, Branhamella catarrhalis* and *Staphylococcus epidermidis.* A strong association was observed between increased numbers of polymorphonuclear leukocytes (PMNLs) in the effusion sample and certain bacteria (*H. influenzae* and *S. pneumoniae*) but not other bacteria (*S. epidermidis* and *B. catarrhalis*). The present study was performed to explore further the relationship between bacteria and PMNLs in the middle ear space of children with chronic OME and to determine whether the PMNLs are the source of lysozyme and subsequent middle ear tissue injury.

MATERIALS AND METHODS

Twenty-five middle ear effusion samples were obtained from 20 children, aged 1 to 12 years, at the time of myringotomy and tympanostomy tube insertion performed because of OME persisting for at least two months before surgery. Each sample was inoculated directly onto chocolate agar and smeared on glass slides for Gram stain examination immediately after collection in the operating room, as previously described.[3] The sample was then frozen at −70°C. Eleven samples of effusion fluid were sterile, ten yielded nontype b *H. influenzae,* and four cultured *S. epidermidis.* Twenty-three samples were mucoid, and two were serous.

Each sample was thawed, diluted 1:3 in Hank's balanced salt solution with 0.1 percent gel, pH 7.4 (gel-HBSS), and homogenized to ensure complete mixing. Chemotactic activity of PMNLs from middle ear effusion fluid was measured using the under-agarose method previously described by Abramson and colleagues.[4] PMNL migration was measured, and the chemotactic activity was calculated by subtracting the distance that the leading PMNL had migrated from the PMNL well edge toward the gel-HBSS (random migration) from the distance that the leading PMNL had migrated toward the effusion sample. Lysozyme content was measured using the Quantiplate Lysozyme Test Kit (Kallestad Laboratories, Inc, Chaska, MN).[5] Lactoferrin content was measured by a double antibody sandwich enzyme-linked immunoabsorbent assay.[6] Serum complement factor C3 was measured by the radial immunodiffusion technique and required a 5 μl aliquot of each sample.[7] Complement C5a concentration was measured by a radioactive (^{125}I) antigen-binding assay using the Human Complement C5a des Arg Radioimmunoassay Kit (Upjohn Diagnostics, Kalamazoo, MI).[8]

RESULTS

The mean (± SE) PMNL chemotactic activity of the 25 effusions (0.85 ± 0.24) was significantly greater than the buffer control (0.14 ± 0.10; $p < .001$); and the mean lactoferrin concentration of the samples (122.2 ± 24.0) was significantly higher than the mean concentration of lactoferrin in serum (0.3 ± 0.1) suggesting the PMNL did indeed contribute to the middle ear inflammation. The mean concentrations of lysozyme and lactoferrin were significantly higher in effusions that cultured *S. epidermidis* or *H. influenzae* than in sterile effusions, and the mean chemotactic activity was significantly greater in *H. influenzae*-, but not *S. epidermidis*-positive effusions, compared with sterile effusions (Fig. 1).

The concentration of lysozyme in effusion was selected as an index of total middle ear inflammation, since this enzyme is found in PMNL granules as well as in mucosal epithelial secretory cells. Lactoferrin concentration in the effusion was used as an indicator for PMNL degranulation. We observed a significant association between lactoferrin and lysozyme content ($p = .002$); however, the weak correlation ($r = .56$) between lactoferrin and lysozyme suggested that cells other than PMNLs contributed a significant amount of lysozyme to the middle ear space in chronic OME. Analysis of covariance was used to determine the effect of bacteria on lactoferrin and lysozyme content of effusion. PMNL degranulation, reflected by the lactoferrin concentration, accounted for 87 percent ($r = .93$) and 17 percent ($r = .41$) of the lysozyme variation in effusions that cultured *S. epidermidis* and *H. influenzae*, respectively, and for 48 percent ($r = .68$) of the lysozyme variation in sterile effusions. These results suggested that non-PMNL sources of lysozyme, such as middle ear mucosal epithelial cells, were more extensively involved in middle ear inflammation in ears that had sterile or *H. influenzae*-positive effusion and that these cells were minimally stimulated by *S. epidermidis*. However, because of the small sam-

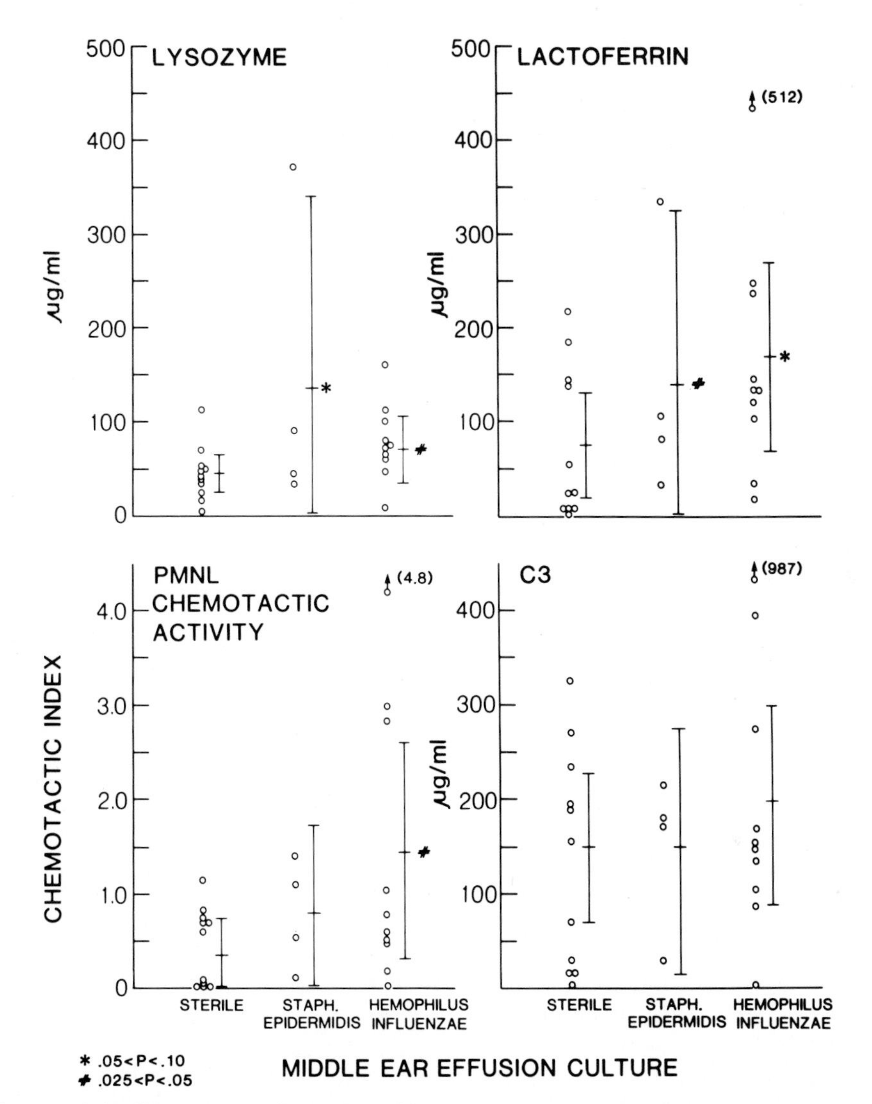

Figure 1 Concentrations of lysozyme, lactoferrin, C3, and PMNL chemotactic activity in 25 chronic middle ear effusion samples.

ple size in each bacteriologic grouping, the three correlation coefficients did not differ significantly. Also, because the slopes of the lines differed, it was not possible to determine the effect of bacteria on lysozyme content independent of the effect of PMNLs.

The source of PMNL chemotactic activity in these effusion samples was examined by studying the relationship between bacteriologic results, PMNL chemotactic activity, and C3 and C5a content. An inverse correlation between chemotactic activity and C3 concentration was observed, as might be expected if chemotaxigenesis was associated with complement activation. However, the association was weak ($r = .23$, $p = .14$), suggesting that most of the chemotactic activity was related to bacterial factors released into the middle ear space and not to complement activation. In support of this conclusion, we observed that the mean C3 concentration of effusions that cultured *H. influenzae* and *S. epidermidis* was similar to the C3 concentration of sterile effusions; and C5a content, which was measured in eight samples, correlated poorly with PMNL chemotactic activity ($r = .02$, $p > .4$).

Analysis of covariance was used to examine the contribution of bacteria to PMNL chemotactic activity in effusion. *H. influenzae* had a greater effect than *S. epidermidis* on chemotactic activity regardless of the lactoferrin content, and sterile effusions showed the lowest level of chemotactic activity at all lactoferrin concentrations. These results indicate that bacteria present in chronic middle ear effusions enhance middle ear inflammation by providing PMNL chemotaxins to the effusion, and these chemotaxins recruit additional PMNL from the circulation, which might maintain the inflammatory process by releasing more lysozyme and lactoferrin.

CONCLUSION

The significant association between lactoferrin and lysozyme concentration observed in our effusion samples supported the hypothesized contribution of PMNLs to middle ear inflammation in chronic OME, since lactoferrin and lysozyme are both contained within the specific granules of PMNL. However, the weak correlation suggested that there was less mucosal cell-derived inflammation in ears that cultured *S, epidermidis* than in sterile effusions or in those that cultured *H. influenzae*.

The action of lysosomal hydrolytic enzymes in the middle ear space would be expected to lead to local tissue injury and capillary permeability with passive diffusion of serum protein into the middle ear space. Consistent with this hypothesis, we observed C3 concentrations in effusions equal to those found in serum. Since complement is activated by a variety of substances, including immunoglobulin, immune complexes, endotoxin, and bacterial polysaccharides, we anticipated that the chemotactic peptide C5a would be demonstrated in these effusions. Although an inverse correlation between PMNL chemotactic activity and C3 concentration was observed, the association was weak, suggesting that most of the chemotactic activity was derived from bacterial factors released into the effusion rather than from complement activation. In addition, the C5a concentration showed no correlation with the degree of PMNL chemotactic activity.

These results support the hypothesis that bacteria and PMNL contribute to chronic middle ear inflammation, perhaps due to the action of lysosomal hydrolases. Eradication of these bacteria from the middle ear space of children with chronic OME might disrupt the host reponses that maintain local inflammation and effusion.

This study was supported in part by grant numbers NS-14538 from the National Institute of Neurological and Communicative Disorders and Stroke; AI-06931 and AI-17160 from the National Institute of Allergy and Infectious Diseases; and a grant from the Minnesota Medical Foundation.

REFERENCES

1. Teele DW, Rosner BA, Klein JO. Epidemiology of otitis media in children. Ann Otol Rhinol Laryngol 89 (Suppl 68):5–6, 1980
2. Schwartz RH, Schwartz DM, Rodriguez WJ. Otitis media with effusion (OME): Natural course in untreated children. Pediatr Res 15:556 (Abstr 687), 1981
3. Giebink GS, Juhn SK, Weber ML, Le CT. The bacteriology and cytology of chronic otitis media with effusion. Pediatr Infec Dis 1:98, 1982
4. Abramson JA, Giebink GS, Mills EL, Quie PG. Polymorphonuclear leukocyte dysfunction during influenza virus infection in chinchillas. Infec Dis 143:836, 1981
5. Osserman EF, Lawlor DP. Serum and urinary lysozyme (muramidase) in monocytic and nonmyelocytic leukemia. J Exp Med 124:921, 1966.
6. Hetherington SV, Spitznagel JK, Quie PG. An enzyme-linked immunoassay (ELISA) for measurement of lactoferrin. To be published
7. Mancini G, Carbonara AO, Heremans JF. Immuno-chemical quantitation of antigens by single radial immuno diffusion. In Immunochemistry, 2:235, 1965
8. Chenoweth DE, Hugli TE. Techniques and significance of C3a and C5a measurement. In *Future Perspectives in Clinical Laboratory Immunoassays*. Nakamura, RM (ed): New York: Alan R. Liss, Inc, 1980

DEFECTIVE PHAGOCYTIC AND ANTIBACTERIAL ACTIVITY OF MIDDLE EAR NEUTROPHILS

J.M. BERNSTEIN, M.D., Ph.D., L.L. MOORE, Ph.D,
and P. OGRA, M.D.

There have been few studies to date on phagocytic activities in exudate material. We have previously reported that phagocytic cells reach the middle ear in adequate numbers and are capable of engulfing and killing a standard test organism, *Staphylococcus aureus* 502A.[1] In those studies we also reported a pronounced defect in phagocytosis of *S. aureus* by neutrophils from seromucinous ear effusions (Fig. 1), as compared with simultaneously studied blood phagocytes. Only a mild microbicidal defect was observed in the purulent exudate neutrophils. No functional defect was seen in phagocytes obtained from serous or mucoid effusions.

The previous study did not allow for distinction between a cellular and a humoral defect, since we used the patients' own serum as opsonin for the test staphylococcus. We now report an extension of this study using two other test organisms, *Candida albicans* and *Streptococcus pneumoniae*, and a standardized opsonin solution to assess the cellular component of phagocytosis of neutrophils simultaneously obtained from ear effusions and blood in 19 children with otitis media.

MATERIALS AND METHODS

Phagocytosis was assessed using the acridine orange supravital stain technique of Pantazis and Kniker.[2] Blood and ear effusion samples were collected at the time of the myringotomy procedure, and the phagocytic cells were deposited on glass coverslips as monolayer preparations. The adherent neutrophils were overlaid with bacteria or yeast suspensions opsonized with 10 percent fresh-frozen AB serum. Neutrophils and microorganisms were allowed to interact for 60 minutes in a moist 5 percent CO_2 incubator at 37° C. Extracellular organisms were rinsed off the phagocytic cells, and their ingested organisms were stained with acridine orange and enumerated under fluorescent light. Acridine orange stains intact DNA green and denatured DNA red; consequently, ingested organisms stain green when they are alive and red when they are dead. All ingested organisms (dead and alive) were counted and expressed as the total number of phagocytized organisms per 100 neutrophils.

RESULTS

Using *C. albicans* as the test organism, we observed a pronounced phagocytic defect in MEE neutrophils (Fig. 2). Blood neutrophils ingested 207 *Candida* per 100 cells, while the ear neutrophils engulfed only 126 yeast per 100 cells. This represents a 40 percent decrease in phagocytosis for the MEE neutrophils. These data represent the pooled mean values obtained in four seromucinous, two serous, and three mucoid effusions, compared with simultaneously obtained blood samples. No purulent exudates were available. The phagocytic defect seemed comparable in all three types of effusion. The percentage of phagocytizing neutrophils (phagocytic avidity) was the same for blood and ear preparations.

When *S. pneumoniae* was used as the test organism, in preparations from ten other children, a phagocytic defect was again seen in the ear effusion neutrophils. This defect was present when the cells were tested with the smooth encapsulated streptococcal organisms (blood neutrophils ingested 580 bacteria per 100 cells, while ear neutrophils ingested 415 organisms, $p < 0.0025$) and when the neutrophils were tested with the rough revertant streptococci (blood neutrophils ingested 782 *S. pneumoniae* per 100 cells, and the ear neutrophils ingested 622 bacteria per 100 cells, $p < 0.05$). When the data were analyzed according to purulent and nonpurulent effusions, the phagocytic defect could be seen in the ear neutrophils regardless of the type of ear effusion.

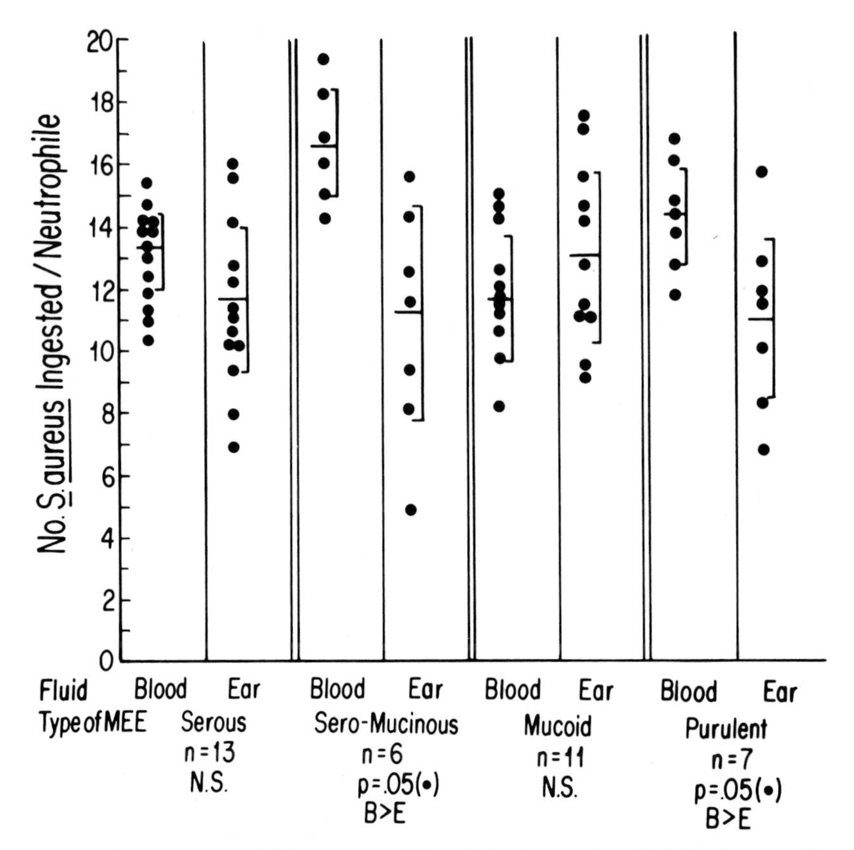

Figure 1 Phagocytosis of *S. aureus* by middle ear neutrophils and simultaneously studied blood neutrophils. A defect in phagocytosis is seen in neutrophils from purulent and seromucinous ear effusions.

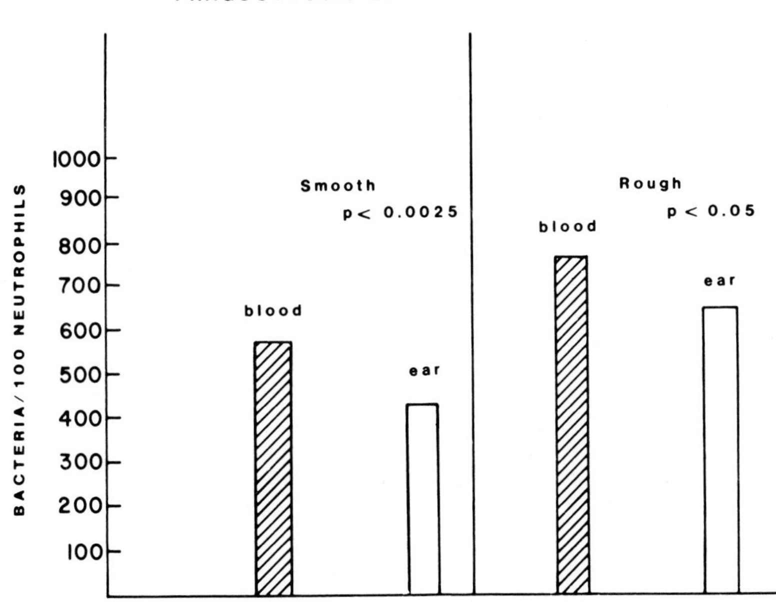

Figure 2 Phagocytosis of *S. pneumoniae* by middle ear neutrophils and simultaneously studied blood neutrophils. A defect in phagocytosis is seen in ear neutrophils when both smooth and rough forms are ingested.

Microbicidal activity toward *C. albicans* and *S. pneumoniae* (smooth and rough strains) was assessed for blood and ear neutrophils in these same patients. Candidacidal activity was similar for ear neutrophils (56 percent of the *Candida* killed) when compared with blood neutrophils (63 percent of *Candida* killed, $p > 0.1$). A mild microbicidal defect was seen in ear neutrophils (46.5 percent organisms killed) as compared with blood neutrophils (58 percent organisms killed) when *S. pneumoniae* type II (smooth strain) was used as the test organism ($p < 0.025$). The small numbers of experiments precluded interpretation of differences observed in samples from purulent and nonpurulent effusions (Table 1). The rough revertant *S. pneumoniae* type II was killed normally in MEE neutrophils (50 percent killed by blood neutrophils compared with 48.4 percent killed by ear neutrophils, $p > 0.1$).

In summary, a cellular phagocytic defect affects ear effusion neutrophils in children with otitis media. The defect is most pronounced in purulent effusions, but depression of phagocytosis exists in ear neutrophils regardless of the ear effusion type. The defect is seen in respect to all organisms examined to date, namely *S. aureus, C. albicans*, and *S. pneumoniae* type II, smooth and rough stains.

A mild microbicidal defect towards *S. aureus* and smooth strain *S. pneumoniae* is also seen in MEE neutrophils.

Further study is required to determine whether this deterioration of phagocytic and microbicidal functions in ear effusion neutrophils is due to an auto-oxidation of cellular membranes[3] or to a loss, blockage, or reorientation of receptor sites for the two essential opsonins, antibody and complement,[4,5] during the passage from the blood compartment to the infected site and after exposure to the infecting organism.

TABLE 1 Phagocytosis of Streptococcus pneumoniae (Organisms/100 PMNs)

	Purulent Ear Effusions (5)		*Nonpurulent Ear Effusions (5)*	
	Smooth	*Rough*	*Smooth*	*Rough*
Blood	578	736	582	810
Ear	342	622	488	622
P	< 0.025	< 0.05	< 0.05	< 0.05

REFERENCES

1. Bernstein JM, Moore L, Cumella J, Ogra P: Phagocytosis and microbicidal killing in middle ear effusion. Presented at the Association for Research in Otolaryngology, St. Petersburg Beach, FL, January 1983
2. Pantazis CG, Kniker WT: Assessment of blood leukocyte microbial killing by using a new fluorochrome microassay. J Reticuloendothel Soc 23:155, 1979
3. Bjorksten B: Autooxidation and neutrophil function. Immunology Today, December 1980, pp 111–112
4. Wilton JMA, Renggli HH, Lehner T: The role of Fc and C3b receptors in phagocytosis by inflammatory polymorphonuclear leukocytes in man. Immunology 32:955, 1977
5. Fearon DT, Collins LA: Increased expression of C3b receptors on polymorphonuclear leukocytes induced by chemotactic factors and by purification procedures. J Immunol 130:370, 1983

MOLECULAR MECHANISMS OF ADHESION OF *STREPTOCOCCUS PNEUMONIAE* TO HUMAN OROPHARYNGEAL EPITHELIAL CELLS

BENGT ANDERSSON, M.D., HAKON LEFFLER, M.D., Ph.D., FINN JØRGENSEN, M.D., SVEN LARSSON, M.D., GÖRAN MAGNUSSON, Ph.D., OLLE NYLÉN, M.D., Ph.D., and CATHARINA SVANBORG EDÉN, M.D., Ph.D.

Bacteria colonizing the nasopharynx need to adhere to components of the mucosa to avoid being eliminated by the flow of secretions.[1] The role of adhesion for pneumococcal colonization of the nasopharynx preceding the onset of acute otitis media (AOM) has been the focus of our studies. Pneumococci isolated from patients with recurrent AOM were found to adhere in larger numbers to human nasopharyngeal epithelial cells than strains from invasive infections such as meningitis or septicemia.[2] In addition, more bacteria attached to epithelial cells from patients with recurrent AOM than to healthy control cells.[3]

Increased virulence in the middle ear for adhering pneumococci, and thus increased susceptibility to infection, might occur in individuals receptive to bacterial attachment.

The biochemical basis for the adhesion of pneumococci is gradually being worked out. The bacterial surface structure-adhesin involved in the binding is probably of a proteinaceous nature[1] (Andersson B, et al, unpublished data), but it has not been identified. This chapter presents evidence that the complementary structures on the epithelial cell, the receptors, are glycoconjugates containing the sequence GlcNAcβ1→3Gal.

MATERIALS AND METHODS

Bacteria

Pneumococcal strains EF 3114 and 10276 were used. The conditions for cultivation have been described elsewhere.[4]

Adhesion Assay

Epithelial cells collected from the oropharyngeal mucosa of a healthy donor were mixed with bacteria. After centrifugation and incubation for 30 minutes at 37°C, the samples were washed free of unattached bacteria in 0.15M saline. The number of bacteria adhering to 40 cells was counted by light microscopy, and the mean number per cell was calculated.[1,4]

Inhibition Experiments

Pneumococci were preincubated with compounds of potential receptor structure. After the bacteria had been washed once in saline, the epithelial cells were added and adhesion was done as described above. When a free saccharide was used the washing step was omitted. Inhibition of adherence compared with the saline control indicated receptor activity of the inhibitor EID_{75}.[4]

Coating Experiments

Epithelial cells were preincubated for 2 hours with the potential receptor structure. After the epithelial cells had been washed once in saline the bacteria were added. An increased adherence to the coated cells indicated receptor activity.[4]

Receptor Analogues

Glycoconjugates. Human plasma fibronectin (Table 1) was isolated according to the methods of Vuento and Vaheri and Simpson and colleagues[5,6] and kindly provided by Dr. W. A. Simpson, Medical Center, VA Hospital, Memphis, TN. The preparation of the glycolipids neolactotetraosylceramide, N-acetylneuraminosylneolactotetraosylceramide, and globotetraosylceramide is described in our previous publication.[4]

Free Saccharides. The tetrasaccharides neolactotetraose and lactotetraose were isolated

TABLE 1 Effect of Glycoconjugates on the Adhesion of Pneumococci to Human Pharyngeal Epithelial Cells

Compound	*Chemical Structure of Characteristic Saccharide Part*	*Inhibition*		*Coating*	
		Concentration (μg/ml)	*Adhesion % of Control (Mean)*	*Concentration (μg/ml)*	*Adhesion % of Control (Mean)*
Fibronectin	NeuNAcα2→4(6)Galβ1→4GlcNAcβ1→2Manα1↘ $^{6}_{3}$Manβ1→4GlcNAcβ1→4GlcNAc-ASN; NeuNAcα2→4(6)Galβ1→4GlcNAcβ1→2Manα1↗	100	42	1000	234
Neolactotetraosylceramide	Galβ1→4GlcNAcβ1→3Galβ1→4Glc-Cer	200	59	200	190
Sialylneolactotetraosylceramide	NeuNAcα2→3Galβ1→4GlcNAcβ1→3Galβ1→4Glc-Cer	200	100	200	94
Globotetraosylceramide	GalNAcβ1→3Galα1→4Galβ1→4Glc-Cer	—	—	200	100

*Bacteria were preincubated with the glycoconjugates before addition of epithelial cells (competitive inhibition, expressed in percentage of a saline control).

†Epithelial cells were preincubated with glycoconjugates, washed, and used for adherence testing (coating, increased adhesion expressed in percentage of saline control).

from human milk[7] and the octasaccharide from the urine of a patient with GM_1-gangliosidosis (Table 1).[8] The disaccharides were synthetic.

RESULTS

Table 1 shows the effect of various glycoconjugates on pneumococcal adhesion to epithelial cells. The active glycoconjugates both inhibited adhesion after bacterial pretreatment and increased adhesion after epithelial cell pretreatment. Fibronectin was most effective, giving an inhibition to 42 percent of the control after bacterial pretreatment at 100 μg/ml and an increase to 234 percent of the control after coating of epithelial cells with 1000 μg/ml. Neolactotetraosylceramide had a similar effect (59 percent of the saline control after bacterial pretreatment and 190 percent of the control after coating, both with 200 μg/ml). The control glycolipids were inactive.

Based on the glycoconjugate results, free oligosaccharides were selected for testing. Table 2 shows the effect of various free saccharides on adhesion. Neolactotetraose and lactotetraose were the best inhibitors, with an EID_{75} of 1.5 and 1.0 respectively. The disaccharide GlcNAcβ1→3Galβ-o-Me completely inhibited adhesion at 10 mg/ml, with an EID_{75} of 4.5 mg/ml. It was thus three times less active than the tetrasaccharides on a weight basis. The specificity of recognition was shown by the lack of inhibitory activity of GlcNAcβ1→4Galβ-o-Me, which differs only in the linkage of the two sugars.

TABLE 2 Inhibition of Pneumococcal Adhesion by Natural Oligosaccharides and Synthetic Disaccharides

Compound Chemical Structure	*Concentration (mg/ml)*	*Adhesion, % of Control (Mean)*	*EID_{75}* (mg/ml)*
Neolactotetraose	10	1	1.5
	5	0	
	1	28	
	0.1	52	
Lactotetraose	5	4	1.0
	1	25	
	0.1	68	
GlcNAcβ1→3Galβ-O-Me	10	4	4.5
	5	15	
	1	105	
	0.1	66	
GlcNAcβ1→4Galβ-O-Me	10	75	>10
	5	73	
	1	72	
	0.1	65	
"Octasaccharide"	5	71	>10
	1	62	
	0.1	141	

*EID_{75} = effective inhibitory dose reducing adherence to 25 percent of the saline control (75 percent inhibition).

DISCUSSION

This study demonstrated specific attachment of pneumococci to glycoconjugate receptors, and the disaccharide GlcNAcβ1→3Galβ was shown to be the main binding site. The high degree of specificity is shown by the lack of activity of GlcNAcβ1→4Galβ-o-Me.

Like *Streptococcus pyogenes*, the pneumococci bound human plasma fibronectin (Andersson B, et al, manuscript in preparation). In contrast to *S. pyogenes*, the pneumococci bound at the collagen-binding region of fibronectin (Andersson B, et al, manuscript in preparation). The partly characterized oligosaccharide sequence at that site contains the octasaccharide, which did not inhibit adhesion. Accordingly, this part of the fibronectin structure probably is not the pneumococcal binding site. The fibronectin binding may involve other adhesin receptor interactions, or a similar specificity to the one described, in a different part of the molecule. Receptor activity of the neolactoseries of glycolipids was indicated by the inhibition of adhesion obtained after pretreatment of pneumococci with neolactotetraosylceramide and the increased binding after coating of epithelial cells. The complete inhibition of neolactotetraose (the sugar part of neolactotetraosylceramide) and lactotetraose suggested that the receptor was a common feature of these tetrasaccharides. The central disaccharide portion, GlcNAcβ1→3Galβ, common to all compounds with inhibitory activity, was found to be inhibitory.

The identification of the epithelial cell receptor(s) for attaching bacteria provides a better basis for the analysis of the role of adhesion in pneumococcal infection, for example, by competitive inhibition of adhesion in vivo. The diagnostic and therapeutic usefulness obviously depends on the outcome of such studies.

This study was supported by grants from the Medical Faculty, University of Göteborg, Sweden; numbers 6561 and 215 from The Swedish Medical Research Council; and the Ellen, Walter and Lennart Hesselman Foundation for Scientific Research.

We thank Britt-Marie Essman for technical assistance and Britta Andersson for secretarial assistance.

REFERENCES

1. Gibbons RJ, van Houte J: Bacterial adherence in oral microbial ecology. Ann Rev Microbiol 29:19, 1975
2. Andersson B, Eriksson B, Falsen E, et al: Adhesion of *Streptococcus pneumoniae* to human pharyngeal epithelial cells *in vitro:* Differences in adhesive capacity among strains isolated from subjects with otitis media, septicemia, or meningitis or from healthy carriers. Infect Immun 32:311, 1981
3. Andersson B, Fogh A, Jørgensen F, et al: Attachment of *Streptococcus pneumoniae* to human pharyngeal epithelial cells *in vitro*—mechanism of binding. Proceedings of the American Academy of Otolaryngology—Head and Neck Surgery, in press
4. Andersson B, Dahmén J, Frejd T, et al: Identification of an active disaccharide unit of a glycoconjugate receptor for pneumococci attaching to human pharyngeal epithelial cells. J Exp Med 158:559, 1983
5. Vuento M, Vaheri A: Purification of fibronectin from human plasma by affinity chromatography under non-denaturing conditions. Biochem J 183:331, 1979
6. Simpson WA, Hasty DL, Mason JM, Beachey EH: Fibronectin mediates the binding of group A streptococci to human polymorphonuclear leucocytes. Infect Immun 37:805, 1982
7. Kobata A: Milk glycoproteins and oligosaccharides. In Horowitz MI, Pigman W (eds): *The Glycoconjugates*. London: Academic Press, 1977
8. Lundblad A, Svensson S: Characterization of a penta- and octasaccharide from urine of a patient with juvenile GM_1-gangliosidosis. Arch Biochem Biophys 188:130, 1978

THE NASOPHARYNGEAL MICROFLORA OF OTITIS-PRONE CHILDREN

ANDERS FREIJD, M.D., SOLGUN BYGDEMAN, M.D., and BRITTA RYNNEL-DAGÖÖ, M.D.

Every clinician who treats children has most certainly encountered so-called otitis-prone children, that is, children who with almost every upper respiratory tract infection develop a purulent middle ear infection requiring antibiotic treatment. These children constitute a major everyday clinical problem.

In November 1979 we initiated a prospective study to investigate different aspects of this condition. One purpose was to investigate nasopharyngeal colonization by different microorganisms compared with control children. Another purpose was to correlate the nasopharyngeal culture findings with the otoscopic middle ear status in order to evaluate the relative importance of different pathogens in middle ear disease.

MATERIALS AND METHODS

Patients

Children who were less than 1 year of age and had diagnoses of acute otitis media were included. The children were subsequently examined at regular intervals. Nasopharyngeal cultures were obtained and otoscopic examination was performed using an operating microscope. The criteria for a normal otologic status included a normally located tympanic membrane with the usual landmarks, no visible fluid in the middle ear in cases of a transparent membrane, and normal membrane mobility as judged with a pneumatic otoscope and an operating microscope. The criteria for otitis media with effusion (OME) included visible fluid, with or without air in the middle ear, or a reduction or an absence of tympanic membrane mobility, with or without membrane retraction. The criteria for acute purulent otitis media (AOM) were a dull red or white-red bulging tympanic membrane or purulent discharge, with or without systemic signs of infection.

Of 150 children initially included, 115 could be monitored up to 30 months of age. The patients were divided into an otitis-prone group and a control group on the basis of the number of AOM episodes that had been recorded during the time of observation. As shown in Table 1, 52 children with a range of AOM episodes from 6 to 17 with a mean of 9 composed the otitis-prone group, and 33 children with a mean number of 2 episodes of AOM (range 1 to 3) formed the control group. These groups have been described in more detail elsewhere.[1]

Microbiologic Procedures

Identification of pneumococci, *Hemophilus influenzae, Branhamella catarrhalis*, and so on was made according to standard laboratory procedures, Biotyping of *H. influenzae* was performed according to the methods of Kilian[2] and Oberhofer and Back.[3]

Statistical Analysis

Statistical analysis was performed using the Chi-square-test with Yates correction.

TABLE 1 Number of Children and AOM Episodes Before 30 Months of Age in the Otitis-Prone and Control Groups

Category	*No. of Children*	*Mean No. (and Range) of AOM Episodes*	*No. of Observations*
Otitis-prone	52	9 (6–17)	854
Controls	33	2 (1–3)	269

RESULTS

The Relationship Between Nasopharyngeal Microflora and Otoscopic Findings

Table 2 shows the distribution of the nasopharyngeal culture findings in relation to otoscopic findings in the otitis-prone and in the control groups. The 53 children in the otitis-prone group had 304 episodes of AOM, at which time simultaneous nasopharyngeal culture had been obtained, and the 33 infants in the control group had 48 episodes.

In the otitis-prone group pneumococci alone were present in the nasopharynx in approximately 30 percent of the subjects, irrespective of otoscopic findings. In the control group, pneumococci were present in 36 percent of the children with a normal tympanic membrance, in 23 percent of the children with OME, and in 46 percent of those with AOM. The differences between observations in connection with OME and AOM were statistically significant ($X^2 = 5.37, 0.05 > p > 0.01$). Regardless of otoscopic findings pneumococci

TABLE 2 Results of Nasopharyngeal Bacterial Cultures and Their Relation to Otoscopic Findings in Otitis-Prone Children and Age-Matched Controls

	*Pn**		*HI**		*Pn+HI*		*BC*		*Other†*		*NF†† or No Growth*		*Total*	
Otoscopic Findings	*No.*	*%*	*No.*	*%*	*No.*	*%*	*No.*	*%*	*No.*	*%*	*No.*	*%*	*No.*	*%*
Otitis-Prone														
normal	*67*	*31*	*28*	*13*	*16*	*7*	*30*	*17*	8	4	70	32	219	100
OME	*97*	*29*	*79*	*24*	*29*	*9*	*43*	*13*	11	3	72	22	331	100
AOM	*103*	*34*	*104*	*34*	*53*	*17*	*17*	*6*	8	3	19	6	304	100
Controls														
normal	57	36	15	9	9	6	12	8	11	7	56	35	160	100
OME	14	23	9	15	10	16	7	11	3	5	18	30	61	100
AOM	22	46	11	23	4	8	2	4	2	4	7	14	48	100

*This group includes findings with the indexed bacterial species as the sole finding or in combination with bacterial species considered nonpathogenic, with species mentioned in "Others", BC, or combinations of these.

†Pathogens referred to this group are *Staphylococcus aureus, Streptococcus pyogenes*, and *Neisseria meningitidis* as the sole finding.

††*Staphylococcus epidermidis*, alpha-hemolytic streptococci, diphtheroids, and nonpathogenic *Neisseria sp.* and *Hemophilus sp.* Pn, *Streptococcus pneumoniae;* HI; *Hemophilus influenzae;* BC, *Branhamella catarrhalis;* NF, normal flora.

were found equally often in the otitis-prone and control groups.

H. influenzae as the sole finding was 2.6 times more common in children with AOM than in those with a normal tympanic membrane. This difference was statistically significant in both groups ($X^2 = 29.84$, $p < 0.001$ in the study group and $X^2 = 5.01$, $0.05 > p > 0.01$ in the control group). In children with AOM, *H. influenzae* was found in 34 percent of the otitis-prone group and in 23 percent of the control group.

Regardless of otologic status, *H. influenzae* was found in 25 percent of all children in the study group, as compared with 13 percent in the control group ($X^2 = 10.49$, $p < 0.01$).

The isolation rates of pneumococci and *H. influenzae* together in the nasopharynx were similar in the two groups, except in cases of AOM, in which it was twice as common in the otitis-prone group as in the control group. However, this difference was not statistically significant. *H. influenzae* as a sole finding or in combination with pneumococci in cases of AOM was found in 52 percent of the otitis-prone and in 31 percent of the control group ($X^2 = 6.10$, $0.05 > p > 0.01$).

The nasopharyngeal culture was sterile or grew nonpathogens in one-fourth to one-third of all children with normal otoscopic findings or OME. However, sterile cultures or nonpathogens were found in 6 percent of otitis-prone cases with AOM and in 14 percent of the controls. Regardless of the otoscopic findings, sterile cultures or nonpathogens were found in 19 percent of the otitis-prone group and in 30 percent of the control group ($X^2 = 6.64$, $p < 0.05$).

Comparison of Nasopharyngeal H. influenzae Biotypes Before and After Treatment of AOM with Different Antibiotics

In 66 children, a total of 80 episodes of AOM with *H. influenzae* isolates from the nasopharynx were recorded. A check-up was done after a mean of 18 ± 7 days (mean ± SD) (Table 3).

TABLE 3 Comparison of *Hemophilus influenzae* Biotypes Before and After Antibiotic Treatment of Acute Otitis Media

	Same Biotype		*Change in Biotype*	
Antibiotic	*No.*	*%*	*No.*	*%*
Amoxicillin	25	59	5	12
Penicillin V	6	37	5	31

Forty-two of the children who had AOM and *H. influenzae* before treatment were treated with amoxicillin. *H. influenzae* of the same biotype as before treatment was isolated from the nasopharynx after treatment in 59 percent of them. In five cases (12 percent) a change in biotype was found in 10 cases (24 percent) *H. influenzae* was not present after treatment, and in two cases the culture was sterile. Penicillin V was given 16 times. In five cases (31 percent) a change in biotype was noted and in six cases (37 percent) the same biotype was found after treatment. Thus, a difference in biotype before and after treatment was found to occur almost three times as often after treatment with penicillin V as after treatment with amoxicillin.

DISCUSSION

The 52 otitis-prone children in this study had six or more recorded episodes of AOM, with a mean of nine up to the age of 30 months. Howie and colleagues[4] define an otitis-prone child as having had at least six episodes of AOM before 6 years of age. In this study the control group was composed of 33 children with one to three episodes of AOM up to the same age, with the first episode occurring early in life. This group can therefore not be regarded as representative of the healthy population of the same age. However, they fulfill the requirements for this study, in which the intention was to compare a group of children with high number of AOM episodes with children suffering from only a few.

A significant difference was observed between the isolation frequency of pneumococci and *H. influenzae*. In contrast to pneumococci, *H. influenzae* were isolated more often in connection with pathologic otoscopic findings, and the otitis-prone group was significantly more often colonized with *H. influenzae* than was the control group. These data imply that *H. influenzae* might have a more pronounced intrinsic ability than pneumococci to cause OME or AOM. An observation that favors this concept has been reported by Giebink and colleagues,[5] *et al.* It was found that, in the chinchilla a significant degree of AOM did not occur unless pneumococci that colonize the nasopharynx were aided by cofactors, such as a concomitant viral infection.

The use of penicillin V seemed to contribute to an increased turnover rate of *H. influenzae* strains. A hypothetical explanation can be based on the fact that *H. influenzae* usually has a reduced susceptibility to penicillin V. Supposing that children are almost constantly exposed to a number of bacterial strains, it is plausible that a new strain that is perhaps less susceptible than the previous may become dominant and take over the colonization. However, since most *H. influenzae* strains are sensitive to amoxicillin, it is less likely that a new strain can establish itself under the "pressure" of this antibiotic. It has been shown that *H. influenzae* strains giving rise to AOM induce an immunologic response with formation of antibodies directed against antigens of that specific strain.[6] From this point of view it seems unfavorable for the otitis-prone child to be subjected to an increased degree of turnover of the colonizing bacteria, since it is known that uncapsulated strains of *H. influenzae* show a high degree of antigenic diversity.[7]

This study was supported by grants from the Swedish Medical Research Council (project B83-17X-06257-02) and from the Swedish Society of Medical Sciences.

REFERENCES

1. Freijd A, Bygdeman S, Rynnel-Dagöö B: The nasopharyngeal microflora of otitis-prone children, with emphasis on *H. influenza*. Acta Otolaryngol, in press
2. Kilian M: A taxonomic study of the genus *Haemophilus*. J Gen Microbiol 93:9, 1976
3. Oberhofer T, Back A: Biotypes of *Haemophilus* encountered in clinical laboratories. J Clin Microbiol 10:168, 1979
4. Howie W, Ploussard J, Sloyer J: The "otitis-prone" condition. Am J Dis Child 129:676, 1975
5. Giebink G, Paolini J, Wright P: Influence of different influenzae A strains on susceptibility to experimental pneumococcal otitis media. Abstract No. 733, ICAAC, 1982
6. Shurin P, Pelton S, Tager I, Kasper D: Bactericidal antibody and susceptibility to otitis media caused by strains of *Haemophilus influenzae*. Pediatr 97:364, 1980.
7. Tunevall G: Otorhinological infections in childhood. Serobacteriological studies of paranasal sinusitits and suppurative otitis with special reference to *Haemophilus influenzae*. Thesis, University of Uppsala, Uppsala, Sweden, 1953

IS THERE A NORMAL MICROFLORA IN THE MIDDLE EAR CAVITY?

MARCOS V. GOYCOOLEA, M.D., Ph.D., EUGENIA M. VALENZUELA, T.M., GUMARO C. MARTÍNEZ, M.D., and AURORA B. MALDONADO, T.M.

Despite the fact that the microbiology of otitis media has been well documented,[1] to our knowledge no studies have established whether there is a normal microbial flora of the middle ear. The purpose of this study was to evaluate and obtain microbial (bacterial and fungal) cultures from human subjects with no known histories of otitis media in an effort to clarify this question.

MATERIALS AND METHOD

Subjects

Between July 1982 and April 1983, 15 adults who were subjected to stapedectomy and had no histories of otitis media were selected for this study.

Samples

The following four specimens were obtained from each patient.

1. Nasopharynx: A specimen was taken immediately before the procedure, using a calcium alginate swab (Calgiswab type 1).

2. External ear canal: The canal was cleansed with an ear curette and filled with povidone-iodine solution, which was left in place for 3 minutes. The solution was aspirated and the canal rinsed with sterile saline. A culture was then obtained using a calcium alginate swab.

3. Middle ear washing: Routine stapedectomy incisions were made. As soon as the middle ear was exposed, the cavity was filled with sterile, nonbacteriostatic saline using a disposable syringe and needle. After 15 seconds it was aspirated and cultured.

4. Middle ear mucosa: By use of a straight pick, mucosa around the round window niche was scraped, removed with cup forceps, and cultured. Small pieces of Gelfoam were placed in the area. The procedure was then completed. Once the flaps were repositioned, a small bed of compressed Gelfoam was placed over the incisions and tympanic membrane. The canal was filled with an antibiotic ointment containing neomycin and bacitracin. Patients were treated with ampicillin for 6 days postoperatively (2 gm/day in 4 divided doses).

All samples were placed in thioglycolate (BBL) enriched with 0.5 μg/ml hemin, 0.5 μg/ml vitamin K, and glucose (without indicator) and processed within 3 hours of obtaining the sample.

Cultures

1. Aerobic bacteria (all samples) were cultured on three types of solid media: (a) 5 percent sheep blood agar incubated in 5 to 10 percent carbon dioxide atmosphere at 35°C; (b) 5 percent sheep blood agar incubated at normal atmosphere at 35°C; (c) Mueller Hinton medium (Difco) enriched with 0.2 ml of sheep blood incubated for 24 hours, after which it was transferred to 5 percent sheep blood agar. Cultures were considered sterile if there was no growth after 72 hours.

2. Fungus (all samples): Each sample was inoculated onto two plates of Sabouraud agar. One was incubated at ambient temperature and kept for one month before being discarded as negative. The other was incubated at 35°C for 48 hours.

3. Anaerobic bacteria (all samples except nasopharynx): Thioglycolate broths were inoculated with samples and incubated in a Gas-Pak system at 37°C for a minimum of 48 hours, after which they were subcultured onto two plates of blood agar (tripticase soy agar, yeast extract, and cistine) with 0.5 μg/ml hemin, 0.5 μg/ml vitamin

K, and 5 percent defibrinated ovine erythrocytes. One plate was incubated in an anaerobic chamber Gas-Pak at 37°C for 48 hours. The other plate was incubated in a candle extinction jar. Simultaneously with incubation a modified Hucker Gram stain was done. If there was no growth on agar after 48 hours, plates were reincubated for an additional 7 days before being discarded. If there was growth, a Gram stained specimen was examined microscopically and colonies inoculated into enriched thioglycolate broth. Once there was growth, subcultures were made on blood agar plates incubated anaerobically and in a candle extinction jar. This was done to determine whether bacteria were strict or facultative anaerobes. Bacteria were cultured in differential media for identification according to the method of Dowell and Lombard.[2]

RESULTS

Table 1 summarizes the results of bacterial isolates from nasopharyngeal and external ear canal specimens. External ear canal cultures revealed no growth in ten cases.

Middle ear washings and mucosal scrapings revealed no bacterial growth except in one case in which *Pseudomonas aeruginosa* was cultured (Table 2). Isolated contaminants were observed in three cases: *Propionibacterium acnes* in two instances and *Micrococcus* sp. in one.

All cultures for fungi were negative.

DISCUSSION

Our method for sterilizing the external ear canal was only partially effective, since isolated bacterial colonies remained present in five of 15 cases. This had no clinical consequences, probably because of the antibiotic ointment used to fill the canal plus the prophylactic antibiotic therapy for six days. At present we sterilize with a mixture of povidone-iodine with hydrogen peroxide and wash with 70 percent alcohol. The effectiveness of this method is being evaluated.

TABLE 1 Results of Bacterial Cultures

Bacterial Isolates	*Nasopharyngeal Swab*	*Ear Canal Swab*
Streptococcus viridans	12	0
Staphylococcus epidermidis	10	2
Micrococcus sp.	7	4
Branhamella catarrhalis	5	0
Staphylococcus aureus	1	0
Pseudomonas aeruginosa	1	1
No growth	0	10

TABLE 2 Bacterial Isolates from Single Exceptional Case

Nasopharynx: *Streptococcus viridans*
Branhamella catarrhalis
Staphylococcus epidermidis
Pseudomonas aeruginosa
External ear canal: *Pseudomonas aeruginosa*
Middle ear washings: *Pseudomonas aeruginosa*
Middle ear mucosa: *Pseudomonas aeruginosa*

Our single case with *P. aeruginosa* isolated from the middle ear was a healthy 40-year-old person with no history of being treated with antibiotics or steroids. *P. aeruginosa* is not part of the normal flora of the upper respiratory tract. The isolated colonies found in the middle ear could have represented contamination from the ear canal; however, we cannot rule out the possibility that these colonies were indeed in the middle ear prior to the procedure, since they were also present in the nasopharynx.

The normal flora of the nasopharynx of Chilean patients does not differ from others reported.[3] Our results suggest that the middle ear cavity of adults has no normal flora and that, even if microorganisms occasionally contaminate the cavity, the middle ear defense system[4] could remove such offenders. Microorganisms in otitis media, where there is an intact tympanic membrane, most probably ascend from the nasopharynx via the eustachian tube if local conditions of defense are debilitated or if the magnitude of the aggression overrides the middle ear defense mechanisms.

We wish to especially thank Carmen G. Valdivieso, M.D., and Julio García, M.D., for their assistance.

Bacteriologic studies were funded by the Instituto Chileno de Salud Pública, Santiago, Chile.

REFERENCES

1. Klein JO: Microbiology and antimicrobial treatment of otitis media. Ann Otol Rhinol Laryngol 90 (Suppl 84):30, 1981
2. Dowell VR, Lombard J: *Laboratory Methods in Anaerobic*

Bacteriology. U.S. Dept. of Health and Human Services, Public Health Services, Center for Disease Control, Atlanta, GA 30333. U.H.S. Publication 81-8272, 1982
3. Isenberg HD, Painter GB: Microorganisms of humans. In Lennette EH (ed): *Manual of Clinical Microbiology*. Washington, DC: American Society for Microbiology, 1980, pp. 27–30
4. Goycoolea MV, Paparella MM, Juhn SK, Carpenter AM: The cells involved in the middle ear defense system. Ann Otol Rhinol Laryngol 89 (Suppl 68):121, 1980

CHILDREN WITH FREQUENT ATTACKS OF ACUTE OTITIS MEDIA: A RE-EXAMINATION AFTER EIGHT YEARS CONCERNING MIDDLE EAR CHANGES, HEARING, TUBAL FUNCTION, AND BACTERIAL ADHESION TO PHARYNGEAL EPITHELIAL CELLS

FINN JÖRGENSEN, M.D., BENGT ANDERSSON, M.D., SVEN Hj. LARSSON, M.D., OLLE NYLÉN, M.D., and CATHARINA SVANBORG EDÉN, M.D.

This chapter describes the follow-up investigation in 1982 of children who had frequent attacks of acute otitis media (AOM) during 1973 and 74.[1]

Kaplan and associates[2] found persistent structural deformities of the tympanic membrane or hearing impairment in about 20 percent of Eskimo children with recurrent AOM. Other investigators have failed to confirm adverse otologic outcomes, even after multiple episodes of AOM.[3–5] With this background, the frequency of structural deformities of the tympanic membrane and the hearing capacity of these Swedish children were examined in relation to their AOM history between 1973 and 1982.

Bacteria reach the middle ear by ascending from the nasopharynx. Children with frequent attacks of AOM have an increased rate of nasopharyngeal carriage of *Streptococcus pneumoniae* and *Hemophilus influenzae* compared with controls with no or few episodes of AOM.[1] The colonization of the nasopharynx is probably determined by the attachment of bacteria to components of the mucosa and by the cell receptivity for attaching bacteria.[6–9] In addition, pressure changes in the nasopharynx with possible insufflation of secretions to the eustachian tube and to the middle ear have been proposed as facilitating infection.[10–13]

In the present study an enhanced epithelial cell receptivity for attaching bacteria and an insufficient tubal protection of the middle ear were found in the few children with persistent ear problems. Most children had no lasting adverse effects from their AOM episodes.

MATERIALS AND METHODS

Patients

Forty-eight children with frequent attacks of AOM who were found to have an increased colonization of *S. pneumoniae*, *H. influenzae*, or *Branhamella catarrhalis* in the nasopharynx in 1973 and 74 were reinvestigated in 1982. Of the 48 who received the questionnaire, 28 of the children, 9 girls and 19 boys, came for an interview and were included in the investigation. The others had moved out of the area. The mean age of the investigated group was 13 years in 1982. The questionnaire considered the number of attacks of AOM per year, otitis media with effusion, hearing impairment, and treatment. At the interview the questionnaire was reviewed and completed.

Ear Examination

All ears were examined using an otomicroscope, and signs of middle ear effusion and structural changes of the tympanic membrane were noted. Hearing was tested with a pure-tone audiometer (Madsen type OB 70) and the mean hearing level was calculated. The impedance of the ear was measured by using an impedance audiometer with a probe tone of 625 Hz.[14] Impedance changes were recorded with an ink recorder (Mingograph, type Elema Schönander, Stockholm) to provide a continuous record of the impedance changes.[13]

The tubal function was tested using the Toynbee test and the impedance audiometer.[15] The subjects were tested in a sitting position and told to swallow against occluded nostrils. When an impedance change was registered this was interpreted as an opening of the tube and the test was noted as positive. Immediately after this test the middle ear pressure was measured.

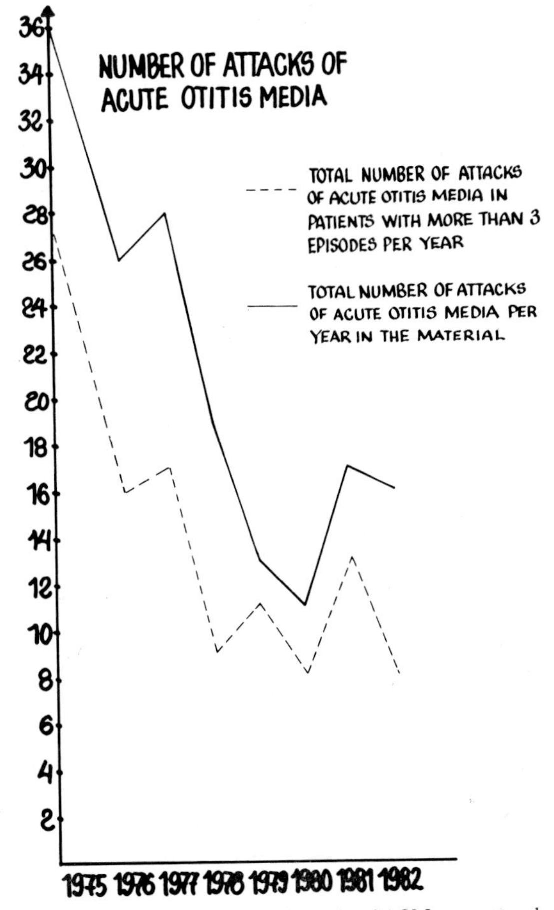

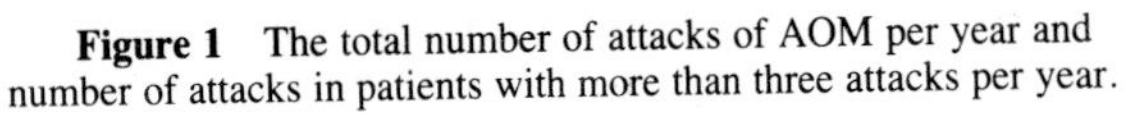

Figure 1 The total number of attacks of AOM per year and number of attacks in patients with more than three attacks per year.

Adhesion Testing

Epithelial cells were scraped from the oropharyngeal mucosa with a brush and suspended in saline. After two washings, the epithelial cells were mixed with a bacterial suspension and centrifuged at 1500g for 10 minutes. The number of bacteria in the test suspension ranged between 10^8 and 10^9 per milliliter. The bacteria and the epithelial cells were incubated without rotation for 30 minutes at 37°C and were then washed twice in saline by differential centrifugation (500g, 10 minutes twice). The number of adhering bacteria per cell were counted using an interference microscope.[6–9]

RESULTS

The total number of attacks of AOM per year, as well as the number of attacks per year in patients with more than three attacks per year, are shown in Figure 1.

Ear Examination

Otomicroscopy revealed 23 ears without pathologic changes in tympanic membrane; 33 ears showed minor structural changes, such as fibrotic scar (12), atrophic scar (11), tympanosclerosis (4), or retraction (4). Six showed signs of middle ear effusion and one had a grommet in the tympanic membrane. At pure-tone audiometry testing we found that the mean hearing level was better than 20 dB in 52 ears; four ears had a mean hearing level between 20 and 30 dB. The impedance audiometry was considered normal in 47 ears, showing a type A curve (32) or a type C curve with middle ear pressure less than -150 mm H_2O (11), or a positive middle ear pressure in four ears. Type C curve with a middle ear pressure more than -150 mm H_2O was found in two ears and five ears showed a type B curve. A patulous tube was found in two ears.

Forty-nine of 56 ears were tested with the Toynbee test; seven were excluded because of otitis media with efffusion. Thirty-four ears showed an opening of the eustachian tube and were registered as positive with the Toynbee test. Fifteen were negative. Of the 34 ears that showed tubal opening, the middle ear pressure was positive in 15. The eustachian tube was patulous in seven ears, while 11 showed a negative middle ear pressure (Fig. 2).

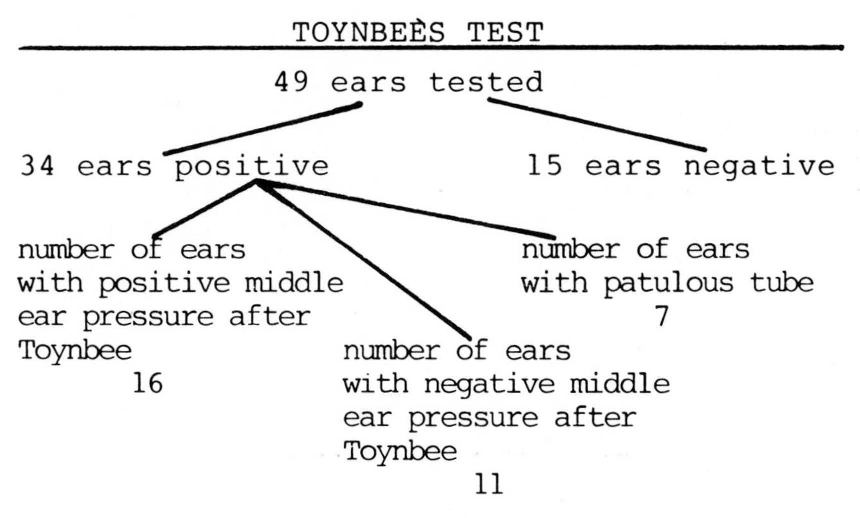

Figure 2 The results of the Toynbee test.

TABLE 1 The Frequency of Attacks of Acute Otitis Media in Relation to the Adhesion of Pneumococci and the Function of the Eustachian Tube

Mean Number of Attacks of Acute Otitis	*Patient No.*	*Tubal Test**	*Adhesion (bact/cell) Mean ± SE*		*Increased Ahesion to Patient Cells*
			Patient Cells	*Control Cells*	
No attacks of acute otitis media	48	+ not tested			NO
	40	− +			Yes
	10	P −			No
	22	P +			Yes
	17	0 +			Yes
	36	0, 0			Yes
	29	−, −	63 ± 17	72 ± 13	No
	9	0 +			Yes
	42	0, 0			Yes
	30	0, 0			No
	43	− +			Yes
	7	−, −			No
	31	−, −			No
1 to 2 attacks of acute otitis media	3	0 not tested			No
	23	0 +			No
	32	+, +			No
	1	P −			No
	28	+, +	88 ± 18	114 ± 19	No
	35	+, +			No
	27	0 +			No
	33	− P			No
	8	0, 0			No
	18	0, 0			Yes
2 or more attacks of acute otitis media	21	− P			Yes
			92 ± 29	56 ± 23	
	41	P, P			Yes
	38	0 not tested			Yes

*+, positive Toynbee test; −, negative Toynbee test; P, patulous tube

Attachment

The receptivity for attaching bacteria to epithelial cells from patients with frequent attacks of AOM compared with healthy controls is shown in Table 1. The results of the Toynbee test are indicated by a + if the middle ear pressure is positive and a − if it is negative. No tubal opening is indicated by 0 and P indicates a patulous tube.

DISCUSSION

In this investigation only three of the 28 children with a history of frequent attacks of AOM during 1973 and 74 had persistent problems with AOM. None developed chronic perforation of the tympanic membrane, and the structural changes of the tympanic membrane were minor. Only one had persistent hearing impairment of more than 20 dB. This is in accordance with findings of Howie,[5] Biles and associates,[16] and Tos,[4] but differs from findings by Kaplan and associates,[2] which showed persistent tympanic membrane perforation in one-fourth and hearing impairment greater than 26 dB in 19 percent of Eskimo children. The populations studied are sufficiently different from ours to make comparison of underlying susceptibility factors impossible. However, it can be concluded that frequent attacks of AOM were not a major long-term problem among the Swedish children studied.

Among host factors that may contribute to increased susceptibility to AOM are those facilitating nasopharyngeal bacterial colonization and decreased tubal protection of the middle ear. The patients with persistent AOM in the present study had increased receptivity for attaching bacteria to the nasopharyngeal epithelial cells compared with cells from healthy controls, and two of three children had patulous tubes. On the other hand, five of the 13 patients without continuing infection problems had both pathologic tubal function and increased adhesion. It may be speculated that other defense mechanisms, such as local immunity, counteract the bacterial virulence in those patients, and the biochemical factors of the mucosal membrane inhibit or promote attachment of pneumococci to nasopharyngeal epithelial cells.[8] It can be postulated that increased adherence contributes to susceptibility to infection in the AOM patients and that agents interfering with bacterial adhesion may have a prophylactic potential, especially in high-risk groups such as patients with pathologic tubal function.

REFERENCES

1. Nylén O. Otitis media acuta. Thesis, University of Gothenburg, Gothenburg, Sweden, 1975
2. Kaplan GJ, Fleshman KH, Bender TR, et al: A ten year cohort study of Alaskan Eskimo children. Pediatrics 52:577, 1973
3. Paradise JL: Otitis media during early life: How hazardous to development? A critical review of the evidence. Pediatrics 68:86, 1981
4. Tos M: Upon the relationship between secretory otitis in childhood and chronic otitis and its sequelae in adults. J Layrngol Otol 95:1011, 1981
5. Howie V: Acute and recurrent acute otitis media. In Jaffe BR (ed): *Hearing Loss in Children*. Baltimore: University Park Press, 1977, pp 14 421–29
6. Andersson B, Pettersson C-M, Nylén O, Svanborg Edén C: Attachment of *Streptococcus pneumoniae* to human pharyngeal epithelial cells in vitro. Ann Otolrhinol Laryngol 89(Suppl 68): 115–16, 1980
7. Andersson B, Eriksson B, Falsen E, et al: Adhesion of *Streptococcus pneumoniae* to human pharyngeal cells in vitro. Differences in adhesive capacity among strains isolated from subjects with otitis media, septicemia or meningitis or from healthy carriers. Infect Immun 32:311, 1981
8. Andersson B, Leffler H, Jørgensen F, et al: Molecular mechanisms of adhesion of *S. pneumoniae* to human oropharyngeal epithelial cells. Submitted for publication, 1953
9. Gibbons RJ, van Houte J: Selective bacterial adherence to oral epithelial surfaces and its role as an ecological determinant. Infect Immun 3:567, 1971
10. Smyth GDL: Middle ear effusions: A consideration of factors involved in their aetiology, maintenance and treatment. Clin Otolaryngol 3:479, 1978
11. Bluestone CD, Paradise JL, Beery QC: Certain effects of adenoidectomy on Eustachian tube ventilatory function. Laryngoscope 85:113, 1975
12. Bluestone CD, Cantekin EI: Current clinical methods and interpretation of Eustachian tube function tests. Ann Otolaryngol 90:552, 1982
13. Jörgensen FR, Holquist J: Toynbee's phenomena and middle ear disease. Svensk Otolaryngol Förh 1:36, 1983
14. Lidén G, Harford E, Hallén O: Automatic tympanometry in clinical practice. Audiology 13:126, 1974
15. Thomsen KA: Investigation on Toynbee's experiment in normal individuals. Acta Otolaryngol Suppl 140:263, 1957
16. Biles R, Buffler PA, O'Donell AA: Epidemiology of otitis media: A community study. AJPH 70:593, 1980

MICROBIOLOGY OF MEDICALLY TREATED CHRONIC OTITIS MEDIA WITH EFFUSION

GEORGE A. GATES, M.D., G. RICHARD HOLT, M.D.,
CHRISTINE A. WACHTENDORF, M.D., ERWIN M. HEARNE, III, Ph.D.,
and JAMES H. JORGENSON, Ph.D.

Before 1958 it was widely assumed that chronic middle ear effusions (MEE) were sterile. The report of Senturia et al,[1] which demonstrated positive cultures in 41 percent of cases of chronic MEE, clearly negated that assumption, and subsequent reports have noted similar results. Current concepts of chronic otitis media with effusion (OME) implicate the presence of microorganisms in the MEE in both the etiology and the continuing pathogenesis of the effusion. Logically, therefore, antibiotic therapy should be used as a treatment of chronic OME and should influence the recovery rate of bacteria from the middle ear.

To test this hypothesis, we have treated all children entered into a prospective, randomized clinical trial of surgical therapy of chronic OME with a 10-day course of erythromycin ethyl succinate and sulfisoxizole (Pediazole) and a 30-day course of decongestant (Novafed). In 48 percent of the children, MEE cleared within 60 days.[2] The children were then completely evaluated according to the protocol, allergies were controlled, and surgical therapy was assigned randomly. Thus, the children undergoing drainage of the middle ear contents had MEE persisting after a fixed course of antibiotics and decongestants. In most instances the MEE was collected within 2 weeks of the end of the 60-day post-treatment period. The children were 4 to 8 years old; none had had prior adenoid or tonsil surgery, and none had evidence of underlying constitutional disease or any anatomic anomaly (such as cleft palate) known to predispose to otitis media.

METHODS

Specimens were collected with the Juhn Tym-Tap via an inferiorly placed myringotomy incision made with the child under general anesthesia. The ear canal had been washed with povidone-iodine solution (Betadine) for 60 seconds and thrice irrigated with sterile saline without preservative in order to remove the sterilizing solution. Control cultures of the tympanic membrane were also obtained. The specimens were plated onto enriched chocolate agar (BBL) and inoculated into Schaedler's broth. Culture plates were interpreted at 24 and 48 hours of incubation by an experienced microbiologist (JHJ) according to standard bacteriologic methods.

The MEE were classified by the operating surgeon as serous, mucoid, purulent, or other, according to their gross physical characteristics. A serous effusion was clear and passed into the collection trap readily. A mucoid effusion was thicker and passed slowly into the collection tubing and could be clear or opaque. Purulent fluids had low viscosity and were opaque.

RESULTS

Of 296 ears undergoing myringotomy and suction aspiration, 75 (25 percent) were dry taps, 38 (13 percent) contained serous fluid, 29 (10 percent) had purulent fluid, and 154 (52 percent) had mucoid effusions. Of the 212 smears that were made: 99 (48 percent) showed bacteria and 90 (42 percent) contained white blood cells. Of the 221 MEE specimens that were cultured, there was no growth noted in 127 (57 percent).

From the 62 middle ear specimens having growth of one or more organisms, the following types were identified: *Streptococcus pneumoniae,* 5; *Hemophilus influenzae,* 32; *Staphylococcus epidermidis,* 9; diphtheroid species, 1; streptococcus, 3; alpha streptococcus, 5; other aerobes, 4; Enterobacter species, 1; Moraxella species, 1; *Staphylococcus aureus,* 8; and Neisseria species, 3. No

TABLE 1 Microbiology of MEE after Medical Therapy

	Number	*Serous*	*Purulent*	*Mucoid*
Total MEE	221	38 (17%)	29 (13%)	154 (70%
Smears	212	36 (17%)	27 (13%)	145 (68%
+ Bacteria	99 (48%)	12 (33%)	10 (37%)	76 (52%
+ Leukocytes	90 (42%)	10 (28%)	12 (44%)	67 (46%
Culture growth	94 (43%)	16 (44%)	11 (41%)	65 (45%
Pathogens only	62 (28%)			
H. influenzae and/or *S. pneumoniae*	37 (17%)			

anaerobes, yeasts, *Branhamella catarrhalis,* or *Neisseria meningitidis* were identified. Only 2 of 31 *H. influenzae* strains were ampicillin resistant; all were susceptible to chloramphenicol. *S. epidermidis* and diphtheroids were found singly or together in 32 additional MEE; we considered these contaminants from the external auditory canal and did not include them in the analysis. Table 1 illustrates the distribution of findings on smear and culture according to the type of effusion. There was little variance in these findings across the three fluid types.

DISCUSSION

We found a lower overall rate of recovery of bacteria from chronic middle ear effusions (28 percent) than reported in previous studies, but similar rates for the two primary pathogens, *H. influenzae* (32/221) and *S. pneumoniae* (5/221).

Liu et al cultured bacteria in 52 percent of 102 specimens from 100 children aged 6 months to 10 years, including 16 *H. influenzae* and 2 *S. pneumoniae*.[3] Healy and Teele cultured organisms from 35 of 96 MEE (36 percent) obtained from 57 children, none of whom had evidence of acute infection of the ears or upper respiratory tract or had had antibiotics in the 2 weeks preceding the surgery.[4] Pathogens were recovered from 11 children and 16 MEI (*S. pneumoniae,* 6 children, 9 MEE; *H. influenzae* 4 children, 6 ears; both, 1 child, 1 MEE). However, discounting the 7 children and 9 MEE in which *S. epidermidis* was the sole organism, 26/9 (27 percent) of MEE contained viable organism and 16/96 MEE (17 percent) grew out the two primary pathogens, *S. pneumoniae* and *H. influenzae*

Thus we conclude that a 10-day course o Pediazole does not influence the rate of recovery o pathogenic bacteria from patients with chroni OME, but does lower the number of positive cultures overall. Interpretation of these findings mus also take into account the narrower age range o our subjects and differences in study methodology

REFERENCES

1. Senturia BH, Gessert CF, Carr CD, et al: Studies concerne with tubotympanitis. Ann Otol Rhinol Layngol 67:44 1958
2. Gates GA, Wachtendorf CA, Holt GR, et al: The history treated persistent otitis media with effusion. In Lim DJ et (eds): *Otitis Media.* Philadelphia, Toronto: BC Decker In 1984
3. Liu YS, Lim DJ, Lang RW, Birck HG: Chronic middle e effusions. Arch Otolaryngol 101:278, 1975
4. Healy GB, Teele DW: The microbiology of chronic midd ear effusions in children. Laryngoscope 87:1472, 1977

IMMUNOLOGY

SECRETORY IgA, SERUM IgA, AND FREE SECRETORY COMPONENT IN MIDDLE EAR EFFUSION

GORO MOGI, M.D., SHOICHI MAEDA, M.D.,
TOYOHARU UMEHARA, M.D., TATSUYA FUJIYOSHI, M.D.,
and YUICHI KURONO, M.D.

Secretory IgA is the chief agent that protects the body against both the invasion of infectious microorganisms and the entrance of inert foreign macromolecules. In previous studies[1] we demonstrated that secretory IgA isolated from middle ear effusions (MEEs) is identical in its subunit structure and antigenicity to secretory IgA in other exocrine secretions, such as nasal secretion, salivary fluid, and colostrum. We also reported that the mean level of concentrations of secretory IgA, determined by radioactive single radial diffusion technique, was 213 μg/ml in serous MEE and 357 μg/ml in mucoid MEE. The calculated percentage of secretory IgA in total IgA was 11 percent in both categories. Recently, Sørensen[2] reported secretory IgA content in MEE, measured by enzyme-linked immunosorbent assay (ELISA), to be 1700 to 2000 μg/ml and the ratio of secretory IgA to total IgA to be 25 percent. In the present study we quantified secretory IgA and serum type IgA in MEE by the electroimmunodiffusion (EID) method.

The mode of action of secretory IgA against bacterial infections is poorly understood. One postulated function is that secretory IgA is capable of blocking bacterial adherence to mucosal surfaces, preventing the colonization of bacteria. It has been suggested that one of the cell wall antigens of *Streptococcus pyogenes,* M protein, participates in its adherence to mucosal surfaces, thereby fostering its colonization. We investigated secretory IgA antibodies of MEE specific for the M protein using the ELISA method.

MATERIALS AND METHODS

One hundred eighteen MEEs were collected, at the time of insertion of a ventilation tube, by Juhn tap (Xomed, Florida) through the eardrums of 98 patients with diagnosed chronic otitis media with effusion (OME). MEEs were aspirated from both ears of 20 of the patients. A total of 77 mucoid MEEs were obtained from 61 patients who ranged from 3 to 68 years of age, with 56 (92 percent) patients being less than 14 years old; 41 serous MEEs were obtained from 37 patients, aged 3 to 73 years, with 16 (43 percent) being under 14. "Chronic," "mucoid," and "serous" were defined as recommended by the 1979 Research Conference on OME.[3] To each MEE specimen was added two to eight times its volume of borate buffered saline (BBS), mixed by a mixer (Vortex-Genie, Bohemia, NY) for 3 minutes and centrifuged at 30,000 g for 20 minutes. The supernatant was used.

Quantitative Analysis of Secretory IgA, Serum Type IgA, and Free Secretory Component

EID techniques, elaborated by Tsukuda[4] for analyses of secretory IgA, serum type IgA, and free secretory component (SC), were adopted. Briefly, for analysis of secretory IgA, after the completion of EID in an agarose gel plate containing rabbit anti-SC antibodies, rocket-shaped precipitates were treated with a solution of goat anti-human IgA conjugated with horseradish peroxidase (HRP). Then the gel plate was washed and stained for HRP. For analysis of serum-type IgA, two equal-sized gel layers were made on a glass plate. The gel on the cathodal side contained anti-SC antibodies, while the gel on the anodal side had anti-IgA antibodies. For analysis of free SC, the cathodal gel had anti-IgA antibodies and the anodal had anti-SC antibodies. After electrophoresis, the gel was dried and stained with Coomassie brilliant blue.

Secretory IgA Antibodies to the M Protein of Streptococcus Pyogenes

To investigate this antibody activity in MEE, an indirect ELISA was employed using partially purified M protein, which was isolated from group A *S. pyogenes* type 3 by the Lancefield and Perlmann[5] method.* Each well of polystyrene microtiter plate was coated with the M protein and then MEE samples diluted 20 to 70 times were applied. After incubation and washing, rabbit anti-SC antibodies conjugated with HRP were added. Incubation and washing were done, and o-phenylnendiamine (as substrate) solution was put into wells and read by a spectrophotometer at 490 nm. To estimate the concentration of secretory IgA antibodies to the M protein, the wells of the first two vertical rows of microtiter plate were coated with goat anti-human IgA antibodies. Then a standard solution of known secretory IgA concentrations was added to the wells, which were incubated and washed. The wells were treated with rabbit anti-SC antibodies labeled with HRP. When the ELISA OD_{490} values of MEE samples were compared with the OD_{490} values developed from known concentrations of secretory IgA, the MEE concentration of secretory IgA specific for the M protein could be estimated.

RESULTS

Concentrations of Secretory IgA and Serum-Type IgA in MEE

Figure 1 shows EID patterns of secretory IgA in MEE and nasal secretions, and EID patterns of serum-type IgA in MEE and sera are exhibited in Figure 2. Table 1 describes mean values of secretory IgA and serum-type IgA in groups of mucoid and serous MME. The mean value of the mucoid category was significantly greater than that of the serous group. There was a significant correlation of concentrations between secretory IgA and serum-type IgA in both categories. Results concerning free SC in MEE will be reported in the near future.

*The M protein was kindly donated by Mr. Sugawara, Research Laboratories of Chugai Pharmaceutical Co, Tokyo, Japan.

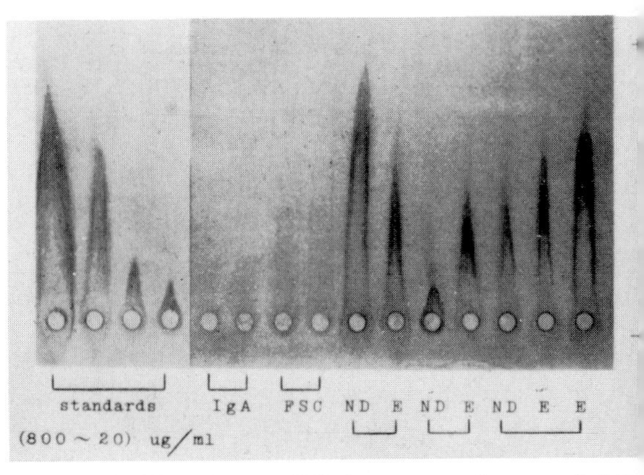

Figure 1 Electroimmunodiffusion patterns of secretory IgA in middle ear effusions (E) and nasal secretions (ND).

Secretory IgA Antibodies of MEE Specific for the M Protein

An appreciable antibody activity of secretory IgA was found in 17 of 77 (22 percent) mucoid MEEs and 5 of 41 (12 percent) serous MEEs. The estimated amount of secretory IgA antibodies against the M protein was 11 to 68 ng/ml in 16 of 22 MEE samples.

DISCUSSION

The value of secretory IgA concentrations of MEE obtained in the present study was found to be

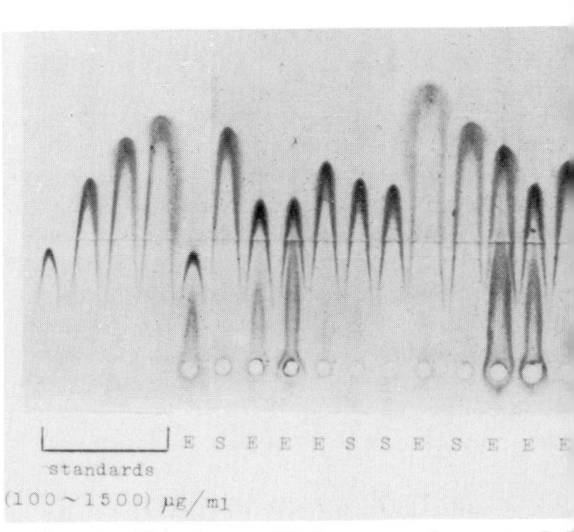

Figure 2 Electroimmunodiffusion patterns of serum-type IgA in middle ear effusions (E) and sera (S).

TABLE 1 Mean Levels of Secretory IgA and Serum-Type IgA in MEE

	Mucoid Group (N = 77)		*Serous Group (N = 41)*	
	MEE	*Serum*	*MEE*	*Serum*
Secretory IgA	2045.5 ± 1560.0*[a]	—	1326.6 ± 1240.0[d]	—
Serum-type IgA	2367.3 ± 1461.0[b]	2867.4 ± 1347.0[c]	2832.7 ± 2011.0[e]	3179.0 ± 1382.8[f]

*mean ± SD, μg/ml
Significant difference: a > d, $p < 0.05$; c > b, $p < 0.01$; e > d, $p < 0.05$
Significant correlation between: a and b, $p < 0.05$, $r = 0.236$; b and c, $p < 0.01$, $r = 0.330$, d and e, $p < 0.005$, $r = 0.527$

2045.5 ± 1560.0 μg/ml (mean ± SD) in mucoid MEE and 1326.6 ± 1240.0 μg/ml in serous MEE. The mean level of secretory IgA in MEE was about six times higher than that reported in the previous study.[1] This discrepancy is probably due to differences in the quantitative methods. The mean value of secretory IgA in MEE, determined by Sørensen using ELISA, was similar to that of the present study.

It is well known that secretory IgA plays an important role in protection against certain viral diseases. Several investigators[6,7] have demonstrated secretory IgA antibodies of MEE specific for poliovirus, RS virus, and parainfluenza. Although more cases of acute otitis media and OME are caused by bacterial infection than by viral infection, little is known about the mode of action of secretory IgA in the protection from bacterial infection. On the other hand, *S. pyogenes* is one of the causative agents of acute otitis media. *S. pyogenes* posseses an array of antigens, but the most important appears to be M protein. This protein is a type-specific surface antigen and essential for virulence. Our study found antibody activity of secretory IgA against M protein in 19 percent of MEEs tested. This evidence suggests that middle ears affected by OME have a mucosal immunity preventing adherence of bacteria and that infection of *S. pyogenes* leads to OME in certain cases.

REFERENCES

1. Mogi G, Maeda S, Yoshida T, et al: Immunochemistry of otitis media with effusion. J Infect Dis 133:126, 1976
2. Sørensen CH: The ratio of secretory IgA to IgA in middle ear effusions and nasopharyngeal secretions. Acta Otolaryngol (Suppl) 386:91–93, 1982
3. Senturia BH, Paparella MM, Lowery HW, et al: Definition and classification. Ann Otol Rhinol Laryngol 89(Suppl 69):4, 1980
4. Tsukuda T: Development of new quantitative methods for assays of sIgA, IgA and FSC and results of the quantitative analyses of these components in oral diseases. Shikoku Acta Med 37:253, 1981
5. Lancefield RC, Perlmann GE: Preparation and properties of type-specific M-antigen isolated from a group A type 1 hemolytic streptococcus. J Expl Med 96:71, 1952
6. Ogra PL, Bernstein JM, Yurchak AM, et al: Characteristics of secretory immune system on human middle ear: Implications in otitis media. J Immunol 112:488, 1974
7. Meurman OH, Sarkkinen HK, Puhakka HJ, et al: Local IgA-class antibodies against respiratory viruses in middle ear and nasopharyngeal secretions of children with secretory otitis media. Laryngoscope 90:304, 1980

IgD AND SECRETORY IMMUNOGLOBULINS IN SECRETIONS FROM THE UPPER RESPIRATORY TRACT OF CHILDREN WITH SECRETORY OTITIS MEDIA

CHR. HJORT SØRENSEN, M.D.

Local secretory immunity primarily mediated by IgA antibodies has been described previously in nasopharyngeal secretions (NPSs)[1,2] and in middle ear effusions (MEEs)[1,3] from children with secretory otitis media (SOM). In MEEs, secretory IgA (SIgA) constitutes only a minor fraction of all IgA antibodies,[1] because a mucosal "leakage" of plasma IgA as well as other plasma proteins is enhanced by the inflammatory reactions found in the middle ear mucosa of children with SOM. As in other external secretions, the second secretory immunoglobulin, secretory IgM (SIgM), should also play an important role in the maintenance of the integrity of the mucosal membranes in the nasopharynx and middle ear cavity.[4] However, in NPS and MEE quantitative data of SIgM are lacking.

During B cell ontogeny, IgD, first discovered in 1965 by Rowe,[5] is located together with IgM on the surface of the majority of human B cells.[6] Nevertheless, only a few of these cells mature into IgD-secreting plasma cells and only trace amounts of this immunoglobulin are normally detected in serum and secretions.[7] However, recently an increased number of IgD immunocytes have been observed in lymphoid tissue from the upper respiratory tract compared with other lymphoid tissues, such as spleen and lymph nodes.[7,8] Moreover, it has been shown that in patients with selective IgA deficiency the majority of B lymphocytes found around the upper respiratory glands belong to the IgD class.[9] Therefore, it seems reasonable to assume that IgD may play a significant role in the humoral immunity of secretions from the upper respiratory tract. The purpose of the present study was to demonstrate the quantitative aspects of the secretory immunoglobulins and IgD in NPSs and MEEs from children with SOM.

MATERIALS AND METHODS

The study was carried out on 45 children (median age 4.7 years, range 0.8 to 8.8 years) whc had suffered from SOM for at least three months. The diagnosis was based on the results of tympanometry and otoscopy and verified at the insertior of the grommets. A medical history of more thar two episodes of acute otitis media (AOM) was recorded in 23 of the children (median age 4.6 years range 0.8 to 7.8 years), but none had had any episodes of AOM within three weeks preceding th operation. After induction of anesthesia, NPS were sucked up from the nasopharynx, and MEEs all of the mucoid type, were aspirated at the tim of myringotomy. All secretions were immediatel frozen at −80°C. Later they were weighed, diluted, shaken with glass beads, and centrifuged a described elsewhere.[2,10] In addition, an EDTA plasma sample was taken from each child durin the operation.

Quantitation of SIgA, SIgM, and IgD wa performed by double sandwich enzyme-linked im munosorbent assays (ELISA).[2,10] All antisera wer raised in rabbits (DAKOPATTS, Copenhagen and the mono-specificity of the various IgG frac tions was proved by crossed immunoelectro phoresis as well as by indirect enzyme immuno histochemical tests.[2,10] A SIgA standard containing 20 gA/L of SIg, was prepared from pool of human colostrum.[2] A pool of naso pharyngeal secretions from children with SOM was used as a working standard for quantitation o SIgM. Arbitrarily, this pool was defined to hav 100 units/L of SIgM, and the total IgM conte was 76 mg/L, as measured by ELISA. Quantita tion of IgD in secretions and in paired plasma sam les was performed by use of a plasma pool made rom 200 healthy blood donors. This plasma pool ontained 24 mg/L of IgD as compared with the ritish Reference Standard 67/37. The albumin ontent in the secretions and in paired plasma samles was measured by routine rocket immunolectrophoresis. The concentration ratio of secreon-albumin/plasma-albumin was used as the ansudation index of plasma proteins through the nucosal surfaces.

Nonparametric statistical analyses were perormed and $p \leq 0.05$ was chosen as the level of ignificance.

RESULTS

Table 1 shows levels of IgA, SIgA, IgM, and IgM in NPSs and MEEs from children with OM. In one child the amount of IgA and SIgA as below the detection limit of the assay (< 50 g/L),[2] and further immunochemical analysis reealed that the patient suffered from IgA and IgD eficiencies without any compensatory increase of gM in the secretions.[4] Another child had undetecble SIgM in his secretions, despite a normal cont of IgM and SIgA. No significant differences in e SIgA and SIgM levels could be calculated beveen children with or without medical histories of OM. As shown in Table 1, significantly reduced tios of SIgA to IgA and SIgM to IgM were found MEEs as compared with NPSs. The quantitative ndings of IgD are listed in Table 2. In MEEs a early three-humped distribution curve was disosed: Most of the children had MEEs–IgD vales ranging between 10 and 300 mg/L, but in eight f 45 MEEs (17 percent), more than 600 mg/L of D could be calculated, and in six MEEs IgD was ndetectable. However, a normal range of IgD was und in the plasma samples.[7] Based on the quantative aspects of albumin in secretions and in aired plasma samples, the median transudation tio was found to be 1:10 in NPS and 1.5:1 in IEEs (Table 2). The corrected median IgD values ere found to be significantly higher in the secreons than in the corresponding plasma samples nd thus indicate a local synthesis of IgD for the cretions, especially in the NPS. In MEEs with ore than 600 mg/L of IgD, between 70 and 98 rcent could be considered locally produced. nally, as shown in Table 3, levels of SIgA, gM, and IgD were correlated. A definitive correlation was found between SIgA and SIgM, both in NPS and in MEE. In contrast, IgD values seemed to be uncorrelated with the SIgA and SIgM values (Table 3).

TABLE 1 Levels of IgA, SIgA, IgM, and SIgM in Nasopharyngeal Secretions (NPSs) and Middle Ear Effusions (MEEs) from Children with Secretory Otitis Media (SOM)

	NPS		*MEE*	
	Median	*(IQR)**	*Median*	*(IQR)*
IgA (g/L)	1.8	(0.8–3.5)	8.6	(4.4–16.3)
SIgA (g/L)	1.4	(0.6–2.2)	1.7	(0.9–3.8)
SIgA/IgA (%)	75	(25–98)	25	(8–65)
IgM (g/L)	0.13	(0.07–0.2)	1.3	(0.8–2.2)
SIgM (units/L)	74	(33–141)	185	(84–313)
SIgM/IgM	1†	(0.6–1.9)	0.2	(0.08–0.3)

Note: SIgM values are expressed arbitrarily in units/L.
*IQR, interquartile range
†Estimated value

DISCUSSION

The secretory immunoglobulins SIgA and SIgM could be detected in all but a few secretions. As shown in Table 1, substantial variations were noted in the ratios of SIgA to IgA and of SIgM to IgM, both within secretions and among them. This means that we must focus on SIgA instead of IgA antibodies and on SIgM instead of IgM antibodies when examining the local immune response in secretions from the upper respiratory tract. In this study a nasopharyngeal secretion pool was used as the standard for the quantitative measurements of SIgM in the secretions, and the concentration of SIgM was defined arbitrarily. Reliable estimates of the true SIgM content are difficult to obtain, mainly because varying amounts of SIgM molecules lose their secretory component during the ordinary purification procedures.[4] A contributory cause is that pentamer IgM combines with secretory component mainly by noncovalent forces.[4] Levels of SIgA in paired plasma samples were found to be negligible compared with the high levels of SIgA in the secretions. SIgM was undetectable in all plasma samples.

TABLE 2 Quantitative Findings of IgD in NPS, MEE, and Paired Plasma Samples

	NPS		*MEE*		*Plasma*	
	Median	*(IQR)**	*Median*	*(IQR)*	*Median*	*(IQR)*
IgD (mg/L)	26	(4–63)	50	(13–289)	16	(6–43)
Transudation ratio of albumin	1:10		1.5:1			
Percentages of IgD locally produced	94%		52%			

*IQR, interquartile range

Brandtzaeg and associates[9] showed that in individuals with selective IgA deficiencies a preponderance of IgM-producing cells is found in jejunal mucosa, whereas nasal, lacrimal, and parotid glands mainly contained IgD-producing cells. In such patients IgD immunocytes seemed to be IgA precursor cells within the upper respiratory tract. However, the results presented in Table 3 do not seem to support these hypotheses. On the contrary, we have demonstrated a correlation between SIgA and SIgM antibodies.

In this study the quantitative data (Table 2) substantiate a local synthesis of IgD for the nasopharynx and middle ear cavity. An active, secretory component-mediated transport of IgD across the mucosal membranes, as a true secretory immunoglobulin, is unlikely to take place as previously suggested.[10] Today we know that IgD and IgM are expressed together on the surface of the majority of human B lymphocytes, but only few of these B cells mature into IgD-secreting plasma cells.[6,7] It is assumed that IgD on the surface of B cells functions as an antigen receptor for transmission of external signals to the cell.[6] However, the function of IgD in the immune response is uncertain and its biologic role in humoral immunity is unknown. An increased number of IgD immunocytes have been observed in the palatine and nasopharyngeal tonsils of children,[7,8] compared with the only occasional occurrence of IgD-producing cells in spleen and lymph nodes. These differences suggest that the maturational pathways of B lymphocytes after antigenic stimulation may differ according to the source of the lymphoid tissue.[9] The pronounced synthesis of IgD to the nasopharynx and to the middle ear cavity thus indicates that IgD plasma cells located in the submucosa of the upper respiratory tract may primarily originate from the palatine and nasopharyngeal tonsils. Further studies are needed to elucidate these assumptions and to confirm the biologic role of these IgD antibodies in the secretions.

TABLE 3 The Correlation Between SIgA, SIgM, and IgD in NPS and MEE

	NPS		*MEE*	
	*Rho**	*Significance*	*Rho*	*Significance*
SIgA–IgD	0.12	NS	0.42	NS
SIgA–SIgM	0.93	P < 0.001	0.61	P < 0.001
IgD–SIgM	0.16	NS	0.25	NS

*Spearmann Rank correlation coefficient

REFERENCES

1. Sørensen CH: The ratio of secretory IgA to IgA in middle ear effusions and nasopharyngeal secretions. Acta Otolaryngol Suppl 386:91, 1982
2. Sørensen CH: Secretory IgA enzyme immunoassay. Application of a model for computation of the standard curve. Scand J Clin Lab Invest 42:577, 1982
3. Mogi G, Honjo S, Maeda S, et al: Quantitative determination of secretory immunoglobulin A (SIgA) in middle ear effusions. Ann Otol 83:239, 1974
4. Hanson LA, Brandtzaeg P: The mucosal defence system. In Stiem ER, Fulginiti VA (eds): *Immunological Disorders in Infants and Children.* London: WB Saunders Co, 198[illegible] p 137
5. Rowe DS, Fahey JL: A new class of human immunoglobulins. I. A unique myeloma protein. J Exp Med 121:171, 1965
6. Parkhouse RME, Cooper MD: A model for the differentiation of B lymphocytes with implications for the biological role of IgD. Immunol Rev 37:105, 1977
7. Rowe DS, Crabbé PA, Turner MW: Immunoglobulin D in serum, body fluids and lymphoid tissues. Clin Exp Immunol 3:477, 1968
8. Korsrud FR, Brandtzaeg P: Immune systems of human nasopharyngeal and palatine tonsils: histomorphometry of lymphoid components and quantification of immunoglobulin-producing cells in health and disease. Clin Exp Immunol 39:361, 1980
9. Brandtzaeg P, Gjeruldsen ST, Korsrud F, et al: The human secretory immune system shows striking heterogeneity with regard to involvement of J chain-positive IgD immunocytes. J Immunol 122:503, 1979
10. Sørensen CH: Quantitative aspects of IgD and secretory immunoglobulins in middle ear effusions. Int J Pediatr Otorhinolaryngol, in press.

IgG SUBCLASS LEVELS IN OTITIS-PRONE CHILDREN

ANDERS FREIJD, M.D., VIVIANNE OXELIUS, M.D.,
and BRITTA RYNNEL-DAGÖÖ, M.D.

The incidence of infections is much higher in infancy than in adulthood. There are distinct periods of proneness to certain infections which might indicate a relationship between the susceptibility to infections and the age-dependent maturation (ontogeny) of the immune system. From the age of 6 months to 2 years, infections due to *Hemophilus influenzae* and *Streptococcus pneumoniae* dominate.[1] It has clearly been shown that recurrent episodes of acute otitis media (AOM) are a major problem during the period from 6 months to 3 to 4 years of age.[2] Physiologic hypogammaglobulinemia might well be one important etiologic factor in recurrent episodes of AOM.

Increased incidence of purulent upper respiratory tract infections is a characteristic feature of antibody deficiency disorders. Recurrent AOM is often an early finding before the development of pneumonia or other more serious infections. The same holds true for individuals lacking IgG2, which is one of four subclasses of IgG.[3] However, the levels of IgG and IgM have been found to be within normal limits in otitis-prone children.[4,5] Since low values of IgG2 may not be revealed by measuring total IgG, we monitored subclass levels in a prospective study of otitis-prone children. We now report data showing reduced levels of IgG2 in children with frequent episodes of AOM.

MATERIALS AND METHODS

Patients and Samples

Heparinized plasma was obtained from children participating in a prospective study of otitis proneness. Children were included who fulfilled the criteria of being younger than 1 year of age and having experienced at least one episode of AOM. Of 150 children included, 115 remained to be evaluated at 36 months of age. Of these, 20 were considered highly otitis prone, having had 8 to 17 recorded episodes up to the age of 30 months. Twenty children who had experienced one or two episodes up to the same age were used as a control group. Blood samples obtained at 12 months of age and at 32 months of age were analyzed.

IgG Subclass Determination

Subclass-specific antisera were raised in rabbits as previously described.[6] Briefly, the animals were rendered tolerant to three of the subclasses and then immunized with the fourth. The quantitative determination of the samples was performed with radial diffusion according to Mancini.[7] WHO reference pool 67/97 was used as standard.

Statistical Analysis

Statistical analyses were performed by using Student's t-test and the Chi-square test.

RESULTS

IgG Subclass Levels in Otitis-Prone Children and Controls

Table 1 shows the IgG subclass levels (IgG1, IgG2, and IgG3) in otitis-prone children and age-matched controls. The IgG1 and IgG3 values were almost identical when the groups were compared at both 12 months and 32 months of age. In contrast, the mean IgG2 value of the otitis-prone children was significantly lower than the values in the control group. This was true at both 12 and 32 months of age ($t = 2.59$, $p < 0.02$; and $t = 3.77$, $p < 0.001$, respectively).

Bacterial Etiology of AOM Episodes in Children with Different Levels of IgG2

To investigate whether the level of IgG2 was related to the bacterial etiology of the AOM episodes of the otitis-prone children, clinical data from the children with an IgG2 level below the mean value at 12 months of age were compared with data from the children with levels above the mean values. The results are summarized in Table

TABLE 1 Serum IgG Subclass Levels in Otitis-Prone and Control Children at 12 and 32 Months of Age

	IgG1		*IgG2*		*IgG3*	
	12 Mo	*32 Mo*	*12 Mo*	*32 Mo*	*12 Mo*	*32 Mo*
Otitis-prone	3.98 ± 1.35	5.38 ± 1.07	0.58 ± 0.3	0.85 ± 0.39	0.44 ± 0.18	0.41 ± 0.16
Controls	3.98 ± 0.77	5.40 ± 1.57	0.82 ± 0.3	1.38 ± 0.49	0.48 ± 0.21	0.41 ± 0.12
			$p < 0.02$	$p < 0.001$		

2. Six children had IgG2 values above the mean and 14 children had values below. The mean number of AOM episodes in the two groups was the same. It was found that AOM episodes with pneumococci as the sole nasopharyngeal finding occurred in 53 percent in the group with IgG2 levels greater than 0.60 g/ml, and in 31 percent of children with IgG2 levels less than 0.60 g/ml ($x^2 = 6.73$, $p < 0.01$). An opposite pattern was noted regarding AOM episodes in which *H. influenzae* was the sole nasopharyngeal finding. The frequencies were 15 percent and 42 percent, respectively, ($x^2 = 9.57$, $p < 0.001$).

DISCUSSION

The present results suggest a humoral IgG2 deficiency as one mechanism contributing to recurrent episodes of AOM in early childhood. As has already been mentioned, purulent infections are rare in infants younger than 6 months old. This is in accordance with the fact that total IgG in full-term neonates is almost the same as in the mother. During the first three to six months after birth serum levels of all subclasses decline due to catabolism of maternal IgG. By six months of age the level of IgG1 is about half of the adult level and it then increases fast. At the age of 6 months the IgG2 level is about one-third of the adult level; it increases more slowly and reaches adult level at about 15 years of age.[8] Furthermore, antibodies to polysaccharide antigens—as, for example, the capsule of pneumococci—are supposed to be of the IgG2 type.[9] The clinical significance of these facts is that children are more susceptible to purulent infections than adults. Still, most children are quite healthy.

Howie[10] defined the otitis-prone condition as more than six episodes of AOM before the child is 6 years old. In our prospective study, 20 children out of 115 turned out to be highly otitis prone, with 8 to 17 episodes of AOM before 30 months of age. The levels of IgG2 in this group were significantly lower than in the control group at both 12 and 30 months of age. It is possible that this group of children will be found to have levels below the mean value even as adults.

The majority of otitis prone children had levels of IgG2 less than 0.6 g/l and suffered from significantly more infections due to *H. influenzae* than children with levels higher than 0.6 g/l. This is in accordance with the pattern of infections in individuals lacking this isotype who are especially prone to *H. influenzae* infections (Oxelius[3]).

The polysaccharide capsule of *H. influenzae* is regarded as a factor of virulence. Ninety percent of *H. influenzae* strains isolated from patients with AOM are uncapsulated and are supposed to be less pathogenic. It therefore seems possible that infections caused by uncapsulated strains affect patients who are immunologically compromised to a high degree.

The high frequency of AOM in early childhood coincides partly with the physiologic period of hypogammaglobulinemia, especially with re-

IgG2 Plasma Level	*No. of (g/l) Children*	*Mean No. of AOM Episodes*	*Nasopharyngeal Culture Finding*				*Unknown Etiology*	*Total No. of AOM Episodes*
			Pn	*Hi*	*Pn + Hi*	*Varia*		
> 0.60	6	10	24	7	8	4	17	60
< 0.60	15	10	29	39	11	15	58	152
			$p < 0.01$	$p < 0.01$				

gard to IgG2. We conclude that some highly otitis-prone children can be regarded as also having an immunologic deficiency of immunoglobulin G subclass that might influence the clinical course and outcome of infections.

REFERENCES

1. Pabst H, Kreth H: Ontogeny of the immune response as a basis of childhood disease. J Ped 97:519, 1980
2. Ingvarsson L, Lundgren K, Olofsson B: Epidemiology of acute otitis media in children. A prospective study of acute otitis media in children. 1. Design, method and material. Acta Otolaryngol (Stockh) Suppl 388, 1982
3. Oxelius V: Chronic infections in a family with hereditary deficiency of IgG_2 and IgG_4. Clin Exp Immunol 17:19, 1974
4. Nylén O: Otitis media acuta. A clinical, bacteriological and serological study of children with frequent episodes of acute otitis media. Acta Otolaryngol (Stockh) 80:399, 1975
5. Gebhart DE: Tympanostomy tubes in the otitis media prone child. Laryngoscope 91:849, 1981
6. Oxelius V: Crossed immunoelectrophoresis and electroimmunoassay of human IgG subclasses. Acta Path Microbiol 86:109, 1976
7. Mancini G, Carbonara AO, Heremans JF: Immunological quantitation of antigens by single radial immunodiffusion. Immunochem 2:235, 1965
8. Oxelius V: IgG subclass levels in infancy and childhood. Acta Pediatr Scand 68:23, 1979
9. Yount W, Dorner M, Kunkel H, Kubat E: Studies on human antibodies. VI. Selective variations in subgroup composition and genetic markers. J Exp Med 127:633, 1968
10. Howie V, Ploussard JH, Sloyer J: The "otitis-prone" condition. Am J Dis Child 129:676, 1975

BACTERICIDAL ANTIBODY TO ANTIGENICALLY DISTINCT NONTYPABLE STRAINS OF *HEMOPHILUS INFLUENZAE* ISOLATED FROM ACUTE OTITIS MEDIA

PAUL A. SHURIN, M.D., COLIN D. MARCHANT, M.D., and VIRGIL M. HOWIE, M.D.

Strains of *Hemophilus influenzae* that are nontypable (NT) in that they do not belong to the known capsular serotypes are isolated from approximately 20 percent of infected middle ear exudates. These organisms are the most prevalent bacterial isolates in cases of chronic or recurrent otitis media with effusion (OME)[1-3] and in cases of therapeutic failure.[4,5] In a recent study we correlated absence of circulating bactericidal antibody directed against a single strain of NT *H. influenzae* with susceptibility to middle ear infection caused by these organisms.[6] Bactericidal antibody directed against the infecting strain was generally absent from sera obtained at the time of diagnosis of acute infection. We interpreted these results as supporting a role for antibody-mediated immunity in OME caused by NT *H. influenzae*. In the present work we have sought further evidence for this role.

MATERIALS AND METHODS

Bacterial Strains

Bacterial strains used were obtained from middle ear effusions of children with acute otitis media who were studied in Boston, Massachusetts (BCH), and Huntsville, Alabama (H). These were employed in bactericidal assays as described previously.[6]

Human Sera

Specimens were from normal individuals of different ages and matched cord and maternal sera. They were stored at −70°C before use.

TABLE 1 Bactericidal Antibody Activity of Rabbit Antisera Against *H. influenzae* NT Isolates from Middle Ear Effusions

			Test Strain Employed in Bactericidal Assay Reciprocal Titers							
Rabbit No.	*Immunizing Strain*	*Serum*	*BCH-37567*	*H-Pr*	*H-Up*	*H-To*	*H-Wi*	*H-Gu*	*H-Po*	*H-Fe*
1	BCH-37567	Preimmune	6	24	< 3	48	24	6	24	24
		Immune	≥ 1536	48	6	≥ 1536	96	192	384	24
3	H-Pr	Preimmune	6	24	48	48	24	6	6	96
		Immune	12	≥ 1536	≥ 1536	768	96	48	384	384

Rabbit Sera

Rabbits were immunized with viable cells of individual *H. influenzae* NT strains. To improve the specificity of some antisera they were absorbed with cells of cross-reacting bacterial strains. Specimens obtained prior to immunization of each rabbit were absorbed and used in individual assays in parallel with the immune serum.

Bactericidal Antibody Assay

The assay was used to quantitate serum antibody in the test specimens. The controls used ensured that nonantibody factors did not contribute to killing of the bacterial inoculum in each test. Results are reported as positive for sera or serum dilutions that killed ≥ 90 percent of the bacterial inoculum. Tests performed with normal human sera gave consistent results when performed with or without addition of absorbed human serum as a complement source.

RESULTS

Classification of NT H. influenzae *Strains with Rabbit Antisera*

Preliminary experiments showed two strains (BCH-37567 and H-Pr) to have different determinants of susceptibility to bactericidal activity of rabbit antisera. Cross-reactions in bactericidal assays were defined by a fourfold or greater increase in titer between preimmune and immune sera. Hyperimmune rabbit antisera to these two strains showed extensive cross-reactions; 4/6 additional strains reacted with anti-BCH-37567 and 6/6 strains with anti-H-Pr (Table 1).

Specificity of these reactions was greatly enhanced by absorption of the immune rabbit sera (Table 2). Absorbed sera gave specific reactions for each of these additional strains. This indicated that each strain carried different specific antigenic determinants of bactericidal susceptibility.

TABLE 2 Bactericidal Antibody Activity of Absorbed Rabbit Antisera Against *H. influenzae* NT Isolates from Middle Ear Effusions

			Test Strain Employed in Bactericidal Assay Reciprocal Titers				
Immunizing Strain	*Absorbing Strain*	*Serum*	*37567*	*H-Pr*	*H-Wi*	*H-Po*	*C-Va*
BCH-37567	Pr	Preimmune	12	< 3	< 3	< 3	< 3
		Immune	≥ 3200	< 3	3	800	< 3
H-Pr	37567	Preimmune	12	24	< 3	< 3	< 3
		Immune	12	≥ 3200	48	48	< 3
H-Wi	Pr	Preimmune	6	< 3	< 3	< 3	< 3
		Immune	12	< 3	1600	< 3	48
C-Va	Pr	Preimmune	< 3	< 3	—	< 3	< 3
		Immune	< 3	< 3	—	< 3	400

TABLE 3 Age Distribution of Human Bactericidal Antibody to *H. influenzae* NT Isolates

Bacterial Strain	*No. With Bactericidal Activity/ No. Tested (%)*		
	Cord	*Age 1–23 Months*	*Age 24 Months*
BCH-37567	2/6 (33)	17/30 (57)	21/22 (95)
H-Pr	1/5 (20)	16/30 (53)	21/22 (95)

Strain Specificity of Human Bactericidal Antibody

To determine whether antibodies in normal human sera also identify antigens of specific *H. influenzae* antigens, we absorbed two sera of normal adults with viable cells of strains BCH-37567 and H-Pr. Only bactericidal activity to the absorbing strain was removed by this procedure.

Age Distribution of Human Bactericidal Antibody

Sera of 59 healthy individuals were tested for bactericidal antibody directed against strains BCH-37567 and H-Pr. Despite the fact that different antigenic determinants are involved, a similar pattern of acquisition of antibody was found for both strains (Table 3).

CONCLUSIONS

Several results of this work will prove useful in further studies of OME caused by *H. influenzae*: First, these bacterial strains may be classified according to their susceptibility to strain-specific absorbed rabbit antisera. Second, a role for antibody as a host defense in otitis media caused by *H. influenzae* is suggested both by the absence of circulating antibody at the time of acute infection and by the inverse relationship in healthy individuals between age of acquisition of antibody and age of greatest incidence of OME. This concept is strongly supported by a recent study of experimental *Hemophilus* OME.[7]

This work was supported by Biomedical Research Support Grant #RR05410 awarded to the Case Western Reserve University School of Medicine and by the Perinatal Clinical Research Center, Cleveland Metropolitan General Hospital, NIH USPHS Grant #5M01RR00210.

REFERENCES

1. Bjuggren G, Tunevall G: Otitis in childhood. Acta Otolaryngol, 42:311, 1952
2. Riding KH, Bluestone CD, Michaels, RH, et al: Microbiology of recurrent and chronic otitis media with effusion. J. Pediatr 93:739, 1978
3. Giebink GS, John, SK, Weber ML, Le CT: The bacteriology and cytology of chronic otitis media with effusion. Pediatr Infect Dis 1:98, 1982
4. Teele DW, Pelton SI, Klein JO: Bacteriology of acute otitis media unresponsive to initial antimicrobial therapy. J Pediatr 98:537, 1981
5. Schwartz RH, Rodriguez WJ, Khan WN: Persistent purulent otitis media. Clin Pediatr 20:445, 1981
6. Shurin PA, Pelton SI, Tager IB, Kasper DL: Bactericidal antibody and susceptibility to otitis media caused by nontypable strains of *Haemophilus influenzae*. J Pediatr 97:364, 1980
7. Pelton SI, Karasic RB, Trumpp CE, Rice PA: Immune response to outer membrane antigens and correlation with protection in experimental otitis media due to nontypable *Hemophilus influenzae* (NTHI). In Lim DJ et al (eds): *Otitis Media*. Philadelphia, Toronto: BC Decker Inc, 1984

SEROLOGIC RESPONSE IN EXPERIMENTAL OTITIS MEDIA DUE TO NONTYPABLE *HEMOPHILUS INFLUENZAE*

STEPHEN I. PELTON, M.D., and RAYMOND B. KARASIC, M.D.

Nontypable *Hemophilus influenzae* is a major pathogen in acute and recurrent otitis media. Despite the clinical importance of this organism few investigations of the immunology of otitis media due to nontypable *H. influenzae* have been reported.

Using a chinchilla model, we measured the immune response to outer membrane protein and lipopolysaccharide antigens derived from nontypable *H. influenzae* and evaluated the role of serum antibody in protection against experimental otitis media.

MATERIALS AND METHODS

Bacterial Strains

The present investigation employed two strains of nontypable *H. influenzae*. The BCH-1 strain was isolated in pure culture by transtracheal aspiration from an adult with lobar pneumonia, and the BCH-2 strain was obtained by tympanocentesis from a child with otitis media.

Experimental Design

Infection was produced in chinchillas by right-sided intrabullar inoculation with 250 to 550 cfu of nontypable *H. influenzae*, strain BCH-1 or BCH-2, on day 0. Six weeks after the first inoculation, following resolution of disease, animals underwent intrabullar rechallenge with the homologous strain of *H. influenzae*. Fourteen weeks after initial challenge, animals were challenged with the heterologous strain. Thus, animals initially infected with the BCH-1 strain were rechallenged during weeks six and 14 with BCH-1 and BCH-2, respectively. Similarly, chinchillas receiving the BCH-2 strain initially were rechallenged six and 14 weeks later with BCH-2 and BCH-1, respectively. Animals were treated with ampicillin for seven days during initial infection with BCH-2 only.

In a separate experiment, 14 animals that had recovered from right-sided otitis due to BCH-1 were rechallenged via the previously uninvolved left bulla with the same strain of *H. influenzae*.

Antigen Preparation

Outer membranes were prepared from whole bacteria by heating in buffered EDTA, mechanical shearing, and differential centrifugation.[1] Outer membrane protein (OMP) was separated from lipopolysaccharide (LPS) by column chromatography in deoxycholate buffer. Lipopolysaccharide was prepared by a modification of the hot phenol water extraction method.

Sodium dodecyl sulfate polyacrylamide gel electrophoresis of the OMP preparations demonstrated the preservation of major protein bands and absence of LPS.

Enzyme-linked Immunosorbent Assay

An enzyme-linked immunosorbent assay (ELISA) was developed to measure serum antibody directed against OMP and LPS antigens from each strain. The ELISA was performed by coating the wells of polystyrene microtiter plates sequentially with antigens in buffer, serum, staphylococcal protein A-horseradish peroxidase, and substrate (o-phenylenediamine).[2] Reactions were read when an internal standard reached a predetermined end point. Appropriate controls were included on each plate.

RESULTS

Results were similar for the two strains. Therefore, data for one strain will be presented in detail and results for the reciprocal experiment briefly reported.

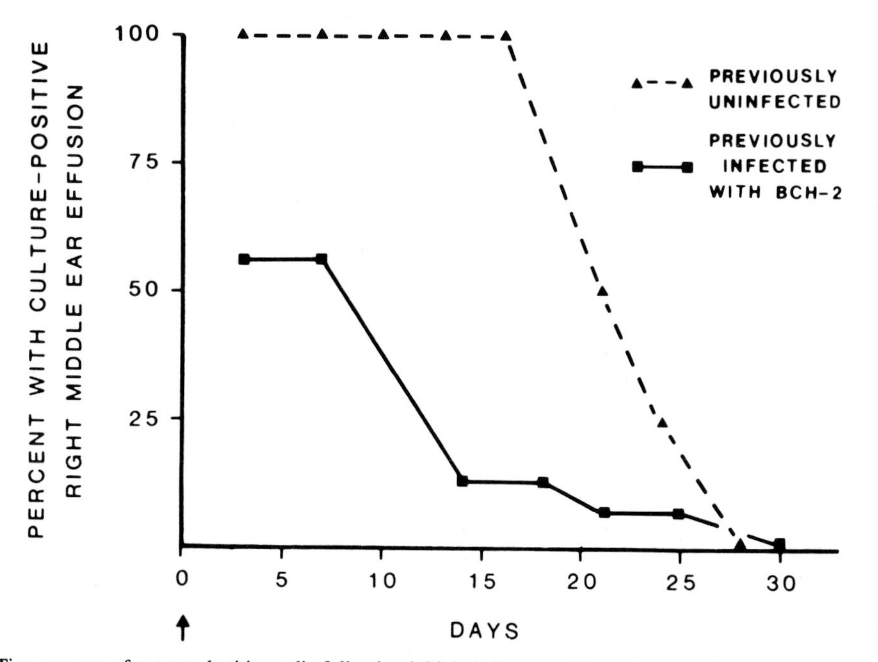

Figure 1 Time courses of untreated otitis media following initial challenge and homologous rechallenge with BCH-2. The natural history of untreated infection was determined in 13 chinchillas undergoing right intrabullar inoculation with BCH-2 on day 0 (▲---▲). A second group of 16 chinchillas that had recovered from otitis due to BCH-2 was rechallenged six weeks later with the same strain (■—■). The rechallenged group had received ampicillin during initial infection.

Homologous Rechallenge

The courses of untreated infection following initial challenge and subsequent rechallenge with BCH-2 are illustrated in Figure 1. Following first inoculation, 100 percent of chinchillas developed culture-positive right-sided otitis media with a mean duration of 20 days. At rechallenge with BCH-2, a reduced incidence (56 percent) and shorter duration of infection (mean, seven days) were observed.

Following homologous rechallenge with the BCH-1 strain, none of six animals developed culture-positive otitis, compared with the incidence of 100 percent observed at initial challenge ($p = 0.001$).

Serologic Response to Homologous OMP and LPS

Animals initially infected with BCH-1 demonstrated a fiftyfold rise in geometric mean titer against OMP derived from that strain. Antibody was undetectable in acute sera at the lowest serum dilution tested, 10^{-2}. The geometric mean titer in early convalescent (five week) sera was $10^{3.7}$ (Fig. 2). No booster response was demonstrated in late convalescent (14 week) sera.

Animals infected with the BCH-2 strain showed a tenfold rise in antibody against homologous OMP in both early and late convalescent sera.

No antibody against homologous LPS was detected at the lowest dilution tested, 10^{-2}.

Serologic Response to Heterologous OMP

Chinchillas infected with BCH-1 had a rise in geometric mean titer against the OMP derived from BCH-2, from $< 10^2$ in acute sera to $10^{2.7}$ in late convalescent sera. Four of six animals developed a fourfold or greater rise in titer by the fourteenth week.

Similarly, seven of 11 animals infected with BCH-2 developed a fourfold rise against the OMP derived from BCH-1.

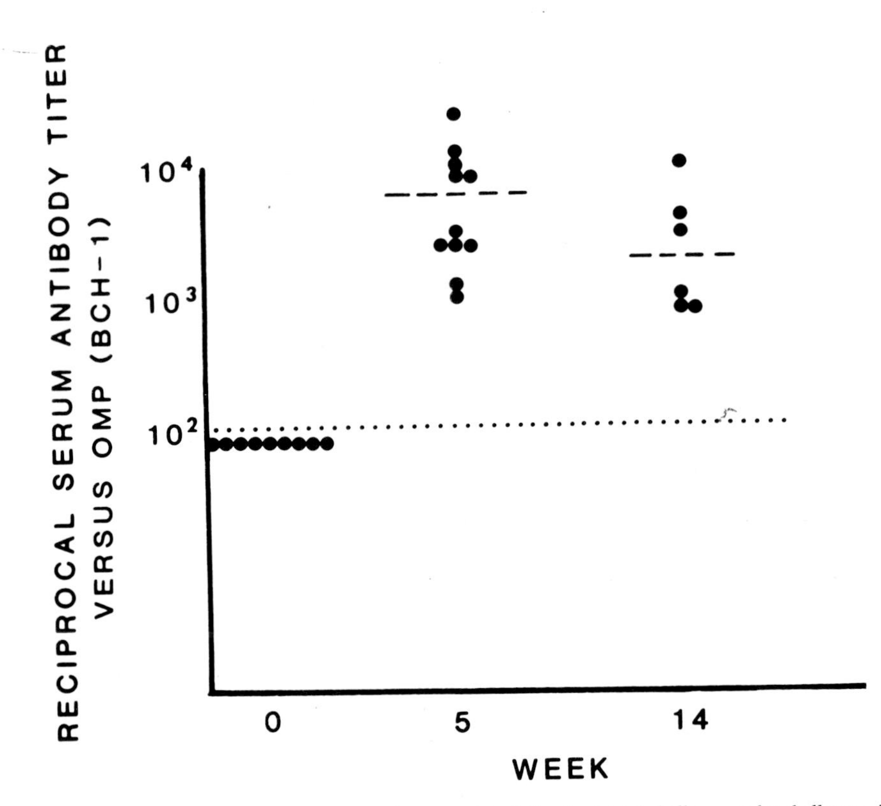

Figure 2 Immune response to homologous outer membrane protein following initial challenge and rechallenge. Animals inoculated on day 0 and rechallenged during week six with BCH-1 are represented by ●. Geometric mean titer is represented by ----. Dotted line (·····) indicates lowest serum dilution tested.

Correlation of Serum Antibody Titer Against OMP and Duration of Infection

The antibody titer against homologous OMP at the time of challenge was compared with the duration of otitis media in two groups of animals inoculated with BCH-2 (Fig. 3). The first group of 15 animals had recovered from initial infection with BCH-2. The second group was composed of five animals that had recovered from two prior challenges with BCH-1. The duration of infection was shortest in chinchillas with the highest antibody titer against the OMP from BCH-2 (Spearman Rank, $p < 0.01$). Only three of nine animals with antibody titers $\geq 10^{3.2}$ developed otitis, compared with all 11 animals with titers below this level.

A negative correlation was also observed between the titer of antibody against OMP from BCH-1 and duration of infection with this strain.

Protection from Contralateral Infection

Only one of 14 animals that had recovered from right-sided otitis media developed left-sided otitis media following left-sided challenge with the same strain. The geometric mean titer against homologous OMP at the time of left-sided challenge was $10^{3.7}$.

DISCUSSION

These results demonstrate the immunogenicity of OMP antigens and support a potential role for systemic antibody in protection against otitis media due to nontypable *H. influenzae*. Previous studies in our laboratory have suggested that OMP is a significant target for bactericidal activity. We observed reduced bactericidal activity in human sera selectively depleted of anti-OMP antibody.[3]

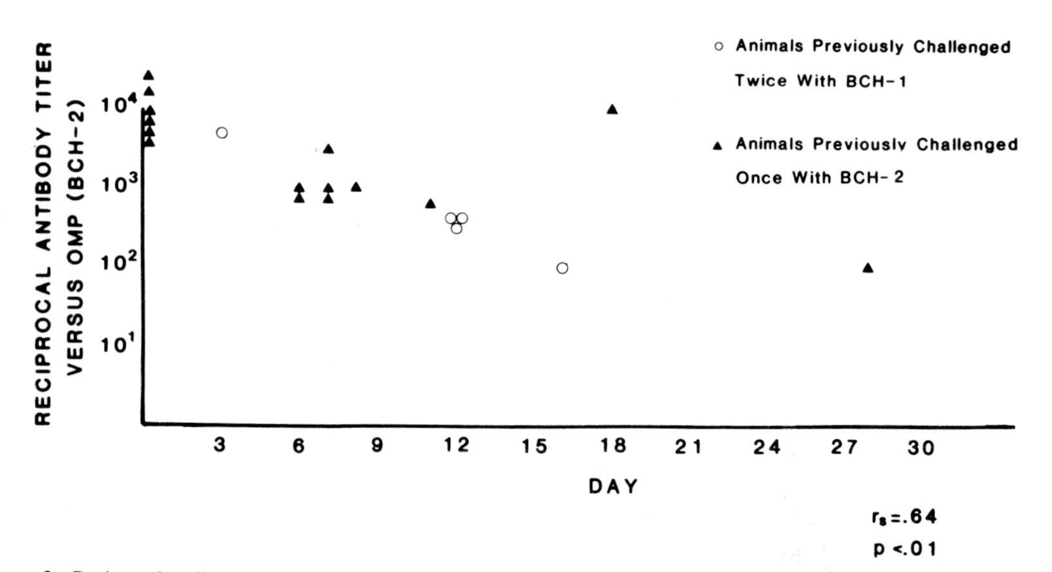

Figure 3 Reciprocal antibody titer against homologous outer membrane protein at challenge versus duration of culture-positive right-sided otitis media following inoculation with BCH-2. Animals challenged previously with the BCH-2 strain are represented by ▲. Animals previously challenged twice with BCH-1 are represented by ○.

Other investigators have demonstrated protection against experimental infection due to *H. influenzae* type b following passive transfer of antibodies against OMP antigens.[4,5]

The absence of a demonstrable antibody response to LPS may indicate that antibody against LPS has a limited role in protection from *Hemophilus* infection. Alternatively, LPS may stimulate classes or subclasses of immunoglobulins that are poorly bound by the staphylococcal protein A-enzyme conjugate. The use of antichinchilla antibody conjugates in future studies may resolve this issue.

The association of high titers of antibody against OMP with protection, and correlation between antibody titer at the time of challenge and duration of infection, suggest that antibody is an important modifier of otitis media due to nontypable *H. influenzae*. However, these data may not distinguish the relative roles of local and systemic antibody. The observed protection of the previously uninvolved contralateral middle ear suggests that systemic antibody may be sufficient to modify the course of otitis due to nontypable *H. influenzae*. However, further studies are necessary to elucidate the relative contributions of local and systemic immunity in protection.

This work was supported in part by Biomedical Research Grant # RR 05569-18 from the Biomedical Research Support Branch, National Institutes of Health, and Grant # AI 18010-03 from the National Institute of Allergy and Infectious Diseases.

REFERENCES

1. Karasic RB, Pelton SI, Trumpp CE, et al: Modification of otitis media in chinchillas rechallenged with nontypable *Haemophilus influenzae* and serologic response to outer membrane antigens. Manuscript in preparation
2. Pelton SI, Karasic RB, Trumpp CE, et al: Immune response to outer membrane antigens and correlation with protection in experimental otitis media due to nontypable *Haemophilus influenzae*. Manuscript in preparation
3. Gnehm HE, Rice PA, Pelton SI, Gulati S: Characterization of antigens from nontypable *Haemophilus influenzae* recognized by human bactericidal antibodies: The role of *Haemophilus* outer membrane proteins. Manuscript in preparation
4. Hansen EJ, Gulig PA, Robertson SM, et al: Immunoprotection of rats against *Haemophilus influenzae* type b disease mediated by monoclonal antibody against a *Haemophilus* outer membrane protein. Lancet 1:366, 1982
5. Shenep JL, Barenkamp SJ, Munson RS Jr, Granoff DM: Role of capsular and noncapsular antibodies against experimental *Haemophilus influenzae* type b infection. Pediatr Res 16:250A, 1982

COMPLEMENT AND PNEUMOCOCCAL ANTIBODIES DURING AND AFTER RECURRENT OTITIS MEDIA

KARIN PRELLNER, M.D., OLOF KALM, M.D.,
and FREDDY KARUP PEDERSEN, M.D.

Streptococcus pneumoniae accounts for 30 to 50 percent of the episodes of acute purulent otitis media (AOM).[1] Types 19, 6, 3, 23, 11, 18 and 14[2,3] have been the most frequently isolated pneumococci. Approximately 5 percent of children have recurrent AOM (rAOM) episodes. The rAOM is often caused by pneumococci and most often by types 19 and 6.[4]

The virulence of pneumococci largely depends on their ability to resist phagocytosis. For phagocytosis to occur the encapsulated pneumococcus must be opsonized by specific antibodies and complement factor C3b.[5,6]

Coupling of specific antibody and the counterpart antigen activates the primary complement (C) factors which, through stepwise activation, form the C3b. The first C factor (C1) is composed of three subcomponents, C1q, C1r, and C1s. C1q binds to antigen-antibody complexes, thus activating C1r and C1s. Aberrations in the C1 factor have been reported in children with rAOM.[7,8]

Antibodies against specific pneumococcal capsular polysaccharides are often present in healthy children, but the levels are lower than those found in adults.[9] During an episode of pneumococcal AOM in children an increased level of specific antibodies is found in 10 to 50 percent of sera samples.[4,10,11]

The aim of the present study was to investigate whether children with rAOM exhibit immunologic aberrations that could explain their relatively higher susceptibility to pneumococcal middle ear infections.

MATERIALS AND METHODS

Patients and Samples

Fifteen children aged 1 to 4.2 years (mean 2 years) with rAOM were investigated in the acute phase of an AOM episode (acute rAOM) and six years later (healed rAOM) (mean age 7.8 years). During the year prior to the acute AOM episode all children had experienced at least five episodes of AOM. During the year preceding the six-year follow-up, all children were free from AOM and were regarded as healthy. Serum and EDTA-plasma (Na_2EDTA 5 mmol/1) samples were obtained in the acute phase of the AOM episode and at the follow-up. Samples were stored in aliquots at −80°C until analyzed. Reference antibody levels were obtained from seven children aged 1.9 to 2.3 years (mean 2 years) and from 12 children aged 7.2 to 8.9 years (mean 7.9 years) with transient acute hematuria whose sera had been referred to the laboratory.

Bacterial Cultures

Middle ear effusions (MEEs) were obtained by aspiration in the acute phase of AOM. *S. pneumoniae* and *Hemophilus influenzae* were identified by conventional methods. Pneumococcal types were determined by the Quellung reaction of Neufeld.[12]

Antibody Determinations

Antibodies against the pneumococcal capsular polysaccharide types 3, 6A, 14, 18C, 19F, and 23F were determined by an enzyme-linked immunosorbent assay (ELISA) as previously described.[13] Antibody concentrations were expressed in arbitrary units representing the optical density corrected for unspecific absorption × 10.[3]

Quantitation of Complement Components

Levels of C1q, C1s, C3, C4, factor B, and properdin were measured by electroimmunoassay.[14] Values were expressed as a percentage of the concentration in a pool of normal adult sera.[14]

C1 Subcomponent Complexes

Complexes of C̄1r-C̄1s-C̄1 inactivator (C̄1-C̄1s-C̄1IA) were quantitated immunochemically. In normal sera levels range between 11 and 25 percent of an all-out activated standard reference.[15] Complexes of proenzyme C1r-C1s were demonstrated by crossed immunoelectrophoresis.[16] C1r-C1s complexes can be detected in 1 percent of normal adult sera and occasionally in low amounts in healthy children.[17]

Statistical Methods

Students' t-test for paired data and the Chi-square-test (the exact method) were used.

RESULTS

Bacteriologic Findings

From the 15 children *S. pneumoniae* type 19F was isolated in pure culture from four aspirated MEEs, and type 6A from two MEEs. *S. pneumoniae* of varying types was isolated from another three MEEs. *H. influenzae* was isolated from five effusions, while in one effusion no pathogen could be isolated.

Levels of Antibody Against Pneumococcal Polysaccharides

The antibody levels for many of the investigated pneumococcal types exhibited an uneven interindividual distribution, as illustrated in Figures 1 and 2 for IgG antibodies against types 6A and 19F. To test the hypothesis that the children with rAOM might include a subgroup of individuals with aberrantly low antibody levels, the Chi-square-test (exact method) was used and the numbers of children with and without rAOM and antibody levels below or above selected limits were statistically tested.

More children with acute rAOM than controls had low IgG antibody levels against the pneumococcal types 6A ($p = 0.020$, Fig. 1) and 19F ($p = 0.038$, Fig. 2). Values used in Figures 1 and 2 are the[10] log values for the arbitrary ELISA units. An IgG antibody level of 1 arbitrary ELISA unit against the pneumococcal type 6A (Fig. 1) was found in eight children (four of them younger and four older than 2 years) and against type 19F (Fig. 2) in five children (three of them younger than 2 years). Four of these children displayed low antibody levels for both types. As to IgA, more children with acute rAOM than contols had low antibody levels ($p = 0.014$) against pneumococcal type 19F. No differences in IgA values were seen for the other pneumococcal types. Children with rAOM more often exhibited low pneumococcal type 3 and 14 IgM antibody levels than control children ($p = 0.005$ and $p = 0.020$, respectively).

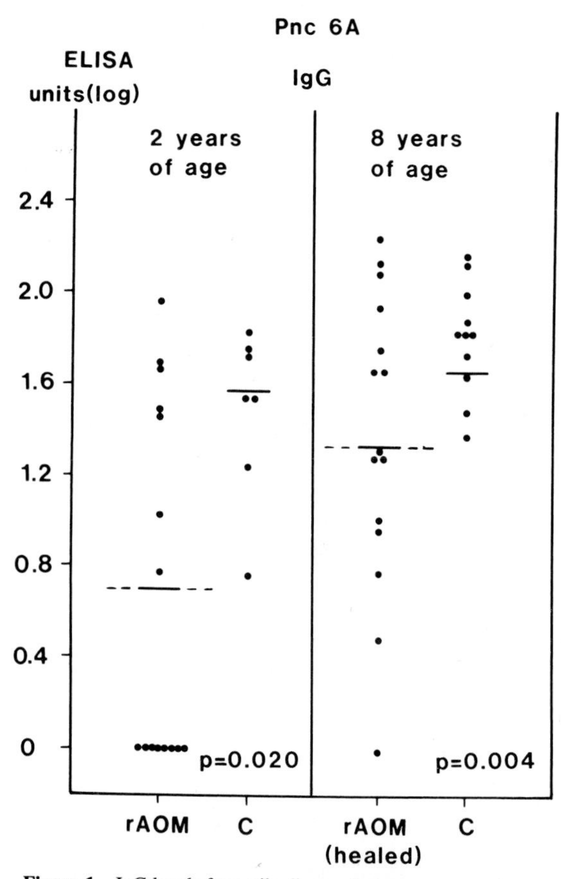

Figure 1 IgG levels for antibodies against pneumococcal capsular polysaccharide type 6A in children with recurrent acute otitis media (rAOM) during an acute episode and at follow-up (rAOM, healed), and in control children (C). Values are given as log values for arbitrary ELISA units. — indicates geometric mean values; --——--indicates the selected limit used in the statistical calculations.

At the six-year follow-up the IgG levels against the various pneumococcal types had generally increased, as illustrated for type 6A and 19F in Figures 1 and 2. For pneumococcal type 3 IgG antibodies, there were more children with healed rAOM who exhibited high levels than control children ($p = 0.04$).

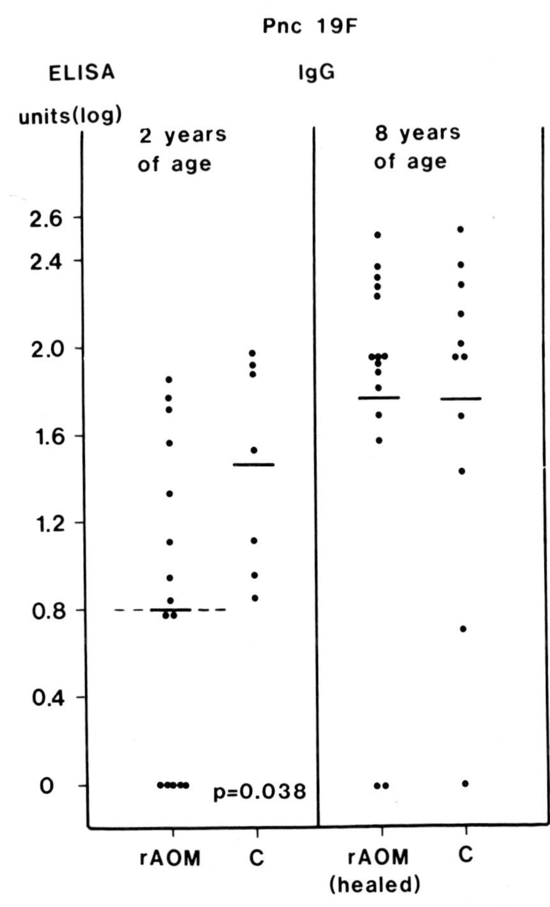

Figure 2 IgG levels for antibodies against pneumococcal capsular polysaccharide type 19F in children with recurrent acute otitis media (rAOM) during an acute episode and at follow-up (rAOM, healed), and in control children (C). Values are given as log values for arbitrary ELISA units. — indicates geometric mean values. --——--indicates the selected limit used in the statistical calculations.

More children with healed rAOM than control children had low IgG antibody levels against pneumococcal type 6A ($p = 0.004$, Fig. 1). As to IgG antibody levels against types 14, 18C, 19F (Fig. 2), and 23F, there was no statistical difference between the groups.

Complement Factor Levels

The C1q and properdin levels were decreased (76 and 82 percent respectively) in cases of acute AOM, while the levels of C1s, C3, C4 and factor B were elevated (Table 1). At follow-up six years later the mean level of C1q was 91 percent and of properdin 102 percent, while C1s, C3, C4, and factor B levels were 97, 101, 92 and 114 percent respectively (Table 1).

C1 Subcomponent Complexes

Amounts above the upper normal limit of C$\bar{1}$r-C$\bar{1}$s-C$\bar{1}$IA complexes were found in six of 15 children with acute rAOM, with a mean of 23 ± 6 percent of the standard reference. At follow-up all 15 children had levels within the normal range (mean ± SD: 14 ± 2, Table 1). In children with rAOM, C1r-C1s complexes were present in 14 of 15 sera samples, often in excessive amounts. At follow-up C1r-C1s complexes were found in two of 15 sera samples and then only in low amounts.

DISCUSSION

Why do some children experience recurrent middle ear infections while others do not? Several theories have been proposed, including various immunologic aberrations.[4,10,11] Since pneumococci are often encountered in rAOM, the present study focused on immunologic factors of importance for phagocytosis of this bacterium, namely, specific antibodies, complement factors, and complement activation.

Although bacteriologic cultures were not performed during the year preceding the current episode, it was reasonable to assume that pnemococci, especially types 19F and 6A, would be common causative agents among the 15 children with rAOM.[2,4] This was substantiated by the fact that pneumococci caused nine of the 15 current AOM episodes.

Among children with rAOM a subgroup exhibiting extremely low levels of IgG antibodies against pneumococcal types 19F and 6A was identified. The corresponding antibody levels in the other rAOM children were on a par with those found in the controls. The children in the subgroup also exhibited pronouncedly low type 19F specific IgA levels.

The specific IgG antibody is not only a prerequisite for the attachment of the pneumococcus to the phagocyte, it is also a major activator of the complement system inasmuch as the coupling between specific antibody and counterpart antigen triggers C1 activation. Six of the 15 children exhibited complement activation during the acute rAOM episode.

However, 14 of the children showed marked aberrations in the first complement factor, that is, low C1q and presence of C1r-C1s complexes, suggesting inadequate prerequisites for optimal complement activation. Why then do the rAOM children have low C1q levels? Do they have inherently

TABLE 1 Serum Levels of Complement Factors and $C\bar{1}r$-$C\bar{1}s$-$C\bar{1}$ Inactivator Complexes in Children with Recurrent Acute Otitis Media in an Acute Phase (Acute rAOM) and at Six-year Follow-up (Healed rAOM)

Complement Factor	*Mean Values ± 1 SD*		*Statistical Difference in Mean Values*
	Acute rAOM	*Healed rAOM*	
C1q	76 ± 25	91 ± 18	Significant increase ($p < 0.01$)
C1s	120 ± 19	97 ± 10	Significant decrease ($p < 0.0005$)
C3	119 ± 25	101 ± 13	Significant decrease ($p < 0.025$)
C4	137 ± 39	92 ± 29	Significant decrease ($p < 0.0005$)
P	82 ± 19	102 ± 14	Significant increase ($p < 0.0005$)
B	154 ± 22	114 ± 25	Significant decrease ($p < 0.0005$)
$C\bar{1}r$-$C\bar{1}s$-$C\bar{1}$ inactivator complexes	23 ± 6	14 ± 2	Significant decrease ($p < 0.0005$)

low C1q or do pneumococcal antigens, not coated with specific antibody, consume the C1q without ensuing activation of the complement system, as has been shown to occur in vitro?[18,19] The fact that the complement profiles were normal six years after the current AOM epsisode does not exclude the concept of inherently low C1q levels at the beginning of the rAOM. However, available data favors the theory that the complement aberrations occur during episodes of infection. The low levels of specific pneumococcal polysaccharide antibodies recorded at the beginning of the rAOM episode could be responsible for the primary establishment of the infection and could also be indirectly responsible for an aberrant C1q consumption, with ensuing low C1q levels which then, together with remaining low antibody levels, further increase the individual susceptibility to recurrent middle ear infections.

REFERENCES

1. Klein, J: Microbiology of otitis media. Ann Otol Rhinol Laryngol 89(Suppl 68):98, 1980
2. Kamme C, Ageberg M, Lundgren K: Distribution of diplococcus pneumoniae types in acute otitis media in children and influence of types on the clinical course in penicillin V therapy. Scand J Infect Dis 2:183, 1970
3. Luotonen J: Studies on the bacteriology of acute otitis media. Thesis, University of Oulu, Finland, 1982
4. Branefors-Helander P, Dahlberg T, Nylén O: Acute otitis media. A clinical, bacteriological and serological study of children with frequent episodes of acute otitis media. Acta Otolaryngol (Stockh) 80:399, 1975
5. Ward H, Enders J: An analysis of the tropic action of normal immune sera based on experiments with the pneumococcus. I Exp Med 57:527,1933
6. Winkelstein JA, Smith MR, Shin HS: The role of C3 as an opsonin in the early stages of infection. Proc Soc Exp Biol Med 149:397, 1975
7. Johnsson U, Kamme C, Laurell A-B, Nilsson NI: C1 subcomponents in acute pneumococcal otitis media in children. Acta Pathol Microbiol Scand (C) 85:10, 1977
8. Prellner K, Nilsson NI: Complement aberrations in serum from children with otitis due to *S. pneumoniae* or *H. influenzae*. Acta Otolaryngol (Stockh) 94:275, 1982
9. Borgoño JM, McLean AA, Vella PP, et al.: Vaccination and revaccination with polyvalent pneumococcal polysaccharide vaccines in adult and infants. Proc Soc Exp Biol Med 157:148, 1978
10. Sloyer JL Jr, Howie VM, Ploussard JH, et al.: Immune response to acute otitis media in children. I. Serotypes isolated and serum and middle ear fluid antibody in pneumococcal otitis media. Infect Immun 9:1028, 1974
11. Branefors-Helander P, Dahlberg T, Nylén O: Study of antibody levels in children with purulent otitis media. Ann Otol Rhinol Laryngol 89(Suppl 68):117, 1980
12. Neufeld F: Über die Agglutinization der Pneumokokken und über die Theorieen der Agglutination. Z Hyg Infektionskr 40:54, 1902
13. Karup Pedersen F, Henrichsen J: Detection of antibodies to pneumococcal capsular polysaccharides by enzyme-linked immunosorbent assay. J Clin Microbiol 15:372, 1982
14. Sjöholm AG: Complement components in normal serum and plasma quantitated by electroimmunoassay. Scand J Immunol 4:25, 1975
15. Laurell A-B, Mårtensson U, Sjöholm AG: Quantitation of $C\bar{1}r$-$C\bar{1}s$-$C\bar{1}$ inactivator complexes by electroimmunoassay. Acta Pathol Microbiol Scand (C) 87:79, 1979
16. Laurell AB, Mårtensson U, Sjöholm AC: Cl subcomponent complexes in normal and pathological sera studied by crossed immunoelectrophoresis. Acta Pathol Microbiol Scand (C) 84:455, 1976
17. Laurell A-B, Nilsoon NI, Prellner K: Immune complex and complement in serous and mucoid otitis media. Acta Otolaryngol (Stockh, 90:290, 1980
18. Prellner K: Bacteria associated with acute otitis media have high Clq binding capacity. Acta Pathol Microbiol Scand (C) 88:187, 1980
19. Prellner K: Clq binding and complement activation by capsular and cell wall components of *S. pneumoniae* type XIX. Acta Pathol Microbiol Scand (C) 89:359, 1981

COMPLEMENT DEPLETION BY COBRA VENOM FACTOR: EFFECT ON IMMUNE MEDIATED MIDDLE EAR EFFUSION AND INFLAMMATION

ALLEN F. RYAN, Ph.D., and CARL-WILHELM VOGEL, M.D.

While eustachian tube dysfunction is regarded as a primary cause of otitis media with effusion (OME), there is extensive evidence to support the concept that immune responses play a role in this multifaceted disease. A variety of immune and inflammatory substances have been identified in middle ear (ME) effusions of patients with OME. In addition, it has been demonstrated that OME can be elicited by a secondary immune response in the ME cavity[1–3] and can be mediated entirely by the IgG immunoglobulin fraction.[3]

The potential for immunologic mechanisms to generate effusion and inflammation in the ME has led to the suggestion that chronic OME may be an immune complex disease, mediated by complement.[4] The evidence regarding this hypothesis is mixed. Laurell and colleagues[5] and Palva and colleagues[6] have reported detecting immune complexes in ME effusions, as well as evidence of complement activation, in chronic OME patients. Mravec and associates injected immune complexes into the ME of animals but detected no middle ear effusion as a result.[7]

The present study was conducted to determine whether activation of the complement system contributes to immune mediated effusion and inflammation in the ME. Cobra venom factor (CVF), which is thought to be the cobra's equivalent of C3b[8] and which nonspecifically activates the complement cascade, was used to decomplement guinea pigs.[9] Experimental OME was then generated by an immunologic mechanism in these animals.

MATERIALS AND METHODS

Subjects were Hartley guinea pigs weighing between 250 and 350 gm. The absence of ME pathologic factors was verified by otoscopic observation and the presence of a normal Preyer's reflex.

Keyhole limpet hemocyanin (KLH), a molluscan blood protein, was used as the antigen. KLH was obtained as an ammonium sulfate slurry (Pacific Biomarine Supply, Venice, CA) and extensively dialyzed against phosphate buffer at pH 6.5. KLH in its associated form was separated by ultracentrifugation for use as antigen. Disassociated KLH was used as a reagent for radioimmunoassay (RIA).[10]

Cobra venom factor (CVF) was prepared from the venom of the cobra *Naja naja Kaouthia* (International Biological Extracts, Sweetwater, Texas). CVF was isolated by sequential column chromatography on Bio-Gel A 0.5 m (Bio-Rad), DEAE-Sephacel (Pharmacia), CM-cellulose (Whatman), and Cibacron Blue Agarose (Bio-Rad). This resulted in a product free of phospholipase A_2. CVF was suspended in phosphate-buffered saline (ph 7.4) for injection.

Three groups of subjects were employed. In the experimental group, 11 guinea pigs were immunized with a single intradermal injection of 1 mg of KLH as an alum precipitate. After 18 days the animals were given an intraperitoneal injection of 300 μg of CVF, followed at 20 days postimmunization by a second injection of 150 μg of CVF. At 21 days postimmunization, a serum sample was obtained and the subjects were challenged in the ME with 1 mg of associated KLH in 0.1 ml of phosphate buffer (pH 6.4). At 22 days, a third injection of 150 μg of CVF was given. At 24 days postimmunization, three days following ME challenge, the animals were bled for serum, killed, and the temporal bones rapidly dissected. A hole was opened in the apex of the bulla and the ME cavity was washed with 0.1 ml of tissue culture medium to recover effusion, cells, and immunoglobulin. Fluid recovered in excess of the 0.1 ml used to wash the bulla was defined as ME effusion. The bulla was then perfused and prepared for histologic study.

In two control groups, animals were treated

identically to those of the experimental group. However, in a positive (secondary immune response) control group of 11 guinea pigs, no CVF was given to ensure that an immune mediated OME was elicited by ME challenge. In a negative (primary immune response) control group of eight guinea pigs, only the alum adjuvant was used for the initial immunization, to ensure that no spurious response to KLH was caused by the CVF treatment.

Complement activity was measured in serum samples by a standard hemolytic titration assay using sensitized sheep erythrocytes. Levels of anti-KLH IgG were assessed in sera and ME effusions by RIA, using the techniques described in Ryan and colleagues[10] and Cleveland and colleagues.[11]

RESULTS

Decomplementation

Serum decomplementation of subjects ranged from complete suppression of hemolytic activity to 6 percent of control activity. In the prechallenge sera, the average hemolytic activity was 2.27 percent of control values. In the postchallenge sera the average value was 3.83 percent.

Middle Ear Effusion

In the negative control subjects, ME effusions evoked by KLH challenge averaged 11 ($\pm$22) μl, and in the positive control group 130 ($\pm$35) μl. These values are similar to those we have previously reported[3,12] at three days postchallenge in primary and secondary ME immune responses, respectively. In the experimental group, effusion averaged 83 ($\pm$60) μl, a value significantly different ($p < 0.05$) from that of either the positive or negative control subjects.

Cellular Content of Effusions

Leukocytic infiltration of the ME cavity is a universal feature of both primary and secondary immune response. In the negative control group, the total leukocyte content of the ME averaged 14 ($\pm$22) $\times$ 10^5 cells. In the positive control group the total averaged 287 ($\pm$247) $\times$ 10^5 cells. In the decomplemented animals, total leukocytes averaged 130 ($\pm$125) $\times$ 10^5 cells. This value was not significantly different from that of the positive control group, although it should be noted that the variability of total ME leukocyte content is always extremely high. The cells recovered from the MEs of decomplemented animals contained a smaller percentage of neutrophils (61 percent) and a greater percentage of eosinophils (20 percent) than was seen in the positive (74 percent neutrophils, 4 percent eosinophils) or negative (87 percent neutrophils, 0.2 percent eosinophils) control groups.

Histology

The ME mucosae of the negative control group subjects were slightly hypertrophic and infiltrated by neutrophils. In the positive control group, the mucosae showed extensive hypertrophy and edema. Infiltration of the mucosae by neutrophils, eosinophils, and lymphocytes was marked, and free erythrocytes were a prominent feature. The mucosae in decomplemented animals were similar to those of the positive control subjects, with exceptions: The number of free erythrocytes was much reduced and, as might be expected from the cellular content of ME effusions, fewer neutrophils and more eosinophils were observed in the mucosae of CVF treated subjects.

DISCUSSION

In summary, decomplementation by CVF treatment resulted in a significant reduction in the amount of effusion generated during a secondary immune response in the ME. Depletion of serum complement also reduced other features of immune mediated ME inflammation, including extravasation of erythrocytes and total leukocytic infiltration of the ME cavity. CVF treatment increased the proportion of eosinophils infiltrating the ME.

These data suggest that complement fixation plays a significant role in immune-mediated OME, although it clearly is not the only mechanism involved. The activation of complement during a secondary immune response to KLH in the ME presumably occurs via the classic pathway, triggered by antigen-antibody complexes. There are a number of ways in which components of the complement system could mediate various aspects of our model of OME.

In addition to the terminal membrane attack complex, the complement cascade generates a number of biologically active compounds. The complement anaphylatoxins C5a, C3a, and C4a, in decreasing order of activity, have been shown to be potent vasoactive mediators.[8] By increasing vascular permeability they could release serum and erythrocytes into the middle ear cavity. C5a and C3a are also chemotactic for leukocytes, primarily neutrophils.[8] C5a stimulates the degranulation of mast cells,[13] which could also increase vasopermeability and leukocyte chemotaxis.

There is no obvious explanation for the increase in the proportion of eosinophils which we observed in the ME of decomplemented animals. This observation may reflect a predominance of eosinophil chemotactic factors in noncomplement-dependent inflammatory pathways that remain intact in the CVF treated animals. The several eosinophil chemotactic factors of the mast cell[13] are potential candidates.

Finally, the fact that even complete suppression of serum complement did not eliminate immune mediated OME suggests that other mechanisms contribute to this phenomen. A variety of other inflammatory pathways can be released by immune recognition of antigen, including mast cell mediators, lymphokines, and various products of arachidonic acid metabolism.

This study was supported by grant #NS14389 and by RCDA NS00176 from the NIH/NINCDS to A.F.R. The technical contributions of Sharon Batcher, Virginia Black, and Ruth Papin are gratefully acknowledged.

REFERENCES

1. Hopp E, Elevitch F, Pumphrey R, et al: Serous otitis media—an "immune" theory. Laryngoscope 74:1149, 1965
2. Miglets A: The experimental production of allergic middle ear effusions. Laryngoscope 83:1355, 1973
3. Ryan AF, Catanzaro A: Passive transfer of immune-mediated middle ear effusion and inflammation. Acta Otolaryngol 95:123, 1983
4. Veltri R, Sprinkle P: Secretory otitis media: An immune complex disease. Ann Otol Rhinol Laryngol 85 (Suppl 25): 135, 1976
5. Laurell A, Nilsson N, Prellner K: Immune complexes and complement in serous and mucoid otitis media. Acta Otolaryngol 90:290, 1980
6. Palva T, Lehtinen T, Rinne J: Immune complexes in middle ear fluid in chronic secretory otitis media. Ann Otol Rhinol Larynol 92: 42, 1983
7. Mravec J, Lewis DM, Lim DJ: Experimental otitis media with effusion, an immune-complex-mediated response. Otolaryngology 86:258, 1978
8. Kohler PF: The human complement system. In Samter M (ed): *Immunological Diseases,* 3rd ed. Boston: Little, Brown, and Co, 1978 pp, 244–280
9. Cochrane CG, Müller-Eberhard HJ, Aikin BS: Depletion of plasma complement *in vivo* by a protein of cobra venom: Its effects on various immunologic reactions. J Immunol 105:55, 1970
10. Ryan AF, Cleveland PH, Hartman MT, Catanzaro A: Humoral and cell-mediated immunity in peripheral blood following introduction of antigen into the middle ear. Ann Otol Rhinol Laryngol 91:70, 1982
11. Cleveland PH, Richman DD, Oxman MN, Ryan AF, Worthen DM: A rapid and simplified radioimmunoassay for small particulate antigens using a filter manifold. J Immunoassay 2:117, 1981
12. Catanzaro A, Ryan AF, Robb J: Immune-mediated and nonspecific inflammatory events in the middle ear. Clin Immunol Immunopath 24:361, 1982
13. Wasserman SI: The mast cell: Its diversity of chemical mediators. Int J Dermatol 19:7, 1980

TRANSFORMATION RESPONSE OF LYMPHOCYTES TO PHYTOHEMAGGLUTININ AND POKEWEED MITOGEN IN PATIENTS WITH SECRETORY OTITIS MEDIA

PEKKA SIPILÄ, M.D., PEKKA KARMA, M.D., PAULI RYHÄNEN, M.D., and ANTTI PALVA, M.D.

In the in vitro assessment of cellular immunity in patients with infectious diseases, immunodeficiency, autoimmunity, and cancer, the transformation response of lymphocytes to mitogens is a commonly used technique. It measures the functional capacity of lymphocytes to proliferate following an antigenic challenge.[1] Sloyer and colleagues used an approach of this kind in acute otitis media, and they observed that the transformation response of lymphocytes to phytohemagglutinin (PHA) in middle ear effusion was approximately one-tenth of that in the peripheral blood of the same patients and control subjects.[2] They hypothesized that there is a paucity of local T cell activity in acute otitis media. Yamanaka and associates reported that the transformation responses of lymphocytes to PHA and pokeweed mitogen (PWM) in middle ear effusions were generally low compared with the responses observed in peripheral blood and adenoidal tissue lymphocytes.[3] They observed that macrophages present in the middle ear effusion have a marked effect on the transformation responses of lymphocytes.

To obtain additional information concerning the role of cellular immunity in secretory otitis media, we decided to study the spontaneous proliferating activity and the transformation responses of lymphocytes in the middle ear effusions and blood of patients with secretory otitis media (SOM) to PHA and PWM. The responses were compared with those of subjects having neither infection nor any systemic diseases.

MATERIALS AND METHODS

Patients

Twenty-nine mucoid middle ear effusions and corresponding blood samples of 23 patients with SOM were studied (14 males and 9 females, ages 6 months to 9 years; mean, 3.3 years). All the patients had symptoms of otitis media with effusion for at least two months. None of them had any signs of acute infection at the time of sampling, nor had they received antimicrobials during the three weeks prior to the procedure. Furthermore, 23 control blood samples were studied from subjects without infection or systemic diseases (13 males and 10 females; ages 5 months to 10 years; mean, 4.8 years).

Separation of Cells

During tympanostomy under general anesthesia and under the control of an operating microscope, the effusion of each patient was collected from the middle ear using a sterile glass suction tip. After washing with RPMI-1640, the cell suspension was stained with trypan blue, and the absolute number and percentage of viable cells were determined in the Bürger's chamber. The mononuclear cells were not separated from the granulocytes. The peripheral blood samples were drawn into heparinized plastic tubes. The cells were layered on methylcellulose-Isopaque solution and the leukocytes were separated.

Cell Cultures

The cells were cultured on round-bottomed, covered microtiter plates. Each sample was cultured in triplicate. Lymphocytes were stimulated by PHA and PWM. The cell cultures were incubated at +37°C in a tissue culture incubator with a humidified gas mixture containing 95 percent air and 5 percent dioxide. Tritiated thymidine was used as the labeling substance.

Immediately after the termination of the cell cultures on the fifth day, the cultures were harvested. The radioactivity of the cells was counted in a liquid scintillation counter for 1 min. The median counts per minute (cpm)/well values of the samples made in triplicate were used for statistical analysis. The spontaneous proliferating activity and the transformation responses to PHA and PWM were expressed as cpm/10^4 lymphocytes in the well.

Using a cytocentrifuge, cell slide preparations were made of the cell suspensions prepared for the cell culture from each effusion and blood sample. One slide was stained with May-Grünwald-Giemsa (MGG) and the percentages of the different inflammatory cell types were counted. Another slide was marked with acid alphanaphthyl acetate esterase (ANAE) stain, as previously described,[4] and the percentage of ANAE-positive cells (T cells) out of all lymphocytes was determined. The statistical analyses were made using the Mann-Whitney U-test.

RESULTS

The mean spontaneous proliferating activity (SPA) was greatest in the effusion samples (282 cpm/10^4 lymphocytes) and smallest in the blood samples of the control subjects (80 cpm/10^4 lymphocytes) (Table 1). The difference between the blood samples of the patients and the controls was not statistically significant, nor was the difference between the effusion and blood samples of the patients with SOM.

The mean transformation responses of lymphocytes to PHA and PWM were greatest in the blood samples of the patients with SOM (12,270 cpm/10^4 lymphocytes and 6946 cpm/10^4 lymphyocytes, respectively) (Table 1). In the blood samples of the control subjects they were somewhat lower, but the difference was not statistically significant. The mean transformation responses of lymphocytes to PHA and PWM in the effusion samples were significantly weaker than in the corresponding blood samples ($p = 0.015$ and $p = 0.004$, respectively).

The numbers of viable cells in the effusion specimens were determined before the cell culture procedures and ranged from 1.0 to 6.0 $\times$ 10^6 (mean, 2.13 $\times$ 10^6; S.D., 1.40 $\times$ 10^6). The percentage of viable cells ranged from 60 to 93 percent, being 77 percent on the average. The percentage of viable cells did not correlate with the spontaneous proliferating activity or the transformation responses to PHA and PWM noted in the specimens.

The percentage of ANAE-positive cells (T cells) of all lymphocytes in the effusion samples ranged from 0 to 71 percent (mean, 30.9 percent; S.D., 16.8 percent).

No or only low response to PHA occurred in the effusion samples that contained less than 20 percent of ANAE-positive lymphocytes of all lymphocytes (Fig. 1). There was a positive correlation between the transformation response to PHA and the percentage of ANAE-positive cells present in the culture medium (correlation coefficient 0.818). When the lymphocytes were stimulated by PWM, no or low response occurred in the specimens containing less than 20 percent of ANAE-positive cells. In the specimens that contained more than 20 percent ANAE-positive cells, higher responses occurred, but the responses were more variable following PHA stimulation (correlation coefficient 0.620).

Figure 2 shows the transformation response of lymphocytes to PHA in correlation with the percentage of monocytes and macrophages out of all mononuclear cells present in the culture medium. As can be seen, low responses occurred in the samples with both low and high percentages of monocytes and macrophages when the samples with less than 20 percent ANAE-positive cells were excluded from the analysis. The same phenomenon could be seen when the cells were stimulated by PWM.

TABLE 1 Spontaneous Proliferating Activity (SPA) and Transformation Responses of Lymphocytes to PHA and PWM (cpm/10^4 Lymphocytes)

	SPA			*PHA*			*PWM*		
	Range	*Mean*	*S.D.*	*Range*	*Mean*	*S.D.*	*Range*	*Mean*	*S.D.*
Effusion	4.0–1315	282	363	9.0–20,446	7532	6389	9.3–13,256	4079	4369
Blood of SOM patients	9.9–1003	132	212	3723–27,928	12,270	6051	937–13,750	6946	2649
Blood of controls	13.2–353	80	86	5365–20,661	10,064	4277	1320–14,986	5757	3095

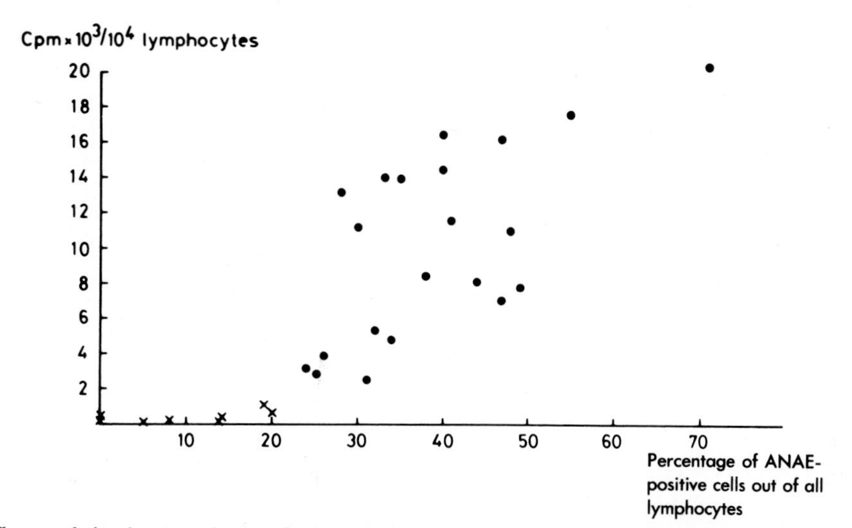

Figure 1 The correlation between the transformation response of lymphocytes to PHA and the percentage of ANAE-positive lymphocytes (T cells) of all lymphocytes in 29 mucoid middle ear effusion samples. The samples marked "X" contained less than 20 percent T cells.

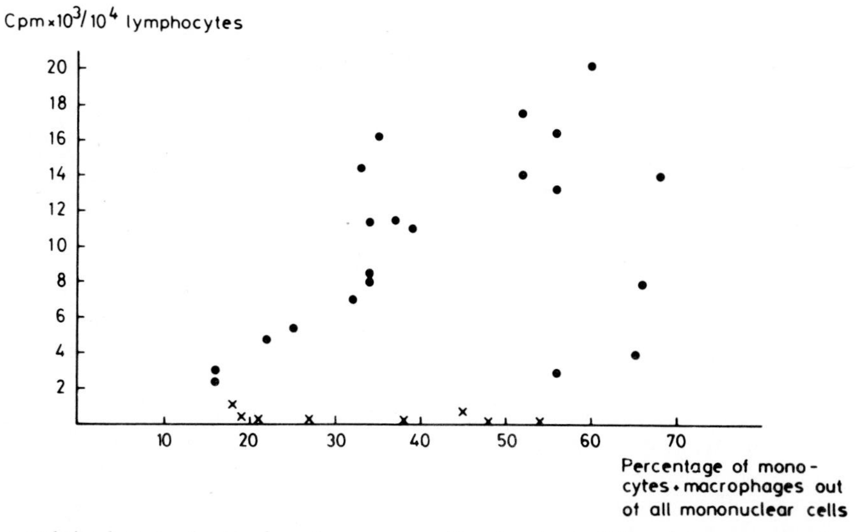

Figure 2 The correlation between the transformation response of lymphocytes to PHA and the percentage of monocytes plus macrophages of all mononuclear cells in 29 mucoid middle ear effusion samples. The samples marked "X" contained less than 20 percent T cells.

DISCUSSION

In the present study, the transformation responses of blood lymphocytes to PHA and PWM in the patients with SOM as compared with the control subjects were not significantly different. Thus, the functional capacities of blood T cells, and probably also B cells, to respond to these mitogens do not differ in patients with SOM and in healthy subjects of the same age.

One aim of this study was to measure the transformation response of the lymphocytes of middle ear effusion to mitogens under conditions reminiscent of those to which the inflammatory cells are subject in middle ear effusions during otitis media. No attempt to separate the cells was made, which the reader should keep in mind in the following discussion.

The transformation responses of lymphocytes to PHA and PWM were significantly lower in the effusion samples than in the corresponding blood samples. The results are in accordance with those reported by Sloyer and colleagues[2] and by Yamanaka and colleagues.[3] The fact that PHA stimulates primarily T cells but not B cells[5,6] may explain the finding of low responses occurring in the samples with a small number of T cells. These samples probably did not contain enough T cells to respond to PHA. In contrast, higher responses occurred in the effusion samples with higher concentrations of T cells.

PHA and PWM stimulate different T cell populations, and PWM also stimulates B cells.[6,7] However, in the effusion samples that contained a small amount of T cells, low responses to PWM occurred as well. The observations support the notion that middle ear effusions form a sliding scale with regard to the relative proportion of T cells.

Monocytes and macrophages are necessary for the transformation response of lymphocytes to mitogens;[8,9] macrophages are even considered an absolute requirement for the T cell response to an antigen.[8]

It was noted that an increasing percentage of monocytes and macrophages had a stimulating effect on the transformation response of lymphocytes. However, in the effusion samples with a very high percentage of monocytes and macrophages, lower responses also occurred. This may be explained by the postulation that macrophages in high concentrations have a capacity to inhibit the T lymphocyte response to mitogen,[9] and this inhibition is even more conspicuous if activated macrophages are present.[8] The effect of activated macrophages on the transformation response in the middle ear effusion samples may be important, because macrophage activation in middle ear effusion is assumed to take place on the basis of morphologic studies.[10] This finding probably reflects the cellular cooperation between macrophages and T cells in the immune responses.[8,9]

It can be concluded that middle ear effusions are basically heterogeneous, containing varying proportions of the different inflammatory cells. The variations in the transformation responses of lymphocytes to PHA and PWM in SOM effusions were in accord with the variations in the proportion of ANAE-positive cells (T cells) and also with the variations in the proportion of macrophages plus monocytes out of mononuclear cells in these effusions. This suggests that the role of the different cellular immune responses may vary in middle ear effusions and that cellular cooperation depends on the proportions of the mononuclear cells present in the effusions.

REFERENCES

1. Stites DP: Clinical laboratory methods of detecting cellular immune function. In Fudenberg HH et al (eds): *Basic and Clinical Immunology,* 2nd ed. Los Altos, CA: Lange Medical Publications, 1978
2. Sloyer JL, Ploussard JH, Howie VM: Immunology and microbiology in acute otitis media. Ann Otol Rhinol Laryngol 85 (Suppl 25): 130, 1976
3. Yamanaka T, Bernstein JM, Cumella J, et al: Immunologic aspects of otitis media with effusion: Characteristics of lymphocyte and macrophage reactivity. J Infect Dis 145:804, 1982
4. Sipilä P, Ryhänen P, Karma P: T cells as marked with acid alphanaphthyl acetate esterase staining in secretory otitis media. Acta Otolaryngol (Stockh) Suppl 360: 216, 1979
5. Daguillard F: The differing responses of lymphocytes to mitogens. *Proceedings of the Seventh Leukocyte Culture Conference.* Daguillard F, ed: New York: Academic Press, 1973, p 571
6. Weksler ME, Kuntz MM: Synergy between human T and B lymphocytes in their response to phytohaemagglutinin and pokeweed mitogen. Immunology 31:273, 1976
7. Douglas SD: Cells involved in immune responses. In Fudenberg HH et al (eds): *Basic and Clinical Immunology,* 2nd ed. Los Altos, CA: Lange Medical Publications, 1978
8. Wing EJ, Remington JS: Delayed hypersensitivity and macrophage functions. In Fudenberg HH et al (eds): *Basic and Clinical Immunology,* 2nd ed. Los Altos, CA: Lange Medical Publications
109, ed. H.H. Fudenberg, D.P. Stites, J.L. Caldwell, J.V. Wells, Los Altos, California
9. de Vries JE, Caviles AP Jr, Bont WS, et al: The role of monocytes in human lymphocyte activation by mitogens. J Immunol 122:1099, 1979
10. Sipilä P, Sutinen S, Sutinen SH, Karma P: Ultrastructural morphology of mucoid effusion in secretory otitis media. Acta Otolaryngol (Stockh) 90:342, 1980

LYMPHOCYTE–MACROPHAGE INTERACTION IN OTITIS MEDIA WITH EFFUSION

T. YAMANAKA, M.D., J.M. BERNSTEIN, M.D., Ph.D.,
J. CUMELLA, M.D., and P.L. OGRA, M.D.*

It is now well established that the inflamed middle ear cavity possesses many attributes of a mucosal immune system,[1] including the presence of secretory IgA and other immunoglobulins, T- and B-lymphocytes, neutrophils, and macrophages, plus an ability to mount a specific antibody response against a number of bacteria and viruses.[2]

Little or no information is available, however, regarding the role of cell mediated immunologic mechanisms in the middle ear effusion and the mechanisms of protection against microorganisms or the pathogenesis of middle ear disease in children. We have studied the interaction of middle ear macrophages with other cellular components in middle ear effusion relative to the expression of antibody and the cell mediated immune response. The present investigations were undertaken to examine the nature of macrophage mediated immunologic modulation of lymphocyte functions in different types of otitis media.

MATERIALS AND METHODS

Middle ear cells were separated on Ficoll-Hypaque gradient and the mononuclear cells harvested. The mononuclear cells were further divided by separating adherent cells (macrophages) from nonadherent cells (lymphocytes) by adherence to Petri dishes. In this way, not only middle ear fluid mononuclear cells but also peripheral blood mononuclear cells and adenoid cells were separated.

These groups of cells were studied for their lymphoproliferative response to a number of mitogens and specific antigens, including purified protein derivative (PPD), herpes simplex virus (HSV), sheep red blood cells (SRBC), and ovalbumin (OVA). Furthermore, the presence of polyclonal immunoglobulin secreting cells was also established using these antigens as well as pokeweed mitogen (PWM) and phytohemagglutinin (PHA).

In addition, co-culture of macrophages from the middle ear, peripheral blood, and the adenoids, with lympocytes from the adenoidal tissue, was undertaken to determine the effect of these adherent cells on the lymphoproliferative response and polyclonal immunoglobulin synthesis of adenoidal lymphocytes. Finally, pooled middle ear fluid was fractionated to determine which fraction was responsible for either depression or augmentation of these immunologic responses.

The processing of the cells and the lymphoproliferative responses and detection of polyclonal immunoglobulin secreting cells was performed with standard immunologic techniques described elsewhere.[3]

RESULTS

The relative proportion of adherent macrophage cells and lymphocytes in the various middle ear classes, peripheral blood, and adenoidal tissue is presented in Table 1. Although the absolute number of cells in different forms of middle ear effusions varies considerably, the highest number was observed in the purulent effusions and lowest in the serous and mucoid effusions. The predominant cell type in middle ear effusion was the macrophage, regardless of the type of effusion. The mean proportion of middle ear mucoid, seromucinous, and serous effusions was 58.6 percent, 63.1 percent, 48.3 percent, and 53.3 percent of total mononuclear cells, respectively. T-cells varied

*Director of Infectious Diseases, Children's Hospital, 219 Bryant Street, Buffalo, NY 14222.

TABLE 1 Distribution of Subpopulations of Mononuclear Cells in MEEs, PBCs, and Adenoidal Tissues of Subjects with Various Types of MEEs Due to Chronic Otitis Media

Type of MEEs (No. of Subjects)	*No. of Cells × 10⁶*	*Middle Ear*		*Peripheral Blood*		*Adenoidal Tissue*	
		Macrophage	*Lymphocyte*	*Macrophage*	*Lymphocyte*	*Macrophage*	*Lymphocyte*
Purulent (9)	2.88 ± 3.43	58.6 ± 12.5	40.7 ± 11.5	24.3 ± 7.6	73.1 ± 8.9	7.3 ± 4.9	92.0 ± 5.3
Mucoid (19)	0.59 ± 0.66	63.1 ± 11.6	36.7 ± 11.6	25.2 ± 6.3	72.8 ± 7.1	9.3 ± 7.8	90.1 ± 6.9
Seromucoid (16)	1.10 ± 2.56	48.3 ± 9.3	51.3 ± 9.1	23.2 ± 5.8	76.1 ± 6.1	8.2 ± 7.5	91.3 ± 6.6
Serous (6)	0.48 ± 0.29	52.3 ± 11.2	46.1 ± 12.1	19.8 ± 4.9	79.3 ± 5.8	7.7 ± 8.3	92.0 ± 7.7

Note: Data are means ± S.D. of the total number of cells and of percentages for each subpopulation.

from 11 to 66 percent of nonadherent cells but did not appear to differ significantly among the types of effusions.

The proliferative response of unfractionated middle ear cells (MEC) and peripheral blood cells (PBC) after *in vitro* stimulation with PHA or PWM is seen in Figure 1. The MECs appear to be hyporesponsive to both PHA and PWM stimulation. Polyclonal immunoglobulin synthesis of IgM, IgG, and IgA isotypes in unfractionated MECs and

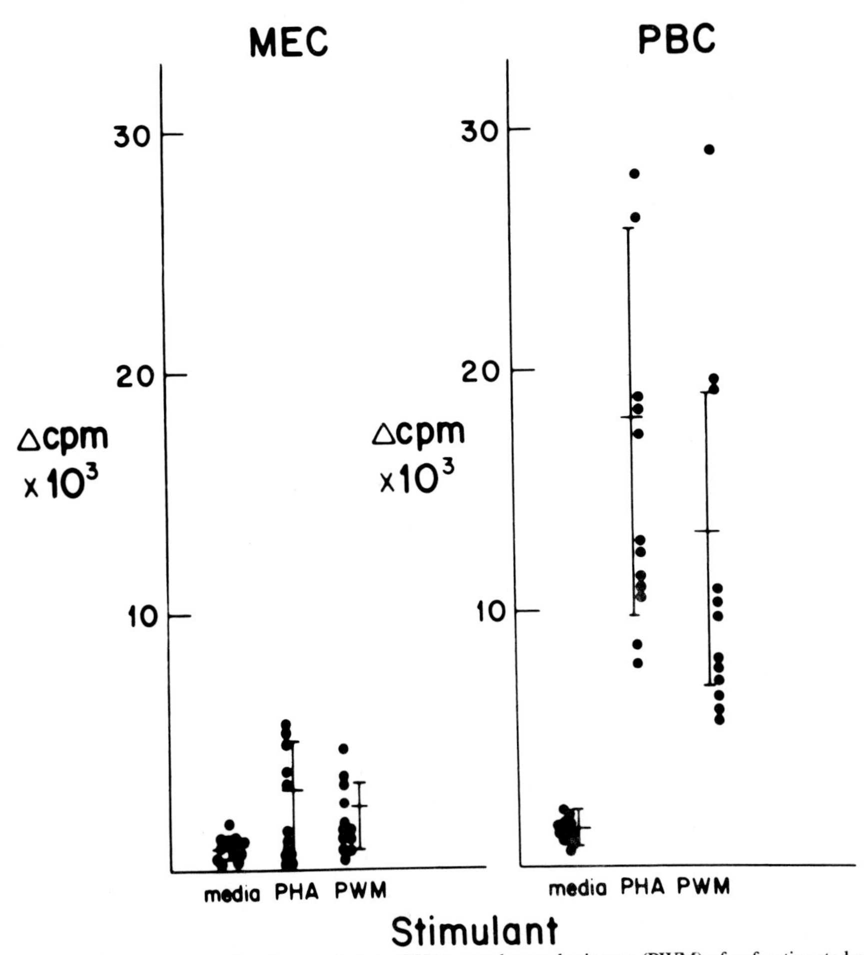

Figure 1 The proliferative response to phytohemagglutinin (PHA) or pokeweed mitogen (PWM) of unfractionated middle ear cells (MEC) and peripheral blood cells (PBC) from patients with chronic otitis media. Data are the differences between the counts per minute (cpm) in cultures stimulated with PHA or PWM and the cpm in unstimulated cultures. Values for the control cultures (media alone) are also shown. Bars = geometric means ± S.D. The total numbers of lymphocytes used for testing MECs and PBCs were similar.

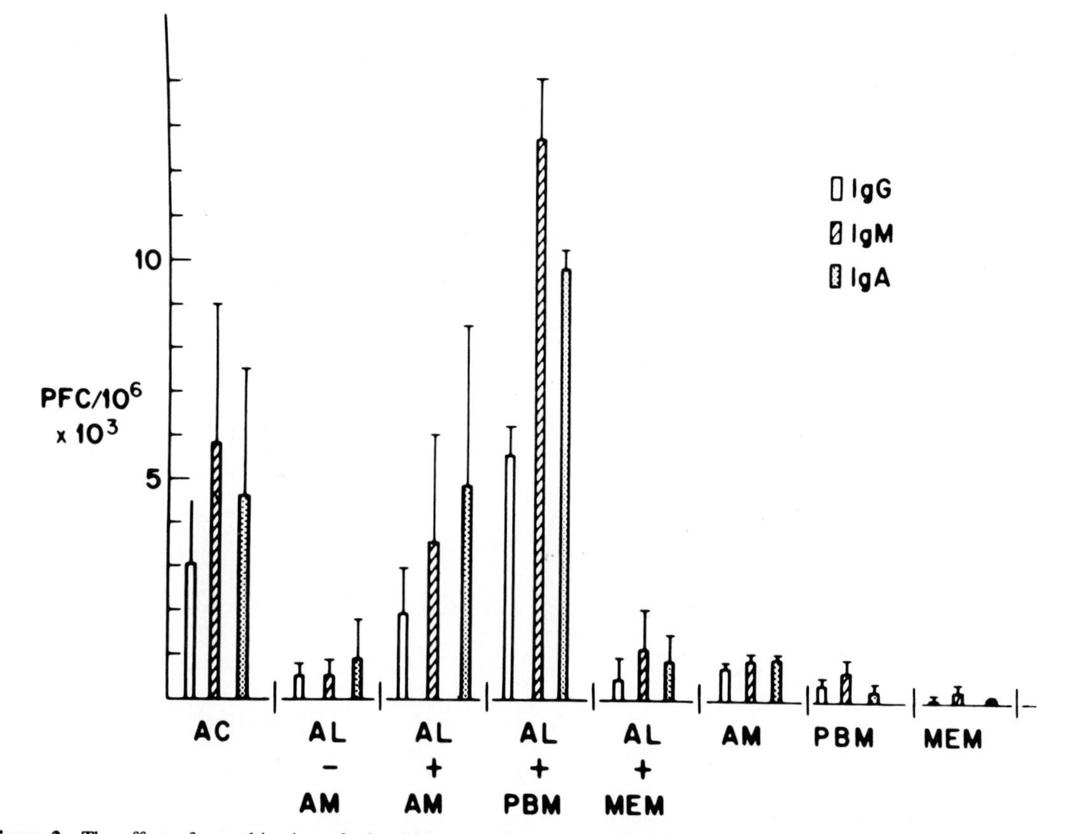

Figure 2 The effect of co-cultivation of adenoidal macrophages (AM), peripheral blood macrophages (PBM), and middle ear macrophages (MEM) from patients with chronic otitis media on the synthesis of polyclonal IgG, IgM, and IgA antibodies by adenoidal lymphocytes (AL) after *in vitro* stimulation by pokeweed mitogen. Data are mean plaque-forming counts (PFC)/10^3 cells. Bars = S.D. AC = adenoidal cells (unfractionated).

adenoidal cells in response to PWM was studied. A significant degree of polyclonal immunoglobulin synthesis is demonstrated in PWM-stimulated cultures of both MEC and adenoidal cells for each immunoglobulin isotype. However, the immunoglobulin synthesis as evidenced by plaque numbers appeared to be significantly higher in the adenoidal cells as compared with the responses in the middle ear cells. When preparations of adenoidal lymphocytes depleted of adherent macrophages were cocultured with macrophages obtained from the middle ear fluid and peripheral blood cells, the plaque-forming assay was studied; the results are described in Figure 2. The responses of adenoidal lymphocytes were significantly depressed in the presence of middle ear fluid macrophage in regard to both plaque-forming cells and lymphocyte proliferation.

In additional studies the effects of different types of middle ear effusions on the peripheral responses of adenoidal lymphocytes to PHA and PWM were examined. The proliferative activity to PHA as well as PWM was found to be consistently lower in the presence of middle ear effusion than in the presence of homologous serum. Middle ear effusion-induced suppression of proliferative activity was significant for PHA response in the serous and seromucinous types of effusions. Significant suppression was also observed for PWM-induced response in the presence of seromucinous middle ear effusion.

Finally, to determine whether the immunosuppressive activity in middle ear effusions was associated with a specific molecular weight protein, pooled middle ear fluid was fractionated and the different molecular weight components were examined. The effects of various fractions tested on the proliferative response of adenoidal lymphocytes to PWM are shown in Figure 3. A significant degree of suppression was observed with the fractions in the molecular weight range 50,000 to 60,000. No suppression was observed for other fractions. Fractions with molecular weights of 13,000 to 15,000 actually elicited an enhancement

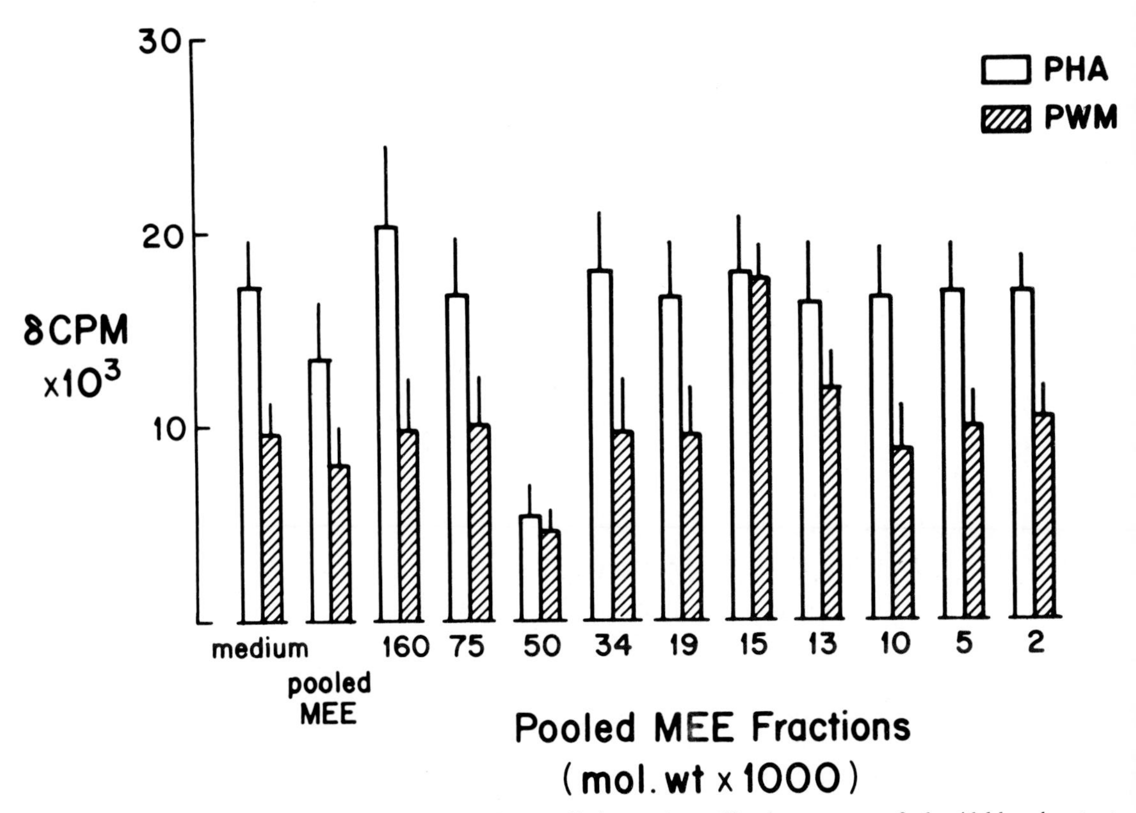

Figure 3 Effects of different fractions of pooled middle ear effusion on the proliferative responses of adenoidal lymphocytes to phytohemagglutinin (PHA) and pokeweed mitogen (PWM). Unfractionated middle ear effusion (MEE) and tissue culture medium are included as controls.

of proliferative response to PWM. In additional studies, proliferative responses to specific antigens, such as tuberculin and herpes simplex virus, and IgM antibody synthesis for SRBC and OVA were observed to be markedly inhibited by the presence of fractions with a molecular weight of 50,000. The effect of preparations of middle ear macrophage supernatants and PBC supernatants on lymphocyte proliferation and polyclonal immunoglobulin synthesis of unfractionated adenoidal cells and macrophage-depleted adenoidal lymphocytes to PWM also showed that the responses were consistently suppressed in the presence of middle ear fluid macrophage culture supernatants compared with the responses obtained in the presence of culture supernatants of peripheral blood monocytes.

DISCUSSION

The data represented in this study suggest that PHA- and PWM-induced proliferative responses of MECs appear to be low, and MECs are generally hyporesponsive compared with the response observed in PBCs and adenoidal cells. Of particular importance is the observation that PWM-induced proliferative responses and polyclonal immunoglobulin synthesis of adenoidal cells are significantly depressed only by middle ear macrophages and not by an equivalent number of peripheral blood monocytes or adenoidal monocytes.

It is known that the optimal number of monocytes will augment proliferative responses to PWM, and reconstitution of macrophage-depleted lymphocytes with syngeneic monocyte population will restore lymphocyte responsiveness to PWM.[4] On the other hand, the presence of an excess macrophage-monocyte cell population appears to inhibit PWM-induced responsiveness of peripheral blood lymphocytes.[5] Thus, the hyporesponsiveness of MECs to PWM and PHA may be a reflection of the relatively large proportion of macrophages observed in middle ear effusion.

The immunosuppressive activity was limited to a soluble factor(s) of a molecular weight of approximately 50,000. The degree of immunosuppression appeared to be most marked with serous or seromucoid forms of middle ear effusion (MEE). Although the proliferative response to both PHA and PWM was affected, the suppression was particularly significant for PHA.

The observation that middle ear macrophages could be induced to generate such suppressive activity after their cultivation *in vitro* is particularly important. The culture supernatants of peripheral blood monocytes failed to exhibit such suppressive effects. This directly relates the immunosuppressive activity found in MEE with soluble products produced by the middle ear macrophages.

Based on the data summarized in this report, we suggest that the cell populations observed in MEEs of the serous and seromucoid types are associated with the production of such suppressive factors. In view of the low molecular weight of the suppressive products, it is unlikely that they represent soluble immune complexes or immunoglobulins. It is more likely that the suppressor activity observed is a function of immunosuppressive cytokines, similar to those that have been shown to be released by a variety of immunoregulatory cells in peripheral blood.

A certain degree of immunologic enhancement was observed with two molecular weight fractions of MEE. These fractions appeared to be of smaller molecular weight (15,000 plus 13,000) than those involved in immunosuppression. These observations suggest that middle ear macrophages may possess a heterogeneous spectrum of immunoregulatory factors. Secretory products of macrophages permit numerous feedback loops, both positive and negative, to affect the inflammatory response. Macrophage–lymphocyte interaction can result in potentiation of the immunologic response, inducing T helper cells, activating cytotoxic effector cells, and enhancing specific immune responsiveness to antigens. Their interaction can also result in immunologic suppression, as noted in several clinical disorders.

Although the precise role of such regulatory effects of middle ear macrophages on the development of chronic otitis media with effusion cannot be defined on the basis of the data, it is suggested that hyporesponsiveness of immunoglobulin and possible specific antibody production in the middle ear may be intimately related to the pathogenesis of otitis media. The depression of specific immunologic responsiveness may favor ineffective elimination of antigens through humoral mechanisms as well as cell mediated mechanisms. This may lead to chronicity of the disease process, persistence of effusions, and irreversible tissue injury.

SUMMARY

On the basis of our observations and previously published data, we propose that at least in certain forms of chronic otitis media with effusion (serous or seromucoid) there is a relative predominance of macrophage–monocyte cells that are actively immunosuppressive for the proliferative response to mitogens and specific antigens as well as for the synthesis of specific immunoglobulins. Such immunologic hyporesponsiveness may be related to the pathogenesis of chronic otitis associated with such effusions.

REFERENCES

1. Ogra PL, Bernstein JM, Yurchak AM, et al: Characteristics of secretory immune system in human middle ear: Implications in otitis media. J Immunol 112:488, 1974
2. Sloyer JL, Howie VM, Ploussard JH, et al: Immune response to acute otitis media in children. III. Implications of viral antibody in middle ear fluid. J Immunol 118:248, 1977
3. Yamanaka T, Bernstein JM, Cumella J, et al: Immunologic aspects of otitis media with effusion is characteristic of lymphocyte and macrophage reactivity. J Infect Dis 147:794–799, 1983
4. Hammarstrom L, Bird AG, Brittan S, Smith CIE: Poke weed mitogen induced differentiation of human B cells: Evaluation by a protein A hemolytic plaque assay. Immunology 38:181, 1979
5. Meyling FG, Waldman TA: Human B cell activation *in vitro:* Augmentation and suppression by monocytes of the immunoglobulin production induced by various B cell stimulants. J Immunol 126:529, 1981

IN VIVO IMMUNOLOGY: SEROUS OTITIS MEDIA IN CHILDREN WITH IMMUNODEFICIENCY DISORDERS

JAN E. VELDMAN, M.D., Ph.D., JOHN J. ROORD, M.D., WIETSE KUIS, M.D., JAN W. STOOP, M.D., and EGBERT H. HUIZING, M.D.

A study of children with different immunodeficiency disorders—as an "experiment of nature"—may help determine the role of the immunologic defense system in the development of otitis media with effusion (OME). Patients with immunodeficiency disorders which express themselves as humoral immunity deficits, still develop OME, suggesting that a key to the events leading to OME does not necessarily lie in the B-cell compartment of the immune apparatus.

After antigen contact, three types of immune responses involving both T- and B-cells occur in peripheral lymphoid tissue. As a consequence of antigenic stimulation, cellular and humoral immunity usually develop, including immunologic memory.

The lymphocytic population of any peripheral lymphoid tissue is not static but is continuously exchanged. It appears that two distinct populations of lymphocytes exist: thymus-derived T lymphocytes (T-cells) and nonthymus-derived B lymphocytes (B-cells). They belong to the two compartments of our immunologic defense system (humoral and cellular immunity). T-cells, although originating in the bone marrow, undergo a proliferation and differentiation process in the thymus; B-cells in mammals seem to lack a comparable structured microenvironment. A preprogrammed (re)circulation route appears to be incorporated in the various B- and T-cell subpopulations of the body.

To develop further the issue of OME in cases of immunodeficiency disorders, we will focus on two important fundamental aspects of lymphoid tissue dynamics: (1) the experimental evidence that leads to the concept of the physiologic role of germinal center reactions (for example, in tonsils and adenoids): sites of B-cell amplification and B-memory cell production; and (2) the auxiliary role, played by so-called interdigitating and/or Langerhans' cells, in both the induction and the expression of T-cell immune reactivity.

GERMINAL CENTER REACTIONS

Sites of Virginal B-Cell Amplification and B-Cell Memory Production

Germinal centers—focal accumulations of proliferating lymphoid cells in the centers of follicles—appear first in draining peripheral lymphoid tissue only three to five days after antigenic stimulation. In tonsils and adenoids these germinal centers are located immediately beneath the cryptal epithelium, strategically located for antigen capture. The phenomenon of antigen transportation to these particular areas is usually described as "antigen trapping." Experimental data indicate that the retained material is an antigen-antibody complex. Much of our present knowledge of germinal centers has come from histologic studies, as early as Flemming's in 1885,[1] revealing a variety of unique microenvironmental features. Immunofluorescence and autoradiographic studies demonstrated that antigens are retained at the outer membrane of the so-called follicular dendritic cells for a prolonged period of time (weeks). In addition to B-cells, a specific T-cell subset, a helper cell, seems to be essential at this site to permit the whole machinery of a germinal center to operate.

In experiments in the rabbit designed to evaluate the contribution of the gut-associated lymphoid tissue to the postirradiation regeneration of B-follicular structures, it has been found that germinal centers may function as sites of virginal B-cell amplification.[2]

At present it is thought that germinal centers contribute to the pool of primary antibody-forming cell precursors through an amplification process by virtue of a surface receptor sensitive to mitogenic factors present in this particular microenvironment. Superimposed on this B-lymphocytopoiesis, germinal center activity seems to add to the production of B-memory cells. In a normally functioning immune system, adenoids and tonsils contribute adequately to such a physiologic role of the body's defense mechanism. In children with various B- (and T-) cell immunodeficiencies it most likely does not operate at all or is inadequate.[3,4]

INTERDIGITATING CELLS, LANGERHANS' CELLS, AND THE T-CELL TERRITORIES

How does the microarchitecture of the lymphoid system promote cellular interactions leading to cellular immunity? As a corollary to the previously mentioned B-cell reactions, pure T-cell reactivity takes place in the thymus-dependent areas (TDAs) of lymphoid tissue. Most types of antigenic stimulation elicit clear immunoblast reactions of T-cell origin in the TDAs. Autoradiographic studies proved that these reactions give rise to a lymphocytic cell progeny. Cellular immunity reactions in the TDAs of any peripheral lymphoid organ reveal a highly characteristic pattern: agglomerates of medium-sized lymphocytes and T-blasts are observed, surrounding nonphagocytic cellular elements, electron microscopically characterized and designated as interdigitating cells (IDCs).[3] IDCs are like Langerhans' cells; however, they generally lack Birbeck granules in their cytoplasm. Recent experimental data reveal that these cells belong to a highly dynamic pool, presumably a product of bone-marrow–derived monocyte precursors.[4] These cells tend to move from the circulation into the body's linings, transform into Langerhans' cells and/or IDCs, and presumably pick up antigenic information to transport into the TDAs.[5] At that specific site T-cell reactivity will start. T-cell reactivity does not need help from the B-cell system to operate.[3]

At a molecular level HLA antigens, normally present and genetically determined on an individual basis, are essential for any immune reactivity of the B-, T- and auxiliary cell (IDC and/or Langerhans' cell) system, including their collaboration.[4] In Waldeyer's ring the regular nasopharyngeal flora of a child will carry on such reactions for a prolonged period of time; even in those children in whom a pure B-cell immunodeficiency is present cellular immune reactions may develop undisturbed.

THE MIDDLE EAR: A T-CELL TARGET IN OME?

Of a group of 22 children with well-documented immunodeficiency disorders, six developed OME during the past two years (Table 1). Patient 1, with a congenital agammaglobulinemia, completely lacks B-cells; immunoglobulins are not produced, but he still has a persistent OME. Patient 2 has a late-onset agammaglobulinemia, normal T-cell function, B-cells, but no specific antibody production of any class. Patients 3 and 4 do have B- and T- cells, cannot produce specific antibody to any antigen, but also have a negative cell-mediated immunity (CMI) reaction *in vivo* and *in vitro.* In patient 4 all HLA antigens are lacking on the membranes of nucleated cells.[7] Patient 5 has a progressive functional deficit in both antibody formation and CMI. However, it is not totally absent, nor is it in patient 6.

In patient 1 a middle ear exploration was performed prior to insertion of a ventilation tube. A mucosal biopsy was taken for immunopathologic surveillance. Immunofluorescence staining for all immunoglobulin classes (IgG, IgM, IgA, IgD,

TABLE 1 OME in Immunodeficient Children

Patient	*Age (yrs)*	*Diagnosis**	*Functional Deficiency*	*Treatment at Time of OME*
1	12	Congenital agammaglobulinemia	Ab formation	IgG 100 mg/kg body weight every 3 weeks
2	6	Late-onset agammaglobulinemia	Ab formation	None
3	8	Combined immunodeficiency (Juvenile chronic arthritis)	Ab + CMI	Prednisone, 1 mg/kg body weight alternate days
4	2	Bare lymphocyte syndrome	Ab + CMI	IgG 100 mg/kg body weight
5	6	Wiskott Aldrich syndrome	Ab† + CMI	None
6	6	IgG_1 deficiency	Ab (IgG_1 subclass)	None

*Classification according to WHO[6]
†Especially to polysaccharides

be demonstrated in the mucosa. However, T-lymphocytes were present in abundance, designated by monoclonal antibodies as helper T-cell and suppressor T-cell phenotype subclasses. No B-cells or plasmacellular elements could be detected.

DISCUSSION

It is most interesting to observe in different well-documented cases of B- and T-cell immunodeficiencies that these children still can develop OME. "Experiments of nature" give us the chance to evaluate the role that B- and T-cells and the auxiliary systems play in the pathogenesis of OME. A functioning B-cell system (antibody formation) or the mere presence of a nonfunctioning B-cell lineage does not seem to be a prerequisite for the development of OME at all. A congenital lack of B-cells still gives rise to OME. Is T-cell reactivity then responsible for a possible release of bioactive substances in the middle ear mucosa? If so, a form of CMI seems to be unlikely, since two of our patients could not develop CMI but still had OME. Therefore, if T-cells play a role in the expression of OME it most likely is a different T-cell subclass from the one that is responsible for CMI. The fact that the child with a bare-lymphocyte syndrome also develops OME should raise the question of whether any part of the immune apparatus at all needs to play a role in the development of the disease. The afferent and efferent limb of the defense system is not functioning in an appropriate way: B-, T- and auxiliary cells lack the HLA-antigens for adequate cooperation.[7] However, the child with that syndrome still develops OME.

Further analyses of identical cases, including detailed immunopathologic surveillance of middle ear mucosa biopsies, should help us to formulate a better answer.

Thea M. Vroom, M.D., Slotervaart Hospital, Amsterdam, performed the clinical immunopathologic studies for this report.

REFERENCES

1. Flemming E: Studien über Regeneration der Gewebe. Arch für Micr Anat 24:355, 1885
2. Nieuwenhuis P: B-cell differentiation in vivo. Immunol Today 2:104, 1981
3. Veldman JE, Keuning FJ: Histophysiology of cellular immunity reactions in B-cell deprived rabbits. Virch Arch B Cell Pathol 28:203, 1978
4. Veldman JE, Kaiserling E: Interdigitating cells. In *The Reticuloendothelial System*, vol 1. Carr I, Daems WT (eds): *Morphology*. New York: Plenum Press, 1981, pp 381–416
5. Veldman JE, Keuning FJ, Lennert K, et al: Interdigitating cells. A guiding cell line in T cell reactivity. In *In Vivo Immunology: Histophysiology of the Lymphoid System*, vol 149. Nieuwenhuis P, Broek AAvd, Hanna MG (eds): New York: Plenum Press, 1982, pp 407–414
6. WHO: Immunodeficiency. Report of a WHO-scientific group. Clin Immunol Immunopathol 13:296, 1979
7. Kuis W, Roord JJ, Zegers BJM, et al: Clinical and immunological studies in a patient with the 'bare lymphocyte' syndrome. In *Bone Marrow Transplantation in Europe*, vol II. Touraine JL, Gluckman E, Griscelli C, (eds): Amsterdam: Elsevier North Holland, 1981, pp 201–208

BIOCHEMISTRY

BIOCHEMISTRY OF MIDDLE EAR EFFUSION: STATE OF THE ART

S.K. JUHN, M.D.

The biochemical characteristics of middle ear effusion (MEE) reflect the inflammatory changes in the middle ear cavity. Several sources provide the constituents of MEE, namely, mucosa, bacteria, inflammatory cells, and plasma. The degree of involvement of each is not easy to identify, because some of the constituents come from different sources. There are several types of MEE: serous, mucoid, purulent, or some combination of these. The characteristics of various types of MEE have been identified to a certain degree by the physical appearance and bacterial, biochemical, and immunochemical characteristics. Several conditions that can produce MEE are known, for example, eustachian tube dysfunction and bacterial or viral infection. Certain predisposing conditions are suggested but not yet confirmed. Therefore, the aims of the biochemical studies of MEE are to identify the biochemical constituents of the various types of MEE, to select certain specific parameters that can serve as an inflammatory index, and to find the means to utilize this information for the proper evaluation of the types of otitis media, the stages of inflammation, efficacy of treatment, and prediction of prognosis.

BIOCHEMICAL PARAMETERS

Protein and Enzymes

Proteins present in middle ear effusions appear to be primarily from the plasma. This is shown in MEE from experimental animals with eustachian tube obstruction. However, in human MEE, total protein concentrations of both serous and mucoid effusions are significantly higher than that of serum.[1] This indicates that local production of enzymes and antibodies contributes to the protein content of MEE. In animal experiments, when purulent otitis media (POM) and serous otitis media (SOM) were compared, different patterns of protein fractionation were observed.[2]

The content of various enzymes in human MEE has been studied by many investigators. It is clear that most of the enzymes studied are higher in MEE than in serum, indicating the local release of enzymes from the various sources, namely, bacteria, inflammatory cells, and inflamed mucosa. Lysozyme has multiple functions. It is a relatively weak agent against bacteria, but it can act synergistically with the complement and specific antibodies.[3] It is also known that lysosomal enzymes, including lysozyme, can enhance the inflammatory changes in the middle ear mucosa by increasing capillary permeability, stimulating chemotaxis, activating plasminogen, activating complement, and possibly leading to chronic inflammation in the middle ear cavity in otitis media with effusion.[4] Levels of lysozyme in recurrent cases of MEE were higher than those in nonrecurrent cases.[5] Therefore, the lysozyme level in MEE appears to be related to the recurrence rate or chronicity of the otitis media.

Recently, Diven and associates[6] studied the content of lysosomal hydrolases in the MEE. They found that the mean specific activity for alpha-glucosidase in mucoid effusions was ten times higher than that in serous effusions. They also found that the activities of alpha-mannosidase, alpha-glucuronidase, hexosaminidase, acid phosphatase, alpha-galactosidase, alkaline phosphatase, and lactate dehydrogenase were three to five times higher in mucoid than in serous effusions. The specific activities of lysosomal hydrolase from purulent effusions were found to be between the activities in serous and mucoid effusions. These investigators could not observe a significant correlation between the specific activities of lysosomal hydrolases and the presence or absence of bacteria in mucoid or serous middle ear effusions. The presence of neuraminidase both in human MEE from patients with chronic otitis media and in chinchilla MEE from cases of acute otitis media induced by *Streptococcus pneumoniae* has been reported by La Marco and colleagues.[7] They could demonstrate neuraminidase activity in 95 percent of effusions that were positive for *S. pneumoniae* and in only 20 to 45 percent of effusions positive for other bacteria.

Proteases also seem to play an important role in middle ear inflammation. The granulocyte proteases are classified according to their pH optima. Proteases active at a neutral pH of the extracellular environment are collagenase, elastase, and cathepsin G. Neutral proteases are capable of degrading collagen, elastin, and proteoglycans of connective tissues, and of cleaving plasma proteins, such as fibrinogen; coagulation factors VII, VIII, XII, and XIII; immunoglobulins; and the complement factors C1, C3, and C5. The proteolytic activity on C3 and C5 results in conversion products, which have a chemotactic effect and can trigger a further release of granulocyte proteases. Carlsson and coworkers[8] studied proteases in MEE extensively. They observed that concentrations of both granulocyte neutral protease and elastase were lower in MEE from cases of serous otitis media of long duration than those of short duration. This can be explained by the fact that the extracellular release of granulocyte proteases increases with increasing inflammatory activity.

Enzyme Inhibitors

The control of proteases involved in biologic processes, including inflammation, is exerted by protease inhibitors, which are characterized by their ability to block the catalytic site of the enzymes. Therefore, the role of the protease inhibitors is essential, because insufficient inactivation of protease will result in an unbalanced free proteolytic activity. The main inhibitors of granulocyte proteases are alpha-1-antitrypsin, alpha-1-antichymotrypsin, alpha-2-macroglobulin, alpha-1-anticollagenase, and antileukoprotease. Protease inhibitors in MEE have been studied by several investigators.[9–12] According to Carlsson's report, the mean concentration of protease inhibitors was higher in MEE from cases of chronic SOM than in MEE from cases of acute POM. Carlsson also reported that albumin in MEE/plasma ratio was higher in cases of chronic otitis media than in acute otitis media. It can be concluded that membrane permeability is increased in chronic otitis media and more plasma protease inhibitors can get into MEE in the chronic stage of otitis media.

The fibrinolytic activity of MEE for the dissolution of fibrin clots has been reported by Bernstein and associates.[13] When the activity was compared in serous and mucoid MEE, they observed a higher level of both general proteolytic activity and fibrinolytic activity in serous effusion than in mucoid effusion. They suggested that plasmin, the active protease of the fibrinolysis system, is capable of activating a number of proteolytic systems, including the intrinsic coagulation system, the vasoactive peptide system, and the complement system. They also speculated that the lack of fibrinolytic activity may promote the development of a fibrin mash, and this may contribute to connective tissue synthesis and progressive fibrosis with eventual development of adhesive otitis media.

Carbohydrate and Mucous Substances

The glucose concentration in the MEE has also been reported on.[1,14–16] A lower concentration of glucose in the MEE than in the corresponding serum was observed. This may be due to increased glucose consumption by the inflammatory cells or microorganisms. Microbial proliferation as well as phagocytosis is accompanied by increased oxygen consumption and an increase in both aerobic and anaerobic glycolysis.

Senturia and associates identified the protein-bound carbohydrates in the MEE.[17] Vered and associates characterized the glycoproteins in the MEE and reported the presence of protein-bound hexosamines, neutral sugars, and sialic acid, which are typically present in glandular excretions.[18] Based on these data, they suggested that MEE may be a mixture of mucus secreted by the glands in the middle ear mucosa and an inflammatory exudate.

Hexosamine levels in MEE were studied by Juhn and coworkers.[19] Mucoid effusions had a higher level of hexosamines than serous effusions. Hyaluronate estimation was also performed using chromatographic separation, and a higher percentage was observed in mucoid effusion than in serous effusion.[20] All these results indicate that the mucoid substances identified in the MEE are responsible for viscosity or stickiness of the effusions.

Inflammatory Mediators

Several inflammatory mediators, including prostaglandins and histamines, have been identified in the MEE. Prostaglandins (PGs) have been found in human MEE at levels higher than corresponding serum or plasma.[21] Mucoid effusions contained higher concentrations of prostaglandins than serous effusions.[22] Recently, Jung and colleagues reported higher levels of PGE_2 and 6-keto-$PGF_{1\alpha}$ in human MEE from cases of mucoid otitis media than from cases of SOM.[23] PGE-like material has also been found in human granulation tissue from cases of chronic otitis media.[24] Recently, the levels of PGE_2 and 6-keto-$PGF_{1\alpha}$ in human granulation tissue and cholesteatoma were reported.[25] In animal studies, the ability of middle ear mucosa to synthesize prostaglandins has been shown.[25] Both PGE_2 and $PGF_{2\alpha}$ were found to be higher in MEE from a chinchilla POM model than from a SOM model.[26] PG-producing cyclo-oxygenase was localized in human and animal middle ear mucosa, granulation tissue, and cholesteatoma.[23]

Dennis and colleagues showed that histamine, bradykinin, and prostaglandins of the E series can induce vasodilation, increased vascular permeability, and edema in the middle ear and eustachian tube mucosa.[27] Recently, Berger and colleagues reported that histamine was found in significant levels above its blood concentration in 62 percent of the effusions.[28] Although a wide scattering of histamine levels exists in different types of effusion from cases of secretory otitis media, the mucoid type has been found to contain a higher level than the serous type. They also reported that a comparison of histamine levels in MEE from allergic versus nonallergic subjects revealed no significant differences between the two groups. In our animal studies, we observed a higher level of histamine in MEE from the POM model than from the SOM model. Based on these data, the mechanisms responsible for histamine release may not be solely type I immediate type of hypersensitivity, but may include type III, which involves immune complexes through activation of the complement system, producing anaphylatoxin and release of histamine by mast cell degranulation.

SUMMARY

The biochemical studies of MEE in various types of otitis media are still incomplete. Further biochemical characterization of MEE at various inflammatory stages is necessary. There are certain limitations in studying the various biochemical parameters, namely, the amount of effusion available is not sufficient to analyze many of these, and it is possible to obtain samples only at the time when therapeutic myringotomy is performed. Therefore, the biochemical data we obtain will represent the status of inflammation at that point. In animal studies, however, it is possible to control the experimental conditions, and serial sampling can provide us the information on the sequential biochemical changes in the MEE. Therefore, parallel animal studies can contribute a great deal to the interpretation of the data we obtain from human MEEs.

In general, activities of various enzymes are higher in mucoid MEE than in serous MEE. The hexosamine content has also been reported to be higher in mucoid MEE than in serous. However, the mechanisms of the production of the mucoid effusions have not been clarified. Further studies are necessary to identify factors that trigger the middle ear mucosa to produce mucoid effusions.

Finally, the incorporation of the laboratory data on MEE with clinical features of otitis media is necessary. Recent attempts to evaluate the biochemical data in relation to the patient's history of recurrence are noteworthy. Retrospective studies of patient histories after obtaining initial biochemical data indicate that certain differences in the levels of enzyme and protein exist between recurrent and nonrecurrent groups. These preliminary data provide some hope that these biochemical characteristics might predict future risk of OME. It is clear that a single parameter may not be sufficient to evaluate the complex inflammatory events taking place in the middle ear cavity. A combination of two or more parameters that are related to specific events may help us to understand and identify the disease processes taking place in the middle ear cavity. Although the concept of inflammatory index should be better defined, the data now available from retrospective studies appear to have predictive value for otitis media morbidity. It must be validated and refined in more extensive longitudinal follow-up studies.

This study was supported by NINCDS grant # NS 14538.

REFERENCES

1. Juhn SK, Huff JS: Biochemical characteristics of middle ear effusions. Ann Otol 85(Suppl 25):110, 1976

2. Juhn SK: Unpublished data
3. Veltri RW, Sprinkle PM: Serous otitis media. Immunoglobulin and lysozyme levels in middle ear fluids and serum. Ann Otol Rhinol Laryngol 82:297, 1973
4. Bernstein JM: The significance of lysozymal enzymes in middle ear effusions. Otolaryngol Head Neck Surg 87:845, 1979
5. Juhn SK: Studies on middle ear effusions. Laryngoscope, 92:287, 1982
6. Diven WF, Glen RH, Bluestone CD: Lysozome hydrolases in middle ear effusions. Ann Otol Rhinol Laryngol 990:14, 1981
7. LaMarco K, Diven W, Glen RH, et al: Neuraminidase activity in middle ear effusions. Ann Otol Rhinol Laryngol, 92(Suppl 107), 1983
8. Carlsson B, Lundberg C, Ohlsson K: Granulocyte proteases in middle ear effusions. Ann Otol 91:76, 1982
9. Kastenbauer ER, Hochstrasser K, Reichert R, et al: Der Nachweis eines niedermolekularen säurestabilen Protease-inhibitors im Ohrsekret bei chronischer Mittelohreiterung. J Laryngol Otol 56:201, 1977
10. Hochstrasser K, Arnold W: Proteinases and proteinase inhibitors in middle ear effusions (Abstr). Third International Symposium on Recent Advances in Otitis Media with Effusion, 1983, p 49
11. Carlsson B, Lundberg C, Ohlsson K: Protease inhibitors in middle ear effusions. Ann Otol 90:38, 1981
12. Carlsson B, Lundberg C, Ohlsson K: Protease-protease inhibitor balance in otitis media with effusion. In Lim DJ et al (eds): *Otitis Media*. Philadelphia, Toronto: BC Decker Inc, 1984
13. Bernstein JM, Steger R, Bock N: The fibrinolysin system in otitis media with effusion. J Otolaryngol 1:28, 1979
14. Lupovich P, Bluestone CD, Paradise JL, Harkins M: Middle ear effusions: Preliminary viscometric, histologic and biochemical studies. Ann Otol 80:342, 1971
15. Juhn SK, Huff JS, Paparella MM: Biochemical analysis of middle ear effusions. Preliminary report. Ann Otol 80:347, 1971
16. Juhn SK, Jung TTK, Giebink GS, et al: Factors involved in the alteration of middle ear effuson composition (Abstr). Third International Symposium on Recent Advances in Otitis Media with Effusion, 1983, p 50
17. Senturia BH, Gessert CF, Carr CD, Baumann ES: Studies concerned with tubo-tympanitis. Ann Otol 67:440, 1958
18. Vered J, Eliezer N, Sadé J: Biochemical characterization of middle ear effusions. Ann Otol 81:394, 1972
19. Juhn SK, Paparella MM, Kim CS, et al: Pathogenesis of otitis media. Ann Ot Rhin Laryngol 86:481, 1977
20. Juhn SK: Unpublished data
21. Jackson RT, Waitzman MB, Pickford L, et al: Prostaglandins in human middle ear effusions. Prostaglandins 10:365, 1975
22. Bernstein JM: Biochemical mediators of inflammation in middle ear effusions. Ann Otol 85(Suppl 25):90, 1976
23. Jung TTK, Huang D, Juhn SK: Prostaglandins in middle ear fluids, cholesteatoma and granulation tissue (Abstr). Third International Symposium Recent Advances in Otitis Media with Effusion, 1983, p 53
24. Gantz BJ, Clancey C, Abramson M: Decalcification factors in granulation tissue and ear canal skin. In McCabe BF, Sadé J, Abramson M: *Cholesteatoma: First International Conference*. Birmingham, AL: Aesculapius, 1977, pp 167–169
25. Jung TTK, Smith DM, Juhn Sk, Gerrard JM: Effect of prostaglandin on the composition of chinchilla middle ear effusion. Ann Otol 89(Suppl 68):153, 1980
26. Smith DM, Jung TTK, Juhn SK, et al.: Prostaglandins in experimental otitis media. Arch Otorhinolaryngol 225:207, 1979
27. Dennis RG, Whitmire RN, Jackson RT: Action of inflammatory mediators on middle ear mucosa. Arch Otolaryngol 102:420, 1976
28. Berger G, Hawke WM, Proops DW, et al: Histamine levels in middle ear effusions (Abstr). Third International Symposium on Recent Advances in Otitis Media with Effusion, 1983, p 51

PROTEINASES AND PROTEINASE INHIBITORS IN MIDDLE EAR EFFUSIONS

KARL HOCHSTRASSER, M.D., W. ARNOLD, M.D., and R. NAUMANN, M.D.

The primary defense system of the human upper respiratory tract is based on interacting mechanical, immunologic, and cellular factors. Polymorphonuclear neutrophilic granulocytes release active proteases in the course of defensive immune and cellular reactions. These enzymes result in an array of pathologic processes demonstrated in many studies.[1,2] Several proteinase inhibitors derived from blood serum or from glands in the mucous membranes counteract the pathogenic effects of these granulocytic proteases. However, the demands on the pool of inhibitors should not be excessive, and their action should not be disturbed by other factors. The relationship between granulocytic protease and proteinase inhibitors in vivo has been evaluated in normal and pathologic nasal or bronchial secretions. Methods to demonstrate free, inactive, or protease-attached inhibitors have been developed.[3–5] By these methods, all inhibitors demonstrable in the secretions of the upper respiratory tract have been shown to participate in the neutralization of proteases. In addition, the activity of these inhibitory systems in a given secretion has been defined by inhibitograms.

To examine the activity of the inhibitory system in the effusions of otitis media, we have developed a detailed assay system. Characteristic findings in individual effusions are presented and discussed.

MATERIALS AND METHODS

Reagents

Trypsin treated with chloro(N-toluene-sulfonyl-L-phenylalanyl)-methane (TPCK) was purchased from E. Merck (D-6100 Darmstadt). Elastase from porcine pancreas (120 U/mg) was obtained from Serva (D-6900 Heidelberg). Elastase and cathepsin G from human polymorphonuclear granulocytes were prepared according to the method of Tschesche and associates.[8] Antibodies directed to human alpha-1-PI* and alpha-2-macroglobulin were obtained from Behringwerke (D-3550 Marburg). BzArgNan† was obtained from E. Merck; Suc(Ala)$_3$Nan, Suc(Ala)$_2$ValNan, and SucPheLeuPheSBz were from Bachem (CH-Bubendorf).

Preparation of Samples

Serous and mucous effusions were collected from 32 children who had histories of secretory otitis media. No case of obviously purulent effusion was included among these 32 ears. From eight ears with clinically purulent effusions the fluid was collected separately for comparison with the first group. The children's ages ranged from 2 to 12 years. Most of them were admitted to the hospital for adenoidectomy and for the insertion of ventilating tubes because of a conductive hearing loss caused by secretory otitis media. The effusions were separated from the cotton strips according to the method of Eichner and colleagues.[9]

*Formerly alpha-1-antitrypsin.

†Synthetic substrates are abbreviated according the IUPAC-IUB rules for abbreviations of amino acid: Bz = benzoyl; Nan = p-nitro-anilide; Suc = 3-carboxypropionyl.

Removal of Alpha-1-PI

One hundred percent of the inhibitory activity against pancreatic elastase in native middle ear effusion (MEE) results from alpha-1-PI. To precipitate alpha-1-PI quantitatively, 20 μl of IgG solution is necessary for a sample of MEE containing 2 mIU antielastase activity. This mixture is incubated at 37°C for 12 hours. The immunocomplexes are then centrifuged off to provide supernatant free of alpha-1-PI.

IgG from Antiserum Directed Against Alpha-1-PI

From commercial antiserum the IgG is isolated by affinity chromatography on protein-A-sepharose and brought to the same starting volume.[10]

Deproteinization

To native MEE 1/10 volume of 70 percent $HClO_4$ was added. After 10 minutes precipitated proteins were removed by centrifugation. The supernatant was neutralized with 4M KOH (insoluble $KClO_4$ centrifuged off) and used for measurements.

Enzyme and Inhibitor Assays

Molarities of trypsin solution were determined by active site titration with p-nitrophenyl-p′-guanodinobenzoate according to the method of Chase and Shaw.[11]

The activities of trypsin, pancreatic elastase, granulocytic elastase, and granulocytic cathepsin and their inhibition were determined with BzArgNan, Suc(Ala)$_3$Nan, Suc(Ala)$_2$ValNan, and SucPheLeuPheSBz as substrates.[12–15]

The molarities of elastase and cathepsin G stock solutions were determined by titration with an inhibitor solution of known molarity (DSI[10] = dog submandibular inhibitor with *two* independent reactive sites, one for trypsin and one for elastases and cathepsin G.)

The activity of individual inhibitors and the amount of inhibitors involved in protease neutralization were determined as follows:

First, the inhibition of the activity of target enzymes such as trypsin, pancreatic elastase, granulocytic elastase, and granulocytic cathepsin G by untreated secretions was measured by using specific enzyme substrates. Since the inhibition of pancreatic elastase is virtually due to alpha-1-PI alone, the assay yields an estimate of the concentration of alpha-1-PI in the effusions. Also, the assay indicates the presence of active inhibitors. Lack of inhibition of enzymatic activity by the effusions indicates an exhaustion of the inhibitory activity: the rate of hydrolysis of the substrates increases measurably.

Second, if the presence of inhibitory factors has been shown in the first step of the procedure, alpha-1-PI may be removed from the effusions by immune precipitation with specific antibodies. Step 1 is then repeated. The difference between the results obtained in untreated effusions and after precipitation of alpha-1-PI indicates the specific inhibitory capacity of alpha-1-PI.

Secretion-specific inhibitors are resistant to protein-precipitating agents. Hence, their activity remains unchanged and measurable upon their release from the inhibitor-protease complex. An increase in inhibitory activity of alpha-1-PI free effusions that have been treated with protein precipitating agents indicates the presence of complexed inhibitors that can be quantitated.

Alpha-2-Macroglobulin–IgG Complexes

Alpha-2-macroglobulin in MEE and serum was determined according to the method of Laurell and colleagues.[20] With serum the amount of antiserum was determined to precipitate alpha-2-macroglobulin quantitatively. MEE and serum were mixed with an amount of antiserum directed against alpha-2-macroglobulin sufficient to precipitate alpha-2-macroglobulin. The mixture was allowed to stand for 12 hours at 37°C. Then the immune complexes were separated by centrifugation and the precipitate washed twice with 0.9 percent NaCl solution. The complexes were incubated with the substrates used for enzyme and for inhibitor measurements. Depending on the enzymatic activities of the complexes, incubation times between 10 min and 1 hour were necessary. Immune complexes were then removed by centrifugation and in the supernatant the rate of substrate cleavage was determined by photometric methods.[12–15]

RESULTS AND DISCUSSION

The protease inhibitors that have been demonstrated in effusions from the middle ear are listed in Table 1, together with their chemical and inhibitory properties. Specific antisera directed against all humoral inhibitors and antisera against leukocytic proteases are currently available and useful for further investigations.[17] However, they do not provide quantitative data on the biologic availability of these inhibitors. Although oxidation[18] or limited proteolysis inactivates alpha-1-PI, the reactivity of this inhibitor with specific antisera re-

TABLE 1 Proteinase Inhibitors in Secretions of the Upper Respiratory Tract and Middle Ear Effusions

	Interaction					
Inhibitor	*Trypsin*	*Chymotrypsin*	*Elastase (From PMN*	*Cathepsin G Granulocytes)*	*Elastase (Pancreatic)*	*Synonyms*
Products of submucous glands						
SI-TE	+	+	+	+	−	Antileukoproteinase
SI-TE*	+	+	+	+	+	
SI-E	−	−	+	−	+	
Humoral inhibitors						
Alpha-1-PI	+	+	+	+	+	Alpha-1-antitrypsin
HI-30†	+	+	+	−	−	
ITI	+	+	+	−	−	Inter-alpha-trypsin inhibitor
alpha-1-X	+	+	−	−	−	Alpha-1-antichymotrypsin
alpha-2-M	+	+	+	+	+	Alpha-2-macroglobulin

*SI, secretory inhibitor
†HI-30, the inhibitory active part of ITI (Mm 30 kDt) released physiologically from ITI

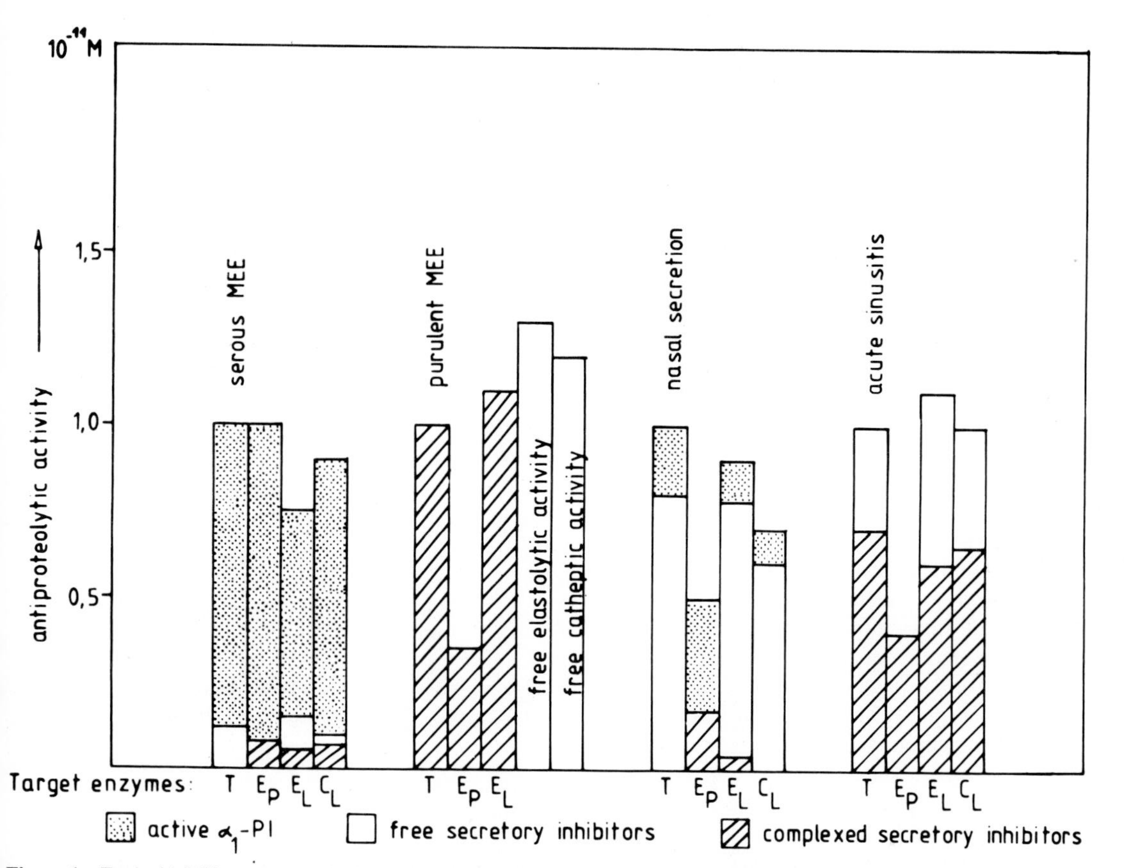

Figure 1 Typical inhibitor patterns obtained with serous and purulent middle ear effusion and normal and pathologic nasal mucus. (T, trypsin; E_P, pancreatic elastase; E_L, granulocytic elastase; C_L, granulocytic cathepsin-G.)

mains intact, as does that of alpha-1-PI-protease complexes.

Typical inhibitograms obtained by this method are shown in Fig. 1. The results obtained in two characteristic secretions obtained from the middle ear are compared with results obtained from nasal secretions and secretions from patients with acute sinusitis.

It is difficult to refer the results obtained following chemical analysis of these secretions to a standard value, since the data indicated in the inhibitograms are expressed in relative units. Absolute values, however, are not informative. All activities refer to 1 pmol of antitryptic activity. Thus, the importance of the various inhibitors for protease neutralization becomes apparent immediately.

The inhibitogram of normal nasal secretion readily shows that the inhibition of the activity of the target enzymes is mainly due to secretion-specific inhibitors. The contribution of alpha-1-PI toward this inhibition is small, and secretory inhibitors bind only small amounts of granulocytic elastase. Active alpha-1-PI cannot be demonstrated in acute sinusitis. The increase in proteases is shown by the large amount of complexed inhibitors.

The pattern is markedly different in serous middle ear effusions. The inhibition of the activity of all target enzymes rests almost exclusively on active alpha-1-PI derived from the blood plasma. Secretion-specific inhibitors represent a small fraction of the pool of inhibitors. They are mainly present in the form of complexes. This finding indicates that proteolytic proteases must have been released in the course of this type of otitis media. As one would expect, there is no active alpha-1-PI in purulent effusions; the concentration of inhibitory substances is low, and the secretion-specific inhibitors form complexes. There are signs of free elastolytic and catheptic activity.

On the basis of these findings, we assume the

release of granulocytic proteases does not play an important pathogenetic role in serous otitis media. However, the exudative changes must have been mediated by factors that enhance vascular permeability. Other proteases that are not derived from granulocytes may be of pathogenetic importance. This hypothesis is supported by the following observations: substantial amounts of alpha-2-M, another protease inhibitor, are found in serous effusions. This substance exerts its inhibitory activity in a way that is quite different from that of other inhibitors. The inhibition rests on the interaction of reactive sites of the inhibitor with the catalytic site of the proteases, resulting in complete abolition of the catalytic effect.

Alpha-2-M forms complexes[19] with all the proteases that have been studied to date. The alpha-2-M molecule (mol wt, 800,000), opened up by the proteolytic action of the protease, incorporates the enzyme, which then loses its capacity for hydrolysis of high molecular weight substrates. However, substrates of low molecular weight, for instance those used to determine the activity of proteases, may penetrate the shield formed by the alpha-2-M molecule, gain access to the protease, and undergo hydrolysis. Proteolytic activity is not reduced by precipitation of alpha-2-M-protease complex with specific anti-alpha-2-M-antibodies.

These findings have been used to determine the role of alpha-2-M in protease neutralization in effusions from the middle ear. Alpha-2-M was precipitated from middle ear effusions by using specific antibodies. The immune complexes were incubated with elastase- and cathepsin-specific substrates. The breakdown of the substrates indicates the presence of active alpha-2-M-protease complexes in the effusions. Upon determination of the protease-binding capacity of alpha-2-M by use of highly purified granulocytic proteases, the amount of proteases bound by alpha-2-M in a given effusion can be measured.

Figure 2 displays typical results obtained from analysis of serous or purulent middle ear effusions as compared with normal serum. In the effusions, very small amounts of granulocytic elastase appear to be bound by alpha-2-M. Serous effusions reveal small amounts of granulocytic elastase associated with alpha-2-M. Conversely, there is a striking activity against cathepsin-specific substrates. In purulent exudates, nearly all of the alpha-2-M is associated with proteases. Again, there is a relatively small amount of elastase, compared with the large amounts of cathepsin G or cathepsin G-like proteases.

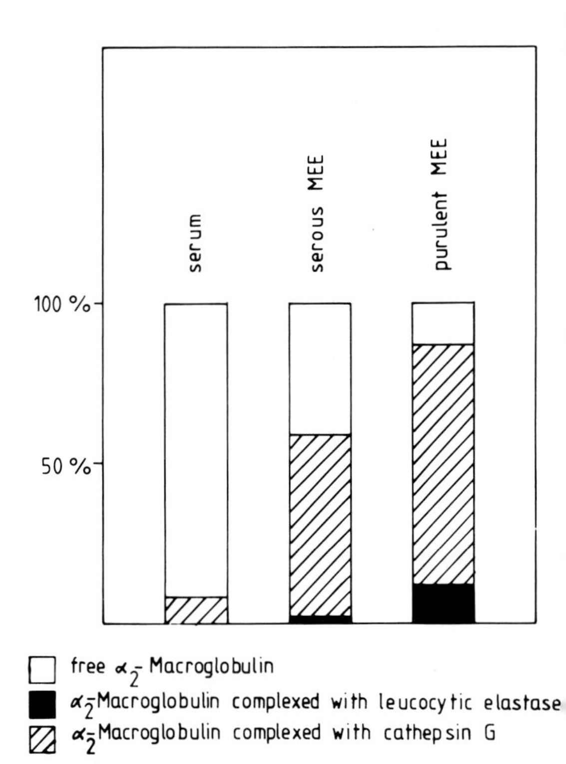

Figure 2 Occupation of alpha-2-macroglobulin in human serum and serous and purulent middle ear effusions by elastolytic and catheptic proteinases.

The findings support the contention that only a few proteases are being released into serous effusions. The high catheptic activity associated with alpha-2-M can only be explained by the release of nongranulocytic proteases. Their origin should be determined in further investigations, since all chymotrypsin-like proteases hydrolyze the substrates that have been used to date. However, the demonstration of protease activity by use of the alpha-2-M complexes helps elucidate the local mechanisms on which the presence of pathologic secretions in otitis media with effusion is based.

REFERENCES

1. Reich E, Rifkin D, Shaw E: Proteinases and Biological Control. Cold Spring Harbor Laboratory, 1975
2. Havemann K, Ianoff A (eds): *Neutral Proteinases of Human Polymorphonuclear Leucocytes*. Munich: Urban und Schwarzenberg, 1978
3. Ohlsson K, Tegner H, Fryksmark U, Polling A: Distribu-

tion of antileucoprotease in upper respiratory mucosa. Ann Otol Rhinol Laryngol 91:268, 1982
4. Hochstrasser K, Naumann R, Albrecht GJ: Neue Methoden zur differenzierten Erfassung des antiproteolytischen Systems des menschlichen Bronchialsekrets. Atemw Lungenkrkh 9:136, 1983
5. Naumann R, Behbehani AA, Eichner H, Hochstrasser K: Simultaneous determination of free and complexed proteinase inhibitors in human nasal secretions. Arch Otorhinolaryngol, in press
6. Hochstrasser K, Albrecht GJ, Schönberger OL, et al: An elastase-specific inhibitor from human bronchial mucus-isolation and characterisation. Hoppe Seyler Z Physiol Chem 362:1369, 1981
7. Wachter E, Hochstrasser K: Kunitz-type proteinase inhibitors derived by limited proteolysis of the inter-alpha-trypsin inhibitor III. Hoppe Seyler Z Physiol Chem 360:1305, 1979
8. Engelbrecht E, Pieper E, Macartueg HW, et al: Separation of the human leucocyte enzymes, alanin aminopeptidase, cathepsin G, collagenase, elastase and myeloperoxidase. Hoppe Seyler Z Physiol Chem 363:305, 1982
9. Eichner H: Eine neue Methode zur Gewinnung von Nasensekret und erste Untersuchungen zur Eiweißzusammensetzung des Nasensekrets mittels Diskelektrophorese. Laryngol Rhinol Otol 53:269, 1979
10. Hjelm H, Hjelm KH, Sjöquist S: Protein A from Staphylococcus aureus: Its isolation by affinity chromatography and its use as an immunosorbent for isolation of immunoglobulins. FEBS Letters 28:73, 1972
11. Chase T, Shaw E: Titration of trypsin, plasmin and thrombin with p-nitrophenyl-p′-guanidinobenzoate HCl. In Perlmann CG, Lorand L (eds): *Methods in Enzymology*. New York: Academic Press, 1970, p 19
12. Fritz H, Trautschold I, Werle E: In Bergmeyer HU (ed): *Methoden der Enzymatischen Analyse*. Weinheim/Bergstr: Verlag Chemie, 1977, pp 1021–1031
13. Bieth J, Spiess B, Wermuth CG: The synthesis and analytical use of a highly sensitive and convenient substrate for elastase. Biochem Med 11:350, 1974
14. Wenzel HR, Engelbrecht G, Reich H, Tschesche H: Synthesis and analytical use of 3-carboxypropionyl-alanyl-alanyl-valyl-4-nitroanilide: A specific substrate for human leucocytic elastase. Hoppe Seyler Z Physiol Chem 361:1413, 1980
15. Harper JW, Ramirez G, Powers JC: Reaction of peptide thiobenzyl esters with mammalian chymotrypsin-like enzymes: A sensitive assay method. Anal Biochem 118:382, 1981
16. Hochstrasser K, Fritz H: Die Aminosäuresequenz des doppelköpfigen Proteinasen-Inhibitors aus der geandula submandibularis des Hundes II. Ein Methionintest als reaktives Hemmzentrum für Chymotrypsin. Z Physiol Chem 356:1859, 1975
17. Carlsson B, Lundberg C, Ohlsson K: Granulocyte proteases in middle ear effusions. Ann Otol 91:76, 1982
18. Ianoff A, Carp H, Lee DK: Inactivation of alpha-1-proteinase inhibitor and bronchial mucous proteinase inhibitor by cigarette smoke in vitro and in vivo. Clin Resp Physiol 16 (Suppl): 321, 1980
19. Barrett AJ, Starkey PM: The interaction of alpha-2-macroglobulin with proteases. Biochem J 133:709, 1973
20. Laurell CB: Electroimmunoassay. Scand J Clin Lab Invest 29(Suppl 124):21, 1972

PROTEASE–PROTEASE INHIBITOR BALANCE IN OTITIS MEDIA WITH EFFUSION

BRITT E.M. CARLSSON, M.D., Ph.D.

The cellular response to inflammatory stimuli in otitis media—in particular, the release of proteolytic enzymes from the granulocytes—poses a great risk to middle ear structures. When not inactivated by protease inhibitors, granulocyte proteases degrade tissues and immunoglobulins and potentiate the inflammatory response. Consequently, the balance between protease release and protease inhibition is of fundamental importance for the prevention of tissue destruction and for the control of the inflammatory process.

MATERIALS AND METHODS

Middle ear specimens were obtained from patients suffering from acute otitis media (AOM) and serous otitis media (SOM). The diagnosis of AOM was established by a history of acute onset of severe pain and a reddened, bulging tympanic membrane seen on otoscopy. The diagnosis of SOM was established by a history, and follow-up, of persistent middle ear effusion (MEE) and a pale tympanic membrane and serous fluid in the middle ear cavity seen at otoscopy followed by myringotomy. Owing to the lack of a suitable method for reliable handling of mucoid specimens, patients with such middle ear effusions were excluded from this study. Patients with SOM were divided into those with a duration of SOM exceeding one year (SOM-1) and those with a shorter duration of SOM which exceeded two months (SOM-s). In all, ten middle ear specimens from nine patients with AOM, 20 specimens from 15 patients with SOM-s, and six specimens from six patients with SOM-1 were studied. Paired plasma specimens were analyzed as controls.

The immunochemical methods used for analysis of the proteins in MEE and plasma have been described in detail previously.[1] Electroimmunoassay and single radial immunodiffusion were used for the quantitative analyses, except for the quantification of granulocyte elastase in plasma, for which an RIA technique was used. Crossed immunoelectrophoresis was used to study complexes between proteases and alpha-1-antitrypsin and alpha-2-macroglobulin. In the latter studies, the analyses were preceded by isoelectric focusing. Gel filtration followed by single radial immunodiffusion was used for assaying complexes between proteases and antileukoprotease. The residual inhibitory capacity of alpha-1-antitrypsin and antileukoprotease was studied by adding purified granulocyte elastase in excess to middle ear specimens, followed by the methods for detecting protease–protease inhibitor complexes, as above.

RESULTS

The proteolytic enzyme granulocyte elastase was demonstrated in all but one MEE. The concentration of this enzyme showed a wide range within the different categories of otitis media (Table 1). In particular, in SOM-s effusions the concentration of elastase varied greatly, and in individual SOM-s specimens the concentration exceeded the upper range of that of AOM effusions. However, the mean concentration of granulocyte elastase within each category of otitis media decreased with increasing duration of illness. When compared with the plasma concentration of elastase, which was normal in each studied case, the mean concentration of elastase in MEE of SOM-1, of SOM-s, and of AOM, respectively, was 1400, 3200, and 5500 times higher than in plasma.

TABLE 1 Granulocyte Elastase in Middle Ear Effusions in Patients with Acute Otitis Media (AOM), Serous Otitis Media of Short Duration (SOM-s) and Serous Otitis Media of Long Duration (SOM-1)

		AOM (*μg/ml*)	*SOM-s* (*μg/ml*)	*SOM-1* (*μg/ml*)
Elastase	Mean ± SEM	660 ± 96.9	315 ± 80.3	170 ± 50.6
	Range	160–1000	43–1420	45–375
	Number	10	19	6

The main plasma protease inhibitors, alpha-1-antitrypsin, antichymotrypsin, and alpha-2-macroglobulin, were demonstrated in all MEE specimens. Antileukoprotease was demonstrated in all but three specimens. Alpha-1-antitrypsin appeared as the dominating protease inhibitor in all the different stages of otitis media, as illustrated in Table 2.

Complex formation, indicating enzyme inhibition, was demonstrated in MEE for all protease inhibitors, except for antichymotrypsin. In AOM effusions, 25 percent of alpha-1-antitrypsin, 60 percent of alpha-2-macroglobulin and 100 percent of antileukoprotease were found in complex with proteases. In SOM-1 effusions, less than 10 percent of alpha-1-antitrypsin, 35 percent of alpha-2-macroglobulin, and 50 percent of antileukoprotease were found in complex (Fig. 1). In SOM-s effusions the findings were similar to those in SOM-1 effusions.

Analyses for residual inhibitory reactivity of antileukoprotease and alpha-1-antitrypsin showed the remaining free antileukoprotease to be able to bind added elastase, whereas the reactivity of free alpha-1-antitrypsin was reduced in AOM as well as in SOM effusions (Fig. 1).

TABLE 2 Molar Concentration of Granulocyte Protease Inhibitors in MEE in Patients with Acute Otitis Media (AOM), Serous Otitis Media of Short Duration (SOM-s) and Serous Otitis Media of Long Duration (SOM-1)

	AOM (*μmole/l*)	*SOM-s* (*μmole/l*)	*SOM-1* (*μmole/l*)
Alpha-1-antitrypsin	15 (55)	27 (69)	21 (48)
Alpha-1-antichymotrypsin	6 (22)	7 (18)	14 (33)
Alpha-2-macroglobulin	1 (4)	2 (5)	2 (5)
Antileukoprotease	5 (19)	3 (8)	6 (14)
Totals	27 (100)	39 (100)	43 (100)

Note: Values in parentheses represent the percentage of the total concentration of the protease inhibitors.

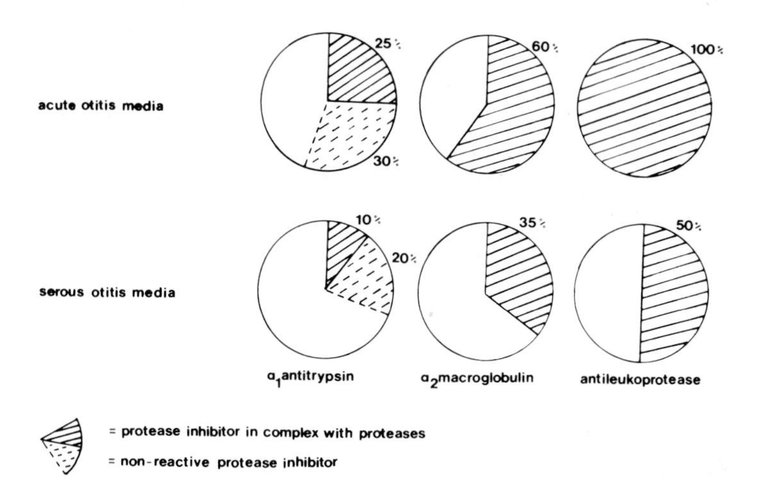

Figure 1 The utilization of the main protease inhibitors in middle ear effusions in patients with acute otitis media and serous otitis media. Striped sections denote the relative amount of each inhibitor in complex with proteases or in a non-reactive form.

DISCUSSION

Despite extensive work on the pathophysiology of otitis media, the etiologic factors in destruction of middle ear structures have not been established. The inflammatory process itself provides several possible mechanisms of tissue destruction. Much attention has been focused on enzymatic degradation of tissue during inflammation.[2] A release of arachidonic acid metabolites,[3] oxygen-derived free radicals,[4] and complement activation[5] are additional possible mechanisms for mediation of tissue injury.

Granulocyte lysosomal proteolytic enzymes are capable of degrading basilar membranes and other connective tissue components.[2] The considerable release of granulocyte elastase in MEE, as shown in the present study, supports the concept that the inflammatory cell products are responsible for tissue degradation in otitis media. Furthermore, the extracellular release of granulocyte proteases represents a mechanism of self-perpetuation of the inflammatory reaction in the middle ear through an interaction with the complement system.[6]

The release of proteases varies with the degree of inflammation, as shown by the higher mean concentration of elastase in AOM than in SOM effusions. The wide range of granulocyte elastase concentrations found within each category of MEE can be regarded as a reflection of the dynamics of otitis media with exacerbation and regression of the inflammatory degree.

The control of proteases is exerted by protease inhibitors, which are characterized by their ability to block the catalytic site of the enzymes. In MEE, the main plasma protease inhibitors are present in high concentrations. Furthermore, the locally produced low molecular weight protease inhibitor, antileukoprotease, is present in MEE. In an earlier study,[7] the production site of antileukoprotease was shown to be confined to the goblet cells of the middle ear mucosa. The large amount of complexes between proteases and protease inhibitors, plasma derived and locally produced, present in MEE provides convincing proof of the biologic role these inhibitors play in the defense of middle ear structures against the action of granulocyte proteases.

The amount of complexes is higher in AOM effusions than in SOM effusions: In AOM effusions, all antileukoprotease and a considerable portion of alpha-1-antitrypsin and alpha-2-macroglobulin have been utilized for protease inhibition, thus indicating a high risk for tissue destruction. The residual inhibitory capacity of the protease inhibitors in SOM effusions suggests the existence of protection against a possible further release of proteases. However, protease release takes place not only during the process of phagocytosis, but also during the migration of the granulocyte through the tissues, with the possibility of a local saturation of the inhibitory capacity. Therefore, an imbalance of the protease–protease inhibitory system, with the occurrence of free proteolytic activity in the middle ear in AOM as well as in SOM, is conceivable. This potentially destructive nature of the middle ear fluid should be considered when the clinician is confronted with patients suffering from any stage of the otitis media syndrome.

REFERENCES

1. Carlsson B, Lundberg C, Ohlsson K: Granulocyte protease inhibition in acute and chronic middle ear effusion. Acta Otolaryngol (Stockh) 95:341, 1983
2. Barrett A: *Proteinases in Mammalian Cells and Tissues.* Amsterdam: North-Holland Biomedical Press, 1977
3. Bernstein JM, Okazaki T, Reisman RE: Prostaglandins in middle ear effusions. Arch Otolaryngol 102:257, 1976
4. Greenwald R, Moy W: Inhibition of collagen gelation by action of the superoxide radical. Arthritis Rheum 22:251, 1979
5. Veltri RW, Sprinkle PM: Secretory otitis media. An immune complex disease. Ann Otol Rhinol Laryngol 85 (Suppl 25):135, 1976
6. Goldstein I, Brai M, Osler A, Weissmann G: Lysosomal enzyme release from human leukocytes: Mediation by the alternate pathway of complement activation. J Immunol 111:33, 1973
7. Carlsson B, Ohlsson K: Localization of antileukoprotease in middle ear mucosa. Acta Otolaryngol (Stockh) 95:111, 1983

FACTORS INVOLVED IN THE ALTERATION OF MIDDLE EAR EFFUSION COMPOSITION

S.K. JUHN, M.D., TIMOTHY T.K. JUNG, M.D., Ph.D.,
G. SCOTT GIEBINK, M.D., and JAMES EDLIN

The biochemical characteristics of middle ear effusion (MEE) differ among various types of otitis media.[1] Factors that contribute to the alteration of the composition of MEE are products of epithelial and subepithelial cells, microorganisms, inflammatory mediators and inflammatory cells, and ventilation. Since most of the factors are present as inflammatory reaction products, it is important to identify those that can yield specific alterations of the component. Animal models can provide an excellent opportunity to obtain information related to the products that are caused by specific conditions imposed. Several factors involved in the alteration of MEE composition are presented, and possible application of these data to the interpretation of human MEE data is discussed.

MATERIALS AND METHODS

Purulent otitis media (POM) was induced in chinchillas by inoculation of type 7 *Streptococcus pneumoniae* (2 × 10) into the bulla. Serous otitis media (SOM) was induced by inserting small silastic sponges into the pharyngeal orifice of the eustachian tube. In the combination model, pneumococci were inoculated at various times (7, 14, 21 days) after SOM was induced. In the penicillin treatment studies, penicillin G, 50,000 U per day i.m., was injected into animals with POM (seven days) for three days.

MEE were aspirated through the bullae at various times after experimental conditions (SOM, POM, SOM + POM, POM + penicillin) were imposed. Temporal bones were removed for histologic sectioning after the MEE samples were collected.

Lysozyme was measured using agar plates containing *Micrococcus lysodeikticus*.[2] Lactoferrin was measured by the immunoelectrophoretic "rocket" technique using 1.0 percent agar gels and rabbit antilactoferrin antiserum at a 0.75 percent concentration. Glucose concentration was measured by the ultraviolet enzymatic method with hexokinase and glucose-6-phosphate dehydrogenase.[3]

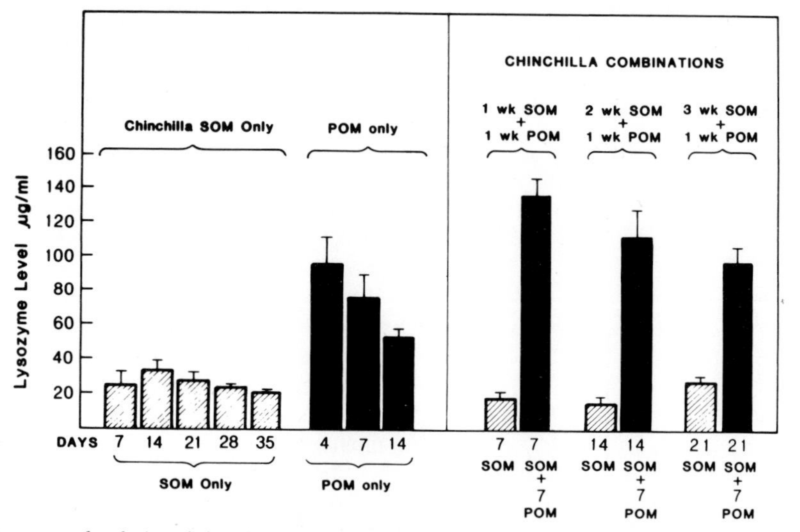

Figure 1 Lysozyme levels (μ/ml) in middle ear effusions (MEE) from serous otitis media (SOM), purulent otitis media (POM), and combination (SOM + POM) models in chinchilla.

RESULTS

Lysozyme levels in MEEs from animals with SOM, POM, and SOM + POM combination are shown in Figure 1. It is obvious that lysozyme levels are higher in MEE from the POM group than from the SOM group. The lysozyme levels in MEE from the SOM + POM combination group were higher than in the animals with POM alone. Glucose levels, on the other hand, were lower in the combination model than in the POM group (Fig. 2). In the penicillin treated group, the MEEs became sterile and the level of lysozyme decreased compared with the untreated animals (Fig. 3).

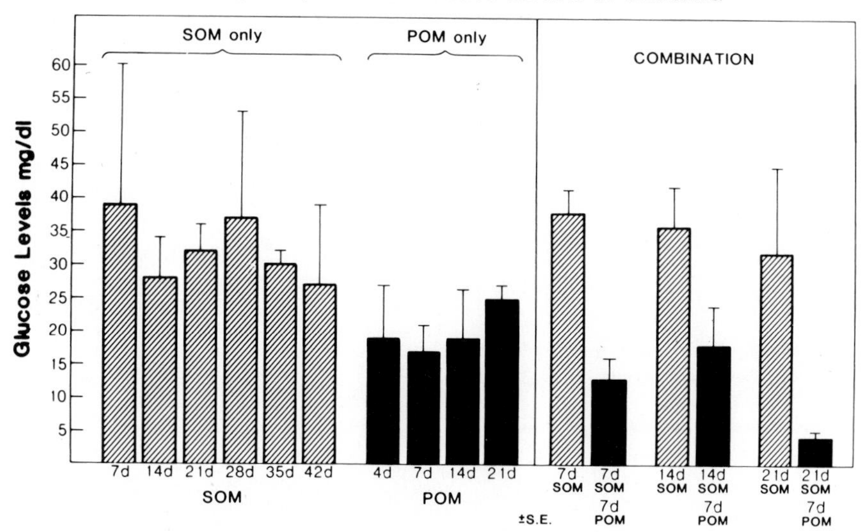

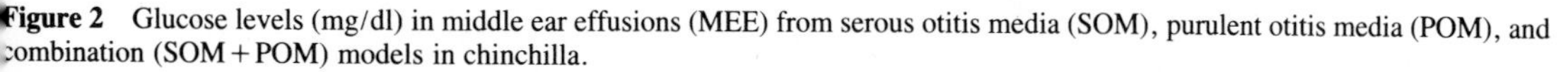
Figure 2 Glucose levels (mg/dl) in middle ear effusions (MEE) from serous otitis media (SOM), purulent otitis media (POM), and combination (SOM + POM) models in chinchilla.

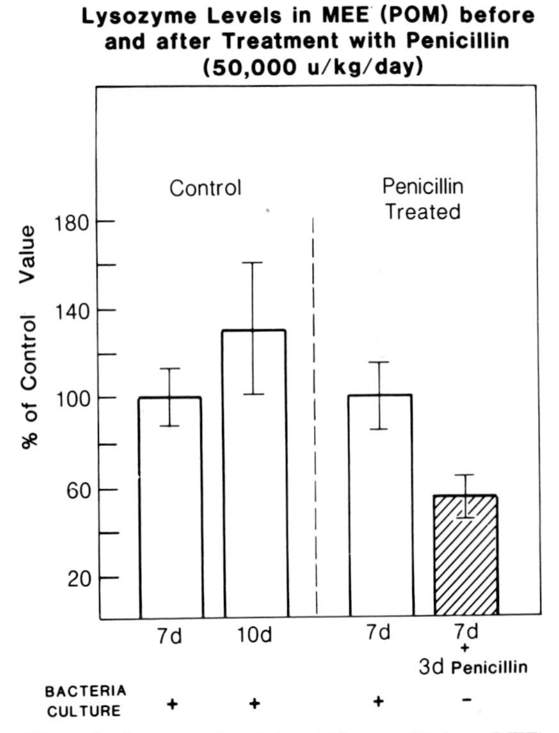

Figure 3 Lysozyme levels in middle ear effusions (MEE) from purulent otitis media (POM) before and after treatment with penicillin.

In preliminary human studies, lysozyme and lactoferrin levels were measured simultaneously. When the lysozyme levels of MEE that had similar levels of lactoferrin were compared, a higher level of lysozyme was observed in the recurrent group (Table 1) and a lower level in the penicillin treated patients (Table 2).

DISCUSSION

The present study clearly demonstrates that certain experimental conditions can alter the composition of MEE. The lysozyme and glucose levels are distinctly different in two animal models of SOM and POM. The results of the biochemical analyses of MEE from the SOM and POM models may represent the contribution of eustachian tube obstruction or inoculated microorganisms *(S. pneumoniae)* to the composition of MEE. It is interesting to observe that the levels of lysozyme in MEE from the SOM + POM combination model were higher than those from the POM model. This may indicate that the obstruction of middle ear ventilation can enhance the inflammatory changes of the middle ear mucoperiosteum to bacterial infection.

Lysozyme is a hydrolytic enzyme located in the neutrophil granules. It is released in the process of phagocytosis. This enzyme has also been identified in the epithelial cells.[4] The level of lysozyme can serve as an index of inflammatory changes in the middle ear cavity. The lowered levels of glucose found in the combination model also support this hypothesis that more intense inflammatory reaction can take place when bacterial infection is superimposed on the obstruction of ventilation. A lower level of glucose concentration in MEE compared with serum was reported previously and was attributed to the increased glucose consumption by the inflammatory cells in the effusion.[1] It is also known that phagocytosis is accompanied by increased oxygen consumption and increase in both aerobic and anaerobic glycolysis.

The results of the penicillin treatment study showed a decrease of lysozyme level after treatment. Although histologically the mucosa showed less inflammatory change, the presence of cuboidal and goblet cells in the epithelial lining two weeks after treatment indicate that complete resolution of the inflammation did not take place. The optimum antimicrobial regimen to eradicate bacteria and induce a complete recovery of the middle ear mucosa needs to be established.

Retrospective studies of patient histories after initial biochemical data have been obtained and in-

TABLE 1 Lactoferrin and Lysozyme Levels in Middle Ear Effusions from Recurrent Otitis Media with Effusion

Age	*Recurrence*	*Lactoferrin (μg/ml)*	*Lysozyme (μg/ml)*
11	5 myr	520	800
6	1 myr	640	116

TABLE 2 Lactoferrin and Lysozyme Levels in Middle Ear Effusions from Patients with Otitis Media with Effusion

Age	*Antibiotic*	*Lactoferrin (μg/ml)*	*Lysozyme (μg/ml)*
6	Penicillin treatment before myringotomy	210	52
6	No penicillin treatment before myringotomy	280	190

dicate differences in the levels of lysozyme between recurrent and nonrecurrent groups.[5] In our present study, lysozyme levels in MEE were higher in the recurrent cases when the lactoferrin level was comparable. Lysozyme level was lower in MEE from the patients who received penicillin before the myringotomy than in MEE from patients who did not receive penicillin treatment. Previous animal studies did indicate that pencillin treatment can reduce the lysozyme level.

Lactoferrin is an iron-binding protein isolated from breast milk[6] and is widely distributed in body fluids. It is also found in cytoplasmic granules of neutrophil leukocytes. A progressive but nonlinear rise in lactoferrin levels with increasing neutrophil counts has been reported.[7] The results of the present study indicate the possibility of simultaneous measurement of two or more parameters in the evaluation of the MEE composition and the disease processes taking place in the middle ear cavity. When we assume that lactoferrin arises only from neutrophils and that lysozyme can be derived both from neutrophils and epithelial lining of the mucosa, the ratio of lysozyme to lactoferrin can reflect the generalized efflux of lysosomal constituents accompanying the inflammatory response in the middle ear cavity. The concept of an inflammatory index created by combining two or more biochemical or immunochemical measurements needs to be further developed and better defined. However, the data currently available from retrospective studies suggest the possibility of the predictive power of MEE analyses for otitis media morbidity.

This research was supported by NINCDS grant #NS-14538.

REFERENCES

1. Juhn SK, Huff JS: Biochemical characteristics of middle ear effusions. Ann Otol 85:110, 1976
2. Shugar D: Measurement of lysozyme activity and the ultraviolet inactivation of lysozyme. Biochim Biophys Acta 8:302, 1952
3. Slein MW: Determination with hexokinase and glucose-6-phosphate dehydrogenase. In Bergmeyher, HY (ed): *Methods of Enzymatic Analysis.* New York: Academic Press, 1963, pp 117–123
4. Lim DJ, Liu YS, Birck H: Secretory lysozyme of the human middle ear mucosa: Immunocytochemial localization. Ann Otol 85:50, 1976
5. Juhn SK: Studies on middle ear effusions. Laryngoscope 92:287, 1982
6. Shafer KM: Elektrophoretische Untersuchungen zum Milcheiweissproblem. Monatsschr Kinderheilkd 99:67, 1951
7. Bennett RM, Skosey JL: Lactoferrin and lysozyme levels in synovial fluid. Arthritis Rheum 20:84, 1977

HISTAMINE LEVELS IN MIDDLE EAR EFFUSIONS

GILEAD BERGER, M.D., MICHAEL HAWKE, M.D., F.R.C.S.(C),
DAVID W. PROOPS, B.D.S., M.B., F.R.C.S.,
NARENDRANATH S. RANADIVE, Ph.D., and DAVID WONG, B.Sc.

There is substantial evidence to suggest that biologic mediators of inflammation may be involved in the pathogenesis of otitis media with effusion. Recent studies confirmed the presence of prostaglandins, chemotactic factors, macrophage inhibitor factor, complement, lysosomal enzymes, and kinins in middle ear effusions.[1–3] It is natural, therefore, to question the role of histamine in secretory otitis media. Since histamine is a potent pharmacologic mediator of inflammation, with influence on smooth muscles and permeability of small blood vessels, it may participate in the production and maintenance of an effusion in the tympanic cavity. It has been shown experimentally that histamine causes vasodilatation and increases the permeability of the middle ear mucosa.[4,5] It has also been demonstrated in rats that an effusion that is rich in histamine accumulates in the attic space after blocking the tympanic isthmus. The histamine is released from mast cells located in the subepithelial layers of the pars flaccida of the eardrum.[6]

A review of the literature revealed only two publications that discussed histamine levels in otitis media with effusion.[7,8] In these papers, histamine was reported to be either absent or present in only small amounts. One of these studies used the biologic assay technique, the second did not detail the technique used.

The purpose of this study was to determine histamine levels in middle ear effusions using a well-established technique not used before in this context.

MATERIALS AND METHODS

Samples of middle ear effusions were taken during the tympanostomy procedure from 131 middle ears of 96 patients (58 males and 38 females) with secretory otitis media. The patients' ages ranged from 1 to 60 years with a mean age of 6.5. Twenty-three of the 96 had a history of allergy. A standard form that included the following parameters was completed for each patient at the time of the myringotomy: (1) sex, (2) age, (3) date, (4) allergic history, and (5) side (right or left); (6) the physical properties of the effusion were assigned to one of the following three categories: (a) mucoid—tenacious consistency, (b) serous—thin and watery consistency, or (c) purulent—watery consistency with a creamy coloration.

The effusion was removed using a 16-gauge blunt cannula attached to the barrel of a 1-ml disposable tuberculin syringe, from which the proximal flange had been removed so that the barrel could be directly attached to the suction tubing. Using this method, the middle ear aspirate remained within the barrel and its volume could be easily measured using the calibration of the tuberculin syringe. The volumes of the aspirated effusions ranged between 50 and 200 microliters. The effusions were thereafter diluted with normal saline to 1 ml of total volume and stored at −20°C.

The histamine content was measured using a modification of the fluorometric assay of Shore and colleagues.[9] This method involves the extraction of histamine into n-butanol from alkalinized perchloric acid tissue extracts, followed by return of the histamine to an aqueous solution and condensation with O-phthalaldehyde (OPT) to yield a product with a strong and stable fluorescence that is measured in a Turner fluorometer Model No. 110, using a 360 nm wavelength for excitation and 450 nm for emission. The fluorescent readings were converted to histamine levels by reference to a standard curve prepared with readings from standardized histamine samples that had been processed in the same way as the effusion samples. A linear relationship was found between relative fluorescence and histamine concentrations in the range of 5 to 100 ng/ml. To compensate for the dilution factor, the measured concentration was multiplied by the volume of the sample (1 ml) and divided by the volume of the aspirated effusion. Histamine concentration in each sample was expressed as nanograms of histamine per 1 ml of middle ear effusion.

Twenty of the effusions that had larger volumes were taken, and each one was assayed for total white cell and differential white cell counts, as well as for histamine concentration.

Three ml of venous blood was obtained from ten patients at the same time the myringotomy was performed, and the histamine levels in the blood were determined by using the same method.

The following statistical techniques were used when applicable: (1) correlation coefficient, (2) Student's t-test, and (3) analysis of variance.

RESULTS

Histamine concentrations in middle ear effusions varied a great deal, ranging from 0 to 3650 ng/ml per sample, with a mean concentration of 449 ng/ml. The mean histamine blood concentration was 49 ng/ml, and this value is comparable to those blood levels reported in the literature.[10] Statistical analysis of the data confirmed that the mean effusion was significantly higher than the mean blood level, and there was no correlation between these two levels (Table 1). There was no significant difference between males and females or between right and left ears. Factors such as age, total white cell, and differential white cell counts were not correlated with the effusion histamine levels. A

TABLE 1 Mean Histamine Concentrations in Effusions and Blood

	Histamine Concentrations ng/ml			
	N	*Range*	*Mean*	
Effusion	131	0–3650	449	Effusion vs. blood $P < 0.001$
Blood	10	3–120	49	
	Correlation coefficient probability Blood			
Effusion	0.3			

significant difference existed between the mucoid and serous variants; the histamine content of the mucoid type was significantly higher than of the serous type, but there was no significant difference between the mucoid and purulent variants or between the serous and purulent types (Table 2).

Comparison between histamine levels in effusions of allergic* versus nonallergic patients failed to disclose a significant difference between the two groups (Fig. 1).

Histamine levels varied with the seasons of the year. The summer levels were the highest, winter, spring, and fall levels followed in decreasing order. Since the study was carried out from August through April, data from the summer and spring are only partially presented. Therefore, the seasonal analysis is limited to some extent.

DISCUSSION

The presence of significant amounts of histamine in most of the middle ear effusions supports the hypothesis that this substance might be involved in the production and maintenance of the inflammatory reactions observed in otitis media with effusion.

The genesis of histamine in the effusion of secretory otitis media poses the following questions: (1) Is it a transudate from the serum or is it locally produced? (2) If locally produced, is it the product of basophils or mast cells? (3) Which mechanisms trigger the release of the histamine?

Histamine appears to be a local product of the middle ear lining rather than a transudate from the serum. The high levels of histamine found in all types of effusion and the dissociation between its blood and effusion levels support this concept.

It seems unlikely that basophils are responsible for the histamine present in the effusions, since they were rarely observed either in the fluid or in the inflamed middle ear mucosa.[11,12] On the other hand, mast cells were reported to be present in the lamina propria of the middle ear lining[13,14] and to increase considerably in certain cases of secretory otitis media.[15] Therefore, we postulate that the histamine is released from mast cells located in the subepithelial layers of the tympanic mucoperiosteum.

*A total of 23 patients had histories of allergy (13 with respiratory allergy, five with drug allergy, and two each with skin and food allergy); one patient had eosinophilia without evidence of intestinal parasites.

TABLE 2 Histamine Concentrations in Various Types of Effusions

	Mucoid	*Serous*	*Purulent*
N	83	37	11
Mean	515	255	467

Mucoid vs. serous, $P = 0.049$
Mucoid vs. purulent, $P = 0.907$
Serous vs. purulent, $P = 0.282$

A clue to understanding the triggering stimuli that activate mast cells to release histamine is obtained by comparing histamine levels in effusions of allergic and nonallergic patients. Histamine levels should be significantly higher in effusions of allergic patients if an immediate-type of hypersensitivity (type I) is responsible for activation of the mast cells. However, the absence of a significant difference between these two groups may indicate that allergy is not the sole mechanism involved in histamine release. Furthermore, the relatively low concentrations of histamine recorded during the seasons usually associated with allergic phenomena lend support to a nonallergic origin. This assumption is supported by the observations of other investigators who failed to find elevated levels of IgE in the effusions.[16,17] An alternative mechanism of mast cell triggering is suggested by the finding of several components of the comple-

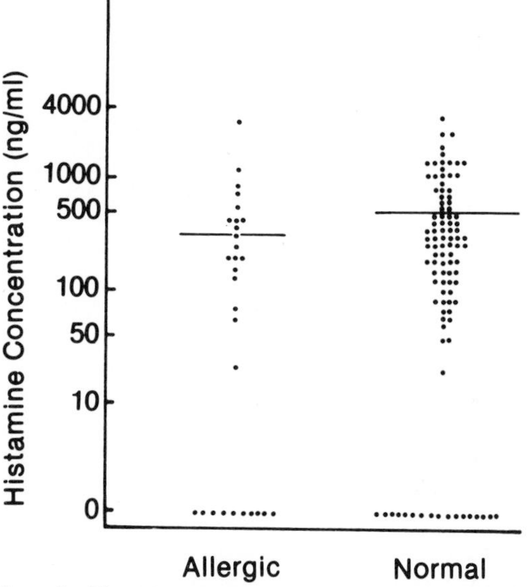

Figure 1 Histamine concentrations in effusions of normal and allergic patients. The horizontal bar is drawn at the geometric mean. Allergic versus nonallergic, $P = 0.25$.

ment system in middle ear effusions.[1,18] It is possible, therefore, that immune complexes, through activation of the complement system, produce anaphylatoxin, which may degranulate mast cells and release histamine.

This research was supported by grants from the St. Joseph's Health Centre Research Foundation and the Ministry of Health of the Government of Ontario, Special Health Studies Grant RD48.

REFERENCES

1. Bernstein JM: Biological mediators of inflammation in middle ear effusions. Ann Otol Rhinol Laryngol 85(Suppl 25):90, 1976
2. Wright I: Lysosomal enzymes in fluids from glue ear. Arch Otorhinolaryngol 208:233, 1974
3. Bernstein JM, Steger R, Back N: The kallikrein-kinin system in otitis media with effusion. ORL 86:249, 1978
4. Dennis RG, Whitmire RN, Jackson RT: Action of inflammatory mediators on middle ear mucosa. A method for measuring permeability and swelling. Arch Otolaryngol 102:420, 1976
5. Frady RP, Parker WA, Jackson RT: Studies in permeability of the middle ear mucosa. Arch Otolaryngol 103:47, 1977
6. Alm PE, Bloom GD, Hellström S, et al: The release of histamine from the pars flaccida mast cells: One cause of otitis media with effusion? Acta Otolaryngol 94:517, 1982
7. Jackson RT: Autonomic stimulation, osmolarity and prostaglandin effects in the eustachian tube. Ann Otol Rhinol Laryngol 85 (Suppl 25):187, 1976
8. Lim DJ: Pathogenesis of otitis media with effusion. Pediat Infect Dis 1(Suppl) 5:14, 1982
9. Shore PA, Burkhalter A, Cohn VH: A method for the fluorometric assay of histamine in tissues. J Pharm Exp Ther 127:182, 1959
10. Vaugman I, Rocha e Silva M: Histamine contents of organs and body fluids. In Rocha e Silva M (ed): Handbook of Experimental Pharmacology 18/1; *Histamine and Anti-histaminics:* 97–115. Berlin, Springer Verlag, 1966
11. Palva T, Halopainen E, Karma P: Protein and cellular pattern of glue ear secretions. Ann Otol Rhinol Laryngol 85(Suppl 25): 103, 1976
12. Sipilä P, Karma P: Inflammatory cells in mucoid effusions of secretory otitis media. Acta Otolaryngol 95:467, 1982
13. Lim DJ, Liu, YS, Schram JL, et al: Immunoglobulin E in chronic middle ear effusions. Ann Otol Rhinol Laryngol 85(Suppl 25): 117, 1976
14. Lim DJ, Shimada T, Yoder M: Distribution of mucus-secreting cells in normal middle ear mucosa. Arch Otolaryngol 98:2, 1973
15. Lim DJ, Viall J, Birck H, St. Pierre R: The morphological basis for understanding middle ear effusions. Laryngoscope 82:1625, 1972
16. Reisman RE, Bernstein J: Allergy and secretory otitis media. Clinical and immunologic studies. Pediat Clin North Am 22:251, 1975
17. Mogi G, Maeda S, Yoshida T, Watanabe N: Radioimmunoassay of IgE in middle ear effusions. Acta Otolaryngol 86:26, 1976
18. Veltri RW, Sprinkle PM: Secretory otitis media, an immune complex disease. Ann Otol Rhinol Laryngol 85(Suppl 25):135, 1976

HYDROLASE ACTIVITY IN OTITIS MEDIA WITH EFFUSION

WARREN F. DIVEN, Ph.D., ROBERT H. GLEW, Ph.D., and KAREN L. LAMARCO, M.S.

Persistent middle ear effusions (MEEs) are a characteristic of otitis media with effusion (OME), and many studies have been conducted in an attempt to learn more about the etiologic and pathophysiologic properties of these fluids. Obstruction of the eustachian tube is the most common cause of MEE.[1] Serous and mucoid MEEs both contain inflammatory cells, polymorphonuclear leukocytes, macrophages, lymphocytes, cell debris, bacteria, hydrolytic enzymes, and plasma proteins.[2–8] A host cellular origin has been suggested for at leas[t] some of the hydrolytic enzymes found in MEE,[9,10] while a bacterial origin has been proposed for neu[raminidase] activity that displays a neutral pH op[timum].[11] It is possible that bacterial enzymes re[leased] into the middle ear cavity may play [a] significant role in inducing inflammation.[11,12]

Since little is known about the biochemistr[y]

and enzymology of MEE, we have extended our earlier work on the hydrolase activity of MEE[10] to include patients with acute OME. We also present the results of quantative analysis of several plasma proteins from MEE obtained from patients with chronic OME. In each group we have compared the biochemical determinations with the microbiological findings in those patients.

MATERIALS AND METHODS

Subjects

The subjects for these studies were children with either acute or chronic OME. There were approximately equal numbers of males and females between the ages of 1 month and 10 years. These patients underwent tympanocentesis as described by Riding and associates.[3] Middle ear effusions were collected and classified with respect to appearance and bacterial flora as described elsewhere.[10]

Enzyme Assays

Neuraminidase activity was measured using a fluorometric assay as described by LaMarco and colleagues.[11] Other hydrolases were measured as described by Diven and colleagues.[10]

Protein Determinations

Total protein was estimated by the method of Lowry and associates[14] using bovine serum albumin as standard. Albumin was determined by the electroimmunoassay technique of Laurell.[15] Alpha-1-antitrypsin activity was determined by the trypsin inhibitory capacity method of Eriksson.[16] The total mass of alpha-1-antitrypsin was determined by the single radial immunodiffusion plate technique of Mancini and associates[17] using purified human alpha-1-antitrypsin as standard. Haptoglobin was determined by the radial immunodiffusion plate technique of Mancini and coworkers[17] using purified haptoglobin as standard.

Antiserum to human albumin was purchased from Miles Biochemical (Elkhart, IN), haptoglobin from Calbiochem-Behring (San Diego, CA), and antiserum to human haptoglobin and alpha-1-antitrypsin from Boehringer Mannheim (Indianapolis, IN).

RESULTS

The results of albumin and haptoglobin determinations in MEE from patients with chronic OME are presented in Table 1. Concentrations are expressed as percentage of total protein, with the standard deviation given for each group. Although there is a broad range of values in both serous and mucoid MEE, the mean albumin concentrations are in the range of normal plasma albumin values. Haptoglobin, a protein considered to be an acute phase reactant and elevated in inflammatory disease, is significantly lower in MEE than in control serum.

The protein concentrations were examined further on the basis of the microbiologic findings. Middle ear effusions were considered to be culture positive when the organism identified was not the same as that identified from the external canal. The organisms identified in culture-positive effusions were *Streptococcus pneumoniae*, *Hemophilus influenzae* untypable, *Branhamella catarrhalis*, diphtheroids, *Staphylococcus epidermidis*, and *Staphylococcus* coagulase negative. The presence of microorganisms in either serous or mucoid MEE does not seem to affect the albumin concentration significantly. Although the mean values are slightly higher for the culture-negative fluids, this difference is not statistically significant. The haptoglobin content in the mucoid culture-positive fluids appears higher than in the mucoid culture-negative effusions, but, because of the wide variation in samples, this difference is not statistically significant. The same appears to be true for the

TABLE 1 Haptoglobin and Albumin Content of Middle Ear Aspirates and Serum from Children with Chronic Otitis Media with Effusion

	Haptoglobin		Albumin	
Effusion Type	*N*	*Total Protein (%)*	*N*	*Total Protein (%)*
Serous				
Culture negative	9	1.67 ± 1.7	9	54 ± 24
Culture positive	2	4.11 ± 2.3	8	50 ± 17
Combined	20	1.86 ± 1.8	17	52 ± 20
Mucoid				
Culture negative	21	1.32 ± 1.7	22	52 ± 18
Culture positive	19	2.11 ± 1.9	35	46 ± 19
Combined	47	1.71 ± 1.8	57	48 ± 18
Serum (control)	20	5.25 ± 5.0	20	64 ± 6

TABLE 2 Alpha-1-Antitrypsin in Middle Ear Aspirates from Children with Chronic Otitis Media with Effusion

Effusion Type	*N*	*Trypsin Inhibitory Capacity (Mean ± S.D. mg/mg Protein)*	*Radial Immuno-diffusion (Mean ± S.D. mg/mg Protein)*	*% Free*
Serous				
Culture negative	15	.0140 ± .024	.033 ± .021	42
Culture positive	7	.0092 ± .0021	.029 ± .008	32
Combined	36	.0110 ± .016	.032 ± .016	34
Mucoid				
Culture negative	28	.0065 ± .0056	.043 ± .019	15
Culture positive	47	.0043 ± .0050	.034 ± .020	13
Combined	105	.0054 ± .0050	.034 ± .019	16
Serum (control)	25		.019 ± .002	

serous effusions, but since there are only two culture-positive effusions one must be cautious in the interpretation of these data.

Determinations of alpha-1-antitrypsin concentration in MEE are presented in Table 2. The trypsin inhibitory capacity (TIC) gives a measurement of the free alpha-1-antitrypsin available to react with protease, while the radial immunodiffusion (RID) concentration is an estimate of the total mass of alpha-1-antitrypsin present in the MEE. It can be seen from the RID values that the mean total mass of alpha-1-antitrypsin present is approximately twice that found in normal plasma and does not vary significantly between the types of effusion or with the presence of microorganisms in either fluid type. In a study of protease inhibitors in MEEs ranging from serous to seromucoid from patients with chronic OME, Carlsson and associates found that in 14 of 22 patients alpha-1-antitrypsin values exceeded the values found in the patients' own plasma.[8] In every measurement the RID value is greater than the TIC determination, indicating that 13 to 42 percent of the alpha-1-antitrypsin is reactive and that 58 to 87 percent of the total has been complexed with protease. The mean TIC of the serous effusions is approximately twice that of the mucoid effusions, indicating that less protease inactivation has occurred in the former effusions. The difference between the TIC in the culture-positive and culture-negative mucoid effusions is small. If, as would be expected, there is bacterial protease present in the culture-positive mucoid effusions, a significant difference in TIC between culture-positive and culture-negative effusions would be expected due to bacterial protease inactivation. Thus, either only small amounts of bacterial protease are present or it does not interact with alpha-1-antitrypsin. For the serous culture-negative effusions a mean of 42 percent of alpha-1-antitrypsin is active, while in the culture-positive MEE this is reduced to 32 percent, suggesting the possibility that a significant amount of bacterial protease has been inactivated in the latter group.

In a previous report, we presented a study of lysosomal hydrolase activities in MEEs from patients with chronic OME.[10] We present here a similar study of patients with acute OME. In Table 3 are the results of enzyme determinations on effusions classified as serous or purulent. The mean activity for each enzyme within the group is presented along with the standard deviation of the group. In every case the mean activity is higher in the serous effusions; however, this difference is not statistically significant due to the large variation within each group.

The enzyme activities were examined further on the basis of the microbiologic findings. Table 3 also presents the results of this analysis. When mean enzyme activities in culture-positive effusions are compared with those of culture-negative effusions, no significant difference is seen.

In an earlier study, we demonstrated the presence of a neuraminidase with optimal activity near neutral pH in MEE from patients with chronic OME.[11] In a similar study of patients with acute OME, effusions were visually classified as purulent or serous, analyzed for the presence of neutral (pH 6.4) neuraminidase, and cultured for bacteria. The distribution of measurable activity by type of predominant organism is shown in Table 4. Fourteen of the 19 specimens (74 percent) that were culture positive for *S. pneumoniae* had demonstrable neuraminidase, ranging from 0.056 to 0.269 units/mg protein. In contrast, this enzyme activity was present in only 26 to 46 percent of the remaining specimens without pneumococcal growth.

Certain strains of *S. pneumoniae* are found more frequently as the causative organisms in OME. The secreted hydrolase activity was measured in growth medium from a number of pneumococcal strains varying in their causative frequency as determined by Austrian and coworkers.[18] The results of this study are shown in Table 5. Although the activities presented here

TABLE 3 Lysosomal Hydrolases in Patients with Acute Otitis Media

	Acid Phosphatase	*Alpha-Mannosidase*	*Beta-Galactosidase*	*Beta-Glucuronidase*	*Hexosaminidase*
Purulent					
N	62	54.0	65.0	62.0	59.0
$\overline{X}$	176	25.3	14.6	92.3	215.0
S.D.	216	24.8	13.6	53.1	137.0
Serous					
N	5	5.0	5.0	7.0	7.0
$\overline{X}$	235	38.6	27.7	101.0	289.0
S.D.	123	26.4	18.6	86.9	174.0
Culture Negative					
N	14	13.0	15.0	13.0	14.0
$\overline{X}$	136	19.0	11.5	87.0	204.0
S.D.	148	23.2	15.5	67.6	142.0
Culture Positive					
N	52	45.0	53.0	54.0	51.0
$\overline{X}$	195	28.3	17.4	93.2	223.0
S.D.	226	25.5	13.7	54.8	140.0

Note: All values are expressed in terms of nanomoles/milligram/hour.

vary significantly, there seems to be no correlation between amount of enzyme secreted and the frequency with which the organism is found to cause OME.

DISCUSSION

The presence of plasma protein constituents such as albumin, haptoglobin, and alpha-1-antitrypsin in effusions suggests that at least part of the MEE from patients with chronic or recurrent OME is a transudate from blood.[5,7,8] The albumin concentrations reported here are consistent with the results of Mogi and Honjo, who reported albumin values essentially the same in serum and either serous or mucoid MEE from patients with chronic OME.[7] Similarly, Carlsson and colleagues reported albumin concentrations ranging from 56 to

TABLE 4 Neuraminidase Activity in Middle Ear Aspirates from Children with Acute Otitis Media with Effusion

*Middle Ear Isolate**	*Purulent*	*Serous*	*n*	*No. of Specimens with Activity*	*Mean Activity††*	*Standard Deviation*
Streptococcus pneumoniae	17	2	19	14 (74)†	0.097	0.121
Hemophilus influenzae	23	—	23	6 (26)	0.0065	0.013
Others§	7	2	9	4 (44)	0.154	0.031
No growth	11	2	13	6 (46)	0.0152	0.270
Total			64	30 (47)	—	—

*If more than one organism was cultured from the middle ear effusion, we have recorded as the culture finding only one of the bacteria present according to the following hierarchical ranking: *S. pneumoniae; H. influenzae;* miscellaneous bacteria.

†Numbers in parentheses indicate percentage.

††One unit of enzyme activity is defined as the release of 1 nm of N-acetylneuraminic acid per hour from the substrate MU-NANA.

§Others include diphtheroids, *Neisseria* sp., *Branhamella catarrhalis,* beta-*Streptococcus, Staphylococcus* coagulase negative.

TABLE 5 Extracellular Hydrolase Activity from Various Strains of *Streptococcus Pneumoniae*

Strain	*Infectivity**	*Neuraminidase*	*Hexosaminidase*	*Beta-Galactosidase*	*Phosphatase*
13	0.1	427	65.7	10.5	26.4
14	0.1	437	25.8	11.8	83.8
5	0.2	790	92.3	5.4	18.9
12F	0.5	1163	753	5.9	39.6
8	1.5	1232	348	10.5	47.2
9V	2.7	1158	436	45.8	90.5
4	3.7	532	26.0	21.1	37.7
3	6.1	147	25.0	8.2	90.5
6A	12.4	1300	108	20.2	56.3
23F	12.8	963	170	11.2	97.3
19F	23.9	216	28.3	8.6	85.1

Note: All enzyme values are expressed in terms of units per milliliter.

*Infectivity is the percentage of total infections caused by a particular strain of *S. pneumoniae* in a study of 1205 cases of pneumococcal otitis media.[18]

267 percent of the patients' own plasma values.[8] Haptoglobin, one of the proteins whose plasma concentration is increased in response to inflammation, is present in significant concentrations in 76 percent of the MEEs examined. The mean concentration is less than that typically found in plasma, which would be expected, since its large size would limit diffusion across cell membranes. In confirmation of the report by Carlsson and associates,[8] we also found that alpha-l-antitrypsin, a major protease inhibitor found in plasma, is also found in significant concentrations in MEEs. The mean absolute mass of alpha-l-antitrypsin is relatively constant in all the effusion types examined, but in serous effusions a larger fraction is available to react with protease. This suggests that mucoid MEEs contain significantly greater amounts of protease. In the culture-negative serous effusions, approximately 40 percent of the total protease inhibitor is available for reaction, while only 30 percent is available in culture-positive effusions. It is possible that this difference is due to the inactivation of bacterial proteolytic enzymes secreted into the middle ear cavity. In the mucoid effusions the level of active protease inhibitor is much lower and there seems to be no significant difference between culture-positive and culture-negative effusions. This suggests that in mucoid effusions a greater amount of protease activity is found, perhaps due to an increased release of granulocyte protease.

In our previous study of acid hydrolases in MEEs from patients with chronic or recurrent OME, we demonstrated ratios of activities in mucoid versus serous effusions of from 3 to 11, depending on the particular enzyme.[10] In this current study of MEEs from patients with acute OME, we found no significant differences in the corresponding ratios between serous and purulent effusions, although in every case the serous effusion mean values were slightly higher. Again, as in the previous study,[10] bacterial hydrolases do not seem to be responsible for the measured activity, since the culture-negative and culture-positive effusion activities are not significantly different.

In this report, similar to our finding in patients with chronic or recurrent OME,[11] we document that neutral neuraminidase is often a component of MEE from patients with acute OME. We find that 74 percent of MEEs containing *S. pneumoniae* also have neuraminidase activity, in contrast to 26 to 46 percent of all other effusions in which there is no pneumococcal growth. Since we have shown that *S. pneumoniae* grown in culture secretes an active neuraminidase, this remains as the most likely source of the enzyme in those MEEs from which that organism can be cultured. It could be that in acute OME in which no pneumococcal growth is detected, a positive finding of neuraminidase is due to a previous infection with *S. pnemoniae*. Another possibility is that under the growth conditions found in the middle ear, organisms produce an enzyme that is not expressed when grown in laboratory culture medium. This raises the question of what role such a secreted enzyme might play in the infectious process. One role might be to help establish the organism at the site of infection, perhaps aiding in bacterial adherence to cells in the middle ear cavity. If such a hypothesis were true, it might be expected that those strains of *S. pneumoniae* that are more frequently implicated in middle ear infections would have higher levels of neuraminidase. Such does not seem to be the case (Table 5), since we find no correlation between the level of neuraminidase and the infectivity of the organism.

Work is in progress in an attempt to identify the source of neuraminidase in those MEEs in which no pneumococcal growth occurs and to determine the role that this enzyme plays in the pathologic processes of OME.

REFERENCES

1. Bluestone, CD: Eustachian tube obstruction in the infant with cleft palate. Ann Otol Rhinol Laryngol 80(Suppl 2):1, 1971
2. Wright I, Kapadia R: The cytology of "glue ear." J Laryngol Otol 83:367, 1969
3. Lim DJ, Lewis DM, Schram JL, Birck HG: Otitis media with effusion: Cytological and microbiological correlates. Arch Otolaryngol 105:404, 1979
4. John SK, Huff JS, Paparella MM: Certain oxidative and hydrolytic enzymes in the middle ear effusion in serous otitis media. Arch Otorhinolaryngol 212:119, 1976
5. Tonder O, Gunderson T: Nature of the fluid in serous otitis media. Arch Otolaryngol 93:473, 1971
6. Juhn SK, Huff JS: Biochemical characteristics of middle ear effusions. Ann Otol Rhinol Laryngol 85:110, 1976
7. Mogi G, Honjo S: Middle ear effusions. Analysis of protein components. Ann Otol Rhinol Laryngol 81:99, 1972
8. Carlsson, B, Lundberg C, Ohlsson K: Protease inhibitors in middle ear effusions. Ann Otol Rhinol Laryngol 90:38, 1981
9. Bernstein JM, Villari EM, Rattazi MC: The significance of lysosomal enzymes in middle ear effusions. Otolaryngol Head Neck Surg 87:845, 1979
10. Diven WF, Glew RH, Bluestone CD: Lysosomal hydrolases in middle ear effusions. Ann Otol Rhinol Laryngol 90:148, 1981
11. LaMarco KL, Diven EF, Glew RH, et al: Neuraminidase activity in middle ear effusions. Ann Otol Rhinol Laryngol 92(107):22, 1983
12. Lowell SH, Juhn SK: The role of bacterial enzymes in inducing inflammation in the middle ear cavity. Otolaryngol Head Neck Surg 87:859, 1979
13. Riding KH, Bluestone CD, Michaels RH, et al: Microbiology of recurrent and chronic otitis media with effusion. J Pediatr 93:739, 1978
14. Lowry OH, Rosebrough NJ, Farr AL, Randall RJ: Protein measurement with the Folin phenol reagent. J Biol Chem 193:265, 1951
15. Laurell CB: Electroimmunoassay. Scand J Clin Lab Invest 29 (Suppl 124):21, 1972
16. Eriksson, S: Studies in alpha-1-antitrypsin deficiency. Acta Med Scand 177 (Suppl 432):1, 1965
17. Mancini G, Carbonara AO, Heremans JF: Immunochemical quantitation of antigens by single radial immunodiffusion. Immunochemistry 2:235, 1965
18. Austrian R, Howie VM, Ploussard JH: The bacteriology of pneumococcal otitis media. John Jopkins Med J. 141:104, 1977

ANIMAL MODELS

EXPERIMENTAL OCCLUSION OF THE EUSTACHIAN TUBE: THE ROLE OF SHORT- AND LONG-TERM INFECTION AND ITS SEQUELAE

W. KUIJPERS, Ph.D., and J.M.H. VAN DER BEEK, M.D.

Based on the assumption that eustachian tube dysfunction or occlusion plays an important etiologic role in secretory otitis media, many experimental studies have been performed in which tubal blockage was induced to settle the effect of tubal obstruction on the middle ear mucosa.[1-5] However, most of these studies are confined to rather short observation periods and to limited areas of the middle ear mucosa. In addition, these observations are largely complicated by the lack of reliable data on the structure of the normal mucosa throughout the middle ear cavity.

This chapter describes a comprehensive morphologic study of the normal mucosa of the rat middle ear and the effect of tubal occlusion on it in short- and long-term experiments, with special emphasis on the role of infection.

MATERIALS AND METHODS

Two groups of Wistar rats were used in this study. One group was born and raised without special hygienic precautions. The second group consisted of specific pathogen-free animals harboring only nonpathogenic symbionts. Tubal occlusion of the left ear was performed under Nembutal anesthesia. The right ear served as control. The tube was reached medially to the posterior belly of the muculus digastricus and coagulated in its extratympanic course. The condition of the middle ear was determined by otoscopy at regular intervals. The animals were killed after periods varying from one day to two years.

Morphologic studies of the middle ear mucosa both of normal ears and after tubal occlusion were performed with the use of light microscopy and scanning and transmission electron microscopy. To search for the presence of microorganisms a small amount of the middle ear content was cultured according to the techniques described by Schade and colleagues.[6]

RESULTS

The normal epithelial lining of the rat middle ear is composed of both squamous and ciliated epithelium; by far the major part is lined with squamous epithelium. It consists of only one cell layer, and the cells vary in shape from cuboidal to flattened. The epithelium is extremely flattened, especially on the promontory and on the tympanic membrane.

The ciliated epithelium, varying from cuboidal to columnar, is pseudostratified and appears to be arranged in two distinct areas, which are continuous with the ciliated epithelium of the eustachian tube. One area forms an elongated tract coursing from the round window niche along the promontory into the orifice of the eustachian tube (Fig. 1). The second area is located in the dorsocranial part of the hypotympanum. Secretory cells are present not only in the ciliated areas, but also in various parts of the squamous epithelium, where their character could be established only with transmission electron microscopy.

The lamina propria is composed of dense connective tissue and varies in thickness at different sites of the middle ear cavity. Blood and lymph vessels of varying size are present in the fibrous strona.

Tubal occlusion induced a large variety of reactions. Because of the evoked underpressure, a serumlike fluid accumulated in the middle ear cleft during the first days, as established by otoscopy.

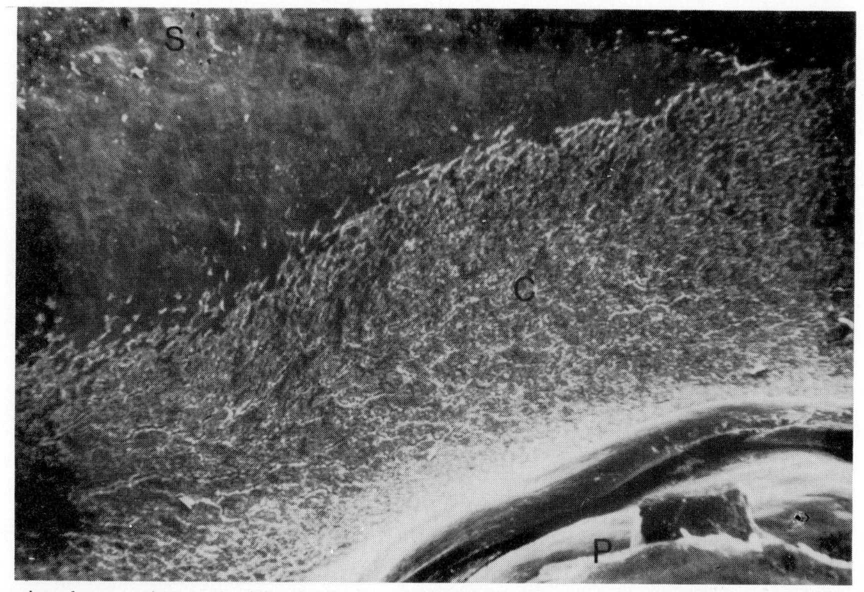

Figure 1 Scanning electron micrograph of the distribution of ciliated (C) and squamous (S) epithelium along the promontory (P). (X80 magnification)

Thereafter, most of the animals raised without special hygienic precautions developed an infective middle ear disease. Culturing of the middle ear content revealed a high number of *Mycoplasma pneumoniae*. This microorganism could also be cultured from the nasopharynx and from most of the control ears. A similar course of events was observed in the group of specific-pathogen-free animals. A notably high number of occluded ears of rats in this group developed an infective middle ear disease. The causal agent appeared to be a nonpathogenic streptococcus, which also was present in the nasopharynx and in many of the unoperated ears.

The course of this induced infection was rather divergent. In some ears a very destructive disease process was established, with bone destruction and labyrinthitis, but in most of the ears the infection was much milder; spontaneous clearing occurred after a short infective period and the ears became serous again.

In the infected ears a tremendous expansion of the ciliated/secretory epithelium often was found, and accumulations of secretory cells, resembling glands, were another common finding. The infective process frequently resulted in a partial or nearly total fibrosis of the middle ear cavity (Fig. 2). After longer survival periods cholesterol granuloma and ectopic bone appeared to develop in this fibrous tissue. This fibrosis can be considered an attempt by the middle ear to encapsulate the infectious focus as part of the healing process and is reminiscent of adhesive processes, which have been suggested to result from chronic middle ear disease.

The original squamous epithelium, which is completely buried in the fibrous tissue, revealed extensive secretory activity; normally this epithelium was not considered secretory (Fig. 3). Occasionally ciliated cells were also observed between these secretory cells. After a prolonged infective period intraepithelial glands appeared to develop, notably in the originally ciliated areas.

Ears that recovered after a limited infective period and become serous again revealed a disturbance of the original arrangement of ciliated and squamous epithelium, as could be seen in the scanning electron micrographs. In addition to the originally ciliated tracts, large isolated islands of ciliated cells interspersed with secretory cells were present in the squamous areas. Furthermore, the surface of the middle ear cavity was very irregular because of local thickenings of varying sizes, in the shape of local protuberances or polypoid formations. Sometimes a considerable part of the middle ear cleft was obliterated. These thickenings were composed of fibrous tissue containing many cysts of buried squamous epithelium. These cells contained many secretory granules and the cyst lumen was filled with secretion. These infection-induced changes appeared to persist for more than eight months after healing.

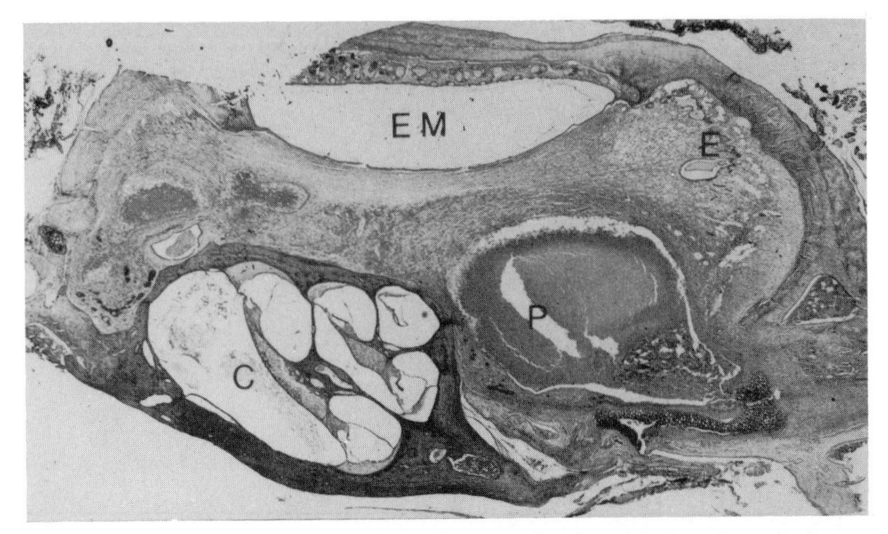

Figure 2 Micrograph of a rat middle ear that had been serous for two weeks after tubal obstruction and subsequently infected for one month. The middle ear cavity is nearly completely filled with fibrous tissue. The remaining part of the lumen contains pus (P). Note the islands of enclosed squamous epithelium (E). C, cochlea; EM, external meatus. (X25 magnification)

DISCUSSION

These observations lead us to conclude that the rat middle ear is supplied by a mucociliary transport system for cleaning the middle ear cavity. Blockade of this transport system by tubal obstruction can be supposed to favor pathogenic behavior of normally harmless inhabitants of the middle ear cavity. Tubal occlusion with supervening infection can lead to transformation of squamous epithelium into ciliated/secretory epithelium and to a varying degree of fibrosis of the middle

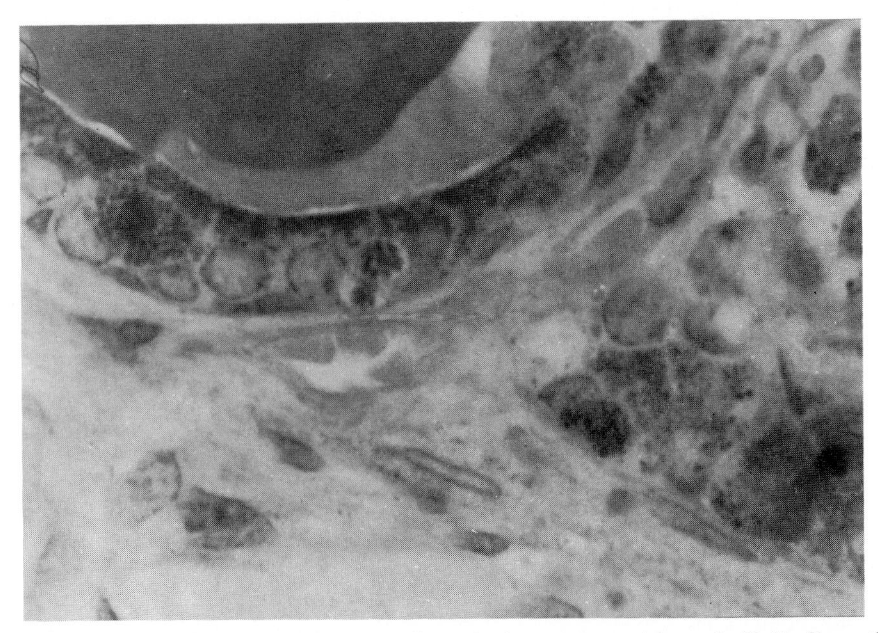

Figure 3 Part of the originally squamous epithelium, revealing extensive secretory activity, embedded in fibrous tissue. This ear had been serous for one week after tubal obstruction and thereafter became infected for six months, resulting in nearly total obliteration of the middle ear cleft. (X800 magnification)

ear cleft. The sequelae of this infective process can persist for a long period after healing.

The observed changes in the middle ear mucosa of the rat after tubal occlusion can be assumed to be essentially the same as those described in the middle ear mucosa of patients with serous otitis media[8–12] and validate the use of this experimental model for a better understanding of the pathogenesis of this disease.

REFERENCES

1. Sadé J, Carr CD, Senturia B: Middle ear effusions produced experimentally in dogs. Ann Otol Rhinol Laryngol 68:1017, 1959
2. Senturia BH, Carr CD, Ahlvin RC: Middle ear effusions: Pathologic changes of the mucoperiosteum in the experimental animal. Ann Otol Rhinol Laryngol 71:632, 1962
3. Lim DJ, Hussl B: Tympanic mucosa after tubal obstruction. Arch Otolaryngol 91:585, 1970
4. Arnold W, Vosteen KH: Die Reaktion der Mittelohrschleimhaut bei Tubenverschluss. Acta Otolaryngol Supp 330:48, 1975
5. Goycoolea MV, Paparella MM, Carpenter AM, Juhn SK: A longitudinal study of cellular changes in experimental otitis media. Otolaryngal Head Neck Surg 87:685, 1979
6. Schade AC, Koopman PJ, Kuijpers W, van Nunen MCJ: The rat as a model for experimental secretory otitis media. Z Versuchstierk 19:228, 1977
7. Beck C: Neue Erfahrungen bei Paukensklerose. HNO 17:234, 1969
8. Zechner G, Tarkkanen J, Holopainen E: Histomorphological and histochemical studies of chronically infected middle ear mucous membrane. Ann Otol Rhinol Laryngol 77:54, 1968
9. Palva T, Palva A: Mucosal histochemistry in secretory otitis media. Ann Otol Rhinol Laryngol 84:112, 1975
10. Tos M, Bak-Pedersen K: Density of goblet cells in chronic secretory otitis media: Findings in a biopsy material. Laryngoscope 85:377, 1975
11. Lim DJ: Normal and pathological mucosa of the middle ear and eustachian tube. Clin Otolaryngol 4:213, 1979
12. Sadé J: Secretory otitis media. New York: Churchill Livingstone, 1979

THE SHORT- AND LONG-TERM EFFECTS OF TUBAL OCCLUSION IN A GERM-FREE ANIMAL MODEL

J.M.H. VAN DER BEEK, M.D., and W. KUIJPERS, Ph.D.

Obstruction or dysfunction of the eustachian tube is generally thought to be the basic pathogenic factor in the onset and continuation of otitis media with effusion (OME). This concept is supported by both clinical observations in patientswith OME[1,2] and by laboratory findings in experimental animals.[3–5] It is not known, however, to what extent tubal occlusion or dysfunction is directly related to the mucosal changes observed in the middle ear epithelium, because signs of infection are a constant finding in the middle ear epithelia of patients with OME and in experimentally occluded ears.[5–7] Previous experiments in our laboratory indicated that the presence of microorganisms (both pathogenic and nonpathogenic) in the upper respiratory tract of the experimental animal inevitably leads to infection of the middle ear after tubal occlusion.[8] To prevent such a complicating infection we developed a germ-free animal model, which guaranteed the absence of microorganisms at the moment of tubal occlusion and thus enabled us to study the isolated effects of eustachian tube obstruction on the middle ear epithelium.

MATERIALS AND METHODS

A total of 115 female Wistar rats were used, which were about 3 months old at the time of operation. These animals were born and raised under completely sterile conditions. They were fed with sterile food and water, housed in sterile balloons, and operated on under completely sterile conditions in a laminar flow cabinet. Under Nembutal anesthesia the tube was reached by a ventral approach and cauterized in its extratympanic course. One week after the operation the animals were transferred into a normal housing unit in the animal department. Otoscopic examination under ether was performed at regular intervals after the operation to assess the efficacy of the operation and the possible interference of infection. The animals were killed after survival times of one day to 24 months; the middle ears were dissected and prepared for light microscopy (LM), scanning electron microscopy (SEM), or transmission electron microscopy (TEM).[9]

RESULTS

One hundred fifteen animals were operated on, 15 of them bilaterally (130 ears). Eleven animals died spontaneously (14 ears) and occlusion failed in 14 ears. Thirty-nine ears showed signs of infection on otoscopic examination and were excluded from the study. It is likely that some infections were due to operative wound infection, whereas in other instances recanalization of the eustachian tube must be held responsible for the infection, as seen in the serial sections.

Sixty-three ears that showed no signs of infection on repeated otoscopic examination during observation periods ranging from one day to 24 months were studied with LM, SEM, or TEM. Bacterial cultures of the middle ear fluid from ten randomly selected ears were negative, and histologic sections of the middle ear epithelia never showed any sign of infection.

The first effects of tubal occlusion were seen in the lamina propria and consisted of an edematous reaction due to dilatation of vessels and transudation of fluid into the intercellular spaces. This process led to a typical cobblestone appearance of the epithelial surface on scanning electron micrographs and severe arcading and bulging of individual cells on TEM sections. This irregularity of the surface persisted throughout the whole observation period. Approximately two days after occlusion, fluid—frequently containing erythrocytes and phagocytotic cells—started to collect in the middle ear cavity. After one week the middle ear cavity was completely filled with faintly staining PAS-positive fluid that showed the same characteristics as the paired serum on electrophoretic examination.

The first signs of fibrosis could be seen in the lamina propria after one week, leading to a denser stroma in the animals surviving longer. At about the same time there was an increase in the periosteal activity at the luminal side of the bony bulla, resulting in apposition of new bone.

This process continued until about eight weeks postoperatively. The reaction was not observed in sham operated animals. After longer survival times the simple squamous epithelium gradually transformed into a two-layered, stratified epithelium consisting of nonsecretory cells and atypical secretory cells. Occasionally squamous metaplasia, as judged by the presence of intracellular tonofilaments, was found. The epithelium in the ciliated areas revealed basal cell hyperplasia. Scattered throughout the whole epithelial lining were large, clear cells that protruded into the lumen and subsequently became detached. In the middle ear fluid they were visible as free-floating cells or clusters of cells, often with signs of degeneration. This process of desquamation was seen throughout the whole observation period (Fig. 1).

The induced abnormalities with respect to hyperplasia, stratification, atypical appearance of secretory granules, and the presence of tonofilaments observed during the first three months were also common findings in the animals surviving longer, but they differed from one ear to another and from site to site in a particular ear. Characteristic changes in animals surviving for very long periods consisted of an increased number of interdigitations of the basal and lateral cell walls and the presence of multivesiculated bodies and siderosome-like structures. No change in the number of secretory elements was observed. The tympanic membrane developed comprehensive changes after longer survival times. After two months scattered white spots could be seen on otoscopic examination, and this process progressed to a nearly total chalky appearance of the tympanic membrane after more than one year (Fig. 2). Microscopic examination demonstrated that this process was due to the deposition of an amorphous "calciferous" substance in the lamina propria of the pars tensa.

With respect to the middle ear fluid, cholesterol clefts were seen after two weeks and persisted in varying amounts, usually intermingled with phagocytotic cells throughout the observation period. These cells, together with the desquamated epithelial cells, were the only cellular components observed in the middle ear fluid (see Fig 1).

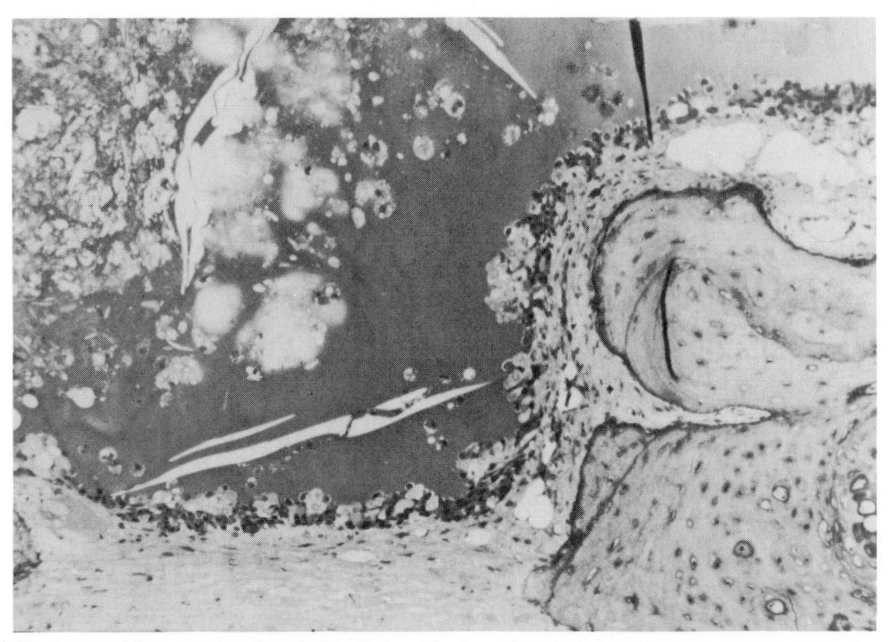

Figure 1 Light micrograph two months after tubal occlusion. The irregular epithelial surface shows stratification and desquamation of epithelial cells. In the lumen cholesterol clefts, desquamated epithelial cells and phagocytotic cells can be seen.

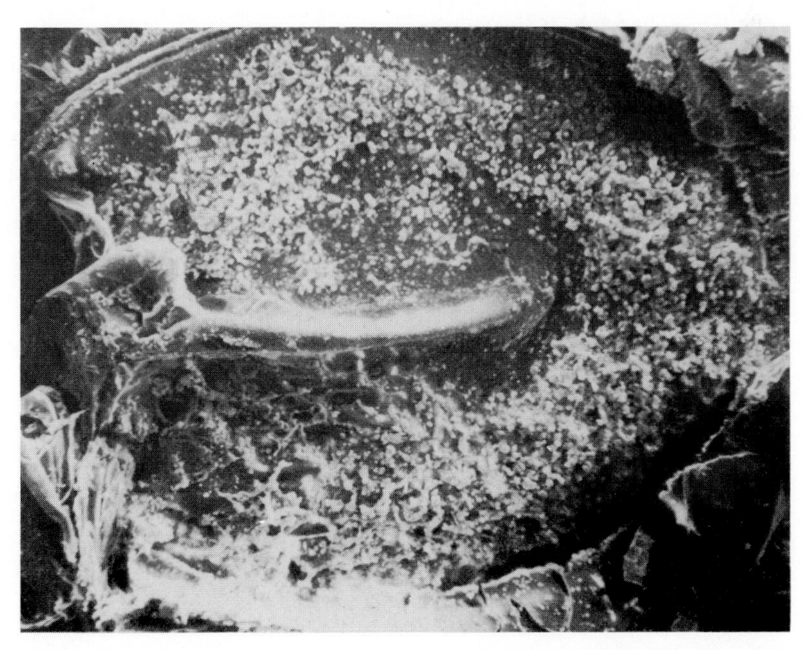

Figure 2 Scanning electron micrograph of irregular medial surface of tympanic membrane 17 months after tubal occlusion.

DISCUSSION

By using germ-free animals it is possible to study the isolated effects of tubal occlusion on the middle ear epithelium without the interference of a complicating infection. Obstruction of the eustachian tube inevitably evokes an underpressure in the middle ear cavity. This results in a retraction of the tympanic membrane and the transudation of fluid from the submucosal vessels into the lamina propria and middle ear cavity. Tubal occlusion without the interference of infection induces changes in the epithelial middle ear lining which include basal cell hyperplasia of the ciliated epithelium, stratification of the squamous epithelium, desquamation of cells, and peculiar cell differentiations as squamous metaplasia and atypical transformation of secretory cells. In comparison with the impressive changes observed in occluded ears with a concurrent infection,[8] the changes in the noninfected epithelium are less conspicuous and quite different.

The present observations in the noninfected ears demonstrate that tubal occlusion per se does not result in an increase of secretory elements and cannot account for the pathologic changes of the middle ear mucosa encountered in patients with OME, as stated by some authors.[4,11] Some observations on the isolated effects of tubal occlusion are of special interest in connection with human middle ear pathology. The observed squamous metaplasia is interesting because of the suggested relationship between OME and aural cholesteatoma.[12] However, it must be noted that in the present study this squamous metaplasia never resulted in a keratinizing squamous epithelium. It is also surprising that phenomena such as formation of new bone, accumulation of cholesterol clefts, and tympanosclerosis-like changes, frequently associated with infectious processes, can be elicited by tubal occlusion alone, that is, without the interference of infection.[13–15] The lack of an increase in the secretory elements in these middle ears indicates the involvement of infectious processes in the opathogenesis of OME. This study convincingly demonstrates that infectious processes must be held responsible for the induced changes in the middle ear epithelium of patients with OME.

REFERENCES

1. Renvall U, Holmquist J: Eustachian tube function in secretory otitis media. Scand Audiol 3:87, 1974
2. Ingvarsson L, Ivarsson A, Lundgren K: Eustachian tube function and volume of the air-filled ear space during the course of serous otitis media in children. In *Physiology and Pathophysiology of Eustachian Tube and Middle Ear*. New York: Thieme Stratton Inc, 1980
3. Proud GO, Odoi H: Effects of eustachian tube ligation. Ann Otol Rhinol Laryngol 79:30, 1970
4. Arnold W, Vosteen KH: Die Reaktion der Mittelohrschleimhaut bei Tubenverschluss. Acta Otolaryngol Suppl 330:48, 1975
5. Goycoolea MV, Paparella MM, Carpenter AM, Juhn SK: A longitudinal study of cellular changes in experimental otitis media. Otolaryngol Head Neck Surg 87:685, 1979
6. Lim DJ: Normal and pathological mucosa of middle ear and eustachian tube. Clin Otolaryngol 4:213, 1979
7. Sadé J, Weissman Z: Middle ear mucosa and secretory otitis media. Arch Otorhinolaryngol 215:195, 1977
8. Kuijpers W, van der Beek JMH, Willart ECT: The effect of experimental tubal occlusion on the middle ear. Acta Otolaryngol 87:345, 1979
9. van der Beek JMH: Experimental obstruction of the eustachian tube. Thesis, University of Nijmegen, Nijmegen, 1981
10. Kuijpers W, and van der Beek JMH: Experimental occlusion of the eustachian tube: the role of short- and long-term infection and its sequelae. In Lim DJ et al (eds): *Otitis Media*. Philadelphia, Toronto: BC Decker Inc, 1984
11. Tos M, Poulsen J, Borch J: Etiologic factors in secretory otitis. Arch Otolaryngol 105:582, 1979
12. Gundersen R, Tonning FM: Ventilating tubes in the middle ear. Arch Otolaryngol 102:198, 1976
13. Friedmann I: The comparative pathology of otitis media experimental and human. J Laryngol Otol 69:588, 1955
14. Ferlito A: Histopathogenesis of tympanosclerosis. J Laryngol Otol 93:25, 1979
15. van der Beek JMH, van der Broek P, Kuijpers W: Effect of tubal occlusion on bone formation in the middle ear of the rat. ORL 45:87, 1983

EXPERIMENTAL LONG-TERM TUBAL OCCLUSION IN CATS: A QUANTITATIVE HISTOPATHOLOGICAL MODEL TO STUDY THE NORMALIZATION OF THE MIDDLE EAR MUCOSA

MIRKO TOS, M.D., MICHAEL WIEDERHOLD, M.D., and PER LARSEN, M.D.

Most of the recent and several of the old experiments on tubal occlusion have shown that serous effusion is produced within 24 hours and that epithelial damage occurs in the form of epithelial cell hyperplasia. In addition, some workers have found transformation of the epithelium into secretory epithelium.[1–3] Others have claimed that the main histologic changes and the production of mucous effusion result from the ensuing infection, and that the tubal occlusion in itself cannot provoke the transformation into secretory epithelium.[4,5] Our previous quantitative investigations have shown that the number of mucous elements increases two to four weeks after tubal occlusion without infection,[3] but the changes were considerably more pronounced in cases of concomitant infection, as often occur in animals with tubal occlusion.

The present study describes the changes of the middle ear mucosa found three to four years after experimental occlusion of the eustachian tube. Such changes have, to our knowledge, not been described before. Senturia and associates,[6] Sala and De Stefani,[7] and Proud and Odoi[8] found granulomatous hyperplasia of the middle ear mucosa, metaplasia of the epithelium into pseudostratified ciliated epithelium with goblet cells, and formation of glands up to 8 months after tubal occlusion. Main and associates found inflammatory reaction and formation of cholesterol granulomas in squirrel monkeys six to 12 months after tubal occlusion.[9]

The main object of this study was to describe the normalization processes of the middle ear mucosa taking place after improvement of the tubal function in experimental animals. These problems have not been discussed before.

MATERIALS AND METHODS

During the period August 1976 to March 1978, the eustachian tubes of ten cats were ligated. The cats were killed in June 1980, so that the longest observation period was 44 months and the shortest 26 months, with an average 35 months. Four methods of ligation were used, as described elsewhere.[10] Throughout the observation period bilateral tympanometry and auditory nerve response were recorded repeatedly.[11] Paracentesis with evacuation of effusion was performed up to eight times under Nembutal anesthesia, and the effusion was examined with respect to viscosity.[12] The last paracentesis was performed shortly before the animal was killed.

After sacrifice, the patency of the eustachian tube was examined with a soft, 0.5-mm thick rubber bougie and the tympanic membrane with otomicroscopy. The entire middle ear mucosa was removed and stained according to the PAS-alcian blue whole mount method[13] for quantitation of goblet cells and mucous glands. Serial sections of characteristic parts of the mucosa from various parts of the middle ear were stained with a combination of hematoxylin-eosin/PAS-alcian blue methods. In each bulla several histopathologic characteristics were evaluated quantitatively and given a score from 0 to 5 (Table 1). The mean histopathologic score was calculated for each cat.

The quantitative investigations of the goblet cells were performed in each cat in a total of 11 localities of the middle ear. In each locality goblet cells were counted in ten 0.01768-mm^2 fields distributed across the locality. Countings were thus done in a total of 110 fields in each middle ear with ligated tube and in the opposite normal ear.

TABLE 1 Quantitative Score of the Histopathologic Changes in the Bulla of the Individual Cases

		Glue			*Thin Effusion*				*Dry*		
		Case No.			*Case No.*				*Case No.*		
Content in the Bulla	*Normal Score*	*1*	*2*	*3*	*4*	*5*	*6*	*7*	*8*	*9*	*10*
Eustachian tube occluded	–	+	+	–	+	–	–	+	–	–	–
Mucosal thickness	0	5	5	4	3	2	2	4	2	2	2
Content in the bulla	0	5	5	0	5	0	0	5	0	0	0
Pseudostratified epithelium	0	5	5	1	1	0	4	4	0	0	0
Leukocytes—neutrophils	0	4	4	1	2	0	0	1	0	0	0
Lymphocytes	0	5	5	5	4	2	2	3	2	2	1
Plasma cells	0	5	5	5	5	2	2	3	2	2	0
Phagocytes—macrophages	0	5	5	5	5	3	2	3	2	2	0
Cellular migration	0	5	5	2	3	0	0	1	1	0	0
Vessel proliferation	0	5	5	5	5	4	4	4	3	2	2
Fibrosis	0	5	5	5	5	4	4	5	4	4	4
Gland number	0	5	5	5	5	3	3	5	3	3	3
Mostly active glands	0	5	5	2	4	0	0	5	0	0	0
Mean score	0	4.9	4.9	3.3	3.9	1.7	1.9	3.6	1.6	1.4	1.0

RESULTS

Based on the presence and viscosity of middle ear effusion at sacrifice, the ten cats were divided into one group of three cats with glue, a group of four with thin effusion, and a group of three with dry middle ears and normal tympanometry findings. The comparison of the mean quantitative histopathologic score of each group allowed us to study the varying degrees of severity of secretory otitis and the course of normalization of the disease.

Ears with Glue at Sacrifice

All 20 repetitive tympanometries showed type B. In one cat the effusion was thin (Table 1, case one) at the first paracentesis and glue at the last three. In two cats the effusion was glue at all 11 paracenteses. The amount of effusion varied from 0.2 to 0.8 cm^3. Anatomically, the eustachian tube was completely closed in two cases (one and two) and heavily stenotic but patent in the third. In this last case the bulla was empty, and the histopathology score was lower than in the other two cases (Table 1). The extension and height of the pseudostratified epithelium were especially small (Fig. 1C); in some parts of the bulla the epithelium was one-layered, and few glands were active. Despite the presence of glue at all paracenteses and the type B tympanogram in case three, there was marked evidence of the epithelium becoming gradually lower cylindric, two-layered cuboidal and one-layered squamous flat. The active mucous glands in cases 1 and 2 are bult up by pseudostratified cylindric epithelium (Fig. 1A), whereas in the glands showing signs of degeneration, the gland epithelium becomes lower two- or one-layered and secretorily inactive (Fig. 1B). The reason for this improvement in case three must be that the tube became patent and a mucociliary clearance could take place.

Ears with Thin Effusion at Sacrifice

In four ears all 32 tympanometries showed type B, and all ears except one (Table 1, case five) had glue at at least one paracentesis. At the remaining 11 paracenteses, the effusion was thin. Case five showed thin effusion at all five paracenteses, and the histopathologic score was lowest in this case. In two cases (four and seven) with anatomically occluded eustachian tubes, the histopathologic score was highest and the bullae were filled with a gel-like mass. Goblet cell density in the bulla, which was extremely high in the group with glue (90 cells/field, Fig. 1E), was 15 cells/field in the group with thin effusion, and in two cases (five and six) all glands were degenerated cystic and covered with one- to two-layered secretorily inactive epithelium (Fig. 1B). Comparison of the histopathologic score in each case within this group clearly demonstrates a low score and signs of improvement in the two cases with patent eustachian tubes: The mucosal thickness and infiltration of neutrophils, lymphocytes, and plasma cells were lower, and there was no cellular migration and no active glands.

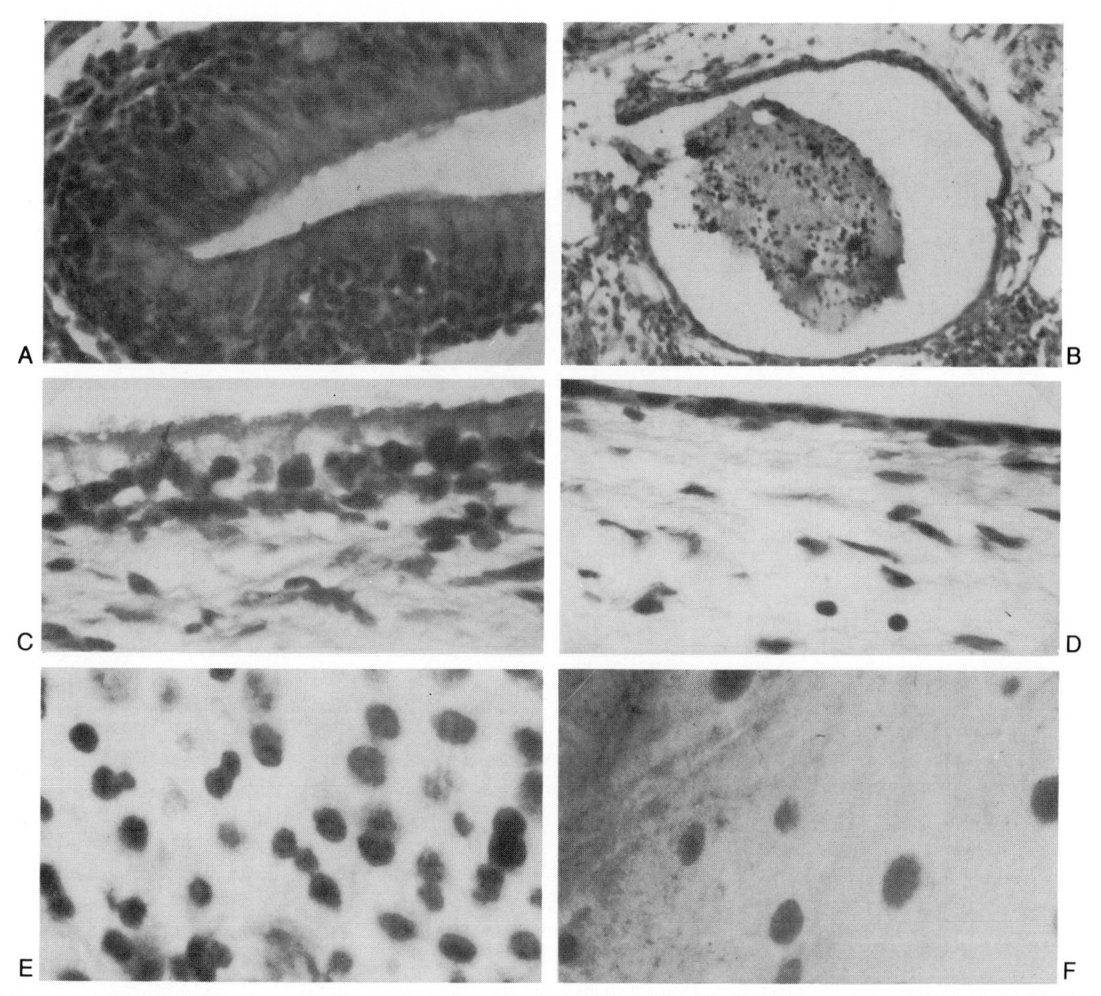

Figure 1 Some examples of mucosal changes in the bulla. A, A part of an active gland tubulus covered with high pseudostratified epithelium with ciliary cells in a thick mucosa with round cell infiltration typical for cases with glue and totally occluded eustachian tube. (Section, X500 magnification.) B, A degenerated gland filled with dead round cells and mucus covered with one-layered cuboidal or flat epithelium, typical for cases with thin effusion and dry ears. (X200 magnification.) C, Low cylindric pseudostratified ciliated epithelium found in ears with glue and thin effusion. (X500 magnification.) D, Flat one-layered epithelium with some fibrosis in the lamina propria found in dry ears after ligation and in normal bullae. (X500 magnification.) E, Highly increased goblet cell density in ears with glue. PAS-alcian blue stained whole mount. (X500 magnification.) F, Several degenerated cystlike glands filled with mucus in a ligated but dry ear, indicating previous secretory otitis (Case ten). Whole mount, X100 magnification.)

Dry Ears at Sacrifice

All three ears had type B tympanograms and glue at paracentesis at the first examinations during the first six months (Table 1); case eight had type B tympanograms all through the first two years. Later the middle ear pressure normalized, and the ears were dry at paracentesis (Fig. 2). At sacrifice the mucosa was thin, and the histopathologic changes were distinct, indicating sequelae changes. The epithelium of the bulla was one- to two-layered, flat to cubic (Fig. 1D). In the lamina propria the round cell infiltration was low, but there was an increase of fibrous elements. The gland number was quite high, but all were degenerated and inactive (Fig. 1F). The median goblet cell density in the bulla was extremely low—3 cells/field—but still higher than in the contralateral normal ears (0 cells/field). Case eight had probably been a severe and long-lasting case with glue at several paracenteses (Fig. 2) and type B tympanograms for two years, but has normalized again. Case ten also had middle ear effusion for about six months.

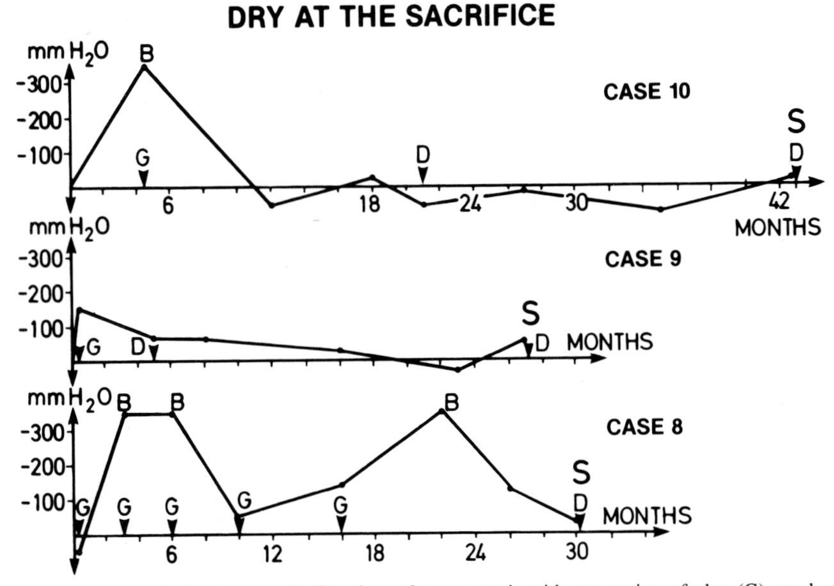

Figure 2 Tympanogram curve including type B (B), time of paracentesis with evacuation of glue (G), or dry ear (D). Time of sacrifice (S) of three cats with dry ears at the last paracentesis.

DISCUSSION

Owing to considerations of space, only the normalization processes of the middle ear mucosa can be discussed here in relation to improvement or normalization of tubal patency and function. Other interesting aspects, such as pathogenesis and etiology and the relationship between glue and thin effusion and histopathology have been described and analyzed elsewhere.[10]

From this experiment it is evident that the patency and function of the eustachian tube is of the greatest importance for the prognosis of secretory otitis, whatever its origin. In our cases with anatomically occluded tubes, the histopathologic changes have been most pronounced, and there was no evidence of improvement. These ears will end up with either total obliteration of the middle ear or with chronic infection. The bullae have been filled with a gel-like mass, and the middle ear mucosae were granulating and hyperplastic. In humans complete anatomic occlusion is rare, and such ears will usually end in obliterative otitis,[14] which is characterized by total obliteration of the middle ear. In cases in which the tube became patent but its function was defective (cases three, five and six), the histopathologic score was significantly lower, showing clear signs of improvement of the disease and of the mucosa. The bullae were empty, indicating the persistence of some degree of mucociliary clearance despite poor function. In ears in which the tubal function became normal, the histopathologic score was significantly lowest (Mann-Whitney test, $p < 0.001$), and the mucosa was nearly normal.

The normalization process of the pseudostratified epithelium is slow and runs over several turnover periods. It is controlled by the division rate of the basal cells.[15] When the division and differentiation rates of the basal cells decrease, fewer cells will differentiate into goblet cells and ciliated cells, and the result will be a lower density and a lower epithelium. During the following turnover periods the goblet cell density further decreases, and the epithelium attains its original premorbid appearance.

Exactly the same processes of normalization of the glandular epithelium take place in the pathologic mucous glands that are formed during the disease.[16] The active epithelium is a pseudostratified epithelium with mucous cells and ciliated cells. This epithelium becomes gradually lower, two- or one-layered, and secretorily inactive, and the glands degenerate. The same processes in human middle ear mucosa have been described by us previously.[16,17]

REFERENCES

1. Arnold W, Vosteen K: Die Reaction der Mittelohrschleimhaut bei Tubenverschluss. Acta Otolaryngol (Stockh) Suppl 330: 48, 1975

2. Lim D, Hussl B: Tympanic mucosa after tubal obstruction. Arch Otolaryngol 91:585, 1970
3. Tos M: Experimental tubal obstruction. Changes in middle ear mucosa elucidated by quantitative histology. Acta Otolaryngol (Stockh) 92:51, 1981
4. Kuijpers W, van der Beek JMH, Willart ECT: The effect of experimental tubal obstruction on the middle ear. Acta Otolaryngol (Stockh) 87:345, 1979
5. van der Beek JMH: Experimental obstruction of the eustachian tube. Thesis., Schrijen-Lippertz, Heerden, 1981
6. Senturia BH, Carr CD, Ahlvin RC: Middle ear effusions: Pathologic changes of the mucoperiosteum in the experimental animal. Ann Otol Rhinol Laryngol 71:632, 1962
7. Sala O, DeStefani G: Modifications caused by the occlusion of the tube on the mucosa of the middle ear; their prevention by corticosteroids. Laryngoscope 73:320, 1963
8. Proud GO, Odoi H: Effects of eustachian tube ligation. Ann Otol Rhinol Laryngol 79:30, 1970
9. Main TS, Shimada T, Lim DJ: Experimental cholesterol granuloma. Arch Otolaryngol 91:356, 1970
10. Tos M, Wiederhold M, Larsen P: Experimental long-term tubal occlusion in cats. Acta Otolaryngol (Stockh), 1983, in press
11. Wiederhold M, Martinez SA, Scott REC, DeFries HD: Effects of eustachian tube ligation on auditory nerve responses to clicks. Ann Otol Rhinol Laryngol Suppl 45:12, 1978
12. Wiederhold M, Zaitchuk JT, Vap JG, Paggi RE: Hearing loss in relation to physical properties of middle ear effusions. Ann Otol Rhinol Laryngol Suppl 68:185, 1980
13. Tos M: Mucous glands of the trachea in children. Quantitative studies. Anat An 126:146, 1970
14. Tos M: Obliterative otitis media. J Laryngol Otol 93:569, 1979
15. Tos M: Middle ear epithelia in chronic secretory otitis. Arch Otolaryngol 106:593, 1980
16. Tos M: Pathogenesis and pathology of chronic secretory otitis. Ann Otol Rhinol Laryngol Suppl 68:91, 1980
17. Tos M: Production of mucus in the middle ear and eustachian tube. Ann Otol Rhinol Laryngol 83:44, 1974

A PRIMATE MODEL OF CLEFT PALATE AND MIDDLE EAR DISEASE: RESULTS OF A ONE-YEAR POSTCLEFT FOLLOW-UP

WILLIAM J. DOYLE, Ph.D., AMY INGRAHAM, B.A.,
MOHAMED M. SAAD, M.D., Ph.D., and ERDEM I. CANTEKIN, Ph.D.

To understand the pathogenesis and sequelae of otitis media with effusion (OME) in the cleft palate population, various animal models have been developed.[1,2] Using juvenile rhesus monkeys, recurrent OME and impaired eustachian tube function (ETF) were shown to develop following surgical clefting of the palate.[2] An abnormal transfer of nasopharyngeal pressures to the middle ear was also documented.[3] In the present study, infant rhesus monkeys were clefted and middle ear status, ETF, and hearing threshold were evaluated during a one-year follow-up.

MATERIALS AND METHODS

Nine rhesus monkeys less than 6 months of age were observed from seven to 12 weeks preoperatively. Tympanometry and otomicroscopy were performed weekly to document middle ear status. ETF was assessed for the left ears of all study animals by means of the inflation-deflation and forced-response tests described previously.[4] The hearing thresholds of the right ears of the animals were estimated using the auditory brain stem response (ABR) with methods and equipment described by Fria and coworkers.[5] Following collection of these baseline data, animals were sedated and an incision was made along the palatal midline from the uvula to the posterior border of the palatine bone. The midline membranous septum was excised. After surgery, middle ear status was monitored weekly. ABRs were elicited on the right ears and ETF tests were conducted on the left ears periodically for a one-year period.

RESULTS

Before surgery the right middle ears of eight of the nine animals remained free of effusions. The usual range of preoperative middle ear pressure was from $-100mm\ H_2O$ to $+100mm\ H_2O$, and of the 114 recordings for the right ears only eight instances of negative and one instance of positive pressure lay outside this range. However, for one animal three weeks of OME and three weeks of high negative pressure were recorded.

After the palatal clefting, the right middle ears of five animals showed evidence of a chronic middle ear disease lasting from nine to 25 weeks. Following this initial period, middle ear disease and OME recurred sporadically over the one-year period of study. In the remaining animals, the right middle ears were characterized by periodic bouts of recurrent OME interrupted by periods of high positive, high negative, or normal middle ear pressures. Overall, 37.5 percent of the observations were characterized by OME.

Twenty-eight middle ear effusions were aspirated and submitted for culture. Of these, 27 were shown to be sterile for pathogenic bacteria. *Streptococcus pneumoniae* was cultured from the effusion of one animal in the chronic OME group.

Sixteen preoperative and 39 postoperative ETF tests were performed. A limitation of these tests is the criterion for an effusion-free middle ear. Therefore, the number of tests and the intervals between tests were not constant among the animals. To avoid undue bias of summary statistics in favor of animals with the greater number of tests, the summary mean values discussed are the mean and standard deviation of the means of tests for the individual animals.

The ability to reduce applied positive and negative middle ear pressures by open nose swallowing was assessed during the inflation-deflation test. The residual pressure following attempted equilibration by swallowing was expressed as a percentage of the applied pressures and was designated SW+ for positive pressure and SW− for negative pressure. The preoperative mean SW+ ranged from 72 percent to 100 percent. For three animals the postoperative means were similar to their preoperative means. For the remaining six animals, the postoperative mean SW+ values were significantly less and ranged from 36 percent to 51 percent. A similar relationship was characteristic of the SW− parameter. However, for this parameter one animal could not equilibrate negative pressure pre- or postoperatively. For the remaining animals, the mean SW− recorded postoperatively ranged from 0 to 82 percent and was always less than the preoperative mean values, which ranged from 82 to 95 percent.

Four parameters of the forced-response test were evaluated at each of five constant flow rates. These parameters are the opening pressure (OP), closing pressure (CP), passive tubal resistance (RO), and active tubal resistance (RA). Summary statistics for the pre- and postoperative values of these parameters at each of the flow rates are presented in Table 1. There were no differences between the pre- and postoperative mean values of OP, CP, and RO when evaluated at any of the flow rates. However, the postoperative mean value of RA was always greater than the preoperative mean

TABLE 1 Pre- and Postoperative Means and Standard Deviations of Four Parameters of the Forced-Response Test Measured at 5 Constant Flow Rates

Flow Rate (cc/min)		*Parameters*			
		OP	*CP*	*RO*	*RA*
6	Pre	313 (97)	152 (62)	35.2 (15.6)	3.9 (1.7)
	Post	309 (30)	176 (31)	37.5 (8.7)	14.8 (10.3)
12	Pre	349 (116)	181 (53)	24.0 (9.3)	5.9 (3.1)
	Post	424 (61)	226 (31)	27.6 (4.8)	16.1 (11.1)
24	Pre	472 (99)	163 (83)	14.3 (5.3)	5.8 (2.3)
	Post	441 (62)	213 (36)	16.8 (2.7)	11.3 (8.4)
48	Pre	455 (137)	155 (61)	9.6 (4.2)	4.4 (2.4)
	Post	465 (54)	156 (29)	9.1 (1.6)	8.5 (5.5)
108	Pre	532 (136)	150 (132)	5.7 (2.1)	4.3 (1.9)
	Post	568 (128)	134 (32)	5.9 (1.7)	6.9 (2.6)

Note: OP = opening pressure; CP = closing pressure; RO = passive tubal resistance; RA = active tubal resistance. Values in parentheses are standard deviations.

value, both for individual animals and for the group. This larger value of active resistance indicated a poorer ETF postoperatively. In 12.8 percent of the postoperative tests the active tubal resistance was greater than or equal to the passive tubal resistance recorded at all flow rates, suggesting that the ET failed either to dilate or to constrict with swallowing. The dilation efficiency of the ET is defined as the ratio of passive tubal resistance to active tubal resistance. The mean values of this ratio are shown for the pre- and postcleft condition in Figure 1. The dramatically reduced values of the tubal dilation efficiency recorded postoperatively emphasize the severe impairment in active tubal function.

The ABR was chosen to evaluate the hearing threshold of animals in the present study because past studies have shown that this test provides unbiased estimates of hearing thresholds and hearing losses in rhesus monkeys.[5] In recent study of the maturation of this response, it was shown that the wave IV/wave I ratio was not dependent on age of the animal, had low interanimal variability, and was sensitive to stimulus intensity.[6] Therefore, this ratio was used to estimate hearing threshold. Each animal had one ABR test prior to clefting. Following production of a cleft, 55 tests were performed. Thirty tests were conducted when the middle ear pressure was considered to be normal ($\pm$100mm H_2O), five when the middle ear pressure was less than $-$100mm H_2O and 20 when a middle ear effusion was present. The mean IV/I wave ratios recorded at 60 dB stimulus intensity are shown for each of these conditions in Figure 2. Also shown is a latency ratio intensity function consisting of mean data previously reported for 44 tests on 23 animals with normal middle ear pressures. The mean value of this ratio for both the nine preoperative tests and the 30 postoperative tests conducted with normal middle ear pressures was 3.00, which is in agreement with the mean value of 3.04 reported for control animals. However, the five tests conducted when high negative middle ear pressure was observed or the 20 done when OME was present had lower mean ratio values of 2.77 and 2.61 respectively. When mapped onto the intensity function, as shown in Figure 2, a mean loss of 10 dB for the ears with high negative pressure and 20 dB for the ears with OME was estimated. In addition, the large standard deviations (0.32 and 0.33) associated with these conditions imply a highly variable degree of hearing loss. The hearing loss was a transient phenomenon and solely determined by the middle ear condition. The resolution

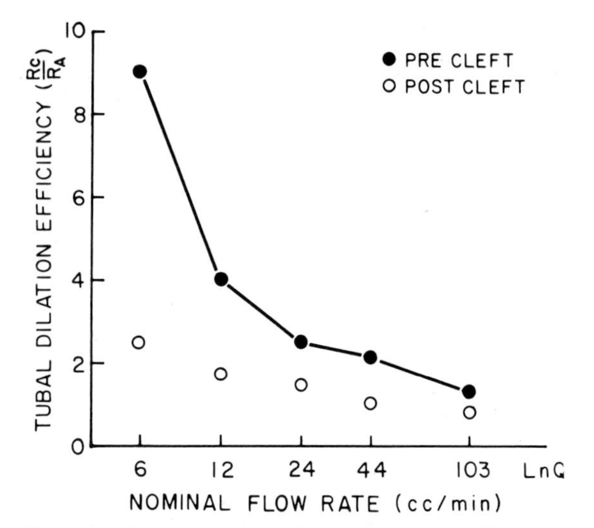

Figure 1 The mean values of the tubal dilation efficiency (ratio of passive tubal resistance to active tubal resistance) recorded pre- and postoperatively as a function of constant flow rate.

of the OME or abnormal pressure resulted in normal hearing without residual effects as measured.

DISCUSSION

In the infant monkeys, the cleft induced a disease condition that was chronic and of significant duration. This is congruent with the chronic OME that purportedly affects children with unrepaired clefts of the plate.[7]

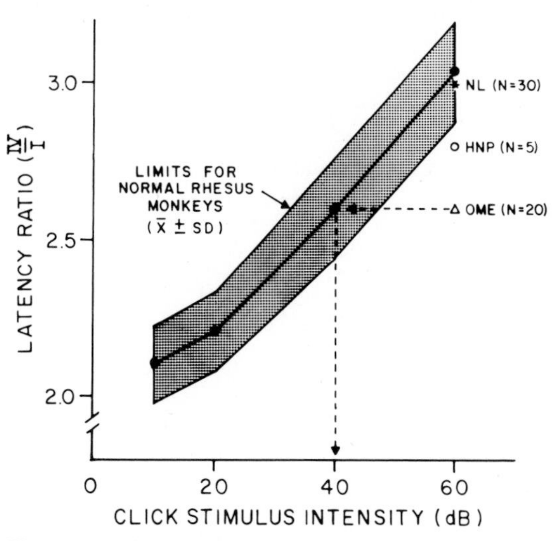

Figure 2 The mean values of the IV/I wave latency ratio as a function of stimulus intensity for a group of control animals. Also plotted are the mean IV/I latency ratios recorded postoperatively for the tests with normal middle ear pressures, high negative middle ear pressures, and OME.

The rather high incidence of positive middle ear pressures reported for the cleft palate monkeys in this and also the previous study was not reported for the clinical population.[2] These abnormal pressures were observed to predominate in the periods immediately following the resolution of an episode of OME. Other studies showed these pressures to be the result of the introduction of a bolus of air from the nasopharynx to the middle ear, probably by a mechanism similar to politzerization.[3] It was suggested that this altered middle ear ventilation may supplement the more usual though deficient mechanism involving muscular assisted tubal dilation and consequently may aid in disease resolution. A similar argument can be developed to explain the abbreviated course of the disease in some animals observed in this study and the recurrent nature of the disease in the remaining animals.

The results of the postcleft ETF tests showed a more extensive debility than that observed in the previously developed monkey model. This debilitated ETF was reminiscent of that reported for children with repaired cleft palates. As with the clinical population, the ability to reduce positive middle ear pressure was deficient and the ability to reduce applied negative middle ear pressure was severely impaired. No significant differences were observed in the forced opening pressure, closing pressure, or passive tubal resistance between the pre- and postoperative states. The active tubal resistance was seen to increase following clefting of the palate. Furthermore, in a significant number of tests the eustachian tube was observed to constrict with swallowing, again mimicking the condition reported for children with repaired palatal clefts.[8] The impaired ability to equilibrate positive and negative middle ear pressure and the increased active tubal resistance and constriction with swallowing suggest that the surgical clefting of the palate in infant monkeys results in a reduced tubal dilation efficiency.

Finally, the results of the ABR testing showed a significant fluctuating conductive hearing loss in these animals that was dependent on the status of the middle ear. Continued study of the hearing loss in similar animal models may contribute significantly to our understanding of the conductive hearing impairment in the cleft palate population and to an evaluation of the possibility of a secondary sensorineural loss associated with a chronic disease state.

This study was supported in part by grant # NS16337 from the National Institutes of Health and DE 01697.

REFERENCES

1. Odoi H, Proud GO, Toledo PS: Effects of pterygoid hamulotomy upon Eustachian tube function. Laryngoscope 81:1242, 1971
2. Doyle WJ, Cantekin EI, Bluestone CD, et al: A nonhuman primate model of cleft palate and its implication for middle ear pathology. Ann Otol Rhinol Laryngol 89(68):41, 1980
3. Doyle WJ, Saad MM, Cantekin EI: Anomalous middle ear gas absorption in a nonhuman model of cleft palate. Cleft Palate J 19:17, 1982
4. Cantekin EI, Saez CA, Bluestone CD, Bern SA: Airflow through the eustachian tube. Ann Otol Rhinol Laryngol 88:603, 1979
5. Fria TJ, Saad MM, Doyle WJ, Cantekin EI: Auditory brainstem response in rhesus monkeys with otitis media with effusion. Otolaryngol Head Neck Surg 90:824, 1982
6. Doyle WJ, Saad MM, Fria TJ: Maturation of the auditory brainstem response in rhesus monkeys (Macaca mulatta). Electroencephalogr Clin Neurophysiol J 56:210, 1983
7. Paradise JL, Bluestone CD, Felder H: The universality of otitis media in 50 infants with cleft palate. Pediatrics 44:35, 1969
8. Doyle WJ, Cantekin ET, Bluestone CD. Eustachian tube function in cleft palate children. Ann Otol Rhinol Laryngol 89(68):34, 1980

LOCAL ANTIBODY IN A MODEL OF OTITIS MEDIA WITH EFFUSION

ANTONINO CATANZARO, M.D., ALLEN RYAN, Ph.D.,
SHARON BATCHER, B.S., VIRGINIA BLACK,
JEFFREY HARRIS, M.D., and STEVE WASSERMAN, M.D.

Clinical studies of otitis media have demonstrated that all the constituents necessary for immunologic injury can be found in middle ear effusion. Further evidence has been presented by our group,[1] as well as by others, that antigens presented to the middle ear can be processed and induce systemic as well as local immune responses. This study further defines the response to antigenic challenge to the middle ear in systemically immunized guinea pigs.

MATERIALS AND METHODS

Healthy Hartley strain guinea pigs weighing 201 to 250 gm were purchased from Charles River and immunized systemically by intradermal injection on the back with 1 mg alum precipitated keyhole limpet hemocyanin (KLH). Animals were allowed three weeks to develop systemic immunity. At the time of middle ear challenge the ear was examined carefully. If there was any evidence of current or past pathologic changes, particularly infection, the ear was not used. If the ear was normal, a transtympanic injection was performed. Soluble associated KLH in the dose selected was injected in 0.1 ml PBS (pH 6.5). Unimmunized guinea pigs served as controls. Three days later middle ear fluid and specimens were harvested as follows: The middle ear was dissected, the bulla entered anteriorly, and 0.1 ml 199 tissue culture medium was instilled. The bulla was gently agitated and free fluid was aspirated (Fig. 1). The volume of fluid recovered was measured, effusion being defined as fluid recovered in excess of the wash volume. The recovered lavage was diluted and centrifuged. The supernatant was stored frozen until assayed. The resuspended cell pellet was counted using a standard hemocytometer. Shannon cytocentrifuge slides were stained with Wright's stain and cytology was carefully defined.

IgG antibody with specificity against KLH was quantified using the radioimmunoassay developed in our laboratory and previously described.[1]

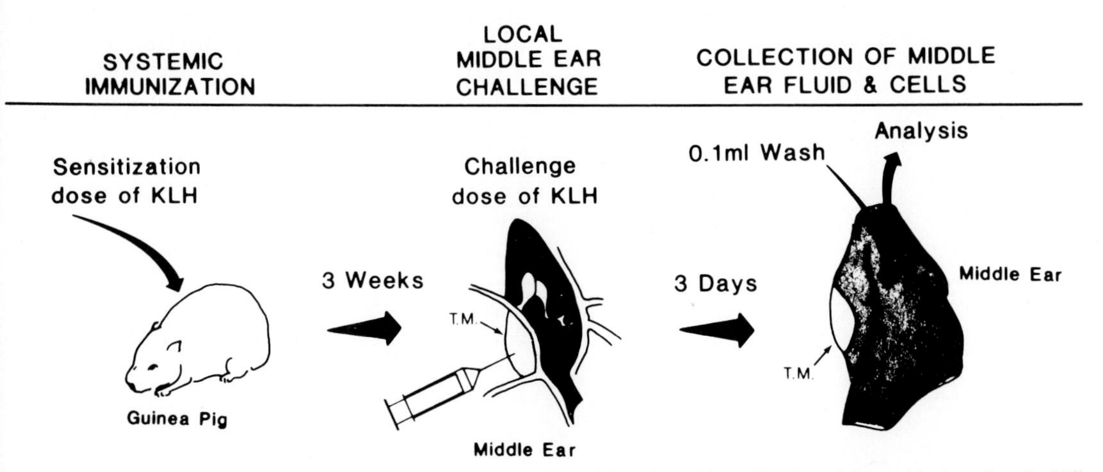

Figure 1 Experimental Design: systemic immunization by intradermal injection of 1 mg KLH precipitate with alum. Local middle ear challenge: selected challenge dose was presented by transtympanic puncture with the middle ear. Collection of middle ear fluid and cells: The middle ear was dissected and the bulla entered anteriorly, 0.1 ml 199 tissue culture medium instilled to wash the middle ear, and all free fluid collected and analyzed.

RESULTS

When the middle ears of the sensitized guinea pigs were challenged with 1000 mcg KLH, eight out of eight developed effusions, with a mean volume of 133 ± 12 μl. In each case, IgG specific against KLH was present in the effusion, the mean being 136 ± 20 mcg/ml. The mean cellular contents of the effusion were as follows: A total of 350 ± 122 × 10^5 leukocytes were recovered; 277 ± 16 × 10^5 were polymorphonuclear cells, 3.7 × 10^5 were eosinophils, 52 ± 0.5 × 10^5 were macrophages, 11 ± 4 × 10^5 were lymphocytes, and 1.6 ± 0.5 × 10^5 were plasma cells. With regard to cellular components, the middle ear effusion recovered from these animals is similar to serous otitis effusion recovered from patients. Control guinea pigs had essentially no effusion, cells, or antibody recovered from middle ear lavage.

A series of experiments was done to explore the response to different challenge doses, ranging from 1000 mcg to 0.3 mcg. The middle ear effusion that developed in response to a range of challenge doses is shown in Fig. 2. The ordinate is the volume of middle ear effusion recovered after subtraction of the wash volume. There was essentially no response to 0.3 or 1.0 mcg KLH, but there is a clearcut response to 3.0 mcg and larger doses. There may be a relationship between the challenge dose and the amount of fluid recoverable, although it is not linear.

The amount of IgG against KLH recovered from middle ear effusion followed a similar pattern (Fig. 3). Very small amounts of antibody were detected in response to 0.3 or 1.0 mcg KLH, with larger amounts present in response to larger doses. Ten or 30 mcg KLH elicited a smaller response

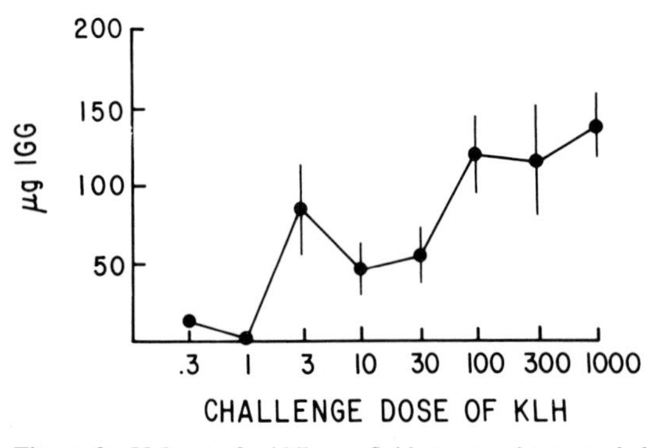

Figure 2 Volume of middle ear fluid recovered versus challenge dose of KLH. A log scale is used to depict the wide range of doses used. Bars indicate standard error of the mean of 4 to 9 animals.

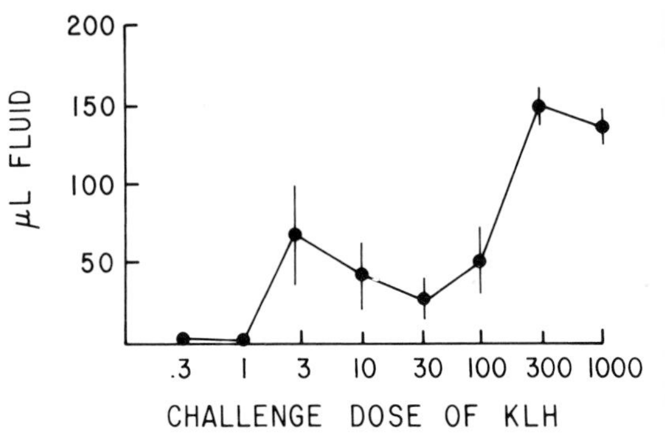

Figure 3 Amount of IgG with reactivity against KLH recovered in middle ear effusions versus challenge dose of KLH.

than doses of 100, 300, and 1000 mcg.

There is a close correlation between the challenge dose of KLH and the number of cells recovered; there were very few cells in response to 30 mcg or less. The correlation coefficient is 0.994, with a standard error of the estimate of only 13.4. A similar relationship exists between dose and polymorphonuclear cells, macrophages, and lymphocytes. The ratio between the cells stays quite constant and is the same as seen in response to 1000 mcg KLH.

DISCUSSION

The report describes middle ear fluid elicited by local antigenic challenge in a sensitized guinea pig. Guinea pigs sensitized to KLH offer an excellent model for the study of immune-mediated phenomena in the middle ear. Middle ear challenge with soluble KLH results in the development of significant amounts of middle ear effusion. The effusion is rich in leukocytes and there is a close correlation between the number of leukocytes and the dose of antigenic challenge over a wide range. The inflammatory response that follows an immune challenge with KLH is very similar to that which follows infection of the middle ear. The middle ear fluid collected contained abundant quantities of IgG reaction against KLH. As little as 3 mcg of KLH elicits an antibody-containing effusion, but 100 mcg was required before the effusion became exudative.

REFERENCE

1. Catanzaro A, Ryan A, Robb JA: Immunologically mediated and nonspecific inflammatory responses in the middle ear. J Clin Immunol Immunopathol 24:361, 1982

THE MONGOLIAN GERBIL AS AN ANIMAL MODEL OF OTITIS MEDIA

RONALD P. HOOGMOED, B.A., ROBERT S. FULGHUM, Ph.D.,
A. MASON SMITH, Ph.D., JACK E. BRINN, Ph.D.,
and HAL J. DANIEL III, Ph.D.

The Mongolian gerbil, *Meriones unguiculatus,* has been shown by us to be microbiologically and anatomically acceptable as an animal model for otitis media.[1,2] The normal gerbil middle ear is lined with a thin layer of stratified squamoid epithelium which we term "mucoperiosteum." The middle ear cavity is subdivided by trabeculae of bone, forming connecting chambers. On otoscopic observation, the normal gerbil tympanic membrane (TM) is slightly yellowish-pink in color and translucent. The tympanic membrane is large relative to the size of the gerbil but requires careful observation for study through the tiny external auditory canal.

We have shown the gerbil to be susceptible to acute otitis media induced by percutaneously inoculating *Streptococcus pneumoniae* type 3, *Hemophilus influenzae* type b, or other aerobic and anaerobic bacteria into the middle ear bulla. Comparison of the response in both gerbils and chinchillas showed similar results. A few gerbils held for chronic studies showed permanent changes, including formation of scar tissue and new bone deposition, when inoculated with a polymicrobic infection flora including anaerobic bacteia.[3] The response to pneumococcal infection in the gerbil was similar to that found in the chinchilla by Giebink and Quie.[4]

The purposes of our present work were to repeat our previous study[3] using a different type of pneumococcus and a nontypable strain of *H. influenzae* in longitudinal studies of ten weeks' duration and to develop a way to cause a brief, mild form of acute otitis media without sequelae. We found the gerbil to be susceptible to *S. pneumoniae* type 23, and *H. influencze* nontypable strain 119. These organisms were found to differ in virulence from the previously used strains. Also, heat-killed type 3 pneumococcal cell preparations produced a very slight inflammation of short duration without sequelae in the gerbil middle ear.

MATERIALS AND METHODS

Healthy young adult gerbils were anesthetized and examined prior to inoculation for any preexisting otitis media.[3] *S. pneumoniae* type 23 was purchased from American Type Culture Collection (ATCC 6323) and passed through mice to enhance pathogenicity. *H. influenzae* nontypable strain 119 was obtained from E.O. Mason, Jr. This strain had been isolated from a case of human otitis media and had been shown to adhere to human buccal epithelial cells.[5] One set of ten gerbils was inoculated with *S. pneumoniae* type 23, and another set of ten gerbils was inoculated with *H. influenzae* strain 119. Gerbils were inoculated with 0.03 ml of a suspension containing 3×10^5 bacteria/ml as in our previous study.[3]

The *S. pneumoniae* type 3 was the same strain used previously.[3] A suspension of approximately 1×10^7 cells/ml was made in sterile 0.85 percent saline and heated for one minute at 100°C to prepare the nonviable pneumococcal cell preparation. It was found to be devoid of living cells by plating on supplemented chocolate agar. Three sets of five, five, and ten gerbils per set were inoculated with the nonviable pneumococcal type 3 cell preparation.

All gerbils were removed from each set weekly, anesthetized, and evaluated for otitis media using behavioral and otoscopic observations.[3] One animal from each group was killed each week. Specimens of middle ear effusions or washings were obtained by tympanocentesis. These were cultured for bacteria and smeared and stained with Wright's stain to detect inflammatory cell types. Each animal was fixed for histopathologic studies by per cardiac perfusion; heads were removed and decalcified, embedded, sectioned, and stained with H&E stain for macro- and microscopic observation.

Specific immunoglobulins were isolated from

gerbils immunized with sheep erythrocytes, polymerized flagellin (POL), *H. influenzae* type b, and *Escherichia coli* lipopolysaccharide. Standard methods of gel filtration, ion exchange chromatography, affinity chromatography, and chromatofocusing were used for immunoglobulin purification. Specific heterologous antisera were made for gerbil IgM, IgA, and IgG.

RESULTS

Following inoculation with *H. influenzae* strain 119, otoscopic observations indicated that otitis media was present from the first and persisted throughout the study. Otoscopic study revealed a grayish, opaque tympanic membrane (TM) with a rough surface texture. In some animals, a yellowish pus was seen either behind the TM or extruding through it. Smears of middle ear washings revealed both polymorphonuclear leukocytes and monocytes present during the first two weeks but not beyond two weeks. *H. influenzae* could be isolated through the third week but not beyond. Secondary invaders, most often a staphylococcus or a gram-negative rod, could be found in some animals during subsequent weeks.

Histopathologic studies of the progression of otitis media due to *H. influenzae* strain 119 revealed an elevated and thickened mucoperiosteum, with large numbers of polymorphonuclear leukocytes and fewer monocytes infiltrating the middle ear cavity at seven days following inoculation. During the second week the mucoperiosteum became further thickened and new bone was laid down in the middle ear cavity. Polymorphonuclear leukocytes and monocytes were still plentiful. Some fibroblasts were seen. More bone was laid down during the third week and the middle ear became filled with a granulomatous-like reactive scar tissue with fibroblasts and collagen fibers found abundantly (Fig. 1). Histopathologic findings similar to those seen in week three were seen in all subsequent weeks of the study. The new bone deposition was of a cancellous type; however, it was about five times as thick as the original compact

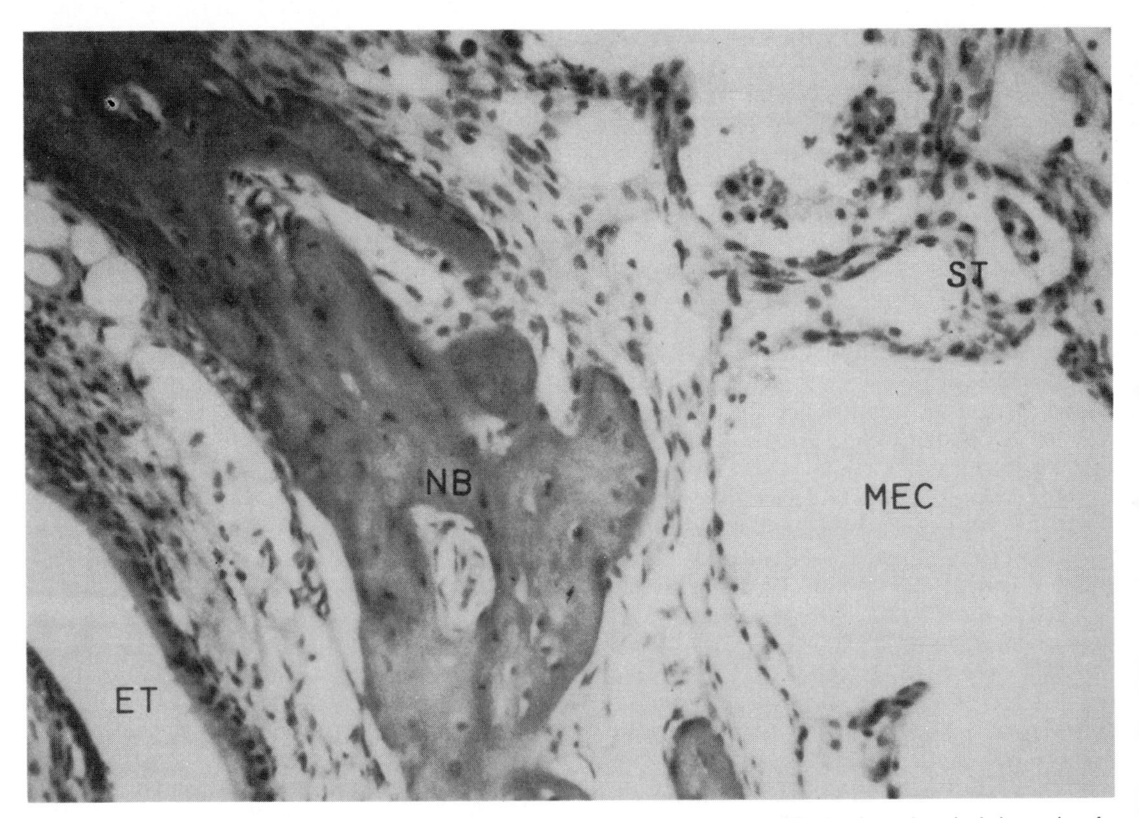

Figure 1 Three weeks after inoculation with *H. influenzae* strain 119 more new bone (NB) has been deposited, increasing the thickness of the temporal bone. Scar tissue (ST), middle ear cavity (MEC), and eustachian tube (ET) are shown. (X125 magnification.)

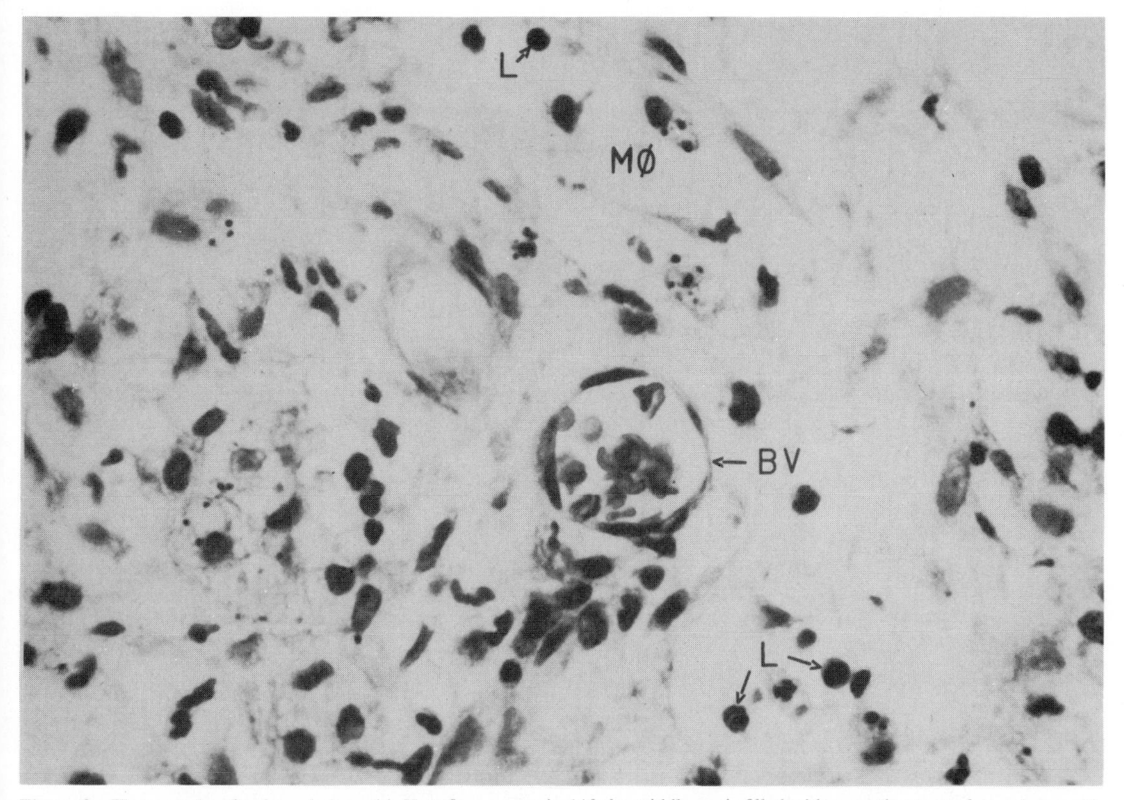

Figure 2 Three weeks after inoculation with *H. influenzae* strain 119 the middle ear is filled with a reactive type of scar tissue with blood vessels (BV) and lymphatics. Lymphocytes (L) may be seen, as may be macrophages (M∅). (X500 magnification.)

bone. The reactive type of scar tissue that filled the middle ear contained blood vessels and lymphatics. Macrophages and plasma cells were seen within the scar tissue (Fig. 2).

Inoculation of the gerbil middle ear with *S. pneumoniae* type 23 produced a mild form of otitis media with remission after the first week. Most TMs were normal or only slightly opaque; however, some had a gray, rough appearance. Histopathologic studies revealed variable changes. At week one, a swollen, elevated mucoperiosteum and an infiltration of polymorphonuclear leukocytes and monocytes were seen (Fig. 3). In subsequent weeks, little evidence of disease could be seen. Only one (week four) animal showed any scar tissue or new bone formation. *S. pneumoniae* was never cultured from the middle ear washings, indicating that this type of pneumococcus may easily be destroyed by the gerbil immune system. Only a staphylococcus was isolated from the week three and week four animals.

Inoculation of nonviable *S. pneumoniae* type 3 caused almost no changes that could be detected otoscopically other than a slight opacity to the TM. Histopathologic study revealed only slight middle ear inflammation. At week one there was a slight amount of exudate with a slightly thickened mucoperiosteum. After week one all middle ears appeared normal, showing no signs of otitis media. Cultures of middle ear washings were almost always sterile, although several staphylococci and corynebacteria were found.

DISCUSSION

The nontypable *H. influenzae* strain 119 produced a serious infection involving striking pathologic changes. Our previous work[3] showed that *H. influenzae* type b produced otitis media; however, no longitudinal study was done. Strain 119, with its ability to adhere to animal cells, produces a more severe disease than the strain of type b we used previously. The disease caused by type b seemed to remit after three weeks in the few animals studied for more than seven days.

S. pneumoniae type 23 produced only a mild infection with remission without sequelae during

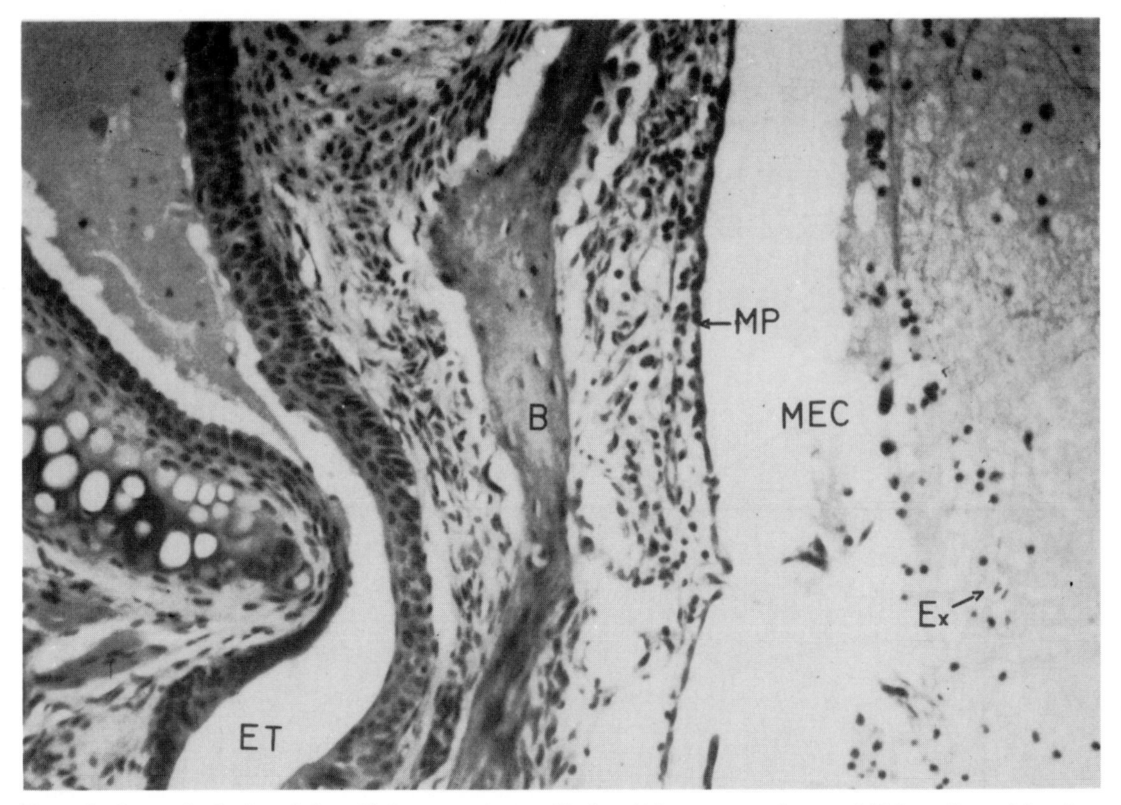

Figure 3 One week after inoculation with *S. pneumoniae* type 23, the middle ear mucoperiosteum (MP) is swollen and there is an exudate containing polymorphonuclear leukocytes. Eustachian tube (ET), bone (B), middle ear cavity (MEC), and exudate (Ex) are shown. (X125 magnification.)

the second week following infection. Histopathologic changes were less pronounced over the same time span than in our previous experiments using *S. pneumoniae* type 3.[3] Thus, type 23 pneumococcus produces a more mild disease in the gerbil middle ear than does type 3 pneumococcus. This agrees with the findings of Giebink and Quie in the chinchilla.[4]

To cause inflammation and to compromise the gerbil middle ear without overshadowing permanent pathologic characteristics that would obscure the subsequent testing of secondary invading bacteria (for example, anaerobic bacteria[6–10]) to cause otitis media, we followed the example of Lowell and colleagues[11] by inoculating gerbil middle ears with heat-killed cultures of pneumococcal cells. We used type 3 pneumococcus. Lowell and colleagues used type 23 pneumococcus.[11] We used a higher temperature to kill the bacteria and found that a much milder response was elicited. The mechanisms of injury from the nonviable cells may be related to bacterial enzymes, and the higher temperature may have affected these enzymes. Some antigenic properties may also have been affected. Further studies must be done to produce a heat-killed preparation with inflammatory properties falling between those found by Lowell and associates[11] and those we found.

Initial inflammatory reactions and the subsequent immune response within the gerbil middle ear will be studied using our isotype-specific antisera conjugated with fluorescent compounds as well as by using enzyme-linked assays for humoral response to various microorganisms.

This work was supported in part by a grant-in-aid from The Deafness Research Foundation. We thank Carolyn Jones, John Worthington, Nicki Smith, and Dr. Paul Strausbauch for their assistance. The East Carolina University School of Medicine provided R.P.H. a scholarship from the Summer Research Program for medical students.

REFERENCES

1. Thompson TA, Gardner, D, Fulghum RS, et al: Indigenous nasopsharyngeal, auditory canal and middle ear bac-

terial flora of gerbils: Animal model for otitis media. Infect Immun 32:1113, 1981
2. Daniel HJ, Fulghum RS, Brinn JE, Barrett KA: Comparative anatomy of eustachian tube and middle ear cavity in animal models for otitis media. Ann Otol Rhinol Laryngol 91:82, 1982
3. Fulghum RS, Brinn JE, Smith AM, et al: Experimental otitis media in gerbils and chinchillas with *Streptococcus pneumoniae, Haemophilus influenzae* and other areobic and anaerobic bacteria. Infect Immun 36:802, 1982
4. Giebink GS, Quie PG: Comparison of otitis media due to types 3 and 23 *Streptococcus pneumoniae* in the chinchilla model. J Infect Dis 136:191, 1977
5. Lampe RM, Mason EO Jr, Kaplan SL, et al: Adherence of *Haemophilus influenzae* to buccal epithelial cells. Infect Immun 35:166, 1982
6. Fulghum RS, Daniel HJ, Yarborough JG: Anaerobic bacteria in otitis media. Ann Otol Rhinol Laryngol 86:196, 1977
7. Jokipii AM, Karama MP, Ojala K, Jokipii L: Anaerobic bacteria in chronic otitis media. Arch Otolaryngol 103:278, 1977
8. Brook I, Anthony BF, Finegold SM: Aerobic and anaerobic bacteriology of acute otitis media in children. J Pediatr 92:13, 1978
9. Brook I, Finegold SM: Bacteriology of chronic otitis media. J Am Med Assoc 241:487, 1979
10. Sugita R, Kawamura S, Ichikawa G, et al: Studies on anaerobic bacteria in chronic otitis media. Laryngoscope 91:816, 1981
11. Lowell SH, Juhn SK, Giebink GS: Experimental otitis media following middle ear inoculation of nonviable *Streptococcus pneumoniae*. Ann Otol Rhinol Laryngol 89:479, 1980

PROVOKING EFFUSION IN EXPERIMENTAL OTITIS MEDIA WITH EFFUSION

STEN HELLSTRÖM, M.D., Ph.D., LARS-ERIC STENFORS, M.D., Ph.D., PER E. ALM, D. MED. SC., GUNNAR D. BLOOM, M.D., Ph.D., BENGT SALÉN, M.D., Ph.D., and LOUISE WIDEMAR, M.D.

As early as 1934, Holmgren reported that ligation of the eustachian tube in dogs caused production of serous effusion in the middle ear.[1] The tubal occlusion was thought to cause a lowering of the pressure in the middle ear and the effusion was developed by a hydrops ex vacuo. Since that time many investigators have been able to reproduce these results with modified techniques and in various animal species.[2–4] Recently Stenfors and associates, in studies on rats, with obstructed eustachian tubes (ETs), noted that the effusion usually started in the attic.[5] The attic in this context refers to the lateral attic compartment, bordered on one side by the pars flaccida and on the other by the ossicular chain with adjacent mucosal folds. The attic communicates with the rest of the middle ear cavity through a small opening, the isthmus tympanicus. At the same time effusion occurs in the attic the pars flaccida changes appearance—it exhibits dilated vessels and becomes discolored and retracted. Histologic studies of this portion of the tympanic membrane have shown that in contrast to the pars tensa and the attic mucosa it is extremely rich in mast cells.[6]

To gain new insight into the possibility that this peculiar attic space is the site of the start of effusion production, we investigated whether experimental procedures not directly interfering with the function of the ET could provoke production of effusion fluid. Furthermore, such experiments might also shed more light on the mechanisms involved. This chapter summarizes some of the data obtained; complete reports have been or will be published elsewhere.[7–9]

MATERIALS AND METHODS

Healthy adult Sprague-Dawley rats were used for the study, and the experimental procedures detailed below were performed on animals anesthetized with a barbiturate administered via a tail vein. The animals were divided into the following groups.

Group One

Through an opened tympanic bulla a piece of Gelfoam was placed in the tympanic isthmus, blocking the passage from the mesotympanum to the lateral attic compartment.

Group Two

The external auditory canals (EACs) of the rats were subjected to mechanical stimulation either by irritating the skin of the EAC by twisting a plastic ear speculum or by exposing the EAC to a stream of chilled air. None of the stimulating procedures lasted longer than 30 minutes.

Group Three

Compound 48/80, a potent mast cell degranulating agent, was instilled drop by drop into the tympanic membrane through the EAC.

Group Four

A polyethylene tube was sealed into a small hole drilled in the tympanic bulla. A pressure of −20 mm H_2O was induced through the tube into the middle ear cavity.

At different time intervals after the initial experimental procedure the tympanic membranes were inspected and photographed through an otomicroscope. In some animals in each group the middle ear cavity was rinsed with a small volume of saline and the rinsing solution was collected for analysis of histamine content. Other rats were injected with a dye, Evans blue, via a tail vein, and 20 minutes later their middle ear cavities were rinsed as described above. The rinsing solutions were subjected to spectrophotometric analysis to establish a possible leakage of blue dye into the middle ear cavity.

After the middle ear fluid was collected for the various analyses, the pars flaccida and pieces of the middle ear mucosa were dissected free, fixed by immersion in various fixatives, and further processed for studies under the light and electron microscopes.

RESULTS

Group One

Within 24 hours after blockage of the tympanic isthmus, an effusion appeared in the attic. The pars flaccida was amber colored and exhibited a network of dilated vessels; it was markedly retracted. No effusion could be seen in the meso- or hypotympanum. At day two the changes in the pars flaccida were more pronounced, and when the tympanic bulla was opened effusion seemed to ooze through the spongy piece of Gelfoam covering the tympanic isthmus. Minute amounts of similar material could be seen below the piece of Gelfoam in the sulcus promontorialis nasalis[10] and the round window niche. The tympanic tubal orifice, however, appeared dry. Rinsing fluid collected at day two showed an increased content of histamine through the middle ear cavity. After injection of Evans blue the rinsing fluid showed a bluish tint, indicative of an increased vessel leakage. Fluid from the contralateral control ear was not colored. Histologically, the pars flaccida, and particularly its lamina propria, appeared edematous and contained granules that apparently are discharged mast cell granules. These granules were found scattered in the proximity of blood vessels (Figs. 1, 2). The sinus-like vessels, which normally characterize the attic mucosa, were greatly enlarged. In contrast, the histologic appearance of the biopsy material from the hypotympanic mucosa was quite normal.

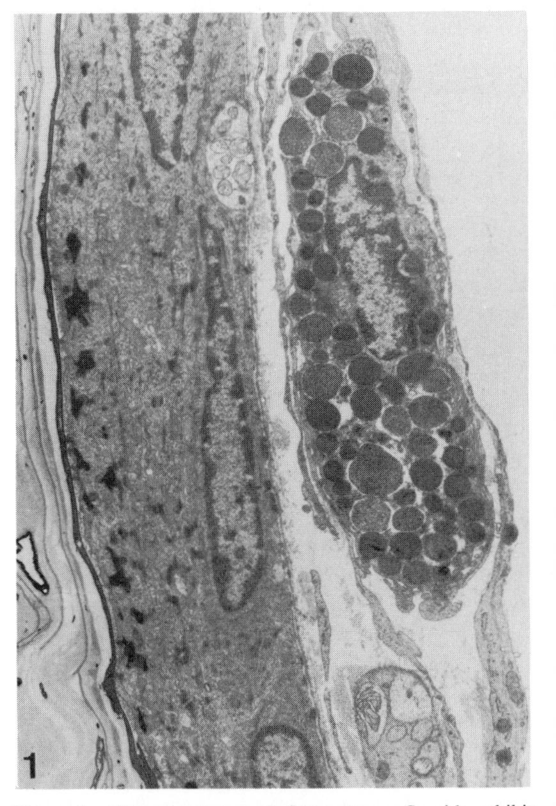

Figure 1 Electron micrograph from rat pars flaccida exhibiting a mast cell located in the lamina propria beneath the keratinizing squamous epithelium. (X10,000 magnification.)

Group Two

As early as 30 minutes after the skin of the EAC was scratched, not touching the tympanic membrane, effusion appeared in the attic. Changes in the pars flaccida, similar to those observed in group one, were noted. Vital staining with Evans blue showed an increased vessel leakage, and the histamine content of the middle ear fluid was markedly increased. Rinsing fluid from the contralateral ear also showed increased levels of histamine.

Histologically, the pars flaccida, and especially its lamina propria, was thickened and had lost its overall organization due to a massive edema. Extravascular inflammatory cells were observed. Twenty-four hours after the mechanical stimulation the attic was still filled with a "muddy" fluid. The pars flaccida was in its normal position but was thickened and discolored. The content of histamine in the middle ear cavity was still increased.

An exposure of the EAC and the tympanic membrane to a stream of chilled air caused changes somewhat similar to those observed after mechanical irritation. The pars flaccida, although edematous, was white and transparent and did not exhibit any dilated vessels.

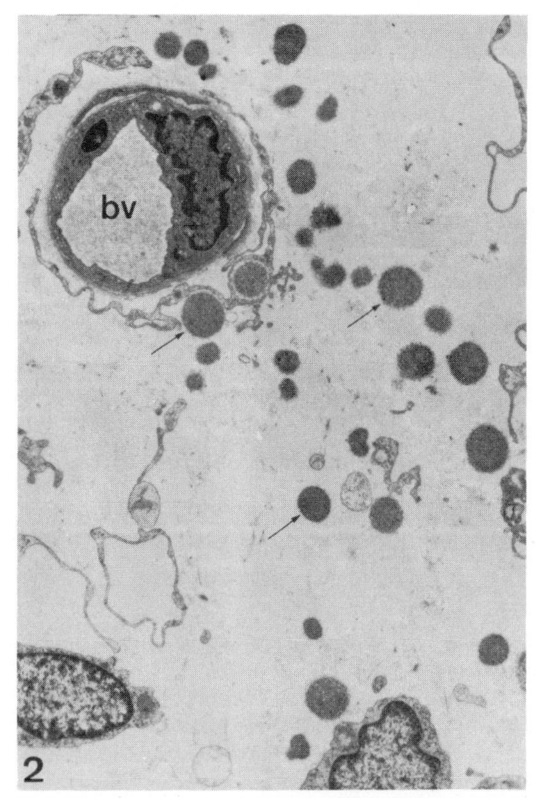

Figure 2 Electron micrograph from pars flaccida after instillation of compound 48/80 onto the tympanic membrane. Granules (arrows) discharged from mast cells are found scattered in the proximity of a blood vessel (bv). (X10,000 magnification.)

Group Three

Twenty minutes after administration of compound 48/80 to the tympanic membrane, effusion had occurred in the attic, behind a discolored pars flaccida with dilated vessels. The administration of Evans blue colored the rinsing fluid of the middle ear cavity. The level of histamine was higher than that determined for the control ear. Histologically, the pars flaccida was edematous and showed degranulation of the normally occurring mast cells.

Group Four

A decreased intratympanic pressure of 20 mm H_2O caused effusion that filled the attic within 10 minutes. The whole middle ear cavity was gradually filled and about 2 hours later the whole middle ear was filled with effusion. The initiation of effusion occurred simultaneously with those changes of the pars flaccida structure which have been described for the other groups.

None of the groups showed any signs of infection of the middle ear cavity.

DISCUSSION

Our studies have shown that effusion can be induced by various procedures that do not directly interfere with tubal function. Regardless of the experimental procedures employed, effusion initially collected in the attic space medial to the pars flaccida. Moreover, the effusion was produced in middle ear cavities without any signs of infection. At the same time as effusion appeared in the attic the pars flaccida changed color, became thickened, and exhibited widely dilated vessels. Histologically, the pars flaccida was edematous and many of its characteristic mast cells were degranulated. The attic mucosa also showed extremely dilated vessels and the Evans blue leakage indicated an increased vascular permeability. The histologic appearance of the pars flaccida and especially its cellular components, together with the increased histamine content of the middle ear cavity fluid that was found, suggests that the effusion may be

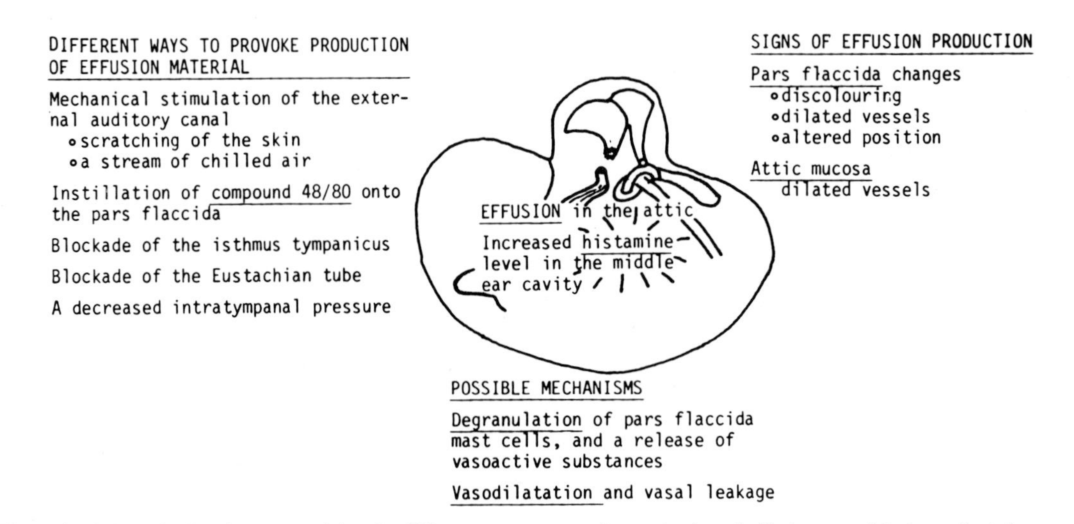

Figure 3 Schematic drawing summarizing the different ways to provoke production of effusion material, the earliest changes of pars flaccida concomitant with effusion production, and some possible mechanisms involved.

caused by vasoactive substances released from the abundant pars flaccida mast cells.

These findings seem to emphasize the importance of the attic region as the initial site of production of effusion.[8] Furthermore, it seems likely that some of the initial cellular events leading to production of effusion take place in the pars flaccida as a marked swelling of the lamina propria accompanies the start of effusion in the attic. A schematic drawing of possible mechanisms is shown in Figure 3. Involvement of the ET in these mechanisms cannot, however, be excluded, since pars flaccida has been shown to react toward minute pressure and volume changes[11] and may thus be connected, neurally or humorally, with the opening process of the ET.

At present we can only speculate about the possibility of otitis media with effusion (OME) in the human being initiated by mechanisms similar to those described in the present study. Pars flaccida, which is a common site of other pathologic conditions of the middle ear for example cholesteatoma, may be involved in the pathogenesis of OME as well. If this proves to be the case the initial localization of the onset of effusion and the proposed mechanisms for its induction must be taken into consideration in future discussions concerning the diagnosis and therapy of OME.

This study was supported by grant # B83-17X-06578-01 from Swedish MRC and a grant from the Medical Faculty, University of Umeå, Sweden.

REFERENCES

1. Holmgren G: Récherche experimentale sur les fonctions de la trompe d'Eustache. Communication préalable. Acta Otolaryngol 20:381, 1934
2. Sadé J, Carr CD, Senturia BH: Middle ear effusions produced experimentally in dogs. Ann Otol 68:1017, 1959
3. Proud GL, Odoi H: Effects of Eustachian tube ligation. Ann Otol 79:30, 1970
4. Paparella MM, Hiraide F, Juhn SK, Kaneko Y: Cellular events involved in middle ear fluid production. Ann Otol Rhinol Laryngol 79:766, 1970
5. Stenfors LE, Carlsöö B, Winblad B: Structure and healing capacity of rat tympanic membrane after Eustachian tube occlusion. Acta Otolaryngol (Stockh) 91:75, 1981
6. Alm PE, Bloom GD, Hellström S, Stenfors LE, Widemar L: Mast cells in the pars flaccida of the tympanic membrane. A quantitative morphological and biochemical study in the rat. Experentia 39:287, 1983
7. Hellström S, Salén B, Stenfors LE: The site of initial production and transport of effusion materials in otitis media serosa. Acta Otolaryngol (Stockh) 93:435, 1982
8. Alm PE, Bloom GD, Hellström S, Salén B, Stenfors LE: The release of histamine from the pars flaccida mast cells—one cause of oititis media with effusion. Acta Otolaryngol (Stockh) 94:517, 1982
9. Alm PE, Bloom GD, Hellström S, et al: Middle ear effusion caused by mechanical stimulation of the external auditory canal. An experimental study. Acta Otolaryngol (Stockh), 96:91, 1983
10. Hellström S, Salén B, Stenfors LE: Anatomy of the rat middle ear. A study under the dissection microscope. Acta Anatomica 112:346, 1982
11. Hellström S, Stenfors LE: The pressure equilibrating function of pars flaccida in middle ear mechanics. Acta Physiol Scand 118:337, 1983

TYPE II COLLAGEN-INDUCED AUTOIMMUNE SALPINGITIS IN RATS

KOICHI TOMODA, M.D., and TAI JUNE YOO, M.D.

Immunity to type II collagen has been found in such human diseases as relapsing polychondritis[1] and rheumatoid arthritis.[2] Type II collagen, which consists of three polypeptide chains linked in triple helices, is genetically distinct from other types of collagen and is found primarily in hyaline cartilage.

Several animals sensitized with type II collagen developed pathologic lesions in the cartilaginous tissues.[3–5] Cremer and colleagues recently reported on an animal model of auricular chondritis induced by immunization with type II collagen and suggested that type II collagen autoimmunity may be the mechanism involved. The purpose of this study was to examine histologically the eustachian tubes of rats immunized with type II collagen, to demonstrate the distribution of type II collagen in the tube, and to evaluate autoimmunity to type II collagen.

MATERIALS AND METHODS

Outbred female Wistar rats were used in this study. Bovine types I, II, and III and rat type II collagen were isolated and purified as previously described.[7,8] Animals were injected with 200 μg of bovine type II collagen with incomplete Freund's adjuvant. Booster injection was given seven days later. Antibody assay against type II collagen was done by the ELISA method.[6] Immune sera for measurement were obtained from two to several weeks after primary injection.

For histopathologic studies, 20 immunized rats were killed two and eight weeks after secondary injection, and 10 untreated rats were prepared as controls. After perfusion with glutaraldehyde, temporal bones were fixed in 10 percent neutral buffered formalin, decalcified with trichloroacetic acid (TCA), and embedded in paraffin. Seven-micron thick sections were routinely stained with hematoxylin and eosin alcian blue.

For immunohistochemical study, indirect fluorescence and peroxidase staining were performed.[9,10] Temporal bones were fixed in cold 95 percent ethanol, decalcified with EDTA for seven days, embedded in paraffin, and sectioned at 7 μ thickness. Nonspecific background was reduced by incubation with normal rabbit serum diluted with 1 percent bovine serum albumin. Endogenous peroxidase was blocked with hydrogen peroxide in methanol. Prepared sections were incubated with goat antirat IgG or C3, followed by an incubation with fluorescein isothiocyanate (FITC) or peroxidase-conjugated rabbit antigoat IgG. Control sections were incubated with normal goat serum or second antibody only.

To study type II collagen distribution in normal eustachian tubes, monoclonal antibody to type II collagen produced in mice[11] was used as a first antibody. As a second antibody, FITC- or peroxidase-labeled goat antimouse IgG was used. Some sections, prior to staining, were treated with testicular hyaluronidase[12] to extract proteoglycans. Control sections were incubated with normal mouse serum, monoclonal antibody to chick type II collagen shown to bind only chick type II collagen or to streptococcus M protein.

RESULTS

Bilateral salpingitis was observed in 17 of 20 rats immunized with bovine type II collagen. The eustachian tubes of these rats were histologically characterized by infiltration of the mucosa and submucosa with an abundance of mononuclear cells, consisting primarily of plasma cells, lymphocytes, and histiocytes; goblet cell hyperplasia on the lining membrane; hypersecretion of mucus; and loss of the usual basophilic staining of the tubal cartilage (Fig. 1). These findings were particularly remarkable in the tympanic side of the tube as compared with the pharyngeal side. In some cases, the numerous mononuclear cells infiltrated into the muscle and glands in the middle part of the eustachian tube. In many instances, a large amount

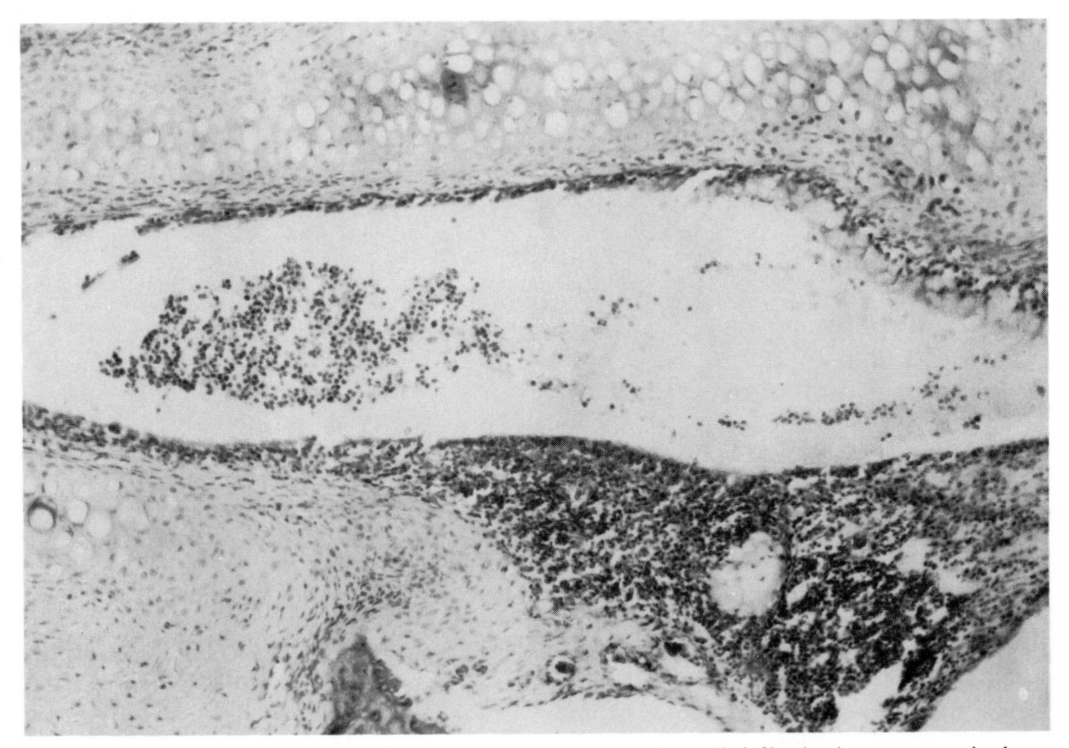

Figure 1 Salpingitis induced with type II collagen. Note abundant mononuclear cells infiltrating into mucosa and submucosa, goblet cell hyperplasia, and loss of the usual basophilic staining of the tubal cartilage. (Hematoxylin & eosin, X60 magnification.)

of seromucinous effusion containing inflammatory cells was observed in the tympanic orifice of the eustachian tube, but less was observed in the tympanic bulla. Spontaneous otitis media and salpingitis were observed in four of the immunized rats and two of the controls.

On the other hand, eustachian tube chondritis was observed in three of the eight rats that were examined eight weeks after secondary injection of bovine type II collagen. The cartilage plate and perichondrium were destroyed and fragmented by inflamed fibrous tissues containing mononuclear cells, fibroblasts, and fibrocytes (Fig. 2).

The animals immunized with other types of collagen, such as bovine types I and III, did not show any changes in the eustachian tube.

Sections labeled with antitype II collagen monoclonal antibody showed positive staining mainly in the perichondrium of the tubal cartilage. When sections were pretreated with hyaluronidase, both perichondrium and intercellular matrix of the cartilage stained prominently. In the cases of salpingitis, positive immune reaction with antirat IgG and C3 antisera were observed in the perichondrium and subperichondrial cartilage matrix. However, these specific stainings were not observed in the rats with spontaneous otitis media and salpingitis. None of the control sections examined in this study showed specific staining.

Antibodies against type II collagen were detected in these rats by ELISA. Mean absorbance of 1:1000 dilution of the sera from ten rats immunized with bovine type II collagen was significantly higher ($p < 0.001$) than that of the controls (Table 1). These antibodies were inhibited with rat type II collagen, but not with bovine type I collagen.

DISCUSSION

Type II collagen distributed within cartilaginous tissue has been demonstrated in the trachea,[13] joints,[14] and intervertebral disc.[15] It is synthesized mainly by chondroblasts and chondrocytes.

In the present study, immunohistochemical examinations using monoclonal antibody to type II collagen revealed the presence of type II collagen in the eustachian tube cartilage, mostly in the peri-

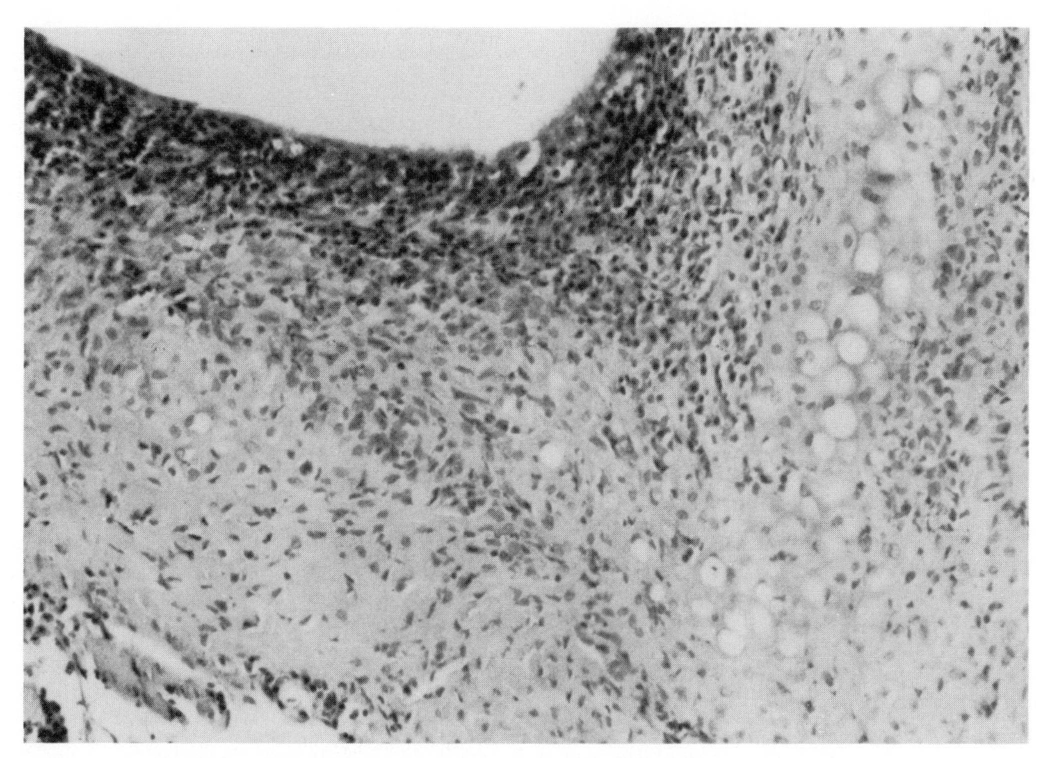

Figure 2 Eustachian tube chondritis induced with type II collagen. Note the deranged cartilage plate and perichondrium by an inflamed fibrous tissue. (Hematoxylin & eosin, X100 magnification.)

chondrium, which contains numerous chondroblasts. When sections were pretreated with testicular hyaluronidase, both perichondrium and intercellular matrix of the cartilage showed type II collagen localization more prominently. Presumably, this is due to the fact that the proteoglycans, which mask the antigenic sites of type II collagen in the cartilage, were extracted by hyaluronidase treatment, as described by Von der Mark and colleagues.[16]

We have shown for the first time that autoimmune salpingitis was induced in 85 percent of rats by immunizing with bovine type II collagen, in which 15 percent of rats developed eustachian tube chondritis eight weeks after secondary injection. These diseases were characterized by inflammatory changes, chondrolysis, immune complex deposition in the perichondrium, and a high titer of antibody against type II collagen that had been inhibited by rat type II collagen.

TABLE 1 IgG Antibody to Type II Collagen Measured by ELISA

		Antibody Level (Absorbance at 450 nm)			
			Inhibition with 50 μg/ml		
Animals	*No. of Sera Studied*	*No Inhibition*	*BII*	*RII*	*BI*
Collagen immunized rats	10	1.196* ± 0.154†	0.126*	0.244	1.094
Control rats	10	0.038 ± 0.008	ND	ND	ND
		$p < 0.001$ (as determined by student's t test)			

Note: BII, bovine type II collagen; RII, rat type II collagen; BI, bovine type I collagen; ND, not done.
*Mean absorbance
†Standard error

It has been already shown that antisera raised in rats against bovine type II collagen extensively cross-reacts with rat type II collagen.[4] Hence, these antibodies suggest "autoimmunity."

How the autoimmunity to type II collagen involves the eustachian tube is not known. However, the high antibody level detected in the immune sera and the presence of immunoglobulins and complement in the tissue suggest type II and/or type III immunologic injuries. Furthermore, the potential importance of cell-mediated immunity and antibody-dependent cytotoxicity as mechanisms of injury cannot be excluded.

On the basis of these data, one can postulate that the eustachian tube could become a target organ in an immune response to type II collagen and that the occurrence of salpingitis without chondritis may be an early manifestation of an autoimmune disorder mediated by immunity to type II collagen, while the eustachian tube chondritis may be a later manifestation in the disease process.

As mentioned at the beginning, autoimmunity to type II collagen has been proven to occur in human relapsing polychondritis. It is known that the auditory system is frequently involved in this disease, with hearing loss observed in about 46 percent of the patients.[17] Cody and Sones[18] reported that the conductive hearing loss occurring in this disease may be due to eustachian tube chondritis, while the sensorineural hearing loss is of the cochlear type, presumably as a result of arteritis. We also have recently found sensorineural hearing loss in rats immunized with bovine type II collagen, as histologically evidenced by the spiral ganglion cell degeneration and perivasculitis of the cochlear artery.[19] Thus, this animal model may well be useful in defining the etiologic factors of deafness which occur in human relapsing polychondritis.

This study was supported by the American Otologic Society, Deafness Research Foundation and the Veteran's Administration.

REFERENCES

1. Foidart JM, Abe S, Martin GR, et al: Antibodies to type II collagen in relapsing polychondritis. N Engl J Med 299:1203, 1978
2. Andriopoulos NA, Mestecky J, Miller EJ, Bradley EL: Antibodies to native and denatured collagens in sera of patients with rheumatoid arthritis. Arthritis Rheum 19:613, 1976
3. Wooley PH, Luthra HS, Stuart JM, David CS: Type II collagen-induced arthritis in mice. J Exp Med 154:688, 1981.
4. Trentham DE, Townes AS, Kang AH: Autoimmunity to type II collagen: An experimental model of arthritis. J Exp Med 146:857, 1977
5. Yoo TJ, Tomoda K, Hernandez A: Type II collagen induced autoimmune inner ear disease in the guinea pig. Abstract No. 50, Research Forum in AAO-HNS and ARO, October 1982
6. Cremer MA, Pitcock JA, Stuart JM, et al: Auricular chondritis in rats: An experimental model of relapsing polychondritis induced with type II collagen. J Exp Med 154:535, 1981
7. Trelstad RL, Kang AH, Toole BP, Gross J: Collagen heterogeneity: High resolution of native $[\alpha 1\ (I)]_2\alpha 2$ and $[\alpha 1\ (II)]_3$ and their component α chains. J Biol Chem 247:6469, 1973
8. Stuart JM, Cremer MA, Dixit SN, et al: Collagen induced arthritis in rats: Comparison of vitreous and cartilage-derived collagens. Arthritis Rheum 22:347, 1979
9. Sainte-Marie G: A paraffin embedding technique for studies employing immunofluorescence. J Histochem Cytochem 10:250, 1962
10. Taylor CR, Burns J: The demonstration of plasma cells and other immunoglobulin-containing cells in formalin-fixed, paraffin-embedded tissues using peroxidase-labeled antibody. J Clin Pathol 27:14, 1974
11. Köhler G, Milstein C: Continuous cultures of fused cells secreting antibody of predefined specificity. Nature 256:495, 1975
12. Sheehan DC, Hrapchak BB: *Theory and Practice of Histotechnology,* 2nd ed. St Louis: CV Mosby Company, 1980, p 174
13. Timple R, Von der Mark K, Von der Mark H: Immunochemistry and immunohistology of collagens. In Viidik A, Vuust J (eds): *Biology of Collagen.* New York: Academic Press, 1980, pp 211–22
14. Gay S, Müller PK, Lemmen C, et al: Immunohistological study on collagen in cartilage-bone metamorphosis and degenerative osteoarthrosis. Klin Wschr 54:969, 1976
15. Wick G, Nowack H, Hahn E, et al: Visualization of type I and II collagens in tissue sections by immunohistologic techniques. J Immunol 117:298, 1976
16. Von der Mark H, Von der Mark K, Gay S: Study of differential collagen synthesis during development of the chick embryo by immunofluorescence. Develop Biol 48:237, 1976
17. Pearson CM: Relapsing polychondritis: Clinical and immunologic features. In Parker CW (ed): Clinical Immunology, vol II. Philadelphia: WB Saunders, 1980, pp 774, 783
18. Cody DTR, Sones DA: Relapsing polychondritis: audiovestibular manifestations. Laryngoscope 81:1208, 1971
19. Yoo TJ, Tomoda K, Stuart JM, et al: Type II collagen induced sensorineural hearing loss and vestibular dysfunction in rats. Ann Otol Rhinol Laryngol 92:267, 1983

APPEARANCE OF EFFUSION MATERIAL IN THE ATTIC SPACE CORRELATED WITH AN IMPAIRED EUSTACHIAN TUBE FUNCTION

LARS-ERIC STENFORS, M.D., Ph.D., STEN HELLSTRÖM, M.D., Ph.D., BENGT SALÉN, M.D., Ph.D., and OVE SÖDERBERG, M.D.

Several investigations have shown that a total blockage of the eustachian tube, which alters the ventilation and/or drainage of the middle ear cavity (MEC), causes liquid to collect. Previous studies have also shown that, whatever the origin of the effusion, its production always starts in the attic.[1-3] Consequently one of the first signs of tubal dysfunction should be appearance of effusion in the attic.

The aim of the present study in the rat was to interfere with the normal tubal function, the paratubal muscles, or nasal ventilation to create dysfunction of the eustachian tube. Particular attention was paid to clarifying whether different parts of the tube have different significance with regard to the development of effusion. The appearance of effusion material in the attic with a retraction and discoloration of the pars flaccida was considered to result from dysfunction of the eustachian tube.

MATERIALS AND METHODS

Healthy adult Sprague-Dawley rats were used for the study. Under aseptic conditions the rats were anesthetized with a hexabarbital (Brietal) through a tail vein, and the animals were divided into the following groups.

Group One

In five rats a small hole was drilled into the wall of the tympanic bulla via a retroauricular approach, and through this a polyethylene plug was hermetically inserted into the tympanic orifice (Fig. 1).

Group Two

In five rats the middle ear cavity was entered through the same approach as in Group One and a polyethylene tube (Intra Medic, ID 0.28 mm, OD 0.61 mm) was inserted into the tympanic orifice. About 80 percent of the eustachian tube was thus blocked but air could still pass through the tube.

Group Three

In five rats the middle ear cavity was entered as described above and the tensor tympani tendon was severed close to the malleus.

Group Four

In five rats the soft palate was split with a scalpel in the midline from the posterior free border to the hard palate.

Group Five

In five rats the nasal airways were completely obstructed by ligatures around both nostrils.

Group Six

In five rats the mandible was excised and the soft palate split. The pharyngeal orifice was inspected and photographed at various tensions and positions of the soft palate (Fig. 2). The surgical procedures in Groups one through three were performed on the right side while the left side was kept as control. In Groups one through five the animals were reanesthetized daily during the first

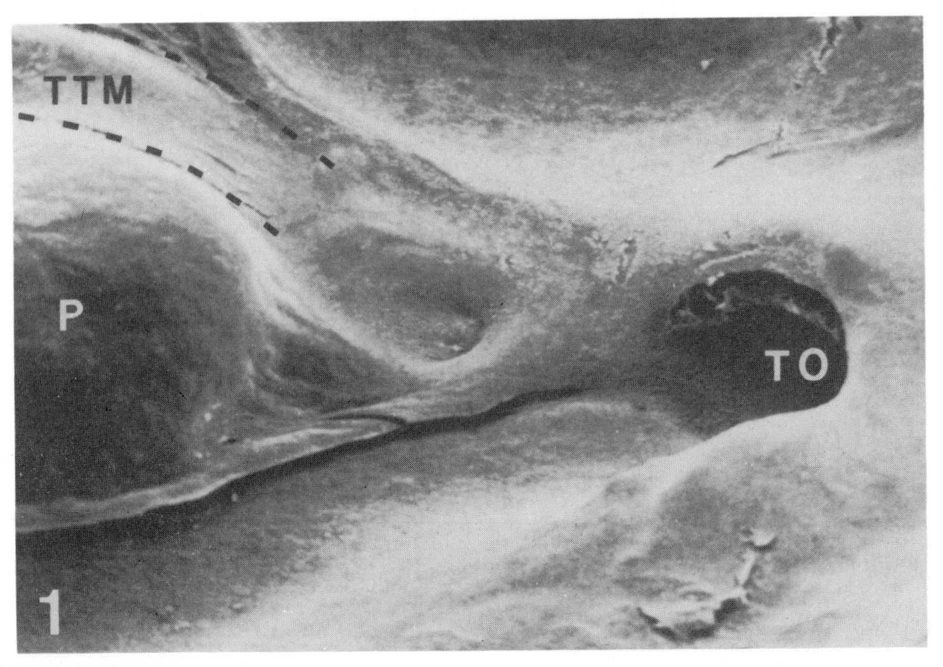

Figure 1 Scanning electron micrograph of the right tympanal orifice (TO). Total blockage of the tympanal orifice caused effusion production. A tube inserted into the orifice allowing air but not effusion material to pass caused no stasis of effusion material around the opening. P, promontory; TTM, tensor tympani muscle. (X10 magnification)

week and every third day thereafter, the tympanic membranes were inspected using an otomicroscope, and the appearance of the pars flaccida was mapped. After various intervals the animals were killed and the middle ear cavities were inspected.

RESULTS

Group One

Total obstruction of the eustachian tube caused almost immediate effusion production. The effusion material first became evident in the attic. If the obstruction was prolonged, effusion also became noticeable in the mesotympanum. Thus, 12 to 24 hours after tubal occlusion, the pars flaccida appeared slightly indrawn and a trace of serous, transparent yellow effusion was noted in the attic. After two to three days the whole attic was filled with fluid that caused a lateral bulging of the pars flaccida. After about ten days, however, the pars flaccida was maximally retracted, forming a "mobile" retraction pocket draping the neck of the malleus. After three to four weeks the middle ear was almost completely filled with a cloudy and highly viscous effusion. The pars flaccida remained indrawn, lacking elasticity, but did not adhere to the neck of the malleus when the effusion was aspirated.

Group Two

A tube inserted into the tympanic orifice caused no effusion to develop. The pars flaccida remained in a normal, relaxed position during the period of observation (four weeks). No effusion was detected around the tubing.

Group Three

Severing the tensor tympani tendon close to the neck of the malleus did not initiate any effusion production in the middle ear cavity. No effusion was noted in the attic or in any other part of the middle ear during the period of observation (eight weeks).

Group Four

In every case splitting of the soft palate caused effusion production within 24 to 48 hours.

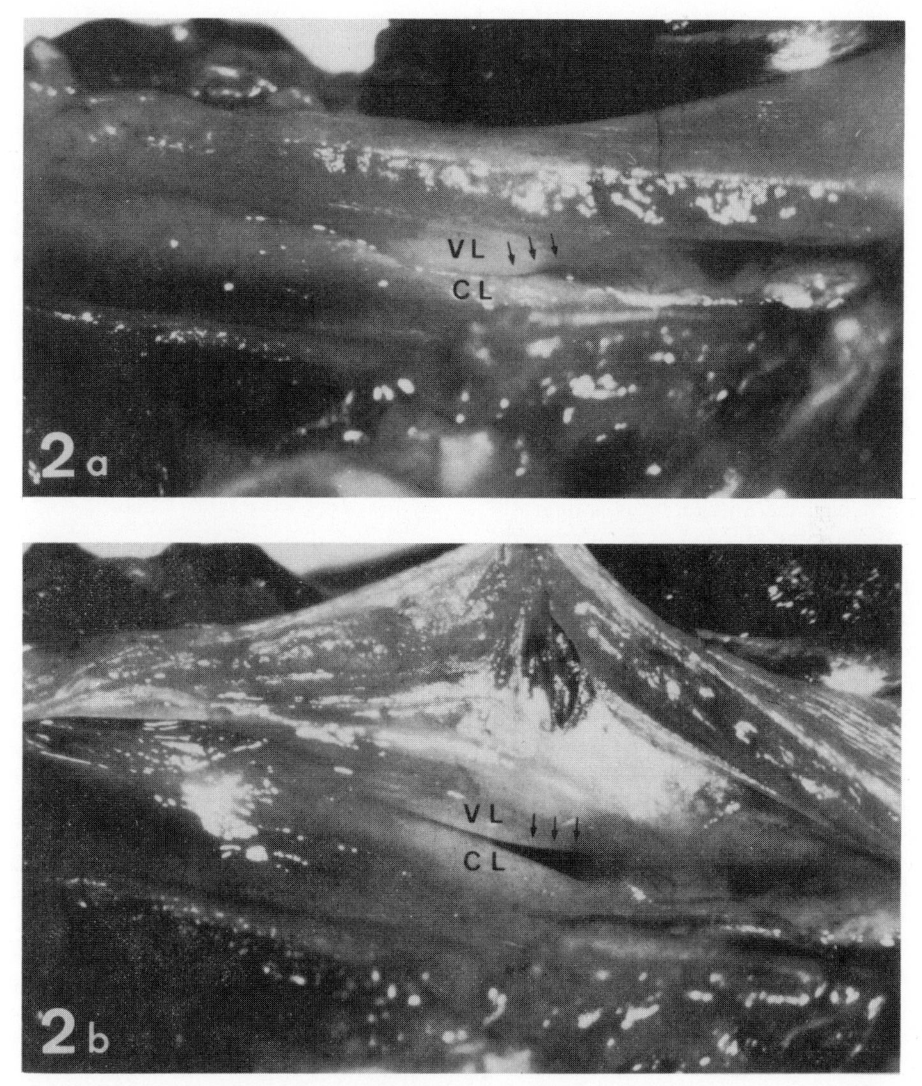

Figure 2 Otomicroscopic pictures of the right nasopharyngeal orifice (arrows), closed (a) and open (b). Ventral lip (VL) covering the pterygoid hamulus and the LVPM and TVPM. Cranial lip (CL) containing the SPM. Opening and closure of the eustachian tube can be controlled by the ventral and cranial lips. (X10 magnification)

The effusion was first evident in the attic concomitant with a discoloring of the medially indrawn pars flaccida. This tympanic membrane part exhibited dilated vessels and formed a retraction pocket. After six days the middle ear cavity was completely filled with effusion and this material was no longer serous but had become flocculent. The pars flaccida was still maximally retracted.

Group Five

Obstruction of the nostrils did not cause effusion to develop in the middle ear cavities.

Group Six

The muscles related to the eustachian tube—the tensor tympani muscle (TTM), the tensor veli palatini muscle (TVPM), the levator veli palatini muscle (LVPM), and the salpingopharyngeus muscle (SPM)—are described in detail in a previous paper.[4] The nasopharyngeal opening makes a slitlike naso-occipital groove on the lateral wall of the nasopharynx. In the ventral fold of the opening the pterygoid hamulus forms a prominence covered by muscle fibers belonging to the TVPM and LVPM and mucosa. The cranial fold of the orifice has no bony prominence but the mucosa covers fibers belonging to the SPM. When the TVPM and LVPM fibers are stretched, a flattening of the ventral prominence occurs, followed by a moderate dilatation of the orifice. A contraction of fibers belonging to the SPM causes an elongated widening of the orifice.

DISCUSSION

In the rat it seems that the most important part of the eustachian tube for ventilation of the middle ear is the nasopharyngeal portion. Thus, the tympanal orifice could be diminished by about 80 percent without eliciting any signs of effusion. Under conditions in which the middle ear is sufficiently ventilated, the draining function of the tube seems to be quite minimal, as a plastic tubing placed in the eustachian tube—allowing air but not effusion material to pass—caused no stasis of effusion around the tympanal orifice. The middle ear mucosa itself seems to have the capacity to resorb desquamated cells and debris from the middle ear mucosa.

Splitting the soft palate, interfering with the TVPM and LVPM but apparently not with the SPM, caused production of effusion in all cases. A normally functioning TVPM and LVPM thus seem to be absolute prerequisites for a normally functioning eustachian tube. One can assume that any condition interfering with the function of the TVPM and LVPM may interfere with the opening of the eustachian tube and with the ventilation of the middle ear cavity.

Although the tensor tympani muscle (TTM) and TVPM undoubtedly have common fibers and both originate from the scaphoid fossa, severing the tensor tympani tendon close to the malleus did not cause effusion in the middle ear. The tensor tympani muscle thus does not seem to take part in the opening mechanisms of the eustachian tube. This has recently been suggested by Honjo and colleagues, based on investigations of the TTM of the cat.[5]

A total blockage of the nostrils did not cause any effusion. Evidently mouth breathing may provide sufficient air to the nasopharyngeal opening and sufficient ventilation to the middle ear.

This study was supported by grant # B83-17X-06578-01 from the Swedish MRC and by a grant from the Medical Faculty, University of Umeå, Umeå, Sweden.

REFERENCES

1. Hellström S, Salén B, Stenfors L-E: The site of initial production and transport of effusion material in otitis media serosa. Acta Otolaryngol (Stockh) 93:543, 1982
2. Alm P, Bloom GD, Hellström S, Salén B, Stenfors L-E: The release of histamine from the pars flaccida mast cells—one cause of otitis media with effusion. Acta Otolaryngol (Stockh) 94:517, 1982
3. Stenfors L-E, Carlsöö B, Hellström S, et al: Structure of the pars flaccida after occlusion of the Eustachian tube or blockade of the tympanic isthmus. Int J Ped Otorhinolaryngol 4:251, 1982
4. Albiin N, Hellström S, Salén B, et al: The anatomy of the eustachian tube in the rat. Anat Rec, in press
5. Honjo I, Ushiro K, Haji T, et al Role of the tensor tympani muscle in Eustachian tube function. Acta Otolaryngol (Stockh) 95:329, 1983

IDENTIFICATION AND DIAGNOSIS

DETECTION OF MIDDLE EAR EFFUSION BY ACOUSTIC REFLECTOMETRY

DAVID W. TEELE, M.D., and JOHN TEELE, M.S.

Accurate detection of middle ear effusion (MEE) is necessary for proper diagnosis and management of both acute otitis media in the symptomatic child and persistent MEE in the asymptomatic child. Because these illnesses account for a large proportion of visits to the pediatrician,[1] much effort has been expended to document the accuracy of existing diagnostic methods. Pneumatic otoscopy is subjective and requires both skill and adequate visualization of the tympanic membrane. Even in experienced hands otoscopy is moderately inaccurate. Otoadmittance measurements require a seal in the ear canal, cooperation of the child, and a period of time to record the output. Finally, the intruments are cumbersome and costly. We recognized the need for a new diagnostic method that would meet the following criteria: safety, accuracy in children of all ages, speed in diagnosis, and freedom from pain. Furthermore, this method would ideally be unaffected by obstructing cerumen, crying, and the need for the child (including not requiring an air seal in the ear canal). One of the authors (JT) then designed and built the acoustic reflectometer to meet these needs.

MATERIALS AND METHODS

Operation of the acoustic reflectometer relies on the principle of partial cancellation of incident sound by sound reflected back from the tympanic membrane. Incident sound is propagated down the external auditory canal (EAC), and a portion of the sound is reflected back from all parts of the EAC, cerumen, and the tympanic membrane. The microphone records net sound pressure produced by both incident and reflected sound. Reflected sounds is variably out phase with the incident sound, resulting in partial decrease in sound pressure as measured by the microphone. A nadir in sound pressure, as measured at the microphone, occurs at a frequency for which the quarter wave length corresponds to the distance from the microphone to the tympanic membrane; at this frequency reflected sound is virtually 180 degrees out of phase with incident sound. At other frequencies reflected sound is partially in phase, resulting in sound pressure amplitudes greater than sound pressure amplitude with probe open to air. The sums of incident and reflected sound generated from 2000 to 5000 Hz are displayed on either the oscilloscope or the X-Y plotter.

The depth of the nadir, or the extent of cancellation of incident by reflected sound (in dB), is calculated as follows:

$$\mathrm{Log}_{10} \frac{\textit{sound pressure amplitude with open probe}}{\text{sound pressure amplitude with probe at external ear canal}} \times 20$$

Presence or absence of MEE was confirmed with two methods. First, we used pneumatic otoscopy employing a sealed diagnostic head. Second, we used measurements of acoustic-admittance (Grason-Stadler, Model 1720B Oto-Admittance Meter at 660 Hz and measuring susceptance).

RESULTS

Table 1 shows the distribution of ears for which the presence or absence of MEE was confirmed by pneumatic otoscopy and measurements of otoadmittance according to whether the reading from the acoustic reflectometer was above or below 4.0 dB. For these ears, with this break point,

TABLE 1 Distribution of Extent of Acoustic Cancellation from Ears with Confirmation of Diagnosis by Acoustic-Admittance Measurements

	Extent of Cancellation	
Diagnosis	*<4 dB*	*4+ dB*
Middle ear effusion	6	101
No middle ear effusion	145	38

Note: $p < 0.001$ by chi-square analysis.

the sensitivity of the acoustic reflectometer was 94.4 percent and the specificity was 79.2 percent.

DISCUSSION

The acoustic reflectometer was designed to detect MEE rapidly and accurately and to be unaffected by crying, cerumen, age, and the need for an air seal in the ear. The data noted here plus clinical experience with prototypes suggest that the technique achieves these goals. Since it employs sound of frequency and intensity that is similar to background noise anywhere but a quiet room, the device is clearly safe. The ability of the device to work properly without insertion into the EAC assures freedom from pain. Obstructing cerumen did not present a problem unless the canal was virtually totally obstructed. In such cases obstruction of the canal was readily apparent by inspection of the output of the device. While a small number of children would not be quiet long enough to record the output, this obstacle has been overcome by inserting circuitry to permit tone generation only in "windows" of silence and recording the results of a single swept-tone over 100 milliseconds. Thus, accurate readings may be obtained independent of both background noise and crying. While the original prototype was not portable, current prototypes are about the size of a large otoscope.

We believe that this technique now offers a valuable adjunct to diagnostic tools currently used to manage disease of the middle ear in children. By overcoming the deficiencies of acoustic admittance, the acoustic reflectometer will add considerably to the ability of both clinician and researcher to detect disease of the middle ear and to follow objectively changes occurring in their patients.

This study was supported in part by Biomedical Research support grant #RR05569-1 from the Biomedical Research Support Branch, National Institutes of Health.

REFERENCE

1. Teele DW, Klein JO, Rosner B, et al: Middle ear disease and the practice of pediatrics: Burden during the first five years. JAMA 249:1026–1029, 1983

ENDOSCOPIC OBSERVATION OF THE EUSTACHIAN TUBE IN OTITIS MEDIA WITH EFFUSION

IWAO HONJO, M.D., KOICHI USHIRO, M.D., and TOKICHIRO MITOMA, M.D.

Observation of the nasopharynx, such as the pharyngeal orifice of the eustachian tube, fossa of Rosenmüller, and adenoid, can be as important as that of the eardrum when treating patients for otitis media with effusion. However, observation of this area is rather difficult, especially in children, because it is located deep in the head.

Using a fine fiber endoscope, we observed the eustachian tube of many patients to determine the presence of characteristic findings in this area.

MATERIALS AND METHODS

Endoscopic observation of the nasopharynx was carried out on 101 patients with otitis media with effusion (OME) and on 46 normal children as controls. The patients with OME included 60 children, 23 adults, and 18 elderly men. Diagnosis of OME was based on ear complaint, otoscopic findings, and tympanograms.

The endoscope used in this study was either an unflexible needle endoscope with a diameter of 1.7 mm or a flexible one with a diameter of 2.7 mm or 3.5 mm. The flexible endoscope with a diameter of 3.5 mm was used for adult patients only. A flexible endoscope of 2.7 mm in diameter was used most frequently. The advantage of this instrument is that its diameter is very small and the angle of its tip is variable, and we were therefore able to observe the eustachian tube from any desirable direction. In some cases the endoscope can be inserted into the tube to see inside the tube. The condition of the pharyngeal orifice of the tube, fossa of Rosenmüller, and the size of the adenoid were observed at rest. Then, during swallowing, movement of the pharyngeal orifice was videorecorded.

RESULTS

In children, a marked hypertrophy of the adenoid tissue, which pressed the pharyngeal orifice of the tube, was frequently observed. Fig. 1 shows typical endoscopic findings in the tube. The adenoid presses the torus tubarius beyond the fossa of Rosenmüller anteriorly and laterally. Consequently, the tubal orifice was closed and did not open even during swallowing. About 83 percent of the 60 children with OME showed passive obstruction of the tube by hypertrophic adenoids.

However, a lateral roentgenogram showed a rather small adenoid that did not completely occupy the nasopharyngeal space. The discrepancy between the endoscopic finding and the roentgenographic one seems to be due to limited hypertrophy of the adenoid only in its upper or nasopharyngeal portion.

Table 1 shows the relationship between the roentgenographic and endoscopic findings of the adenoids. Among the patients who were judged by the endoscopic method to have a marked adenoid that closed the orifice, more than half were judged to have no hypertrophy by the roentgenographic method. Thus, an inconsistency between the endoscopic and the roentgenographic findings was noted.

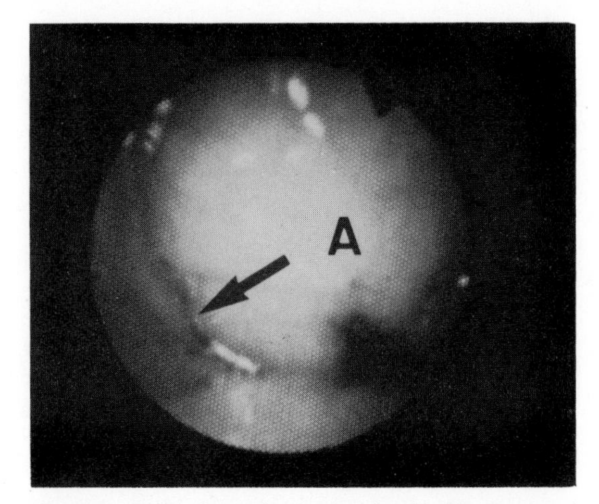

Figure 1 Tubal obstruction by the adenoid. The pharyngeal orifice of the tube (arrow) is closed by hypertrophic adenoid (A).

Table 2 summarizes the endoscopic findings of the children with OME. Forty-six normal children were examined as a control group. In about 83 percent of the patients, the adenoid caused obstruction of the tube, which was seen in only 20 percent of the control group. However, air inflation of the tube by a catheter was successful in 54 percent of the patients, indicating that passive ventilative ability is kept within the normal range in about a half of the patients.

The so-called tubal tonsil that closes the orifice was found to be relatively uncommon in children as compared with adenoid hypertrophy. Only five cases among 70 were judged to have tubal tonsil.

In adult patients edematous swelling around the tubal orifice was frequently noted especially at the posterior lip. Inside the tube the mucosa was anemic and edematous, closing the slitlike lumen of the tube. Therefore, the tube did not open during swallowing. Some adult patients had brownish discharge from the orifice. The fluid was judged to be excretion from the middle ear, because the aural discharge had the same color and viscosity.

TABLE 1 Relationship Between Roentgenographic and Endoscopic Findings

	Roentgenography	
Endoscopy	*Nonhypertrophic*	*Hypertrophic*
Open	9 (90%)	1 (10%)
Closed	26 (52%)	24 (48%)

TABLE 2 Endoscopic Findings in the Pharyngeal Orifice in Children With or Without OME

	Endoscopy	
	Open	*Closed*
OME	10 (17%)	50 (83%)
Normal	38 (80%)	8 (20%)

The aged patients, however, often showed abnormal patency of the tube with marked atrophy at the pharyngeal orifice and inside the tube. The tube of an aged person differs greatly from those of children and adults.

DISCUSSION

Dysfunction of the eustachian tube has been regarded as one of the important factors responsible for OME. However, a controversy has existed as to whether the adenoid has any influence on OME. Using a more direct means for observation, we investigated the relationship between them.

In children with OME current endoscopic techniques revealed frequent obstruction of the tube by adenoid tissue, even though they were judged to have no adenoid hypertrophy by other methods, such as roentgenography. It seems that obstruction of the tube by adenoid hypertrophy may be one of the predisposing conditions for OME.

Our research suggests that the influence of adenoids on tubal function or the effect of adenoidectomy on otitis media can be correctly evaluted on the basis of the endoscopic findings in relation to the tube.

Through endoscopic observation of adult or aged patients, it was found that the tube of an aged person differs greatly from that of children and adults, suggesting a different pathogenesis of OME in each age group.

PREVALENCE OF MIDDLE EAR DYSFUNCTION AND OTITIS MEDIA WITH EFFUSION IN ATOPIC CHILDREN

SUSAN G. MARSHALL, M.D., CLIFTON T. FURUKAWA, M.D., WILLIAM E. PIERSON, M.D., GAIL G. SHAPIRO, M.D., and C. WARREN BIERMAN, M.D.

Many etiologic factors are involved in ear disease in children. Allergy appears to be significant in the initiation of middle ear effusions in the pediatric population.

Appropriate diagnostic measures and environmental control will affect both long-term medical and surgical management and should have an impact on patients' hearing, speech, and language development.

The epidemiology of serous otitis media was recently studied by Kraemer and coworkers.[1] Seventy-six children with persistent middle ear effusions (PMEEs) referred for tympanostomy tube insertion were matched for age, sex, and date of admission with a control group of 76 children admitted for other elective surgery. Patients and controls were similar in all socioeconomic and demographic categories.

Nasal congestion occurred more often and was more persistent in children with PMEE. With more persistent catarrh, the risk of PMEE increased from threefold to fivefold.

Exposure to two or more household cigarette smokers increased the risk for PMEE nearly threefold. With household exposure to smoke of more than three packs of cigarettes per day, the risk increased fourfold.

Atopic disease was assessed by determining whether seasonal rhinitis (spring or summer sneezing, nasal itching, rhinorrhea, or nasal congestion), asthma (recurrent wheezing that improved with use of bronchodilators), and/or eczema (recurrent pruritic dermatitis that improved with topical steroid therapy) had been present during the preceding 12 months. Atopic disease occurred twice as often in children with PMEE. The risk for PMEE increased nearly fourfold in children with persistent atopic symptoms.

These factors were additive. Nasal congestion alone elevated the risk nearly fourfold. When exposure to cigarette smoke or atopy was added to nasal congestion, the risk was slightly higher than fourfold. Children with all three factors of nasal congestion, exposure to cigarette smoke, and atopy were more than six times as likely to manifest PMEE.

Since atopy appeared to be a major factor, we examined the prevalence of middle ear disease in children with documented atopic diseases.

Four hundred eighty-eight children referred for allergy evaluation were studied sequentially. The diagnostic work-up involved two phases: (1) allergic evaluation, including history, physical examination and laboratory data; and (2) otologic evaluation, including history, physical examination, and laboratory data.

A detailed history, including thorough environmental history, helped identify allergic or irritant factors in the home, school, or work environment.

Physical examination included attention to mouth breathing, facial configuration and speech abnormalities, careful examination of the nares, and special attention to proper otoscopic examination.

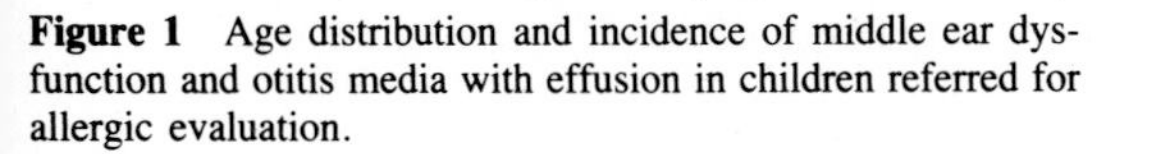

Figure 1 Age distribution and incidence of middle ear dysfunction and otitis media with effusion in children referred for allergic evaluation.

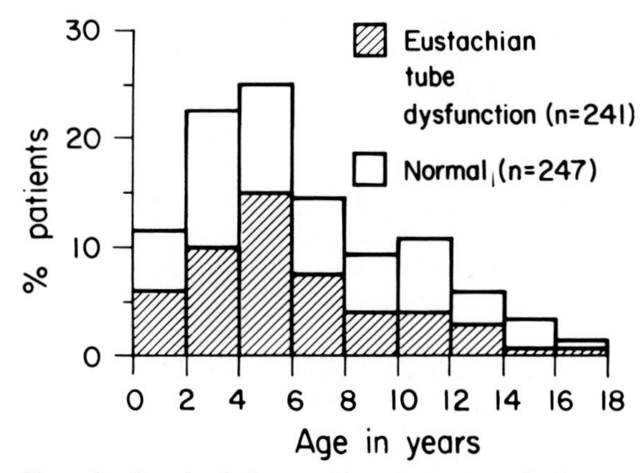

Figure 2 Cross-hatched areas represent percentage of patients in given age group referred for allergic evaluation with middle ear dysfunction.

Laboratory data included ear tests (impedance audiometry, tympanometry, and pure-tone audiometry) and allergy tests (cytologic examination of nasal secretions, quantitative analysis of serum immunoglobulins, and allergy skin tests or RAST tests). Allergic diagnoses included allergic rhinitis diagnosed in 464 (95 percent) of patients; atopic dermatitis, diagnosed in 78 (16 percent) of patients; and asthma, diagnosed in 278 (57 percent) of patients. Otologic diagnoses included (1) abnormal middle ear function by tympanometry, diagnosed in 241 (49 percent) of patients; (2) conductive hearing loss (defined as failure to respond to one or more tones of 20 Hz intensity), diagnosed in 132 (27 percent) of patients; and (3) evidence of OME (type B tympanogram with conductive hearing loss), diagnosed in 98 (20 percent) of patients.

Most children with middle ear dysfunction and otitis media with effusion were between 2 and 8 years of age, with a peak incidence between 4 and 6 years (Fig. 1). This reflects the distribution noted in the literature.

However, if one corrected for the ages of patients referred for allergic evaluation, all age groups appeared to be at substantial risk for middle ear disease (Fig. 2).

We conclude that middle ear dysfunction and otitis media with effusion are common in patients with respiratory allergy and that the risk of middle ear problems in pediatric patients with allergic disease is high at all ages.

REFERENCE

1. Kraemer MJ, Richardson MA, Weiss NS, et al. Risk factors for persistent middle-ear effusions. JAMA 249(8):1022, 1983

THE EFFICACY OF SCHOOL SCREENING FOR OTITIS MEDIA

CHRISTINE A. WACHTENDORF, M.D., LINDA L. LOPEZ, B.S.N., R.N., J. C. COOPER, Jr., Ph.D., ERWIN M. HEARNE, Ph.D., and GEORGE A. GATES, M.D.

The appropriateness of mass hearing screening to detect middle ear effusion (MEE), a major cause of hearing loss in preschool-age children, is controversial.[1,2] Some argue that, because of the lack of information about the natural history and sequelae of untreated middle ear effusion, the lack of acceptable criteria for the diagnosis of MEE, and continuing controversy over treatment methods, mass screening of children should not be recommended until more research is done. Others have shown that 16 to 20 percent of the children who have type B tympanograms indicative of MEE retain this type of tympanogram for three to 12 months.[3-5] Screening programs have been designed primarily to identify these children with persistent MEE, who are probably at higher risk for auditory complications and associated developmental abnormalities.

Controversy also exists over which screening techniques best detect middle ear disease. These techniques include tympanometry, acoustic reflex, pure-tone audiometry and pneumotoscopy, both singly and in combination.[1-14] Specific criteria for referral of children with abnormal screening results have not been universally established, although multiple schemata have been proposed.[1,2,7,13,15,16]

All investigators agree that more data are necessary to determine which screening techniques are most effective and which referral criteria should be used. Until results of such studies are available, it seems advisable to evaluate the mass screening programs currently in use and attempt to guide their efforts toward more productive screenings, that is, to identify and eliminate areas of over-referral.

We present the screening methods and referral patterns of six hearing screening programs established independently in a large metropolitan area and identify the techniques that resulted in the greatest number of over-referrals. This evaluation is from the point of view of the recipient of the referrals and in this regard representative of the role of the private physician. As in most mass screening programs, several weeks elapsed between the screening examination and the diagnostic examination by the physician.

MATERIALS AND METHODS

San Antonio, Texas, a metropolis of over a million people, is served by 13 independent school districts. Five of these districts plus one private hearing screening program were chosen for evaluation based on the screening methods employed, the socioeconomic groups served, and the number of patients referred to the Otitis Media Study Center (OMSC). Table 1 outlines the screening methods and referral patterns of these six programs. The four programs utilizing tympanometry in their screening methods classified tympanograms as A, B, or C using the criteria described by Jerger.[17] A− indicated type A tympanogram with absent acoustic reflex. Type C tympanograms were subdivided into types C_1, those with peak pressure between -100 and -200 mm H_2O; and C_2, those with peak pressure ≤ -200 mm H_2O.

The evaluating agency is the NIH-funded Otitis Media Study Center staffed by certified audiologists and otoscopists trained and validated in pneumotoscopy. The otoscopists' ability to detect fluid by pneumotoscopy as confirmed by myringotomy was excellent with a sensitivity ranging between 95 and 99 percent and a specificity between 80 and 85 percent.

The Madsen Electro-acoustic Impedance Bridge ZO-73 with automatic plotter was used to obtain all tympanograms. Tympanograms were classified into 15 variants by the method described by Cantekin and associates.[13] The impedance bridge was validated against myringotomy findings. Ipsilateral acoustic reflex thresholds were ob-

TABLE 1 Methods and Referral Patterns of Six Screening Programs

Program	Screening Method	Disposition A	Disposition B	Disposition C
1	Tympanometry and pure-tone audiometry for Cs	0	Refer	Refer if audiogram abnormal (PTA ≥ 30 dB)
2	Tympanometry and pure-tone audiometry for A − s	Recheck at 4 wks, refer if still A − and audio abnormal (2 frequencies ≥ 25 dB)	Refer	Recheck at 4 wks, refer if peak pressure ≤ −250 mm H_2O
3	Tympanometry and otoscopy	Recheck, refer if still A −	Refer	Recheck at 6 wks, refer if still C and otoscopy abnormal
4	Tympanometry	Recheck, refer if still A −	Refer	Recheck at 2 wks, refer if still C
5	Pure-tone audiometry	Refer all with 2 frequencies ≥ 30 dB		
6	Otoscopy	Refer all otoscopic abnormalities		

tained at 1000 Hz between 80 and 115 dB SPL. Reflexes obtained at levels ≥ 100 dB were considered abnormal.

Each child was evaluated by pneumotoscopy and tympanometry. An algorithm, modified from that described by Cantekin and colleagues,[13] was formulated using pneumotoscopic results and tympanometric variants to determine the presence of middle ear disease.

Pure-tone audiometry was performed using a Grason Stadler 1705 audiometer to rule out a sensorineural hearing loss in the few cases of absent reflex and normal tympanogram. Hearing levels > 20 dB at any two frequencies were considered abnormal.

RESULTS

Among the 483 children studied, 227 (39 percent) had no evidence of disease at OMSC examination and 356 (61 percent) were appropriate referrals.

Impedance data from all six programs were analyzed by ear across the tympanogram types B, C_1, C_2, and A − and were compared with the OMSC findings (Table 2). The abnormal ears were further divided into three categories: (1) those with evidence of MEE, (2) those with no evidence of middle ear effusion but with peak pressure ≥ −200 mm H_2O, and (3) those with wax impaction.

One hundred thirteen ears were found to have type A tympanograms and absent acoustic reflex (−AR) at school screening (SS) examination. Ninety-five (84 percent) of these ears had type A tympanograms and +AR at OMSC examination. Five (4 percent) had A tympanograms, −AR, but normal pure-tone audiometry, yielding a total of 100 normal ears (88 percent) at OMSC examination. Median time between SS examination and OMSC examination was four weeks.

Eighty-four ears (59 percent) that were C_1 at SS examination were normal at OMSC examination and 48 (34 percent) had evidence of MEE. Of these 48 ears with effusion 47 (98 percent) had

TABLE 2 Appropriate and Inappropriate Referrals by Ear

Findings at OMSC Examination	Tympanogram Type at SS Examination: Type B N %	Type C_1 N %	Type C_2 N %	Type A − N %
Normal	95 (29)	84 (59)	142 (48)	100 (88)
Retracted without fluid	17 (5)	10 (7)	37 (12)	3 (3)
Middle ear disease	191 (59)	38 (26)	101 (34)	7 (6)
Cerumen impaction	22 (7)	11 (8)	17 (6)	3 (3)
Total no. of ears	325	143	297	113
Median time between examinations (weeks)	3	4	3	4

TABLE 3 Appropriate and Inappropriate Referrals by Screening Method

Findings at OMSC Examination	*Program 1* *N %*	*Program 2* *N %*	*Program 3* *N %*	*Program 4* *N %*	*Program 5* *N %*	*Program 6* *N %*
Normal	0 (0)	18 (26)	17 (35)	153 (44)	10 (31)	29 (47)
Retracted without fluid	2 (10)	6 (9)	7 (15)	24 (7)	2 (6)	2 (3)
Middle ear disease	16 (80)	43 (62)	23 (48)	149 (42)	19 (60)	30 (48)
Cerumen impaction	2 (10)	2 (3)	1 (2)	26 (7)	1 (3)	1 (2)
Total no. of children	20	69	48	352	32	62

converted from C_1 to C_2 or B at OMSC examination. Median time between SS examination and OMSC examination was three weeks.

One hundred forty-two ears (48 percent) that were C_2 at SS examination were normal at OMSC examination and 138 (46 percent) had evidence of MEE. Of these 138 with fluid, 55 (40 percent) had converted from C_2 to B at OMSC examination. Median time between SS examination and OMSC examination was three weeks.

Using the normal approximation to the binomial (Z test), the proportion of ears with C_1 tympanograms at SS examination and disease at OMSC examination (0.41) was compared with the proportion of ears with C_2 tympanograms at SS examination and disease at OMSC examination (0.52). The proportions are different at $p = 0.02$. (Significance is defined as $p \leq 0.05$.)

Table 3 outlines the percentages of children from the six screening programs who were found to have normal ears, retracted tympanic membranes without fluid, middle ear disease, and wax impaction. Program 1 made no inappropriate referrals. False-positive results (normal ear) for each program are shown in Table 3, the highest being in programs 6 and 4 and the lowest being in program 2.

Omitting program 1, which had the lowest rate of referral of normal patients, the percentages of normal and abnormal children were compared across the five remaining screening methods, 2 through 6. Using the global chi-square test, the percentages across methods are significantly different at $p \leq 0.05$.

DISCUSSION

Two important issues concerning hearing screening are addressed by this study. First is the use of the acoustic reflex as an indicator of middle ear disease. Cantekin and associates[13] and Renvall and Lidén[7] found the acoustic reflex to have low specificity. Similarly, our study shows a high rate of false-positive results, that is, 88 percent of the ears with normal tympanograms and absent acoustic reflex had no evidence of middle ear disease. The children in this program should have been screened further with pure-tone audiometry, which, being normal, would have precluded referral.

The second issue concerns the referral of type C tympanograms. Of the proposals for the disposition of children with type C tympanograms, three are supported by our results. First, Beery and colleagues[14] and Renvall and Lidén[7] suggest rescreening all children with type C tympanograms whose peak pressure is ≤ -150 mm H_2O. In our present study, referral of 226 normal children would have been prevented if children with C_1 and C_2 tympanograms had been rescreened at a reasonable interval, for example, six weeks. Second, Renvall and Lidén[7] and Northern[8] suggest subdividing type C tympanograms into two categories based on the degree of negative pressure and referring only the children with severely retracted tympanic membranes. In the present study 41 percent of the ears that had C_1 tympanograms at SS examination had evidence of disease at OMSC examination. However, 98 percent of the ears that had C_1 at SS examination and effusion at OMSC examination had converted at OMSC examination to C_2 or B. Fifty-two percent of the ears that had C_2 tympanograms at SS examination were abnormal at OMSC examination, significantly different from C_1 with $p = 0.02$. In addition, only 40 percent of these with fluid at OMSC examination had converted from C_2 to B. Screening program 2, which had the most acceptable proportions of accurate referrals (74 percent) and false-positive referrals (26 percent), incorporated both these aspects into their program, that is, the rescreening of children with type C tympanograms and the referral of children with C_2 but not C_1 tympanograms. Third, Northern,[8] Paradise and Smith,[1] and Renvall and Lidén[7] suggest using pure-tone audiometry to determine which children with C tympanograms with high negative peak pressure have a concomitant hearing loss. Only those with abnormal audiograms would be referred. Of the 32 children in program 5 who had been tested by pure-tone audiometry only 31 percent were normal at OMSC examination, a much lower proportion of false-positive results than seen in the C_1 (59 percent) and C_2 (48 percent) groups. By referring only children with C_2 tympanograms and abnormal pure-tone audiometry a significant decrease in the rate of false-positive referrals could be anticipated.

In reviewing the results of the screening methods it is seen that program 1 had the lowest rate of over-referrals, with no false-positive referrals. This program incorporated two of the methods found to be useful in decreasing over-referrals, namely, not referring children with type A tympanograms with −AR and referring only children with type C tympanograms who also failed pure-tone audiometry. However, if the sensitivity and specificity of this method could have been checked, it would probably have had an unacceptably low sensitivity, that is, a high level of false-negative results. Children with mild disease or early disease would not have been identified. A provision for rescreening children with C_1 and C_2 tympanograms should be made.

Program 2 had the most acceptable level of over-referrals (26 percent). This method incorporates the rescreening of ears with C_1 and C_2 tympanograms at four weeks, the referral of C_2 tympanograms only, and the performance of pure-tone audiometry on type A tympanograms with −AR. This method is similar to that suggested by Renvall and Lidén,[7] who had a 19 percent over-referral rate. In addition, Renvall and Lidén's method utilizes pure-tone audiometry for children with C_2 tympanograms and refers only pure-tone failures.

Programs 3 and 4 had 35 percent and 44 percent over-referrals, respectively. Both groups rescreened C tympanograms but referred all children with C_1 and C_2 on rescreening. Pure-tone audiometry was not used to assess ears with C_2 tympanograms, nor was it used for A tympanograms with −AR to identify real sensorineural losses. Program 3 used pneumotoscopy in addition to tympanometry, but this method did not improve the results significantly.

Program 5 with 31 percent over-referrals used only pure-tone audiometry. The problems inherent in mass screening by pure-tone audiometry are outlined by McCurdy and associates[12] and Bluestone and associates.[10] However, this method, used in conjunction with tympanometry in selected cases, will decrease the number of over-referrals.

Program 6, using only otoscopy as the screening technique, had the highest rate of over-referrals (47 percent), again demonstrating the difficulty in detecting middle ear disease by otoscopy alone.

In conclusion, the drawback of mass screening of children for ear disease, using the currently accepted method of impedance audiometry, is the unacceptably high rate of referrals of children with minimal or no disease. To decrease the rate of over-referrals we recommend the following: First, do not refer children on the basis of absent acoustic reflex alone. Confirm a suspected hearing loss with an audiogram. Second, rescreen all type C tympanograms at six weeks and refer only children with C_2 tympanograms whose audiograms are also abnormal. It is agreed that more research is necessary to validate these test batteries and to determine the most reliable indicators of normal and abnormal states. However, until better guidelines are available, those who initiate mass screening programs must take the responsibility of identifying real disease states rather than placing that burden on the physician and causing a financial burden for the parents. Investigators in the field of middle ear disease could assist in decreasing the number of over-referrals by evaluating the existing screening programs in their communities and by helping these programs keep abreast of the newest findings in the area of mass hearing screening.

This study was supported by NINCDS/NIH contract NS-NO-1-02328 and a grant in kind from Ross Laboratories.

REFERENCES

1. Paradise JL, Smith CG: Impedance screening for preschool children—state of the art. Ann Otol Rhinol Laryngol 88:56, 1979
2. Bess FH, Bluestone, Harrington DA, et al: Use of acoustic impedance measurement in screening for middle ear disease in children. Ann Otol Rhinol Laryngol 87:288, 1978
3. Tos M, Poulsen G: Screening tympanometry in infants and two-year-old children. Ann Otol Rhinol Laryngol 68:217, 1980
4. Fiellau-Nikolajsen M: Tympanometry in three-year-old children—prevalence and spontaneous course of MEE. Ann Otol Rhinol Laryngol Suppl 68:233, 1980
5. Brooks DN: School screening for middle ear effusions. Ann Otol Rhinol Laryngol 25:223, 1976

6. Freyss GE, Manach Y, Narcy PP: Acoustic reflex as a predictor of middle ear effusion. Ann Otol Rhinol Laryngol Suppl 68:196, 1980
7. Renvall U, Lidén G: Screening procedure for detection of middle ear and cochlear disease. Ann Otol Rhinol Laryngol Suppl 68:214, 1980
8. Northern JL: Impedance screening—an integral part of hearing screening. Ann Otol Rhinol Laryngol Suppl 68:233, 1980
9. Brooks DN: Auditory screening—time for reappraisal. Public Health 91:282, 1977
10. Bluestone CD, Beery QC, Paradise JL: Audiometry and tympanometry in relation to middle ear effusions in children. Laryngoscope 83:594, 1973
11. Orchik DJ, Morff R, Dunn JW: Impedance audiometry in serous otitis media. Arch Otol 104:409, 1978
12. McCurdy JA, Goldstein JL, Gorski D: Auditory screening of preschool children with impedance audiometry—a comparison with pure tone audiometry. Clin Pediatr 15:436, 1976
13. Cantekin EI, Bluestone CD, Fria TJ: Identification of otitis media with effusion in children. Ann Otol Rhinol Laryngol Suppl 68:190, 1980
14. Beery QC, Bluestone CD, Cantekin EI: Otologic history, audiometry and tympanometry as a case finding procedure for school screening. Laryngoscope 85:1976, 1975
15. American Speech and Hearing Association: Guidelines for acoustic immittance screening of middle-ear function. ASHA 283, 1978
16. McKenzie E, Magian V, Stokes R: A study of the recommended pass/fail criteria for impedance audiometry in a school screening program. J Otolaryngol 11:1,40, 1982
17. Jerger J: Clinical experience with impedance audiometry. Arch Otolaryngol 92:311, 1970

IMPEDANCE MEASUREMENTS IN THE DIAGNOSIS OF OTITIS MEDIA WITH EFFUSION

HAROLD PETER FERRER, M.D., F.F.C.M., D.P.H.

An integrated hearing conservation program for children must consider the routine use of impedance tympanometry. Following an extensive research project in the Worcester and Malvern districts, a program has been devised that takes into account the current practices in impedance measurements. The previous pilot study had indicated that the correlation between the results of sweep testing and impedance measurement was poor.[1]

The research project was conducted with the same cohort of children as in the previous study.[1] Approximately 1100 children were involved and they were followed through in three phases: phase 1, before school entrance; phase 2, at school entrance; and phase 3, about 12 months after school entrance.

The Worcester and District Health Authority has a well-integrated program, for the screening, diagnosis, and further treatment, including education assessment and development, of children with impaired hearing. The service has been described by various visitors and by the Department of Health as one of the best in the United Kingdom. It is jointly managed by the Education and Health departments and screens infants and young children from the age of 8 months throughout school life. Apart from taking diagnostic measurement, the service can develop programs for treatment of and remedial assistance for children with hearing problems. The question arose as to how current practices in tympanometry could be integrated into such a program, and the research project described above was started with a grant from the Regional Health Authority. The possibility of a large number of false-positive results that could not be followed through in the hospital made a staged program essential at each phase of the research. Stages were as follows: stage 1, all children screened using tympanometry; stage 2, positive results from stage 1 rescreened; stage 3, positive results from stage 2 referred for assessment by audiometrician and clinical medical officer. A decision as to whether referral to the outpatient department was necessary was made.

The guidelines for the program were discussed in some detail elsewhere,[2,3] and although it was decided that there are useful guidelines regarding the negative middle ear pressure and the gradient, in practice and with training the audiometrician began to recognize tympanograms that should be referred for further testing. A provisional cutoff point of −150 mm H_2O and compliance on the AP62 of less than 1.5 was set.

RESULTS

At the preschool screening (Table 1), eleven cases were referred to the hospital outpatient department. Nine cases were operated on and found to have otitis media with effusion (OME). Grommets were inserted.

At this phase the auditory reflex was also screened for and a correlation sought between the results of tympanometry and the presence or absence of auditory reflexes at thresholds of 95, 100, and 110 dB. The frequencies used were 500 Hz and 2000 Hz. All the patients with abnormal tympanograms and OME at operation passed the auditory reflex testing at 500 Hz, but all failed at 2000 Hz. Both frequencies were retained for the additional phases of the program but it was found that the correlation between auditory reflex testing at 2000 Hz was over 95 percent, whereas the 500-Hz auditory reflex carried less than 10 percent correlation. Six of the cases operated on with OME had type C tympanograms.

At phase 2 testing, 15 cases were referred to the outpatient department following stage 3 (Table 2). Ten cases were operated on and found to have gross OME. A review of the phase 1 test of the ten cases operated on was then undertaken to see if these were new cases or cases that had been missed at phase 1. Seven of the ten patients with OME at phase 2 were found to have had clear evidence of OME at phase 1, and the question was then asked, "Why had the system failed at phase 1?" It was found that all seven cases had been referred to stage 3, that is, referral to the clinical medical officer and audiometrician, but a decision had been made by this group not to refer for further treatment. A discussion revealed that these clinicians considered that the OME would resolve. Eight months later it had not; or possibly it had recurred.

TABLE 1 Phase 1: Preschool Screening

	Failed	*Passed*
	No. (%)	*No. (%)*
Stage 1	224 (20.4)	876 (79.6)
Stage 2	31 (2.8)	193 (14.7)

At Stage 3 11 cases referred for E.N.T. opinion.
Note: Test was attempted on 1156 children, of whom 56 were unable to cooperate.

TABLE 2 Phase 2: School Test

	Failed	*Passed*
	No. (%)	*No. (%)*
Stage 1	135 (11.9)	999 (88.1)
Stage 2	16 (1.4)	119 (10.5)

At Stage 3 15 cases referred for E.N.T. opinion.
Note: 1134 children were tested.

One of the cases of OME found at this stage had an early cholesteatoma, the only one found throughout the series. If this represents a true prevalence rate, that is, one cholesteatoma per 1000 children, this would make such a program worthwhile from clinical and cost benefit points of view.

At phase 3 testing, ten cases were referred to the outpatient department following stage 2 (Table 3). Five were subsequently operated on, and OME was found in all cases. Review was then undertaken as described above and it was found that two cases were referred to stage 3 in phase 1 of the program, but the decision not to refer again was taken at the clinical assessment stage.

DISCUSSION

These results indicate that of the 25 cases found to have OME at operation, nine were passed through phase 1 and persisted into phases 2 and 3 of the test series, so in fact 18 cases were already present at preschool screening, and of these nine did not resolve during the subsequent 18 months. This result, inadvertently obtained, showed that

TABLE 3 Phase 3: School Test (Twelve Months after School Entrance)

	Failed	*Passed*
	No. (%)	*No. (%)*
Stage 1	112 (12.1)	810 (87.9)
Stage 2*	23 (2.5)	86 (9.3)

At Stage 3 10 cases referred for E.N.T. opinion.
Note: 922 children were tested.
*Three grommets (0.33%) were present.

the majority of cases were present at the preschool phase and the condition was likely to persist for the next two to three years.

The importance of this finding in the administration of a routine hearing conservation program cannot be overestimated. What is believed to be the first integrated program for both sweep testing and impedance screening using Grason-Stadler equipment is now underway in the Worcester and District Health Authority. The practical implications of this program are that staging will be retained but, owing to the difficulties of contacting a preschool population, the first opportunity of administering this test at present will be at school entrance. It may be possible in the near future, however, to reconsider and include staging at a preschool phase.

REFERENCES

1. Ferrer HP: Use of impedance audiometry in schoolchildren. Public Health 88:153, 1974
2. Møller A: An experimental study of the acoustic impedance of the middle ear and its transmission of the pressure in the auditory meatus. Acta Otolaryngol (Stockh) 60:129, 1965
3. Lildholdt J, Courtois B, Kortholm B et al: The correlation between negative middle ear pressure and the corresponding conductive hearing loss in children. Scand Audiol 8:117, 1979

PREVENTION AND MANAGEMENT

IMMUNIZATION AGAINST PNEUMOCOCCAL OTITIS MEDIA: STATE OF THE ART

JAMES C. HILL, Ph.D.

In 1974, the National Institute of Allergy and Infectious Diseases (NIAID) began trials of pneumococcal polysaccharide vaccine for the prevention of pneumococcal pneumonia in adults. The vaccine had been developed and tested for safety and antigenicity under an Institute-supported program that began in the late 1960s. Based on the availability of the vaccine and the results of studies by Howie[1] in the United States and Kamme[2] in Sweden indicating that 40 to 70 percent of acute cases of otitis media are due to pneumococci, the Institute decided to conduct efficacy trials of polyvalent pneumococcal polysaccharide vaccines for the prevention of pneumococcal otitis media.

Although project proposals were solicited in 1974, it was not until 1975 that the trials began. The delay resulted from the concern of the NIAID human studies committee that the benefit to be gained with these vaccines might not outweigh the risk. Although the vaccines had been shown to be safe in infants in studies by Amman and his coworkers,[3,4] they also demonstrated, using the indirect hemagglutination assay, that the antibody response of these infants was poor. There was also concern about the safety of the myringotomy procedure that was considered essential for confirmation of pneumococcal type-specific disease. After many meetings of NIAID advisors and the human studies committee, a decision was made to proceed with the trials. It was reasoned that lack of good serum antibody responses may not necessarily predict failure of the vaccine to protect. Stimulation of secretory antibody in the middle ear fluid might be induced by vaccination to a greater degree than serum antibody. The trials were modified so that only children considered to be at high risk of repeated episodes of otitis media by virtue of having already had one or more episode were vaccinated. The benefit-to-risk ratio was not considered sufficient for vaccination of healthy children. In addition, the human studies committee required the Institute to do further studies on the antibody responses of infants using the radioimmune assay and various dosage levels and vaccination regimens.

Following the initiation of NIAID-sponsored studies in 1975, two trials supported by Merck Sharp and Dohme were performed in Finland beginning in 1977. An additional study in Sweden was also carried out. I will describe the various trials briefly, give the results, and make some summary conclusions about the value of immunization with pneumococcal polysaccharides.

The Vanderbilt study[5,6] was designed to evaluate vaccine safety and antigenicity in infants. It was not designed as an efficacy trial; however, disease incidence was recorded. Two hundred children were given various vaccine doses at 6 months, 12 months or both. Both the Lilly 8-valent (containing types 1, 3, 6A, 7F, 14, 18C, 19F, and 23F polysaccharides) and the Merck 14-valent (types 1, 2, 3, 4, 6A, 7F, 8, 9N, 12F, 14, 18C, 19F, 23F, and 25) vaccines were used. It was learned that reactions to the vaccines are mild and brief. Only an antibody response to type 3 polysaccharide is seen at 6 months, while responses were observed at 12 months to types 3, 6, 7, 8, 14, 18, and 23. The levels obtained in almost all cases, however, were not considered protective (about 300 ng of antibody N/ml).[7] Vaccination had no effect on disease incidence or on nasopharyngeal carriage.

The Boston trial[8] was a double-blind efficacy trial in which 124 children, 5 through 21 months old, received either the Lilly octavalent vaccine containing polysaccharides of pneumococcal types implicated in otitis media or a control vaccine containing polysaccharides of seven types not responsible for otitis media (Lilly heptavalent vaccine, types 2, 4, 5, 8, 9N, 12F, and 25). In this trial, children must have had three episodes of otitis media before being enrolled and vaccinated.

The results demonstrated that there were fewer cases of type-specific acute otitis media (AOM) in the group receiving the octavalent vaccine than in the controls. There was no difference in the overall clinical experience with AOM. Antibody responses to the polysaccharides were poor; with most types they were below the estimated protective level.

In the trial at Huntsville Hospital in Alabama,[9] 179 children between the ages of 6 months and 21 months who had had one or more episodes of otitis media were given either the octavalent or the heptavalent vaccine. No significant protection was seen in children over 12 months of age, but the number of cases in this age range was very small. The investigators did report fewer episodes in vaccinees under age 12 months than in controls, but the difference was not statistically significant. There was an indication that fewer recipients of octavalent vaccine continued to have episodes (became "otitis prone") than did recipients of control vaccine. Immunization did appear to increase the level of antibody in middle ear effusion, perhaps to a level above that seen in serum.

The first trial in Finland[10,11] also had an enrollment criterion of one or more episodes of otitis media. Eight hundred twenty-seven children from 3 to 6 years of age received either Merck 14-valent vaccine or Merck *Hemophilus influenzae* type b polysaccharide vaccine. Vaccination of children 7 to 83 months old caused a 50 percent reduction of type-specific pneumococcal otitis media during the subsequent six months. If type 6A disease (the polysaccharide is nonimmunogenic) is eliminated from the calculations, the reduction figure becomes 67 percent. All AOM, however, was reduced by only about 10 to 15 percent. There was no protection in infants under 7 months of age, and even in the older children there was no protection for longer than six months after vaccination. This correlates with a drop in antibody level at about the same time.

In the second Finnish trial healthy, non-"otitis prone" infants 6 through 8 months of age were vaccinated. Data are available on 3332 children who received the first of two doses between 6 and 8 months and a second dose five months later. The Merck 14-valent vaccine was also used for this trial; however, saline was used as a control. Vaccination of these infants did not offer significant protection. There was only a slight reduction (3.4 percent) in the overall number of cases of AOM among vacinees compared with the placebo group.

A Swedish trial was conducted with 405 children from 6 months to 5 years of age. Healthy children in day care nurseries received either Merck 14-valent vaccine or a saline control. Vaccination reduced the episodes of AOM by 35 percent in children 2 years of age or older for the first year following vaccination, but the protection did not last through a second year of follow-up. No protection was provided children younger than 2 years of age.

Some general conclusions can be made from the results of these various trials.

The ability of infants to respond to pneumococcal polysaccharides with the production of serum antibody is very poor. This ability to respond improves with age and the improvement varies with the individual polysaccharides.

Once a child is capable of mounting a strong antibody response (attaining a level estimated at around 300 ng antibody N/ml) against a particular polysaccharide, protection against a pneumococcus of that type can occur.

Vaccination of children over 2 years of age offers approximately 50 percent protection against type-specific disease but only about 10 percent protection against overall incidence of otitis media. In this case, protection lasts only about six months to one year following vaccination.

Most children under 2 years of age, certainly those under 1 year of age, receive no protection from pneumococcal polysaccharide vaccines.

There may be some protection conferred by vaccination against repeated episodes—the "otitis-prone" condition—in older children.

Vaccination does appear to stimulate production of antibody in middle ear effusion (predominantly IgA), perhaps to levels slightly higher than in serum (predominantly IgG and IgM).

Effective and practical vaccination against pneumococcal otitis media will await development of vaccines that are more immunogenic in infants.

REFERENCES

1. Howie VM, et al: Otitis media: A clinical and bacteriological correlation. Pediatrics 45:29, 1970
2. Kamme C, et al: The etiology of acute otitis media in children. Scand J Infect Dis 2:217, 1971

3. Amman AJ: Clinical evaluation of octavalent pneumococcal polysaccharide vaccine and antibody response in infants and children. Final Report on Contract #NO1-AI-42518 from the National Institute of Allergy and Infectious Diseases, 1975
4. Cowan MJ, et al: Pneumococcal polysaccharide immunization in infants and children. Pediatrics 42:721, 1978.
5. Sell SH, et al: Clinical studies of pneumococcal vaccines in infants. I. Reactogenicity and immunogenicity of two polyvalent polysaccharide vaccines. Rev Infect Dis 3:S97, 1981
6. Wright PF, et al: Clinical studies of pneumococcal vaccines in infants. II. Efficacy and effect on nasopharyngeal carriage. Rev Infect Dis 3:S108, 1981
7. Landesman SH, Schiffman G: Assessment of the antibody response to pneumococcal vaccine in high-risk populations. Rev Infect Dis 3:S184, 1981
8. Teele DW, et al: Use of pneumococcal vaccine for prevention of recurrent acute otitis media in infants in Boston. Rev Infect Dis 3:S113, 1981
9. Sloyer JL, et al: Efficacy of pneumococcal polysaccharide vaccine in preventing acute otitis media in infants in Huntsville, Alabama. Rev Infect Dis 3:S119, 1981
10. Mäkelä PH, et al: Pneumococcal vaccine and otitis media. Lancet 2:548, 1980
11. Mäkelä PH, et al: A study of the pneumococcal vaccine in prevention of clinically acute attacks of recurrent otitis media. Rev Infect Dis 3:S124, 1981

RECURRENT PNEUMOCOCCAL OTITIS MEDIA: PRESENCE OF PNEUMOCOCCAL ANTIGEN AND ANTIBODY IN MIDDLE EAR EFFUSION COMPARED WITH ANTIBODY LEVELS IN SERUM

MARKKU KOSKELA, M.Sc., and JUKKA LUOTONEN, M.D.

Recurrent acute otitis media (AOM) is a common and recalcitrant problem in otolaryngology and pediatrics. However, why some children are otitis prone—that is, have many repeated attacks of AOM—is not understood. *Streptococcus pneumoniae* is the most common pathogen in AOM, verified both by bacteriologic culture[1,2] and by detection of pneumococcal capsular polysaccharide antigen[2,3] from the middle ear effusion (MEE). During an attack of pneumococcal AOM the pathogen-specific antibody levels increase,[4,5] but the responsiveness is highly dependent on the age of the child and on the serologic type/group of the pneumococcus causing the infection.[6] Pneumococcal antibodies have also been detected in the MEE of patients with AOM.[4,7] The presence of the homologous antibodies in the MEE is associated with both an accelerated rate of clinical clearing of otitis[8] and a reduced incidence of new attacks caused by the same pneumococcal type.[9] Serum antibodies can also be induced by parenteral vaccination with purified pneumococcal capsular polysaccharides.[7,10–13] Such vaccination could protect children from homologous attacks of pneumococcal AOM, but the effect lasts only for a short period of time.[12]

To gain further insight into the relationships between AOM and pneumococcal antibody levels in serum and MEE in frequently recurring otitis media, we have carefully followed up a number of such otitis-prone children clinically, bacteriologically, and serologically. Our data suggest that the immunologic defense against recurrent pneumococcal infection in the middle ear is a complicated process in which both specific pneumococcal antibodies derived from serum and those produced locally are involved. To illustrate these events we present our observations in several individual cases.

MATERIALS AND METHODS

Seven children were selected for this study from among 558 children included in a vaccination program and followed up at the pediatric and/or otolaryngologic outpatient departments of the University Central Hospital in Oulu, Finland, from

1977 to 1980.[14] The children were selected on the basis of the following criteria: They had received the 14-valent pneumococcal capsular polysaccharide vaccine at the beginning of the study; they had the greatest number of visits (≥10) to the clinic because of recurring middle ear infections; and they had acute pneumococcal otitis media, verified bacteriologically, at least once during the follow-up.

The follow-up started when the child was enrolled in the vaccination program. The child was considered to have an acute attack of otitis media when he had acute ear or upper respiratory tract symptoms and effusion could be aspirated from behind an intact tympanic membrane. An episode of recurrent AOM is defined as repeated attacks of otitis media with effusion for up to five months and secretory otitis media (SOM) with constant mucous effusion in the middle ear and without acute symptoms or signs. The children were treated for their ear problems according to the established practice of the departments. Thus, AOM was treated with tympanocentesis and penicillin V; if the disease was prolonged the treatment was amoxicillin and repeated tympanocenteses or, in more prolonged cases, adenotomy and/or tympanostomy.

Tympanocentesis was performed whenever effusion was suspected in the middle ear. The MEE thus aspirated was cultured aerobically,[2] and pneumococcal capsular polysaccharide antigens were looked for by countercurrent immunoelectrophoresis and latex agglutination methods as described by Leinonen,[3] with the exception that before the assays the MEE was kept for 3 minutes in boiling water to release pneumococcal polysaccharides from bacteria or from possible immune complexes.

Antibodies of IgG, IgM, and IgA classes to the serologic type/group of pneumococci isolated from the middle ear were measured from all the serum and MEE samples by enzyme-linked immunosorbent assay (ELISA), as described earlier.[6] The serum antibody levels were expressed as endpoint titers, but the presence or absence of antibodies in the MEE was determined only qualitatively.

RESULTS

The clinical, bacteriologic, and serologic findings in the seven children studied are presented in Figures 1 and 2.

Clinical Follow-Up

At the beginning of the follow-up four of the children were younger than 1 year of age (patients 1–3, 6), and only one of them had experienced otitis before (2 AOM in patient 3). The three other children (patients 4, 5 and 7) were about 2½ years old when enrolled in the program, and all of them had previous histories of several attacks of AOM.

During the follow-up the children experienced two to eight attacks of AOM. Three (patients 5–7) finally developed SOM, which persisted at the end of the study.

Bacterial Etiologic Factors in AOM

On the basis of bacteriologic cultures and/or detection of pneumococcal capsular polysaccharide antigens in the MEE, all of the pneumococcal attacks of AOM in the same child were found to be caused by the same serologic type/group of pneumococci. In five of the children this was group 6; in one child, group 18; and in one, group 23. In all, 18 of the 27 attacks of AOM from which MEE samples were available could be shown to be caused by pneumococci. *Hemophilus influenzae* was cultured alone or together with pneumococci from the MEE in three children (patients 3, 4, and 7) and *Staphylococcus aureus* in two others (patients 2 and 6).

Pneumococcal Antibodies in Serum and MEE

The acute attacks were often but not always followed by an increase in the homologous pneumococcal antibodies of the IgG and IgM classes in the serum, whereas IgA class responses were rare. The pneumococcal vaccine usually caused an increase of serum IgM antibodies, often in younger children, accompanied by a decrease of IgG (patients 1, 2, and 6).

Each episode of recurrent pneumococcal AOM showed a common pattern of MEE findings. At the time of the first attack the infecting pneumococci and the corresponding capsular polysaccharide antigen could usually be demonstrated in the MEE. Later the polysaccharides disappeared and homologous antibodies became detectable in the MEE. IgG and IgM class antibodies were, as a rule, found in the MEE when their levels in the serum were high, whereas homologous IgA class antibodies were often found in the MEE but not in the serum. Although these findings were common to most of the cases, interesting details are illustrated by each individual patient (Figs. 1, 2).

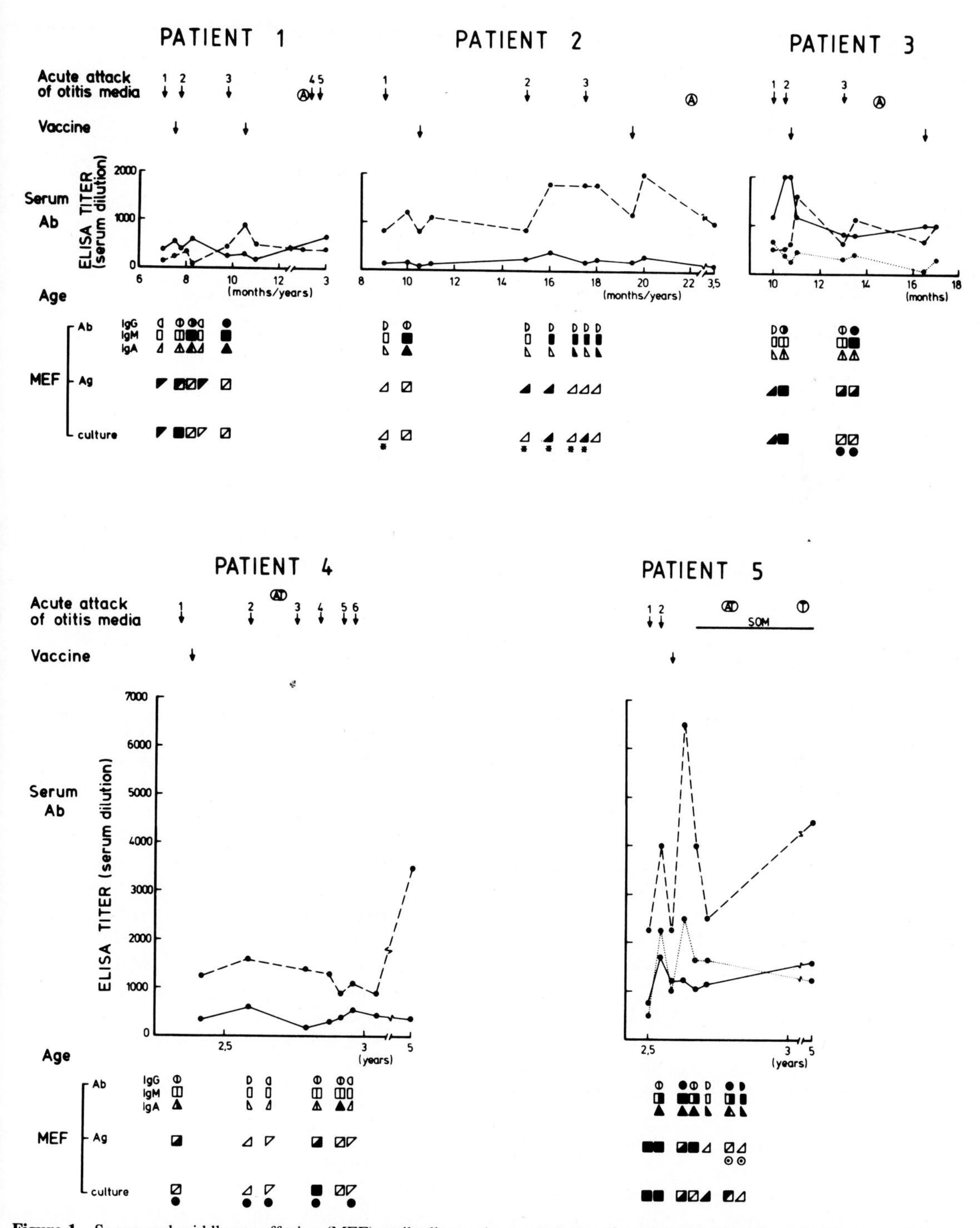

Figure 1 Serum and middle ear effusion (MEE) antibodies to the group 6 pneumococcal capsular polysaccharide in five children with recurrent acute otitis media caused by group 6 pneumococci. Secretory otitis media was diagnosed after two acute attacks of otitis media in patient 5. All of the children were vaccinated with 14-valent pneumococcal capsular polysaccharide vaccine.

Symbols for serum antibodies: solid line, IgG; broken line, IgM; dotted line, IgA class antibodies.

Symbols for MEF results: Findings in the right ear are shown left in the symbols and vice versa. Positive findings are indicated by solid symbols and negative findings by open symbols.

Other symbols: Ⓐ, adenotomy; Ⓣ, bilateral tympanostomy; ⊛, culture grew *Hemophilus influenzae*; *, culture grew *Staphylococcus aureus*; †, culture grew bacteria and/or yeast presumed to be contaminants; ⊙, group 19 pneumococcal capsular polysaccharide detectable.

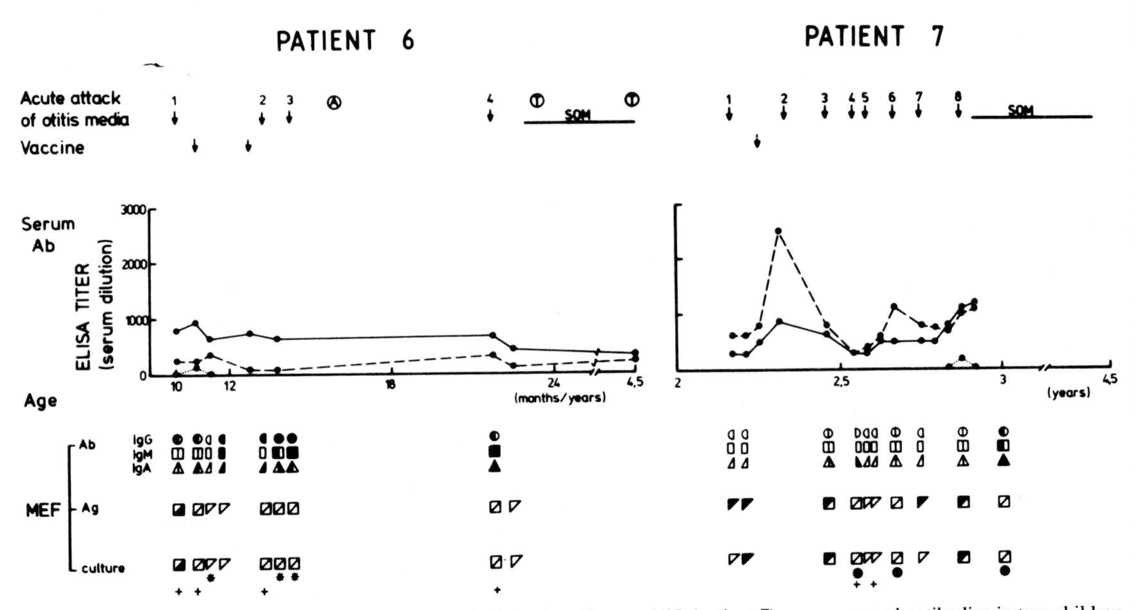

Figure 2 Serum and middle ear effusion (MEE) anti-18 (patient 6) or anti-23 (patient 7) pneumococcal antibodies in two children with recurrent acute otitis media caused by group 18 or 23 pneumococci, respectively. Secretory otitis media developed in both of the children. Symbols same as in Figure 1.

In the youngest child (patient 1) the initial, group 6, pneumococcal attack of AOM recurred once. Thereafter antibodies to the pathogen appeared in the MEE, and pneumococci as well as the polysaccharide antigens disappeared. During the third attack, the increase of the homologous IgM antibodies in the serum indicated a pneumococcal origin, although no pathogen could be found in the MEE. At the same time, the MEE contained antibodies of all three Ig classes to the homologous group 6 pneumococcal polysaccharide.

Patient 3 responded well to his first attack by IgG class serum antibodies. After vaccination, IgM class antibodies also appeared in the serum. IgG was detected in the MEE during his second attack. At the time of the third attack, only the pathogen-specific polysaccharide antigen could be found in the MEE, followed in a short time by the appearance of IgG and IgM. This child had IgA class antibodies in serum samples, but none in the MEEs.

The histories of patients 4 and 7 resembled each other. Both children experienced several attacks of AOM. Only IgA class antibodies were found in the MEE samples, although IgG and IgM class antibodies were present in the serum.

Patient 5 differed from the other children studied in that he responded very strongly by forming serum antibodies of all three Ig classes. Although the homologous antibodies were also frequently present in the MEEs, they could not prevent new infections caused by pneumococci. Two months later he was diagnosed as having SOM, which continued for at least three years.

Patient 6 had a spontaneous perforation in his right tympanic membrane when enrolled in the vaccine program. At the same time AOM caused by group 18 pneumococci was diagnosed in his left ear. Thereafter pneumococci or pneumococcal polysaccharide antigens were no longer detectable in the MEEs, which, however, continued to contain the homologous antitype 18 antibodies. A year later effusion was continuously present in his middle ear, a state resembling secretory otitis media. During the whole period his serum antitype 18 levels were low, without detectable specific IgA.

DISCUSSION

Six of the seven children suffered from recurrent pneumococcal AOM caused by pneumococci of groups 6 or 23, which are very poor immunogens in young children.[6,10,12] Repeated contacts with the pathogen seemed to have a booster effect in the development of antibodies in the youngest children with group 6 pneumococcal otitis (patients 1–3). In one child (patient 6), the pneumococcus was of group 18, which is usually a good immunogen. However, the anti-18 polysaccharide antibody levels in his serum remained relatively low, and he had a prolonged course of AOM, complicated by a spontaneous perforation of the tympanic membrane. Thus, a characteristic feature of these six children was a low level of serum antibodies to the infecting pneumococcus. Yet the responses of these children to the other pneumococcal types in the vaccine were comparable to the responses seen in other children during this project.

Each episode of pneumococcal AOM seemed to follow a general time course: First, the infecting bacteria and the corresponding polysaccharide antigen were present in the MEE. Next, homologous IgG and IgM class antibodies appeared in both the serum and the MEE. However, this did not necessarily result in the disappearance of the pathogen; this seemed especially marked for IgM, the antibody class most often produced as a response to the vaccine (see, for example, patient 2). Finally, IgA class antibodies appeared in the MEE, and both the bacteria and the antigen disappeared. Such IgA was most probably produced locally in the middle ear, because IgA was usually not detectable in the serum of these children. These findings agree with earlier reports of the clinical clearing of the middle ear fluid after AOM.[8] The local IgA class antibody response might also explain why there was no correlation between serum antibody levels and the healing of chinchillas after experimental type 6A otitis.[15]

Even though an IgA response in the middle ear was often accompanied by clearing of the infection, three children developed secretory otitis media at the time of persistent IgA in the MEE. An extreme example may be patient 5, who had a history of several episodes of AOM and developed SOM after an exceptionally strong serum and MEE antibody response to the pathogen.

As illustrated by these case reports, a systemic immune response to the infecting pneumococci does not alone prevent the recurrence or prolongation of otitis media. However, the data suggest that a pathogen-specific secretory IgA response in the middle ear may also be associated with prolongation of the infection and the possible development of secretory otitis media.

This study was supported in part by a grant from Merck Sharp and Dohme Research Laboratories, West Point, Pennsylvania. We thank Mrs. Tarja Kaijalainen and Miss Raili Liukko for their excellent assistance.

REFERENCES

1. Klein JO: The epidemiology of pneumococcal disease in infants and children. Rev Infect Dis 3:246, 1981
2. Luotonen J, Herva E, Karma P, et al: The bacteriology of acute otitis media in children with special reference to *Streptococcus pneumoniae* as studied by bacteriological and antigen detection methods. Scand J Infect Dis 13:177, 1981
3. Leinonen M: Detection of pneumococcal capsular polysaccharide antigens by latex agglutination, counterimmunoelectrophoresis and radioimmunoassay in middle ear exudates in acute otitis media. J Clin Microbiol 11:135, 1980
4. Sloyer JL Jr, Howie VM, Ploussard JH, et al: Immune response to acute otitis media in children. I. Serotypes isolated and serum and middle ear fluid antibody in pneumococcal otitis media. Infect Immun 9:1028, 1974
5. Branefors P, Dahlberg T, Nylén O: Study of antibody levels in children with purulent otitis media. Ann Otol Rhinol Laryngol 89(Suppl 68):117, 1980
6. Koskela M, Leinonen M. Luotonen J: Serum antibody response to pneumococcal otitis media. Pediatric Infect Dis 4:245, 1982
7. Sloyer JL Jr, Ploussard JH, Howie VM: Efficacy of pneumococcal polysaccharide vaccine for preventing acute otitis media in infants in Huntsville, Alabama. Rev Infect Dis 3 (Suppl):S119, 1981
8. Sloyer JL Jr, Howie VM, Ploussard JH, et al: Immune response to acute otitis media: Association between middle ear fluid antibody and the clearing of clinical infection. J Clin Microbiol 4:306, 1976
9. Howie VM: Natural history of otitis media. Ann Otol Rhinol Laryngol 84(Suppl 19):67, 1975
10. Borgóno JM, McLean AA, Vella PP, et al: Vaccination and revaccination with polyvalent pneumococcal polysaccharide vaccines in adults and infants. Proc Soc Exp Biol Med 157:148, 1978
11. Koskela M, Leinonen M: Comparison of ELISA and RIA for measurement of pneumococcal antibodies before and after vaccination with 14-valent pneumococcal capsular polysaccharide vaccine. J Clin Pathol 34:93, 1981
12. Mäkelä PH, Leinonen M, Pukander J, Karma P: A study of the pneumococcal vaccine in prevention of clinically acute attacks of recurrent otitis media. Rev Infect Dis 3(Suppl):S124, 1981
13. Teele DW, Klein JO, Greater Boston Collaborative Otitis Media Study Group: Use of pneumococcal vaccine for prevention of recurrent acute otitis media in infants in Boston. Rev Infect Dis 3(Suppl):S113, 1981
14. Karma P, Luotonen J, Timonen M, et al: Efficacy of pneumococcal vaccination against recurrent otitis media. Preliminary results of a field trial in Finland. Ann Otol Rhinol Laryngol. 89(Suppl 68):357, 1980
15. Marshak G, Cantekin EI, Doyle WJ, et al: Recurrent pneumococcal otitis media in the chinchilla. A longitudinal study. Arch Otolaryngol 107:532, 1981

PNEUMOCOCCAL VACCINATION AND OTITIS MEDIA IN INFANTS AND CHILDREN

PEKKA KARMA, M.D., JUHANI PUKANDER, M.D., MARKKU SIPILÄ, M.D., MATTI TIMONEN, M.D., SEPPO PÖNTYNEN, M.D., ELJA HERVA, M.D., PAUL GRÖNROOS, M.D., MAIJA LEINONEN, Ph.D., and HELENA MÄKELÄ, M.D.

The frequent occurrence[1] and the nature[2] of otitis media make it important to look for ways to prevent this disease. The established efficacy of polyvalent pneumococcal vaccines against pneumococcal pneumonia and bacteremia in adults[3–5] has suggested that acute otitis media (AOM), most commonly caused by pneumococci of types/groups present in the vaccines,[6,7] might be affected by the pneumococcal vaccine. However, the concentration of AOM in the youngest age groups,[1,2] in whom the immunogenicity of polysaccharides might be unsatisfactory,[8,9] and the location of the infection superficially in the mucous membranes make the situation different from systemic adult infections. Encouraged by the results of animal experiments[10] and a preliminary study in a small population of children,[11] investigators in the United States and Finland have carried out clinical field trials.[12] We summarize the results of the Finnish studies, which have been performed in two phases: 1977 to 1979[6,12,13] and 1979 to 1981, including a total of 4167 infants and children.

MATERIALS AND METHODS

As Table 1 shows, the age distribution of children was rather wide in study 1 (1977–1979), but in study 2 (1979–1981) all were younger than 1 year (95 percent were 7 to 9 months old). In study 1 all the children had recently experienced AOM and over 60 percent of them had had three or more earlier attacks of AOM. Only 20 percent of infants in study 2 had previously had AOM. In study 1 the children were given intramuscularly either the 14-valent (Danish types 1, 2, 3, 4, 6A, 7F, 8, 9N, 12F, 14, 18C, 19F, 23F, 25) pneumococcal (P) vaccine (25 μg of each capsular polysaccharide per 0.25 ml) or *Hemophilus* influenzae type b vaccine (5 μg capsular polysaccharide per 0.25 ml) as a control. In study 2 14-valent P vaccine was used and saline given as the control. In study 1 children younger than 2 years received two 0.25-ml doses two or six months apart; after the age of 2 they received only one 0.5-ml dose. In study 2 all the infants received a second 0.25-ml dose approximately five months later. In both studies the children were randomly allocated to the vaccination groups. Study 1 was single-blinded and study 2 double-blinded.

After vaccination the children were observed for up to two years by the same project doctors and clinics, to which the children were invited to return every time they had ear trouble. Myringotomy was always done when effusion in the middle ear was suspected. Clinical data were carefully recorded at each visit. Aspirated ear samples were analyzed by standard culture methods; all pneumococcal isolates were serotyped.[14] In some children antibody responses to the vaccine-type polysaccharides were observed using the RIA method.[15] The treatment regimen for otitis media—the same throughout the studies—also included antimicrobials and control visits until the ear was completely healed.

In both studies the clinical efficacy of the P vaccine was analyzed by comparing the numbers and the bacteriologic studies from postvaccination visits with effusion in the middle ear. A child was clinically defined as forming AOM if, in addition

TABLE 1 Numbers of Vaccinated Children

Vaccination Age (Months)	*Study 1 (1977–1979)*		*Study 2 (1979–1981)*	
	P-Vaccinated	*Control*	*P-Vaccinated*	*Control*
3–5	19	18	—	—
6–8	50	31	1276	1255
9–11	57	30	416	393
12–23	100	67	—	—
24–83	274	181	—	—
Total	500	327	1692	1648

TABLE 2 Antibody Responses and Rate (per 100 Vaccinated) of Pneumococcal AOM after Vaccination

Pneumococcal Type/Group	*Antibody Response**		*Study 1 (1977–1979)†*		*Study 2 (1979–1981)‡*	
	<1 Year Old	*>2 Years Old*	*P-Vaccinated*	*Control*	*P-Vaccinated*	*Control*
19	Poor	Good	1.3§	4.7	3.5	4.0
6	Poor	Poor	2.4	1.7	4.6‖	2.9
23	Poor	Poor	1.5	2.3	2.7	3.2
14	Poor	Intermediate	0.2§	2.0§	1.4	1.5
3	Good	Good			0.2	0.7
9	Good	Good			0.5	0.8
4	Good	Good	0.6	2.0		
7	Intermediate	Good			0.8	0.7
8	Good	Good				
18	Intermediate	Good				
All pneumococcal AOM			7.3§	13.4§	17.0	17.4

*Good response—most children having ≥ two-fold rise of antibody titer; poor response—most children not having ≥ two-fold rise of antibody titer

†Within six months among those aged 7 to 83 months when vaccinated

‡Before the second dose of the same vaccine (within approximately five months) among those aged 6 to 10 months when vaccinated

§$p < 0.01$

‖$p > 0.05$

to effusion in the middle ear, there was at least one of the following signs of an acute infection: fever, otalgia, tugging or rubbing of the ear, irritability, vomiting, or diarrhea. Only visits at least 14 days after vaccination or at least 14 days apart were included. Statistical analyses were done with the X^2-test or the Fischer's exact test.

RESULTS

The adverse reactions to the vaccines were mild and transient, and only slightly more common among the P-vaccinated children than among the controls. Among the P-vaccinated children, mild local reactions (redness, swelling, or pain) were found in one-half of those older than 2 years, in a quarter of those younger than 2 years, and in only 4 percent of those younger than 1 year. A rectal temperature over 38.5°C was found in less than 2 percent of children in both studies. There were no severe reactions, and approximately one-half of the vaccinated had no reactions at all. The second dose of the vaccine did not increase the number or the severity of adverse reactions.

The serum antibody responses to the pneumococcal polysaccharides present in the vaccine varied greatly from type to type. Generally, in respect to their immunogenicity the polysaccharides could be divided into three categories: (1) types 3, 4, 8, and 9N yielded good responses throughout the age range studied (6 months to 6 years); (2) types 1, 6A, 12F, and 23F yielded poor responses in all age groups; and (3) the responses to types 2, 7F, 14, 18C, 19F, and 25 were age dependent, being poor to moderate among infants less than 1 year old but generally good from 2 years on (Table 2). In study 2 (infants) the antibodies were usually reduced to the control level in five months, when the second dose of vaccine yielded a weaker but more stable response. The type-specific protection from postvaccination otitis attacks seemed to correlate to the immunogenicity of specific types, especially among older children (Table 2). Unfortunately for the usefulness of the vaccine, the four most common types of AOM, which made up at least two-thirds of pneumococcal attacks, all belonged to those with the poorest immunogenicity in infants (Table 2). The overall distribution and bacteriologic factors of postvaccination attacks of AOM are shown in Table 3. In study 1 infants who were 3 to 6 months old when vaccinated showed no protection and were excluded from analysis. Among older children (7 to 83 months), during the first 6 months after vaccination the reduction of pneumococcal attacks was almost 50 percent as compared with the controls. Attacks caused by other bacteria were equally common in both groups; those with a negative culture were slightly but not significantly more common among the P-vaccinated. The overall reduction of recurrence of AOM was 13 percent. There was no protection

TABLE 3 AOM within Six Months after Vaccination (Study 1, 1977–1979) or before the Second Dose of the Same Vaccine Approximately Five Months Later (Study 2, 1979–1981)

	*Study 1 (1977–1979)**		*Study 2 (1979–1981)*	
	P-Vaccinated (467)	*Control (299)*	*P-Vaccinated (1922)*	*Control (1648)*
Rate of attacks per 100 children	33.2	38.1	56.6	59.3
with:				
Streptococcus pneumoniae	7.3†	13.4†	17.0	17.4
of nonvaccine types/groups	1.3	2.0	2.0	2.6
group 6	2.4	1.3	4.6§	2.9§
other vaccine types/groups	3.6‡	10.0‡	9.1	10.9
Hemophilus influenzae	5.6	5.4	9.9	9.6
Other bacteria only	7.9	7.7	14.6	16.3
Negative culture	12.4	11.7	15.1	16.1

*Seven to 83 months old when vaccinated
†$p < 0.01$
‡$p < 0.001$
§$p < 0.05$

from pneumococcal recurrence more than six months after the vaccination.

The results of the first study were encouraging, but, considering the usefulness of the vaccination, there were limitations in the study design. So we continued into study 2 with the purpose of vaccinating children before the age when AOM usually begins and is most prevalent.[2] In this way we tried to test the efficacy of the vaccine just at the critical age, considering its potential use. In this way the possible sensitizing effect of AOM itself to further attacks[16] was also avoided. An effort was also made to prolong the duration of protection by giving the second dose of vaccine five months later. Unfortunately, the total reduction of AOM after the primary vaccination in this study was only 5 percent, and pneumococcal attacks were almost equally common in both vaccination groups (Table 3); group 6 attacks were even more common among the P-vaccinated children. The protective effect of the second dose of vaccine was also minor.

The number or bacteriologic agent of prevaccination attacks of AOM did not affect the efficacy of the vaccine in either study. The effect of the vaccine on episodes of otitis media with different grades of clinical severity was rather similar.

DISCUSSION

It is evident that otitis media can be affected by parenteral immunization. However, in infants the preventive efficacy of the vaccine studied seems to be poor. This corresponds to the generally poor immunizing capacity of the vaccine in infants. The antibody responses were poor, particularly to the types that were most common in AOM. Later on the immunogenicity of the vaccine, although variable from one pneumococcal type to another, generally increased with age. Thus, after infancy about one-half of the pneumococcal recurrences were prevented, but, consistent with the short duration of the polysaccharide antibody responses, this preventive effect lasted only for six months after vaccination. Type 6A polysaccharide showed especially poor immune responses at all ages until school age and clinically was also an especially problematic component of the vaccine.

The second dose of the vaccine, given two to six months after the initial vaccination, was not serologically or clinically beneficial. Like the first dose, it was very well tolerated.

The efficacy of the vaccine studied was not affected by the number (even if none) or microbial origin of otitis attacks before vaccination. The effect also seemed to be similar on attacks of AOM of varying clinical severity.

Finally, it can be concluded that the vaccine studied (vaccines available) cannot be recommended for prevention of acute otitis media in infants, although after the age of 2 years the vaccine may be of some benefit in children suffering from recurrent episodes of otitis media. Before further otitis trials are undertaken among infants the immunogenicity of the vaccine must be improved. The other ways of administering the vaccine should also be studied.

The study was supported by a grant from the Merck Sharp and Dohme Research Laboratories, West Point, Pennsylvania, who also supplied the vaccines.

REFERENCES

1. Pukander J, Luotonen J, Sipilä M, et al: Incidence of acute otitis media. Acta Otolaryngol (Stockh) 93:447, 1982
2. Pukander J, Karma P, Sipilä M: Occurrence and recurrence of acute otitis media among children. Acta Otolaryngol (Stockh) 94:479, 1982
3. Austrian R, Douglas RM, Schiffman G, et al: Prevention of pneumococcal pneumonia by vaccination. Trans Assoc Am Physicians 89:184, 1976
4. Amman AJ, Addiego J, Wara DW, et al: Polyvalent pneumococcal-polysaccharide immunization of patients with sickle-cell anemia and patients with splenectomy. N Engl J Med 297:897, 1977
5. Smit P, Oberholzer D, Hayden-Smith S, et al: Protective efficacy of pneumococcal polysaccharide vaccines. JAMA 283:2613, 1977
6. Karma P. Luotonen J, Timonen M, et al: Efficacy of pneumococcal vaccination against recurrent otitis media. Preliminary results of a field trial in Finland. Ann Otol Rhinol Laryngol 89(Suppl 68):357, 1980
7. Austrian R, Howie VM, Ploussard JH: The bacteriology of pneumococcal otitis media. Johns Hopkins Med J 141:104, 1977
8. Borgono JM, McLean AA, Vella PP, et al: Vaccination and revaccination with polyvalent pneumococcal polysaccharide vaccines in adults and infants. Proc Soc Exp Biol Med 157:148, 1978
9. Sloyer JR Jr, Ploussard JH, Karr LJ, Schiffman GD: Immunologic response to pneumococcal polysaccharide vaccine in infants. Ann Otol Rhinol Laryngol 89(Suppl 68):352, 1980
10. Giebink GS, Schiffman G, Petty K, Quie PG: Modification of otitis media following vaccination with the capsular polysaccharide of Streptococcus pneumoniae in chinchillas. J Infect Dis 138:480, 1978
11. Howie VM, Ploussard JH, Sloyer JL: Immunization against recurrent otitis media. Ann Otol Rhinol Laryngol 85(Suppl 25):254, 1976
12. Klein JO, Teele DW, Sloyer JL Jr, et al: Use of pneumococcal vaccine for prevention of recurrent episodes of otitis media. Sem Infect Dis 4:305, 1982
13. Mäkelä PH, Sibakov M, Herva E, et al: Pneumococcal vaccine and otitis media. Lancet ii:547, 1980
14. Henrichsen J: The pneumococcal typing system and pneumococcal surveillance. J Infect 1(Suppl 2):31, 1979
15. Schiffman G, Douglas RM, Bonner MJ, et al: A radioimmunoassay for immunologic phenomena in pneumococcal disease and for the antibody response to pneumococcal vaccines. I. Method for the radioimmunoassay of anticapsular antibodies and comparison with other techniques. J Immunol Methods 33:133, 1980
16. Howie VM, Ploussard JH, Sloyer J: The "otitis-prone" condition. Am J Dis Child 129:676, 1975

EFFECT OF PNEUMOCOCCAL VACCINATION ON ACUTE OTITIS MEDIA IN CHILDREN ATTENDING DAY CARE NURSERIES

CHRISTER ROSÉN M.D., POUL CHRISTENSEN, M.D., BIRGITTA HOVELIUS, M.D., and KARIN PRELLNER, M.D.

It has been well established that vaccination against pneumococci prevents septicemia and pneumonia caused by these bacteria in adults.[1,2] There are few studies of the effect of pneumococcal vaccination on infections in children. Reduced mortality rates in cases of lower respiratory tract infection as well as reduced frequency of recurrent acute pneumococcal otitis media have been demonstrated in children following vaccination.[3–6] Most cases of acute otitis media (AOM) are caused by pneumococcal types included in the currently available vaccines.[7,8]

The present report concerns vaccination of children attending day care centers. The study was designed as a double-blind trial in children aged 6 months to 5 years and compared the effect of Pneumovax against that of placebo injections on the overall incidence of upper respiratory tract infections. This evaluation concerns AOM and was performed 1½ years after the immunization.

MATERIALS AND METHODS

The parents of approximately 4000 children in day care centers were informed about this double-blind study and had to decide if their children would take part in it. Children with chronic or progressive diseases or with immunologic deficiences were excluded, as were children with cleft palate. After written informed consent was obtained from the parents, 405 children entered the trial. They were matched in pairs with respect to age and absence or presence of previous attacks of AOM and allocated to one of the following groups:

Group 1, children less than 2 years of age with no previous episode of otitis (40 children).

Group 2, children less than 2 years of age with previous episode(s) of otitis (52 children)

Group 3, children older than 2 years of age with no previous episode of otitis (94 children)

Group 4, children older than 2 years of age with previous episode(s) of otitis (219 children)

The study was designed as a double-blind matched study in children 6 months to 5 years of age to determine the effect of a 14-valent pneumococcal polysaccharide vaccine (Pneumovax, supplied by Merck Sharp and Dohme, West Point, Pennsylvania) on upper respiratory tract infections. The vaccine contained capsular type antigens from types 1, 2, 3, 4, 6A, 7F, 8, 9N, 12F, 14, 18C, 19F, 23F, and 25 (Danish nomenclature) and was administered subcutaneously in the lateral upper part of the arm. One child in every pair, if older than 2 years, received 0.5 ml vaccine (50 μg of each pneumococcal polysaccharide), and the other child received saline containing thiomersalate as placebo. Children younger than 2 years were given 0.25 ml (25 μg of each pneumococcal polysaccharide). In all, 198 children were vaccinated and 207 served as controls. The demographic data by group for vaccinees and controls are given in Table 1.

When the children needed medical care during the follow-up period, they were requested to attend a special clinic where ENT specialists were available daily. Nasopharyngeal and throat specimens were taken at every consultation sought as a result of respiratory tract infections. Middle ear effusion was aspirated when myringotomy was performed. All therapy, including prescriptions of antibiotics, was given as generally recommended.

TABLE 1 Age and Sex Distribution of Controls (C) and Vaccinees (V)

Group	*Status*	*Number*	*Mean Age (Years)*	*Age Range*	*Percent Male*
1	C	22	1.46	0.89–1.92	55
	V	18	1.38	0.67–1.87	56
2	C	26	1.50	0.74–1.97	73
	V	26	1.50	0.73–1.90	54
3	C	47	3.82	2.07–5.85	40
	V	47	3.67	2.11–5.85	51
4	C	112	3.81	2.00–5.76	54
	V	107	3.77	2.04–5.98	58
Total	C	207	3.27	0.74–5.85	54
	V	198	3.23	0.67–5.98	55

RESULTS

The incidence of side effects to vaccination/placebo injection were 31 percent in those vaccinated and 1.5 percent in the controls. No severe reactions were registered.

During the first 18 months of the follow-up period 517 visits from 228 children were registered. Two hundred ten of the visits among 120 children were made because of AOM. In children younger than 2 years, AOM episodes were almost as frequent among those vaccinated (48 episodes) as among the controls (41 episodes). In children older than 2 years, episodes of AOM were less frequent among those vaccinated than among the controls (Table 2).

During the first postvaccination year the incidence of AOM, regardless of etiologic agent, in children older than 2 years with or without previous otitis was reduced by 33 percent in those vaccinated as compared with the controls (39 and 58 episodes, respectively; $p < 0.05$).

Pneumococcal types included in the vaccine were found in 12 episodes of AOM in vaccinated children older than 2 years, compared with 19 in the controls. In 26 otitis episodes no pneumococci were isolated in vaccinated children older than 2 years, whereas the corresponding figure for the control was 37 episodes.

TABLE 2 Number of Acute Otitis Media Episodes among Vaccinees (V) and Controls (C) during 18 Months Follow-up

Children < 2 Years When Vaccinated (n = 92)		*Children > 2 Years When Vaccinated (n = 313)*	
V	48	V	52
C	41	C	69

DISCUSSION

Children attending day care centers were chosen for this study for several reasons. They constitute a homogeneous population in which those vaccinated and controls mix daily and therefore are exposed to the same microbial agents. Several investigators have reported a higher frequency of respiratory tract infections among children attending day care centers than in those cared for at home or in family day care homes.[9,10] Furthermore, small children cared for daily outside homes are more likely to develop AOM.[11,12]

The present trial is unique in that it was undertaken in a well-defined group of children and estimated the effect of vaccination on AOM regardless of etiologic agents.

The reduction of the total incidence of AOM in children older than 2 years partly resulted from a reduction of episodes due to pneumococcal types included in the vaccine and is in accordance with other studies.[3,5,6] One important finding in our study was that AOM caused by other pathogens did not increase parallel to the reduction of episodes caused by pneumococci.

We were unable to demonstrate protection after vaccination against AOM in children younger than 2 years.

In conclusion, the present study has shown that pneumococcal vaccination has a beneficial effect on the incidence of AOM in children older than 2 years.

REFERENCES

1. Austrian R, Douglas RM, Schiffman G, et al: Prevention of pneumococcal pneumonia by vaccination. Trans Assoc Am Physicians 89:184, 1976
2. Smit P, Oberholzer D, Hayden-Smith S, et al: Protective efficacy of pneumococcal polysaccharide vaccines. JAMA 238:2613, 1977
3. Mäkelä PH, Herva E, Sibakov M, et al: Pneumococcal vaccine and otitis media. Lancet ii:547, 1980
4. Riley ID, Everingham FA, Smith DE, Douglas RM: Immunization with polyvalent pneumococcal vaccine. Effect of respiratory mortality in children living in the New Guinea highlands. Arch Dis Child 56:354, 1981
5. Sloyer JL Jr, Ploussard JH and Howie V: Efficacy of pneumococcal polysaccharide vaccine in preventing acute otitis media in infants in Huntsville, Alabama. Rev Infant Dis 3:S119, 1981
6. Teele DW, Klein JO, et al: Use of pneumococcal vaccine for prevention of recurrent otitis media in infants in Boston. Rev Infect Dis 3:S113, 1981
7. Austrian R, and Gold J: Pneumococcal bacteremia with especial reference to bacteremic pneumococcal pneumonia. Ann Intern Med 60:759, 1964
8. Klein JO: The epidemiology of pneumococcal disease in infants and children. Rev Infect Dis 3:246, 1981
9. Hesselvik L: Respiratory infections among children in day nurseries. Acta Paediatr Suppl 74, 1949
10. Ståhlberg MR: The influence of form of day care on occurrence of acute respiratory tract infections among young children. Acta Paediatr Scand Suppl 282, 1980
11. Ingvarsson L, Lundgren K, and Olofsson B: Epidemiology of acute otitis media in children. A prospective study of acute otitis media in children. 1. Design, method and material. Acta Otolaryngol (Stockh) Suppl 388, 1982
12. Strangert K: Infections in young children attending day care centers. Thesis. Department of Pediatrics, Karolinska Sjukhuset, Stockholm, Sweden, 1976

MEDICAL TREATMENT WITHOUT ANTIBIOTICS

NONANTIMICROBIAL MANAGEMENT AND PREVENTION OF OTITIS MEDIA WITH EFFUSION: STATE OF THE ART

JACK L. PARADISE, M.D.

There are a variety of approaches to the management and prevention of otitis media, all subsumed under one or another of four headings—medical, mechanical, surgical, and skeptical. In this discussion attention is focused on nonsurgical approaches, that is, medical and mechanical treatments, to the exclusion of antimicrobial drugs, whose use is considered elsewhere in this volume.

The purely *medical*, but nonantimicrobial, treatments of current interest are decongestants and antihistamines (used either singly or, more often, in combinaion), corticosteroids, and mucolytic agents. *Mechanical* treatment refers to a direct attack on negative middle ear air pressure by nonsurgical means, that is, by some type of inflation technique—autoinflation, politzerization, or so-called controlled middle ear inflation—or by the injection of a heavy gas.

In the report of the Research Conference that followed the Second International Symposium in 1979,[1] emphasis was placed on a number of critical requirements in the design and execution of research concerning the management and prevention of otitis media. These requirements were (1) explicit definition of the disease state being studied; (2) valid identification of the presence, or confirmation of the absence, of the disease; (3) enrollment of study populations large enough to factor out confounding variables, either by stratifying according to such variables or by depending on randomization to distribute them equitably between treatment groups; (4) enrollment of study populations large enough to detect small differences in outcome where small differences might be important, as, for example, in challenging the efficacy of an established mode of treatment; and (5) use of follow-up periods long enough to avoid potential confounding of results by the inherent variability of the short-term course of otitis media with effusion.

Several critical reviews concerning medical treatments of otitis media have been published since the Second International Symposium,[2–4] and therefore this review will be confined to recent reports not encompassed in those reviews.

Regarding *decongestants and antihistamines*, these drugs have been used for three discrete purposes: (1) to treat acute suppurative otitis media, generally as adjuncts to antimicrobial drugs; (2) to treat nonsuppurative (secretory or serous) otitis media; and (3) to prevent otitis media. With regard to acute suppurative otitis media, Moran and coworkers recently reported that a decongestant-antihistamine combination was efficacious, but not significantly so, in reducing the persistence of middle ear effusion.[5] On the other hand Bhambani and coworkers, testing a similar drug combination, found no evidence of efficacy.[6] Both studies were limited by small sample sizes and uncertain comparability of treatment groups. Whether these drugs are effective adjuncts in acute suppurative otitis media thus remains an unsettled question.

Decongestants and antihistamines have undoubtedly been used most extensively for the treatment of nonsuppurative otitis media. Investigators in the late 1970s had concluded that the drugs lack efficacy for this purpose, but the supporting data were not convincing. Three more persuasive, recent studies, by O'Shea and colleagues,[7] Haugeto and colleagues,[8] and Sorri,[9] also suggest lack of efficacy, but again the designs of the studies and the limited numbers of enrolled subjects preclude unqualified confidence in the studies' conclusions.

Most recently, Cantekin and others of our group in Pittsburgh reported the results of a double-blind trial involving 553 children evaluated after four weeks of treatment with either a decongestant-antihistamine combination or a placebo.[10] The subjects had been stratified according to age, duration of effusion, and previous administration of antimicrobial drugs. The number of subjects was large enough to provide, on the basis of a type I error of 0.05, a probability of 0.98 of detecting a difference of 15 percent between the proportions of effusion-free subjects in the placebo treated and drug-treated groups. No appreciable differences in outcome between the two groups were found. Among subjects with unilateral effusion at entry, 37.5 percent of those treated with placebo and 33.8 percent of those treated with drug became free of effusion; of subjects with bilateral effusion at entry, the corresponding values were 18.5 percent and 20.7 percent. Thus, the study demonstrates that the drug combination used has no efficacy in the treatment of nonsuppurative otitis media.

The Pittsburgh study identified three important prognostic variables in addition to laterality: duration, prior history of otitis media, and the presence or absence of concurrent upper respiratory tract infection. Poorer outcomes were found in children with effusions of long, rather than short, duration, and in children with, rather than without, prior histories of otitis media. Children who had upper respiratory tract infection at the four-week end point had twice the rate of effusion as those without such infection. It follows, in keeping with the research principles discussed above, that studies of otitis media in which the treatment groups are not balanced in regard to these four variables may give misleading results.

Only one recent study, by Randall and Hendley, has reported on the efficacy of decongestant-antihistamine in preventing the development of otitis media in children with upper respiratory tract infection.[11] In a group of 104 such children, the drug combination was found to be ineffective in preventing episodes considered to be acute ear infections. However, the study did not incorporate monitoring for asymptomatic effusions and it had certain other limitations. We do not know whether decongestants and antihistamines have any effect on the development of otitis media in children with simple upper respiratory tract infection.

Regarding *corticosteroids,* at the Second International Symposium Schwartz and colleagues reported limited efficacy for prednisone in a somewhat complex cross-over study that was not immune to the influence of potentially confounding variables and that therefore cannot be considered conclusive.[12] More recently, Macknin and Jones reported no significant differences in efficacy between a two-week tapering course of dexamethasone and placebo in subjects stratified according to age and duration of effusion.[13] The study was terminated on advice from an independent statistical monitor after analysis of data from 49 subjects.

Regarding *mucolytic agents*, the efficacy of one such orally administered drug, S-carboxymethylcysteine, was studied by Khan and colleagues.[14] The drug was given following myringotomy and, in some instances, grommet insertion and was believed to have brought about modestly improved auditory acuity. However, specific effects on middle ear effusion were not reported. For this reason, and because of small sample sizes and various confounding variables, the findings cannot be considered conclusive.

I have found in the literature no recent studies concerning the efficacy of eustachian tube or middle ear *inflation*; I believe that no satisfactorily controlled study of this mode of treatment has ever been reported.

In summary, uncertainty about the nonsurgical, nonantimicrobial management of otitis media has been reduced during the four years since the Second International Symposium, but many important questions remain unanswered.

REFERENCES

1. Palva T, Gates GA, Paradise JL, et al: Report of research conference on recent advances in otitis media with effusion. Ann Otol Rhinol Laryngol 89 (Suppl 69):23, 1980
2. Paradise JL: Otitis media in infants and children. Pediatrics 65:917, 1980
3. Bluestone CD: Otitis media in children: To treat or not to treat? New Engl J Med 306:1399, 1982
4. Bluestone CD, Klein JO: Otitis media with effusion, atelectasis, and eustachian tube dysfunction. In Bluestone CD, Stool SE (eds): *Pediatric Otolaryngology*. Philadelphia: WB Saunders Co, 1983, pp 356–512
5. Moran DM, Mutchie KD, Higbee MD, Paul LD: The use of an antihistamine-decongestant in conjunction with an anti-infective drug in the treatment of acute otitis media. J Pediatr 101:132, 1982
6. Bhambani K, Foulds DM, Swamy KN, et al: Acute otitis media in children: Are decongestants or antihistamines necessary? Ann Emerg Med 12:13, 1983
7. O'Shea JS, Langenbrunner DJ, McCloskey DE, et al: Diagnostic and therapeutic studies in childhood serous otitis media: Results of treatment with an antihistamine-adrenergic combination. Ann Otol Rhinol Laryngol 89 (Suppl 68):285, 1980
8. Haugeto OK, Schrøder KE, Mair IWS: Secretory otitis media, oral decongestant and antihistamine. J Otolaryngol 10:359, 1981
9. Sorri M, Sipilä P, Palva A, Karma P: Can secretory otitis media be prevented by oral decongestants? Acta Otolaryngol Suppl 386:115, 1982
10. Cantekin EI, Mandel EM, Bluestone CD, et al: Lack of efficacy of a decongestant-antihistamine combination for otitis media with effusion ("secretory" otitis media) in children. New Engl J Med 308:297, 1983
11. Randall JE, Hendley JO: A decongestant-antistamine mixture in the prevention of otitis media in children with colds. Pediatrics 63:483, 1979
12. Schwartz RH, Puglese J, Schwartz DM: Use of a short course of prednisone for treating middle ear effusion: A double-blind crossover study. Ann Otol Rhinol Laryngol 89 (Suppl 68):296, 1980
13. Macknin ML, Jones PK: Oral dexamethasone for persistent middle ear effusion: A double-blind placebo controlled study. Pediatr Research 17:225 A, 1983 (Abstr)
14. Khan JA, Marcus P, Cummings SW: S-carboxymethylcysteine in otitis media with effusion (a double-blind study). J Laryngol Otol 95:995, 1981

REDUCTION OF ARTIFICIALLY INCREASED MIDDLE EAR AIR PRESSURE

ULF RENVALL, M.D.

In a middle ear with a retracted tympanic membrane, with or without fluid, the major symptom is hearing impairment. Immediate normalization of the hearing can be achieved by a successful Politzer maneuver. Is this procedure still something to recommend? For how long a time will the favorable result last?

MATERIALS AND METHODS

In 16 patients undergoing medical treatment because of serous or mucoid otitis media (mean age, 31) a middle ear air pressure more negative than − 150 mm H_2O was found in 20 ears by tympanometry. A Politzer maneuver was performed in these 20 ears and the pressure was again recorded. In 12 ears new pressure recordings were made after 30 and 60 minutes and in 8 ears pressure was recorded 15, 30, and 60 minutes following the Politzer procedure.

RESULTS

In 11 ears a positive pressure was created by the Politzer maneuver and in nine ears the negative pressure recorded before the maneuver was changed to a less negative pressure or to atmospheric pressure (Table 1). The major pressure drop occurred within the first 15 to 30 minutes after the procedure. However, a continuous air pressure decrease was recorded during the whole 60-minute period in all but four ears. Table 2 shows the air pressure changes occurring during the 60 minutes in these four ears. There was a less negative pressure at 60 minutes compared with the pressure recorded after 30 minutes. From Table 3 it is evident that the major change of the middle ear air pressure occurred within 15 minutes after the Politzer maneuver. After the major pressure drop within the first 15 minutes, a less pronounced pressure decrease followed during the next 45 minutes. Tympanometry showed a positive pressure at all recordings in only one ear.

DISCUSSION

The findings in the present study accord well with those of Schwartz and colleagues,[1] who also recorded a rapid pressure decrease following the Politzer maneuver. In a normal middle ear, pressure decrease caused by gas absorption is calculated to be about 50 mm H_2O per hour.[2] In another study of ears with tubal occlusion[3] there was a pressure decrease only from atmospheric level down to − 80 mm H_2O during a 4-hour observation period.

The data from the present study of ears with tympanometrically measured middle ear air pres-

TABLE 1 Results from Preset Pressure Recordings in 20 Ears from 17 Patients after Politzer Maneuver

Ear No.	*Before Politzer*	*After Politzer*	*15 Min*	*30 Min*	*60 Min*
1	< − 400	+ 130		+ 50	+ 30
2	− 370	+ 10		− 300	− 330
3	− 340	+ 90		− 250	− 230*
4	− 230	+ 60		− 50	− 150
5	− 350	− 150		− 310	
6	− 250	− 130		− 220	
7	− 170	+ 20		− 160	− 170
8	− 270	+ 180		− 120	− 170
9	− 160	+ 30		− 140	− 160
10	− 190	− 20		− 130	− 220
11	− 350	− 90	− 290	− 320	− 360
12	− 280	− 20		− 180	− 230
13	− 330	− 260		− 340	− 350
14	− 250	− 20	− 220	− 240	− 200*
15	− 175	± 0	− 75	− 120	− 60*
16	− 180	+ 100	− 175	− 175	− 75*
17	− 280	+ 50	− 200	− 250	− 275
18	− 275	− 120	− 225	− 250	− 275
19	− 275	+ 30	− 180	− 220	− 250
20	− 200	+ 50	− 150	− 160	− 200

Note: Pressures are given in mm H_2O.

sure < -150 mm H_2O are not totally comparable with those of the investigation of Koch and colleagues.[3] In this study the pressure in the middle ear was changed artificially. In ear number 15, however, the initial pressure of -175 mm H_2O was raised to 0 mm H_2O, or atmospheric level. In 30 minutes a pressure drop of 120 mm H_2O was recorded compared with 80 mm H_2O during 4 hours in the investigation by Koch and associates.[3] Tympanometrically measured middle ear air pressure is not equivalent to the directly measured pressure,[4] but even if this is taken into account pressure decrease seems to be faster than calculated by Koch and associates[3] in ears with serous or mucoid otitis media.

Is a voluntary act of sniffing then a plausible explanation for the recorded pressure decrease in the 20 ears in the present study? In sniffing, the pressure change is acquired in approximately 20 seconds,[5] whereas in 16 of the 20 ears in the present study a gradual pressure decrease was recorded during 1 hour. Since the act of sniffing is sometimes a valid explanation for retraction of the tympanic membrane, sniffing may be the explanation for the rapid pressure decrease during the first 15 minutes in some cases. Another plausible explanation for the data obtained may be spontaneous elimination of the created overpressure via the eustachian tube in those ears in which the Politzer maneuver resulted in positive middle ear air pressure. The possibility of increased gas absorption from the mucous membrane in ears with serous or mucoid otitis media over that in normal ears could also be argued.

In conclusion, there is only a short beneficial effect from the Politzer maneuver. Knowledge of this short advantageous effect is also of great value in the treatment of ears with serous or mucoid otitis media. If, for instance, a Valsalva maneuver is recommended to a patient, it is important to instruct the patient to do this once every hour. The data from the present study indicate that there may be an accelerated gas absorption from the mucous

TABLE 2 Ears in Which a Pressure Increase Was Found Between the 30- and 60-Minute Tympanometric Recordings

Ear No.	*Before Politzer*	*After Politzer*	*15 Min*	*30 Min*	*60 Min*	
3	−340	+90		−250	−230	
14	−250	−20	−220	−240	−200	
15	−175	0	−75	−120	−60	Same patient
16	−180	+100	−175	−175	−75	Same patient

Note: Pressures are given in mm H_2O.

TABLE 3 Pressure Difference Between the Preset Tympanometric Recordings

Ear No.	*After Politzer*	*Pressure Difference*					
		15 Min		*30 Min*		*60 Min*	
1	(+130)			80	(+50)	30	(+30)
2	(+10)			310	(−300)	30	(−330)
3	(+90)			340	(−250)	20	(−230)*
4	(+60)			110	(−50)	100	(−150)
5	(−150)			160	(−310)		—
6	(−130)			90	(−220)		—
7	(+20)			180	(−160)	10	(−170)
8	(+180)			300	(−120)	10	(−170)
9	(+30)			170	(−140)	20	(−160)
10	(−20)			110	(−130)	90	(−220)
11	(−90)	200	(−290)	30	(−320)	40	(−360)
12	(−20)			160	(−180)	50	(−230)
13	(−260)			80	(−340)	10	(−350)
14	(−20)	200	(−220)	20	(−240)	40	(−200)*
15	(0)	75	(−75)	45	(−120)	60	(−60)*
16	(+100)	275	(−175)	0	(−175)	100	(−75)*
17	(+50)	250	(−200)	50	(−250)	25	(−275)
18	(−120)	105	(−225)	25	(−250)	25	(−275)
19	(+30)	210	(−180)	40	(−220)	30	(−250)
20	(+50)	200	(−150)	10	(−160)	40	(−200)

Note: Pressures are given in mm H_2O.
*Less negative pressure than at the 30-min recording.

membrane in ears with serous or mucoid otitis media compared with normal ears. The act of sniffing may be an explanation in a few cases in which a fast pressure decrease was recorded.

I wish to thank Dr. B. Dahlberg for a valuable review of the manuscript.

REFERENCES

1. Schwartz D, Schwartz R, Redfield N: Treatment of negative middle ear pressure and serous otitis media with Politzer's technique. Arch Otolaryngol 104:487, 1978
2. Elner Å: Quantitative studies of gas absorption from the normal middle ear. Acta Otolaryngol 83:25, 1977
3. Koch U, Middendorf F: Direkte kontinuierliche Bestimmung des Mittelohrdruckes. Laryngol Rhinol Otol 58: 424, 1979
4. Renvall U, Lidén G, Björkman G: Experimental tympanometry in human temporal bones. Scand Audiol 4:135, 1975
5. Magnusson B: Tubal opening and closing ability in unilateral middle ear disease. Academic dissertation No 104, Department of Otorhinolaryngology, Linköping University, Linköping, Sweden.

BROMHEXINE IN THE TREATMENT OF OTITIS MEDIA WITH EFFUSION

NOEL ROYDHOUSE, Ch.M., F.R.C.S., F.R.A.C.S.

Bromhexine hydrochloride (Bisolvon) is an oral mucolytic agent derived synthetically from the alkaloid vasicine. It has been found to reduce the viscosity of mucous secretions in chronic chest diseases. As one of the causes of persistent otitis media with effusion (OME) is reputed to be the viscidity of the mucoid effusion in the middle ear, it was decided to carry out a double-blind drug trial with this mucolytic agent. Wing reported that bromhexine in combination with pseudoephedrine and triprolidine hydrochloride (Actifed) yielded excellent results (90 percent success rate) in an open study in patients with OME.[1] Elcock and Lord, in a previous double-blind trial with bromhexine hydrochloride alone at a lower dose for four weeks, had found no clinical improvement using pure-tone audiometry as a measurement of success.[2] Thus, it seemed important to attempt to confirm Wing's findings in a carefully controlled double-blind study.

MATERIALS AND METHODS

From August 1978 to September 1979, every patient 14 years and under seen at the ENT clinic at Middlemore Hospital, South Auckland, diagnosed as having OME was entered in the trial after formal consent was obtained from the parents. There was a total of 239 cases (Table 1), and of the 59 cases lost to the trial 12 were from the bromhexine groups, 15 from the placebo group, 27 patients withdrew before the end of the first two months, and 5 patients were lost for other reasons. Diagnoses were made on clinical grounds and always confirmed with impedance audiometry. A patient was considered to have OME if he had a flat or "B" curve or a "C" curve with a peak pressure more negative than −300mm of water. The adenoids were x-rayed and the adenoid shadow was sized: 1, none or minimal; 2, small; 3, moderately enlarged; and 4, large. This sizing was carried out by measuring the total thickness of the soft tissue mass in the adenoid region in a standardized lateral x-ray of the nasopharynx. At each monthly visit impedance audiometry was carried out. Failure of patients to take their medicine (four cases) was de-

TABLE 1 Distribution of 239 Cases Entered in Trial

Cured with initial treatment	67
Bromhexine group	57
Placebo group	56
Cases lost to trial	59
Total	239

termined by the hospital pharmacist, who examined the bottles brought back for refills, and by the clinician, who questioned the parents. Most cases were lost to the trial as a result of nonattendance (42) and incorrect diagnosis (12), which was determined by reviewing the criteria for diagnosis to ensure standardization between examiners.

The procedure was divided into three two-month periods. During the first two months patients were given specific measures to improve the health of the nose and sinuses and nonspecific measures to improve general resistance to infection. These and other measures have been previously described.[3,4] The purpose of these measures was to remove from the trial those patients who might spontaneously recover or would recover with minimal treatment.

After this period, during which 67 patients (37 percent) recovered, the group of resistant cases of OME then began the double-blind randomized drug trial. The hospital pharmacist provided the drug bromhexine or the placebo according to the random code for one month in the following doses: age 7 years and over, bromhexine, 16 mg thrice daily; 6 years and under, bromhexine elixir (4 mg/5 ml), 10 ml thrice daily. The patients also obtained from their own pharmacists the two other medicines: age 7 years and over, long-acting chlorpheniramine maleate, 8 mg twice daily, pseudoephedrine, 30 or 60 mg twice daily; 6 years and under, chlorpheniramine maleate elixir (2 mg/5 ml) combined with pseudoephedrine elixir (30 mg/5 ml), 5 ml thrice daily.

After one month the patients returned for impedance audiometry and a refill of the bromhexine or placebo, and at the end of the fourth month in the survey they were examined again. If there was no effusion present in the middle ear, they were given two monthly follow-up appointments, but if OME persisted they were given bromhexine for the fifth month and for the sixth month if necessary. At the end of the six-month period those children with OME were entered for early surgery. This protocol was approved by the Middlemore Hospital ethical committee.

RESULTS

Of the 239 cases enrolled in the survey, 140 cases were admitted to the double-blind trial, and of the remaining 99 cases 32 were lost to the trial and the other 67 cases recovered in the initial two-month period. In a controlled study of adenoidectomy for OME,[4] the recovery rate in the first two months with the same treatment was 42 percent. Their sex, age, and ethnicity are given in Table 2.

TABLE 2 Age, Sex, and Race of the Three Groups

	Sex			*Race*	
Groups	*Male*	*Female*	*Age (SD)*	*Caucasian*	*Polynesian*
Bromhexine	31	26	6.7 (2.5)	32	25
Placebo	34	22	6.5 (1.9)	36	20
Cured initially	37	30	7.6 (2.8)	39	27

Because some cases had only one ear involved (17 in the bromhexine group and 14 in the placebo group) the results were given as related to the 195 ears of the 113 patients who completed the trial. As to distribution of one- or two-ear patients in the groups, there was a nonsignificant *chi*-square value of 0.132. Thus, there was no evidence of either group having significantly more or less of either type of patient. The results of treatment showed more than double the number of successes in the bromhexine group compared with the placebo group (Table 3). There were 48 successful ears in the bromhexine group and only 21 in the placebo group. The success rate of 50 percent in the bromhexine group (total ears, 97) compared with 21 percent in the placebo group (total ears, 98) gives a corrected *chi*-square value of 15.58, which is significant at the 0.005 level. That is, the bromhexine group was 3.6 times more likely to be cured in this two-month period on bromhexine, chlorpheniramine maleate, and pseudoephedrine than on chlorpheniramine maleate and pseudoephedrine alone. These results were for the double-blind drug trial, and after these two months of treatment all cases with persistent OME were openly given bromhexine. A further 10 of the 31 failed cases in the bromhexine group were cured and 11 of the 50 failed cases in the placebo group

TABLE 3 Failure and Success Rates at End of Double-blind Drug Trial

	Failed	*Successful*
Bromhexine	49	48
Placebo	77	21
Total	126	69

were cured. Although the bromhexine group appeared to do better than the placebo group, this difference was not significant (*chi*-square = 0.28).

Because there seemed to be some seasonal effect on the spontaneous recovery from OME, the effect of the season was examined in two ways. First, it was determined whether the allocations into the bromhexine and placebo groups were made consistently on a 50-50 basis and whether there was any evidence of seasonal differences in case accrual. The *chi*-square value to test the former hypothesis was 1.55 with 3 df, indicating a close 50-50 randomization, and for the latter it was 9.25, having $0.025 < p < 0.05$. Thus, there is evidence to suggest that patients did not enter the study at a uniform rate. This could reflect a true seasonal trend, since the highest accrual rate was in October–December and the lowest was in January–March. Secondly, to test whether the advantage of bromhexine over placebo was at all seasonally dependent, the season in which the effusion cleared was examined for the two groups. Although most children recovered in the January–March season, this was similar in both groups. There was a *chi*-square value of 3.79 with 3 df, which is not significant. Thus, the relative success rate of bromhexine is not seasonally dependent.

The effect of the size of the adenoids was compared with the results of treatment. The distribution of the successful and unsuccessful cases was plotted according to the size of the adenoids for both groups. Using a table of the overall successful cases comparing the observed results with the expected results based on adenoid size gave a *chi*-square value of 3.64, which is not significant. For the bromhexine group alone the value was 3.09 and for the placebo group the value was 1.37, neither showing any significance. Thus, there is no evidence to suggest that the size of the adenoids has any influence on recovery from OME.

DISCUSSION

There is a world-wide problem concerning how OME should be treated. A previous study showed that an initial 42 percent of cases presenting at Middlemore Hospital ENT clinic can resolve if medical measures are complied with.[4] In the past, the remaining cases of OME have required surgery, the best form of which, according to the previous study,[4] was myringotomy, drainage, and insertion of aeration tubes. However, there are complications from surgery and the waiting time at Middlemore Hospital is excessive. Accordingly, further medical treatment was investigated. Previously the cause of OME had been believed to be malfunction of the eustachian tube—either functional, through lack of swallowing, as in the mouth breather; obstructional due to nasal congestion; or because of increased viscidity of the middle ear mucus collection.

Treatment was directed toward relieving all three causes of malfunction. First, patients were converted to nose-breathing habits to encourage swallowing, since the eustachian tube is actively opened on swallowing and a mouth-breather does not swallow very often. Second, chlorpheniramine maleate and pseudoephedrine were given to decrease nasal congestion. The third form of treatment was the introduction of the oral mucolytic agent bromhexine to counter the viscidity of the middle ear mucus. Although our results are not as good as those of Wing,[1] who claimed 90 percent success, the success rate of bromhexine was 3.6 times that in the placebo group. This effect was not related to the season or to the size of the adenoids. Therefore, we believe that bromhexine is a valuable adjunct in the treatment of OME in children 14 years old and younger.

I wish to acknowledge the assistance of Mr. C. Treadgold, the hospital pharmacist, Middlemore Hospital, in handling the bromhexine and checking its consumption. The statistical analysis was carried out by Mr. P. Mullins, Department of Community Health, University of Auckland. Supplies of bromhexine hydrochloride (Bisolvon) were provided by Boehringer Ingelheim (NZ) Ltd.

REFERENCES

1. Wing L: Bisolvon and Actifed in the conservative management of glue ear. Med J Aust 1:289, 1978
2. Elcock HW, Lord IJ: Bromhexine in chronic secretory otitis media—a clinical trial. Br J Clin Pract 26:276, 1972
3. Roydhouse N: Middle ear problems in children: Rational treatment. Drugs 15:393, 1978
4. Roydhouse N: Adenoidectomy for otitis media with mucoid effusion. Ann Otol Rhinol Laryngol 89(Supp 68):312, 1980

EFFECTS OF IBUPROFEN, CORTICOSTEROID, AND PENICILLIN ON THE PATHOGENESIS OF EXPERIMENTAL PNEUMOCOCCAL OTITIS MEDIA

TIMOTHY T. K. JUNG, M.D., PH.D., G. SCOTT GIEBINK, M.D., and S. K. JUHN, M.D.

The primary therapy for acute purulent otitis media is administration of antibiotics. Recently a short course of corticosteroid medication has been recommended for the treatment of chronic otitis media with effusion.[1,2] Since it has been suggested that prostaglandins (PGs) play an important role in the pathogenesis of otitis media,[3–9] we wished to study the effects of a cyclo-oxygenase inhibitor (ibuprofen), of a corticosteroid, and of pencillin treatment on the pathogenesis of experimentally induced purulent otitis media (POM) in chinchillas. The results of this study could help to determine the role of prostaglandins and lipoxygenase products on the pathogenesis of otitis media and to determine the best mode of therapy for POM.

MATERIALS AND METHODS

Thirty-eight healthy chinchillas, each weighing approximately 500 gm, were used for this study. Freshly mouse-passed type 7F *Streptococcus pneumoniae* were grown to early stationary phase and were frozen in aliquots in a glycerol-buffered albumin suspension at $-70°C$. An aliquot of the frozen pneumococcal suspension was thawed and diluted in sterile saline to contain 2×10^3 colony-forming units of pneumococci per milliliter immediately before injection into the animals. Under anesthesia induced by intramuscular ketamine hydrochloride (10 mg/kg) fur was removed from the dorsal bullae. Following aseptic preparation of the skin, 0.1 ml of diluted inoculum (200 pneumococci per ear) was injected using a tuberculin syringe (day 0). After three days the presence of POM was verified by otoscopy and the bulla was aspirated to obtain effusion fluid for culture. The POM animals were randomly assigned to six equal treatment groups. The various treatment regimens were given from days 4 to 10 (Table 1).

On day 11 the animals were anesthetized and the dorsal portion of the bulla was opened. Middle ear fluid was aspirated for culture and biochemical assay. Animals were perfused first with normal saline, then with Heidenhain's susa. Temporal bones were removed, fixed in buffered 10 percent formalin, decalcified with 5 percent trichloroacetic acid, dehydrated in a graded series of alcohol, embedded in celloidin, and sectioned at a thickness of 20μ. Every tenth section was stained with hematoxylin and eosin for microscopic examination.

Microbiologic, biochemical, and morphologic parameters, including culture results; presence or absence of effusion; concentrations of lysozyme, 6-keto-$PGF_{1\alpha}$ and PGE_2; and temporal bone histopathology were studied (Table 1).

Lysozyme concentrations were determined using Lysozyme Test Kit (Kallestad Co, Chaska, MN),[8] and PGs were measured by a double-antibody radioimmunoassay method.[9] Data were analyzed using the analysis of variance method.

TABLE 1 Treatment Regimens and Factors Tested

Experimental Regimens	*Factors Tested*
Saline control	Cultures at 3 and 11 days
Procaine penicillin G, 100,000 U/kg/day IM	Presence of effusion
Hydrocortisone (Solu-Cortef), 4 mg/kg/day in 2 doses q 12 h IP	Lysozyme
Ibuprofen 30 mg/kg/day in 2 doses q 12 h IP	6-keto-$PGF_{1\alpha}$
Penicillin plus hydrocortisone	PGE_2
Penicillin plus ibuprofen	Temporal bone histopathology

TABLE 2 Summary of Results

Experimental Groups	Culture Positive Day 3	Culture Positive Day 11	No. Ears with Fluid at Day 11	Average Volume of Fluid (μl)	Lysozyme (μg/ml)	6-Keto-$PGF_{1\alpha}$ (ng/ml)	PGE_2 (ng/ml)
1. Saline	12/12*	10/10	10	452.5	113.8	2.99	34.65
2. Penicillin	12/14	2/10	1	100	63	18.00	70
3. Hydrocortisone	9/14	8/10	7	405	104.3	1.54	69.51
4. Ibuprofen	10/12	11/12	9	415	99.8	4.62	72.38
5. Penicillin + hydrocortisone	6/12	0/12	2	575	80	.33	0
6. Penicillin + ibuprofen	7/12	0/10	4	587.5	85.5	.37	1.45

*Number positive/number tested

RESULTS

Results are summarized in Table 2. Statistical analysis of data is summarized in Table 3.

Culture Results

Three days after inoculation most ears were culture positive. After treatment all of the saline control group's ear cultures (ten of ten) remained positive, as did most of those from animals treated with hydrocortisone or ibuprofen. Conversely, most cultures from animals in the three groups treated with penicillin were sterile. The differences between the treated versus control, "pure" (hydrocortisone or ibuprofen alone) versus "mixed" (pencillin plus hydrocortisone or penicillin plus ibuprofen), and "penicillin" versus "non-penicillin" were statistically significant ($p < 0.001$) (Tables 2 and 3).

TABLE 3 Analysis of Variance

Contrasts	Variables: *a*	*b*	*c*	*d*	*e*	*f*
A	S ($p < 0.001$)	S ($p < 0.001$)	S ($p < 0.001$)	NS	S ($p < 0.05$)	NS
B	NS†	NS	NS	NS	NS	NS
C	NS	NS	NS	NS	NS	NS
D	NS	S ($p < 0.001$)	S ($p < 0.01$)	NS	S ($p < 0.02$)	S ($p < 0.05$)
E	NS	S ($p < 0.001$)	S ($p < 0.01$)	NS	S ($p < 0.02$)	S ($p < 0.05$)

Contrasts: A, Treated (2, 3, 4, 5, 6) versus control (1)
B, Hydrocortisone (3) versus ibuprofen (4)
C, Penicillin + hydrocortisone (5) versus penicillin + ibuprofen (6)
D, "Pure" (3, 4) versus "mixed" (5, 6)
E, "Penicillin" (2, 5, 6) versus "Nonpenicillin" (3, 4)

Variables: a, Culture results at 3 days
b, Culture results at 11 days
c, Presence of fluids
d, Lysozyme level
e, 6-Keto-$PGF_{1\alpha}$
f, PGE_2 level

Experimental Groups: 1, Saline control
2, Penicillin
3, Hydrocortisone
4, Ibuprofen
5, Penicillin plus hydrocortisone
6, Penicillin plus ibuprofen

*S, significant difference
†NS, no significance

Presence of Fluids

Fluid was present in all ears of saline control animals, in 70 percent of those treated with hydrocortisone, and in 75 percent of the ibuprofen group. In the three groups in which penicillin was given, from 10 to 40 percent had fluid in the middle ear (Table 2). The difference between treated and control animals was significant ($p < 0.001$). Significant differences were also found between "pure" and "mixed" and between "penicillin" and "nonpenicillin" groups ($p < 0.001$) (Table 3).

Lysozyme Concentrations

The lysozyme concentrations were largest in control ears, followed by the hydrocortisone, ibuprofen, penicillin plus ibuprofen, penicillin plus hydrocortisone, and penicillin groups in order of decreasing amount; however, the differences were not statistically significant.

6-Keto-PGF$_{1\alpha}$ Concentration

Short-lived prostacyclin (PGI_2) is measured by the stable end product 6-keto-PGF$_{1\alpha}$. The largest amounts of 6-keto-PGF$_{1\alpha}$ were found in the penicillin group and the lowest in the two combination therapy groups. The difference between treated and control groups was significant ($p < 0.05$), as was that between "pure" and "mixed" ($p < 0.02$).

PGE$_2$ Concentrations

The PGE_2 concentrations were smallest in the specimens from animals treated with penicillin and either hydrocortisone or ibuprofen. The differences between "pure" versus "mixed" and "penicillin" versus "nonpenicillin" were significant ($p < 0.05$).

The histopathologic findings are summarized in Table 4. The degree of inflammation was the greatest in animals that were not treated with penicillin. More metaplasia was seen in the ibuprofen group than in any other treatment group.

DISCUSSION

Penicillin therapy, with or without an anti-inflammatory agent, sterilized all but two ears. By

TABLE 4 Histopathology of Temporal Bones

Middle Ear Mucosa Pathologic Findings

Experimental Group	Hyperemia	Edema	Leukocytes: PMN	Leukocytes: Mono	Metaplasia	Focal Hemorrhage
Saline	++	++	++	+	+	+
Penicillin	0	0	+	+	0	0
Hydrocortisone	+++	+++	+	+	+	+
Ibuprofen	++	++	++	++	+++	+
Penicillin + hydrocortisone	0	0	0	0	0	0
Penicillin + ibuprofen	+	+	+	+	+	+

Middle Ear Space Pathologic Findings

Experimental Group	Effusion	Leukocytes: PMN	Leukocytes: Mono	Granulation Tissue	Osteoneogenesis	Hemorrhage
Saline	+++	+++	++	++	+	+
Penicillin	0	0	0	0	0	0
Hydrocortisone	+++	+++	++	0	+	++
Ibuprofen	+++	+++	++	++	+	+
Penicillin + hydrocortisone	+	0	0	0	0	0
Penicillin + ibuprofen	+	++	++	0	0	0

0, none
+, scant
++, moderate
+++, diffuse

chance, there were more culture-positive ears in control animals than in treated animals on day 3, before treatment was initiated.

Presence of fluid closely paralleled the culture results. Untreated and ibuprofen-treated animals had the largest number of fluid-filled ears, suggesting that ibuprofen stimulated fluid production in the middle ear mucosa by promoting production of a lipoxygenase product, such as mono-hydroxy-eicosatetraenoic acid (HETE), which has been shown to increase mucus release in cultured human lung tissue.[10] These findings correlate well with histopathologic observations, which showed the largest degree of metaplasia and increased goblet cell population in the ibuprofen-treated group. It is possible that lipoxygenase products of AA in the middle ear are partly responsible for the pathogenesis of chronic otitis media with effusion (OME). Thus, lipoxygenase inhibitors may have a role in the treatment of chronic OME.

We previously reported that lysozyme concentrations were greatest in culture-positive middle ear fluids (MEEs) and in cases of recurrent OME, and the concentrations decreased after penicillin treatment.[8] The present study showed the largest amount of lysozyme in control animals and the smallest amount in penicillin-treated animals.

It was surprising that neither corticosteroid nor ibuprofen therapy alone blocked PG synthesis despite administration of therapeutic doses of each drug based on studies in humans. However, the combination of pencillin with either hydrocortisone or ibuprofen inhibited PG synthesis significantly compared with either drug alone. As such, the anti-inflammatory agents have proportionately less PG synthesis to inhibit when given with penicillin than when given without penicillin.

Although PG synthesis was inhibited with the combination of penicillin and an anti-inflammatory drug, none of the regimens had a significant effect on lysozyme concentrations.

The results of our study may be summarized as follows: Penicillin is the single most important factor in the treatment of POM.

A combination of penicillin plus corticosteroid is the best mode of therapy, followed by penicillin only and penicillin plus ibuprofen.

Corticosteroid or ibuprofen alone is not adequate for the treatment of POM.

Ibuprofen seems to induce fluid secretion by causing metaplasia of middle ear mucosa. This is probably caused by increased lipoxygenase products due to inhibition of cyclooxygenase.

However, caution should be exercised in translating these data to the clinical setting.

This study was supported by a grant from the Upjohn Company, Kalamazoo, MI, and Grant # NS-14538 from the National Institutes of Health.

We gratefully acknowledge Dr. Chap Le for statistical analysis of data, Dr. Dan Hwang of Louisiana State University for providing PG antibodies, Sherry Lamey for photomicrography, Mary Lou and Jim Edlin for excellent technical assistance, and JoAnn Knox for typing this manuscript. We are grateful to the Upjohn Company, Kalamazoo, MI, for providing funds in partial support of this study.

REFERENCES

1. Schwarz RH, Puglese J, Schwarz MD: Use of a short course of prednisone for treating middle ear effusion. A double-blind crossover study. Ann Otol Rhinol Laryngol 89 (Suppl 68): 296, 1980
2. Persico M, Podoshin L, Fradis M: Otitis media with effusion. A steroid and antibiotic therapeutic trial before surgery. Ann Otol Rhinol Laryngol 87:191, 1978
3. Jackson RT: Autonomic stimulation, osmolarity and prostaglandin effects in the eustachian tube. Ann Otol Rhinol Laryngol 80:313, 1971
4. Bernstein JM, Okazaki R, Reisman RE: Prostaglandin in middle ear effusions. Arch Otolaryngol 102:257, 1976
5. Smith DM, Jung TTK, Juhn SK, et al: Prostaglandins in experimental otitis media. Arch Otorhinolaryngol 225:207, 1979
6. Jung TTK, Smith DM, Juhn SK, Gerrard JM: Prostaglandins and otitis media: Studies in the chinchilla. Otolaryngol Head Neck Surg 88:316, 1980
7. Jung TTK, Juhn SK, Gerrard JM: Identification of prostaglandins and other arachidonic acid metabolites in experimental otitis media. Prostaglandins Leukotrienes Med 8:249, 1982
8. Juhn SK, Huff JS, Paparella MM: Certain oxidative and hydrolytic enzymes in the middle ear effusion in serous otitis media. Arch Otorhinolaryngol 212:119, 1976
9. Hwang DH, Mathias MM, Dupont J, Meyer DL: Lino/eate enrichment of diet and prostaglandin metabolism in rats. J Nutr 105:995, 1975
10. Marom Z, Shelhamer JH, Kaliner M: Effects of arachidonic acid and prostaglandin on the release of mucous glycoprotein from human airway in vitro. J Clin Inv 67:1695, 1981

A COMPARATIVE TRIAL OF STEROIDS VERSUS PLACEBOS FOR TREATMENT OF CHRONIC OTITIS MEDIA WITH EFFUSION

LEO G. NIEDERMAN, M.D., MPH, VALRE WALTER-BUCHHOLTZ, M.S.N., and THERESA JABALAY, M.A.

Few pediatric conditions are as prevalent and yet as therapeutically frustrating as otitis media with effusion. No treatment, either medical or surgical, has clearly been shown to be efficacious. Several reports to date have suggested that a short course of systemic steroids alone or in combination with antibiotics clears up effusion.[1–5] We report the results of a double-blind study comparing steroid treatment and placebo in children with middle ear effusion persisting for eight weeks or longer.

MATERIALS AND METHODS

Children 2 years of age or older seen in the Ambulatory Care Clinics at Michael Reese Hospital and Medical Center between December 1980 and May 1982 were eligible for participation in the study. All children had referring diagnoses of either acute otitis media or nonsuppurative (serous) otitis medial. All were otherwise in good health and had no craniofacial abnormalities (such as cleft palate), no systemic condition predisposing to middle ear disease (for example, immunodeficiency, Down's syndrome), and no history of previous otologic surgery.

Children were seen within three weeks of referral and if middle ear effusion was present at this visit, they were seen subsequently at twenty-one-day intervals. At the initial visit a standardized history was obtained, a standardized pneumo-otoscopic examination was conducted, and tympanometry was performed using a Grason-Stadler automated otoadmittance meter (model 1722). The diagnosis of middle ear effusion was based on the tympanogram using a "peak" versus "no peak" classification as described by Fria and colleagues.[6] When this classification and instrument are used, tympanometry has been shown to be sensitive (0.87) and specific (0.81) for middle ear effusion when compared with myringotomy.[6]

Children with tympanometric evidence of unilateral effusion persisting in the same ear for eight weeks or bilateral effusion persisting for eight weeks were eligible for randomized entry into the study. All children had three or more tympanograms during this pre-entry period. Children meeting these criteria were randomized (using a list of preselected random numbers) to receive either dexamethasone or placebo. Parental informed consent was obtained.

Dexamethasone (0.1 mg/ml or 0.75 mg/tablet) and placebo, both provided by the manufacturer (Merck Sharp and Dohme), were identical in appearance and taste and contained the same inactive ingredients. All medications were dispensed by a hospital pharmacist in a double-blind design. Parents were given an individualized calendar with daily dose recorded and instructions to dispense the medication at the same time each morning. Adverse effects and compliance were assessed from alternate-day telephone contact and measurement of medication at the two-week follow-up visit.

The dexamethasone dosage was 0.15 mg/kg per day up to a maximum of 6 mg per day on days 1 and 2; 0.075 mg/kg per day up to a maximum of 3 mg per day on days 3 and 4; 0.0375 mg/kg per day up to a maximum of 1.5 mg per day on days 5 through 7; and 0.0375 mg/kg per day to a maximum of 1.5 mg per day in children over 40 kg and to a maximum of 0.75 mg per day in children less than 40 kg on days 9, 11, and 13.

Children were examined at two weeks after entry just after medication was completed and again at five weeks after entry. Presence of middle ear effusion was determined by tympanometric criteria, as previously described. Statistical analysis was performed using Fisher's exact test for frequency counts and Student's *t* test for comparison of means.[7]

RESULTS

Twenty-seven children were eligible for randomization. One declined entry into the study and four children were randomized but did not comply either with medication or with follow-up appointments. Twenty-two children with persistent effusion complied with the medical regimen and returned for a two-week follow-up visit. Two of these participants, one in each treatment group, failed to return for the five-week follow-up examination.

Some characteristics purported to influence the persistence of middle ear effusion and their distribution by treatment groups are shown in Table 1. Although sampling was not stratified by any characteristic, there were no significant differences between treatment groups except for duration of effusion. Children randomized to the placebo group had a longer mean duration of effusion—78 days compared with 66 days for the steroid treated children ($p = 0.02$). Other historical characteristics, including family size, personal and family history of allergy, number of episodes of middle ear disease, and symptoms at initial examination, though not shown in Table 1, were similar between the two groups.

Table 2 shows the outcomes in the groups at two-week and five-week follow-up evaluations. At two weeks five of 12 steroid-treated children had resolution of effusion in one or both middle ears compared with none of ten children in the placebo group ($p = 0.040$). The other comparisons in Table 2 are not statistically significant, although steroid-treated children showed relatively better outcomes. However, no persistent effect of steroid treatment was seen at the five-week evaluation in the five children with previous resolution at the two-week evaluation. Three of these children had recurrent effusion at the five-week examination, one remained free of effusion, and the fifth failed to keep the five-week appointment. He was seen two months later and had recurrent middle ear effusion.

None of the factors listed in Table 1 explains the response in the dexamethasone treatment group at two weeks. In particular, the mean duration of effusion was similar for children with resoluton of effusion (71.8 days) and children with no resolution (72.2 days). At the five-week evaluation, however, the mean duration of effusion was shorter in children with resolution in any ear compared to children with persisting effusion (64.3 days versus 75.1 days, $p = 0.045$).

All twenty-two participants were contacted by phone on alternate days and were judged compliant; that is, at least 70 percent of medication doses were correctly given. No significant adverse effects were seen in any study participant. One steroid-treated child had acute otitis media when seen at the two-week examination and was treated with antibiotics.

TABLE 1 Characteristics of Children with Middle Ear Effusion Persisting Eight Weeks or Longer by Treatment Groups

Characteristics	*Dexamethasone Group*	*Placebo Group*
Number	12	10
Mean age in months (minimum–maximum)	46 (26–84)	75 (29–171)
Males	9	7
Mean duration of effusion in days (minimum–maximum)	66 (55–83)*	78 (64–99)*
Bilateral OME	8	9
Antibiotics in previous 2 months	9	7
Fall-winter entry	7	5
Abnormal hearing (no./no. tested)	6/6	5/6

*$p = 0.02$

DISCUSSION

Although published studies have shown some beneficial effect of steroids on middle ear effusion, experimental design, case definition, and control for confounding clinical and demographic characteristics have differed among reports or have not been clearly stated. This report has addressed some of these methodologic issues by using a previously validated definition of middle ear effusion; by using a randomized double-blind, controlled experimental design; and by choosing a rigorously defined study group.

The results of this study do not support the clinical efficacy of short-term systemic steroids for children with middle ear effusion persisting for longer than eight weeks. Although by the most liberal response criteria (resolution of effusion in any involved middle ear) there was a marginally statistically significant effect ($p = 0.04$) at the two-week evaluation, no enduring effect was found three weeks after steroids were discontinued. Further follow-up of these children (from two to 14

TABLE 2 Status of Effusion at Two and Five Weeks by Treatment Groups

	At Two Weeks		*At Five Weeks*	
	Dexamethasone (N = 12)	*Placebo (N = 10)*	*Dexamethasone (N = 11)*	*Placebo (N = 9)*
Number of children with resolution:				
In any ear	5 (42%)*	0 (0%)*	5 (45%)	2 (22%)
In all ears	3 (25%)	0 (0%)	4 (36%)	1 (11%)

*$p = 0.04$

months) showed that only four children, two in each treatment group, had prolonged resolution of effusion. Two of these children had shown no response during the study period.

The small sample size of this study raises the question of a type II error and militates against inferring that there may be no efficacious effect from steroids. Our data suggest, however, that any effect is transient and temporally related to steroid administration. In view of the known risks involved with long-term steroid treatment,[8] and in view of the still unclear detrimental effects of chronic middle ear effusion,[9] the clinical use of steroids for chronic effusion appears unfounded.

This project was supported in part by grant #BRSG S07 RR05476 awarded by the Biomedical Research Support Grant Program, Division of Research Resources, National Institutes of Health.

REFERENCES

1. Oppenheimer RP: Serous otitis—a review of 922 cases. Eye Ear Nose Throat Mon 54:316, 1975
2. Oppenheimer P: Short-term steroid therapy. Arch Otolaryngol 88:46, 1968
3. Persico M, Podoshin L, Fradis M: Otitis media with effusion: A steroid and antibiotic therapeutic trial before surgery. Ann Otol Rhinol Laryngol 87:191, 1978
4. Heisse JW Jr: Secretory otitis media: Treatment with depomethylprednisolone. Laryngoscope 54:54, 1963
5. Schwartz RH, Puglese J, Schwartz DM: Use of a short course of prednisone for treating middle ear effusion. Ann Otol Rhinol Laryngol 89 (Suppl 68): 296, 1980
6. Fria TJ, Cantekin EI, Probst G: Validation of an automatic otoadmittance middle ear analyzer. Ann Otol Rhinol Laryngol 89:253, 1980
7. Statistical Analysis System: *SAS Users Guide*. Carey, NC: SAS Institute Inc, 1979
8. Chamberlin P, Meyer WJ: Management of pituitary-adrenal suppression secondary to corticosteroid therapy. Pediatrics 67:245, 1981
9. Bluestone CD, Klein JO, Paradise JL, et al: Workshop on effects of otitis media on the child. Pediatrics 71:639, 1983

MEDICAL TREATMENT USING ANTIBIOTICS

ANTIMICROBIAL MANAGEMENT AND PREVENTION OF OTITIS MEDIA WITH EFFUSION

JEROME O. KLEIN, M.D.

Prior to the introduction of antimicrobial agents, otitis media either resolved spontaneously or came to medical attention. The physician could manage the patient with warm compresses and analgesia or could incise and drain the middle ear abscess. Suppurative otitis media was a frequent reason for admission of children to the hospital. In 1932 otitis media, mastoiditis, and intracranial complications accounted for 27 percent of pediatric admissions to Bellevue Hospital in New York City.[1] Today we are in the enviable position of choosing among many effective antimicrobial agents. Questions remain, however, about optimal usage of drugs for acute and chronic infection and for prevention of disease. In addition, we must be alert for new or newly important microbial pathogens (such as *Branhamella catarrhalis* and *Chlamydia trachomatis*) and changes in susceptibility of bacteria to drugs of established value (ampicillin-resistant strains of *Hemophilus influenzae*). New drugs with features of potential value for patients with otitis media must be compared with older drugs. New uses of old drugs are identified (prophylaxis for children with recurrent episodes of otitis media). This chapter deals with selected aspects of assessing the efficacy of antimicrobial drugs for treatment of this disease.

ASSESSMENT OF EFFICACY OF ANTIMICROBIAL AGENTS

The efficacy of antimicrobial agents may be assessed in terms of clinical, microbiologic, and immunologic results (Table 1). Clinically, we expect effective drugs to produce a significant decrease in signs and symptoms of disease in 48 to 72 hours, to prevent the disease from extending to adjacent tissues, and to prevent complications. Recent studies by Mandell and colleagues suggest that we should also consider the effect on time to resolution of middle ear effusion.[2] More children who received cefaclor were free of effusion at 14 days after onset of therapy than children who received amoxicillin. The basis for this effect is unknown, but the data suggest that time to resolution of middle ear effusion should be included in assessment of antimicrobial agents evaluated for use in otitis media.

The major microbiologic criterion for efficacy of antimicrobial drugs is sterilization of the middle ear infection. Studies by Howie and Ploussard attest to the value of the information provided by this "in vivo susceptibility test."[3] Recent studies indicate that bacterial antigens are frequently found in middle ear fluids. Pneumococcal polysaccharide has been identified in the vast majority of fluids in which the organism is isolated and in many specimens that have no bacterial growth.[4,5] The role of these bacterial products in disease and the effect of antibacterial drugs in processing and eliminating the antigens are unknown but may be important in dealing with the problem of effusion that persists after acute infection.

TABLE 1 Efficacy of Antimicrobial Agents for Treatment of Otitis Media

Clinical Efficacy:
Resolution of acute signs
Decrease in duration of middle ear effusion
Prevention of complications
Microbiologic Efficacy:
Sterilization of infection
Elimination of microbial antigens
Immunologic Efficacy:
Development of local and systemic immunity

The immunology of otitis media is incompletely understood, and very little information is available about the effect of antimicrobial agents on the development of local and systemic immunity after acute or chronic otitis media. Does the use of antibiotics limit the immune response to infection in the middle ear? Do antimicrobial agents differ in their effect on development of immunity? Will the time of usage of drugs affect immunity? How will these features affect the duration of fluid in the middle ear and protection against recurrences of type-specific infection? These and other questions are currently under investigation.

ARE ANTIMICROBIAL AGENTS NECESSARY FOR TREATMENT OF OTITIS MEDIA?

It has been postulated that the use of antimicrobial agents is not necessary for initial management of acute otitis media. This is most likely correct with regard to selected children; many with signs of acute otitis media do not need antimicrobial agents. The reasons for resolution of disease without drugs are given in Table 2. Nevertheless, the limited incidence of suppurative complications of otitis media in areas where antimicrobial agents are used extensively, when compared with the period of time when these drugs were unavailable or with areas of the world where drugs are not available today, speaks for their beneficial effects.

ANALYSIS OF STUDIES OF EFFICACY OF ANTIMICROBIAL AGENTS

The current literature does not answer all our questions about the optimal use of antimicrobial agents. Questions about the efficacy of drugs based on clinical, microbiologic, and immunologic parameters need to be answered. We must critically review studies to determine that they are of appropriate design: Are the criteria for enrollment of patients provided; is the disease defined; are appropriate techniques used for observation of end points; is the sample size adequate for evaluation; was a control group necessary, and, if so, were the criteria for the group adequate? Studies of appropriate design are needed so that unanswered questions will not remain so.

TABLE 2 Reasons for Resolution of Otitis Media with Effusion Without Usage of Antimicrobial Agents

Effusion is due to a nonbacterial organism
Effusion is due to a noninfectious cause
Effusion persists from a prior episode of otitis media with effusion
Effusion clears by:
Drainage through eustachian tube
Drainage through perforation of tympanic membrane
Absorption by middle ear mucosa

REFERENCES

1. Bakwin H, Jacobinzer H: Prevention of purulent otitis media in infants. J Pediatr 14:730, 1939
2. Mandel EM, Bluestone CD, Rockette HE, et al: Duration of effusion after antibiotic treatment for acute otitis media: Comparison of cefaclor and amoxicillin. Pediatr Infect Dis 1:310, 1982
3. Howie VM, Ploussard JH: The "in vivo sensitivity test": Bacteriology of middle ear exudate during antimicrobial therapy in otitis media. Pediatrics 44:940, 1969
4. Ostfeld E, Altmann GL: Evaluation of countercurrent immunoelectrophoresis as a diagnostic tool in bacterial otitis media. Ann Otol Rhinol Laryngol 89 (68):110, 1980
5. Luotonen J, Herva E, Karma P, et al: The bacteriology of acute otitis media in children with special reference to *Streptococcus pneumoniae* as studied by bacteriological and antigen detection methods. Scand J Infect Dis 13:177, 1981

PENICILLIN TREATMENT FOR ACUTE OTITIS MEDIA IN CHILDREN: WHEN, HOW MUCH, HOW FREQUENTLY, HOW LONG?

JENS THOMSEN, M.D., KAREN-INGER MEISTRUP-LARSEN, M.D., NIELS MYGIND, M.D., HENNING SØRENSEN, M.D., NIELS JON JOHNSEN, M.D., and JØRGEN SEDERBERG-OLSEN, M.D.

In a previous placebo-controlled investigation on the effect of penicillin on acute otitis media in children we demonstrated that penicillin has a rapid pain-relieving and therapeutic effect. However, after two or three days of treatment there was no difference between the penicillin- and placebo-treated patients.[1] The same investigation showed that the spontaneous course was so favorable that only half the placebo-treated children had symptoms for more than 12 hours. Nothing in the trial indicated that penicillin treatment given for more than two days had any effect on the subsequent course of the disease. We have, therefore, conducted a double-blind trial comparing two and seven days of penicillin treatment in children with acute otitis media. A more complete account of the results has been given elsewhere.[2]

MATERIALS AND METHODS

Patients

One hundred three children between the ages of 1 and 10 with acute otitis media and earache for 1 to 48 hours were included in the trial. The diagnosis of otitis was made if the child was crying with pain and the tympanic membrane, as studied with a pneumatic otoscope, was red and inflamed. The exclusion criteria were (1) other treatment apart from acetylsalicylic acid; (2) antibiotic treatment within the last month; (3) acute otitis media within the previous month; (4) suspected chronic otitis media; (5) treatment for secretory otitis media within the previous 12 months; (6) concurrent disease requiring antibiotics, for example, pneumonia or tonsillitis; and (7) suspected allergy to penicillin. All children fulfilling the inclusion criteria entered the trial with the exception of two whose parents refused to give informed consent.

Treatment

A granulate of the potassium salt of penicillin V (Primcillin) was used. The penicillin and placebo granulates were supplied in coded bottles by Astra Pharmaceuticals, Södertälje, Sweden. The patients were given a daily average dose of 55 mg/kg, half in the morning and half in the evening. All children were supplied with two bottles; the first to be used contained enough penicillin V for two days (four doses), and the second contained active drug or placebo. The second bottle was coded and its contents were given for the next five days. Acetylsalicylic acid tablets were supplied as the only analgesic treatment permitted. The maximum permitted dosage was 50 mg/kg/per day for three days.

Symptom Monitoring

Rating scales for pain, fever, and common cold symptoms were filled out by the parents every day. The number of aspirin tablets as well as drainage of secretion from the ear were recorded. Otoscopy and tympanometry were performed after two weeks.

Statistical Methods

One-sided chi-square test with Yates correction and a 5 percent significance level was used for all calculations.

RESULTS

The results of the pain score are given in Figure 1. Pretreatment symptoms and symptoms on the first treatment day (when both groups received penicillin) were more pronounced in the "penicillin-2-days" group, but the differences were not significant. Most patients were without symptoms after two days of penicillin treatment, and there was no difference between the two groups. Furthermore, there was no difference between the two groups with regard to other factors concerning the acute course of the disease and recovery, tympanometry and follow-up after two weeks, and fever (Fig. 2) or common cold symptoms (Table 1).

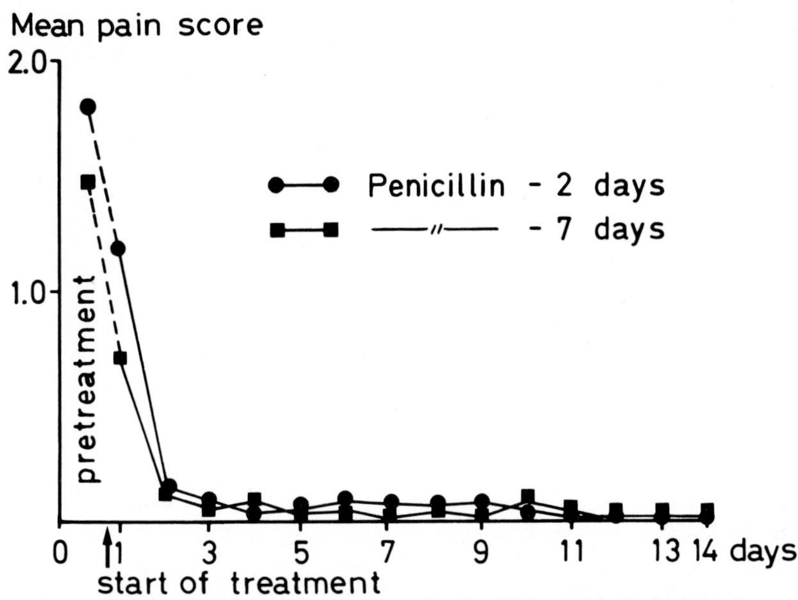

Figure 1. Mean symptom scores for earache. A score 1 indicates that the child complained of pain, and score 2 that it cried from pain. "Day 1" of treatment is the time from the first visit until midnight: the average duration of this "day" was 8 hours.

DISCUSSION

We have previously demonstrated the benign course of acute otitis media in most children,[1] and this has been confirmed by Buchem and associates.[3] The latter authors found no substantial differences between penicillin- and placebo-treated children, whereas we demonstrated a pain relieving effect of penicillin within the very first days.

In acute otitis media a maximum penicillin V concentration of 6 μg/ml has been reported in middle ear secretions 1 hour after oral intake of 25 mg/kg body weight.[4] This penicillin concentration is sufficient to eliminate pneumococci, susceptible *Branhamella catarrhalis,* and the majority of *Hemophilus influenza* strains.[5] In addition, it has been shown by Rundkrantz and Sundför that a simplified dispensation with only two doses is as ef-

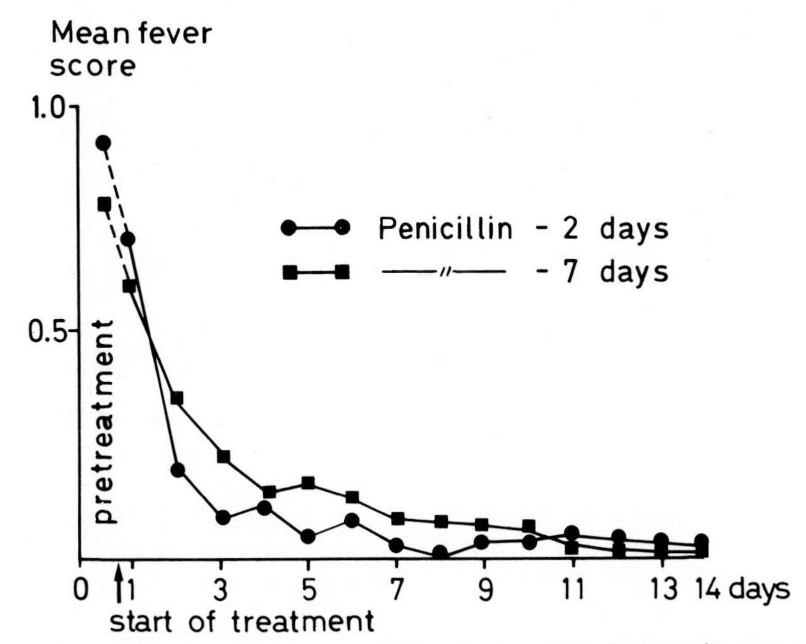

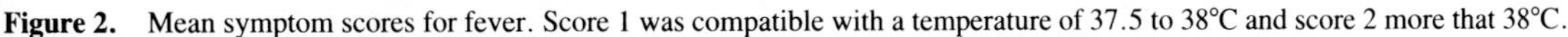
Figure 2. Mean symptom scores for fever. Score 1 was compatible with a temperature of 37.5 to 38°C and score 2 more that 38°C.

TABLE 1 Results of Some Parameters Depicting the Acute Course of the Disease and Healing in the "Penicillin-7-Days" Group and in the "Penicillin-2-Days" Group

		Penicillin-7-Days Group	*Penicillin-2-Days Group*
Contralateral otitis	Days 1, 2	2*	6*
	Days 3–7	5	2
	Days 8–14	1	1
Myringotomy	Days 1, 2	1	0
	Days 3–7	1	0
	Days 8–14	0	0
Spontaneous perforation	Days 1, 2	0*	6*
	Days 3–7	2	2
	Days 8–14	1	1
Amoxicillin		2	4
Average days of otorrhea		2.3 (N = 8)	3.5 (N = 12)
Relapses of otitis media		3	5

*Days one and two both groups received penicillin

fective as three doses daily.[6] Therefore, two divided doses (half in the morning and half in the evening) seems to be a reasonable choice.

Ingvarsson and Lundgren, comparing the results of five days and ten days of penicillin treatment in acute otitis media, concluded that reduction of the treatment time does not lead to increased risk of complications in the form of recurrence, treatment failure, or development of secretory otitis media.[7] In our earlier investigation we raised the question of whether penicillin treatment for more than two days had any advantages compared with a two-day treatment, and we believe we have demonstrated by the present trial that this is not the case. The number of patients in this study is small, and care must be taken in drawing conclusions, but it appears that the advantage of continuing treatment beyond the first two days is, at most, marginal.

There are several advantages of a shortened treatment period. The treatment modality is very simple, fewer side effects from the drugs should be encountered, and the cost of the treatment is reduced. Possibly there is a reduced risk of developing resistant bacterias.

The results of our study, supported by those of Buchem and associates,[3] have influenced our attitude toward treatment of acute otitis media. In children who have not had severe pain resistant to previously administered analgesics we apply masterful inactivity for 6 to 8 hours and give one or two doses of analgesics. If earache persists we give penicillin V, 55 mg/kg per day divided b.i.d. for two days. If symptoms persist the patient is again evaluated by the otologist. Myringotomy is performed in patients with severe pain, and amoxicillin is given when necessary. The implication of such graduated treatment is a significant reduction in the use of penicillin in acute otitis media. This reduction must be considered advantageous, provided it does not entail an increased risk of serious complications of acute otitis media. Based on the available information, there is nothing to indicate such an increased risk. We are confident that instructing the parents to call upon the otologist again if symptoms persist prevents complications better than a routine seven to ten days of penicillin therapy.

REFERENCES

1. Thomsen J, Meistrup-Larsen K-I, Sørensen H, et al: Penicillin and acute otitis media: Short and long-term results. Ann Otol Rhinol Laryngol. Suppl 68:271, 1980
2. Meistrup-Larsen K-I, Sederberg-Olsen J, Johnsen NJ, et al: Two versus seven days penicillin treatment for acute otitis media. A placebo controlled trial in children. Acta Otolaryngol, 1983, 96:99, 1983
3. Buchem FL, Dunk JHM, Hof MAH: Therapy of acute otitis media: Myringotomy, antibiotics, or neither? A double-blind study in children. Lancet 2:883, 1981
4. Ingvarsson L, Kamme C, Lundgren K: Concentration of penicillin V in serum and middle ear exudate during treatment of acute otitis media. Ann Otol Rhinol Laryngol Suppl 68:275, 1980
5. Kamme C: Susceptibility in vitro of *Haemophilus influenzae* to penicillin G, penicillin V and ampicillin. Acta Pathol Microbiol Scand 75:611, 1969
6. Rundcrantz H, Sundför A: Förenklad dosering av penicillin. Läkartidn 71:71, 1974
7. Ingvarsson L, Lundgren K: Penicillin treatment of acute otitis media in children. Acta Otolaryngol 94:283, 1982

TWICE DAILY ANTIMICROBIAL THERAPY FOR ACUTE OTITIS MEDIA

COLIN D. MARCHANT, M.D., PAUL A. SHURIN, M.D., JOAN C. WILTSHIRE, R.N., P.N.A., CANDICE E. JOHNSON, Ph.D., M.D., VIRGINIA A. TURCYZK, R.N., P.N.A., DIANA E. WASIKOWSKI, R.N., P.N.A., LINDA J. KNAPP, M.D., and MIMI A. TUTIHASI, M.D.

Comparative trials of antimicrobial agents for treatment of acute otitis media are required to meet the challenge of emerging antimicrobial drug resistance and to determine the efficacy of simplified treatment regimens. To assess the efficacy of twice daily antimicrobial therapy for acute otitis media we performed two randomized double-blind controlled trials.

MATERIALS AND METHODS

Details of the methods will be described elsewhere.[1] Briefly, two partially concurrent double-blind trials were performed. In the first trial, trimethoprim-sulfamethoxazole (TMP-SMZ), 4 mg TMP + 20 mg SMZ per kilogram twice daily, was compared with cefaclor, 20 mg/kg twice daily, in 129 children less than 2 years of age. In a second trial performed under the identical protocol, bacampicillin, 25 mg/kg twice daily for ten days, was compared with amoxicillin, 13.3 mg/kg thrice daily for ten days, in 69 children less than 2 years of age. Diagnosis of acute otitis media was determined by pneumatic otoscopy and confirmed by tympanocentesis. Middle ear exudates were streaked on chocolate and sheep blood agar plates and inoculated into Levinthal broth within 30 minutes of tympanocentesis. To determine in vivo antibacterial efficacy, middle ear exudates were cultured again three to six days later in patients whose original isolates contained bacterial pathogens. Overall success was defined as eradication of all pathogens from the middle ear exudate(s). Success against a specific pathogen was defined as eradication of that pathogen from the middle ear exudate(s) even if other pathogens persisted in cases of mixed etiology.

Patient compliance was monitored by bioassay of serum and urine at the three- to six-day visit.

RESULTS

The treatment groups were comparable in terms of age, sex, race, number of ears involved, and initial body temperature. Follow-up cultures were obtained in 90 percent of patients in the first trial. The overall success rate of 95 percent for TMP-SMZ was significantly different from the 70 percent observed with cefaclor (Table 1). The success rate for cases caused by *Hemophilus influenzae* was significantly lower in the cefaclor group. When analysis of overall success is restricted to those patients with positive serum or urine assays at the three- to six-day visit, success rates were 34/36 (94 percent) for TMP-SMZ compared with 25/34 (74 percent) for cefaclor (p = 0.027).

In the second trial, 83 percent of patients with pathogens had follow-up tympanocentesis. Success rates for bacampicillin- and amoxicillin-treated patients were not significantly different. The lower 95 percent confidence limit indicates that bacampicillin was at least 72 percent effective and amoxicillin at least 79 percent effective.

DISCUSSION

Our findings demonstrate that twice daily trimethoprim-sulfamethoxazole is a highly effective agent for treatment of acute otitis media. The prolonged half-life of TMP-SMZ and good penetration of both TMP and SMZ into middle ear fluid[2] may be important factors.

In contrast, cefaclor given twice daily failed to eradicate pathogens in 30 percent of cases. Moreover, the success rate of 56 percent for cefaclor treatment of otitis media caused by *H. influenzae* was similar to the 52 percent reported for placebo-treated patients.[3] Factors responsible for the higher failure rates with cefaclor may include

TABLE 1 Eradication of Pathogens from Middle Ear Exudate after Three to Six Days of Therapy

	No. Cures/No. Treated with Antimicrobial Therapy			
	Trial 1		*Trial 2*	
All Bacterial Cases	*Cefaclor 28/40 (70 ± 14)**	*Trimethoprim-Sulfamethoxazole 35/37 (95 ± 07)**	*Bacampicillin 14/16 (88 ± 16)*	*Amoxicillin 20/22 (91 ± 12)*
Streptococcus pneumoniae	16/20 (80)†	19/19 (100)†	10/10 (100)	12/12 (100)
Hemophilus influenzae	10/18 (56)‡	12/13 (92)‡	6/6 (100)	4/5 (80)
Branhamella catarrhalis	8/8 (100)	9/9 (100)	2/3 (67)	7/8 (88)
Streptococcus pyogenes (Group A)	———	0/1 (0)	1/1 (100)	———
Staphylococcus aureus	———	———	0/1 (0)	———

Note: ( ) = percentage, (±) = percentage with 95% confidence intervals
*$p = 0.017$
†$p = 0.12$
‡$p = 0.047$
All others, $p = 0.2$

the short half-life (30 to 60 minutes)[4] or an inadequate total daily dose of 40 mg/kg.[5] Cefaclor has been shown to penetrate middle ear fluid in from 42 percent[6] to more than 75 percent[4] of patients with chronic otitis media. It is unclear whether inadequate tissue penetration might explain the results of twice daily cefaclor treatment.

A previous study comparing twice daily with thrice daily cefaclor in 60 patients found no differences in clinical response with these regimens.[7] Although cefaclor has produced clinically satisfactory results when given three times a day in a number of trials,[8,9] no systematic bacteriologic data have been reported.

Bacampicillin given twice daily appears to be effective therapy, but large sample sizes are required to demonstrate high (> 90 percent) efficacy with more certainty. Our results with amoxicillin are similar to those reported by others.[10]

It may be argued that status at the end of therapy (usually ten days) is a more appropriate indicator of efficacy, but at present there are no systematic data regarding bacteriologic outcome after ten days of therapy. Since patients often fail to take the full prescribed course of therapy, it is our view that an antibacterial agent or regimen that eliminates pathogens more rapidly should be considered superior. This may be particularly important in patients with otitis media and bacteremia,[11,12] who may be at risk for complications.

Our investigation relies on bacteriologic outcome. Differences between agents or regimens in terms of bioavailability, tissue penetration, antibacterial spectrum, and interaction with other host factors are all reflected in success or failure as measured by in vivo efficacy. This outcome, pioneered by Howie and coworkers,[13] is also the most sensitive for detecting differences between antibacterial agents.[14] The feasibility of this outcome has been amply demonstrated by others.[3,10,13,15–17] Comparative trials of antibacterial drugs for urinary infections, streptococcal pharyngitis, gonococcal urethritis, and pulmonary tuberculosis all require bacteriologic proof in the assessment of efficacy. Acute otitis media should be added to this list.

This work was supported by Biomedical Research Support grant # RR05410 awarded to the Case Western Reserve University School of Medicine and by the Perinatal Clinical Research Center, Cleveland Metropolitan General Hospital, NIH USPHS grant # 5M01-RR00210.

REFERENCES

1. Marchant CD, Shurin PA, Turcyzk VE, et al: How should efficacy of antibacterial drugs for acute otitis media be measured? Results of a randomized trial of cefaclor compared to trimethoprim-sulfamethoxazole. Manuscript in preparation, 1983
2. Klimek JJ, Bates TR, Nightingale C, et al: Penetration characteristics of trimethoprim-sulfamethoxazole in middle ear fluid of patients with chronic serous otitis media. J Pediat 96:1087, 1980
3. Howie VM, Ploussard JH: Efficacy of fixed combination antibiotics versus separate components in otitis media. Clin Pediat 11:205, 1972
4. Ginsburg CM, McCracken GH, Nelson JD: Pharmacology of oral antibiotics used for treatment of otitis media and

tonsillopharyngitis in infants and children: Ann Otol Rhinol Laryngol 90(Suppl 84):37, 1981
5. Nelson JD, Ginsburg CM, Clashen JC, Jackson LH: Treatment of acute otitis media with cefaclor. Am J Dis Child 132:992, 1978
6. Lildholdt T, Cantekin EI, Marshak G, et al: Pharmacokinetics of cefaclor in chronic middle ear effusions. Ann Otol Rhinol Laryngol 90(Suppl 84):44, 1981
7. Tarpay M, Marks MI, Hopkins C, et al: Cefaclor therapy twice daily for acute otitis media. Am J Dis Child 136:33, 1982
8. Mandel EM, Bluestone CD, Cantekin EI, et al: Comparison of cefaclor and amoxicillin for acute otitis media with effusion. Ann Otol Rhinol Laryngol 90(Suppl 84):48, 1981
9. Berman S, Lauer BA: A controlled trial of cefaclor versus amoxicillin for treatment of acute otitis media in early infancy. J Pediat Infect Dis 2:30, 1983
10. Howie VM, Ploussard JH, Sloyer J: Comparison of ampicillin and amoxicillin in the treatment of otitis media in children. J Infect Dis 129(Suppl):181, 1974
11. Bratton L, Teele DW, Klein JO: Outcome of unsuspected pneumococcemia in children not initially admitted to the hospital. J Pediat 90:703, 1977
12. Marshall R, Teele DW, Klein JO: Unsuspected bacteremia due to *Haemophilus influenzae:* Outcome in children not initially admitted to hospital. J Pediat 95:690, 1979
13. Howie VM, Ploussard JH: The '*in vivo* sensitivity test': Bacteriology of middle ear exudates during antimicrobial therapy in otitis media. Pediatrics 44:940, 1969
14. Marchant C, Shurin PA: Antibacterial therapy for acute otitis media: A critical analysis. Rev Infect Dis 4:506, 1982
15. McLinn SE, Daly JF, Jones JE: Cephalexin monohydrate suspension: Treatment of otitis media. JAMA 234:171, 1975
16. McLinn SE: Cefaclor in treatment of otitis media and pharyngitis in children. Am J Dis Child 134:560, 1980
17. McLinn SE, Goldberg F, Kramer R, et al: Double-blind multicenter comparison of cyclacillin and amoxicillin for the treatment of acute otitis media. J Pediat 101:617, 1982

SUSCEPTIBILITY OF BETA-LACTAMASE–PRODUCING STRAINS OF *BRANHAMELLA CATARRHALIS* TO SELECTED, ORALLY ADMINISTERED ANTIMICROBIAL AGENTS

PAUL A. SHURIN, M.D., CHEE HOON KIM, DORIS FULTON, B.S., and COLIN D. MARCHANT, M.D.

In recent studies we have isolated *Branhamella catarrhalis* from the middle ear fluid of 20 percent of 243 infants with acute otitis media (AOM) and have found that 79 percent of the strains produce beta-lactamase. Thus, resistant strains of this bacterial species occur in 16 percent of infants with AOM and are the most prevalent antibiotic-resistant organisms in this infection. A similar epidemic rise in infection with this organism has been reported in Pittsburgh, Pennsylvania.[1] Apparently similar strains of *B. catarrhalis* have been isolated in many geographic locations.[2] It therefore appears likely that resistant strains of *B. catarrhalis* will be encountered with increasing frequency as agents of AOM. As a guide in planning optimal therapy and future drug trials, we have performed antimicrobial susceptibility tests of *B. catarrhalis* strains using tube-dilution methods.

MATERIALS AND METHODS

We tested 20 strains of *B. catarrhalis* isolated from tympanocentesis specimens and identified as producing beta-lactamase as described previously.[2] Tube-dilution susceptibility testing was performed in Mueller-Hinton broth in microtiter plates inoculated with appropriate concentrations of selected antimicrobial drugs. The minimal inhibitory concentration (MIC) was defined as the lowest concentration of each drug that prevented visible growth of the test organism after incubation (37°C) for 24 hours.

TABLE 1 Antimicrobial Susceptibilities of Beta-Lactamase–Producing *Branhamella Catarrhalis*

	Minimal Inhibitory Concentrations (mcg/ml)	
Drug	*Geometric Mean*	*Range*
Ampicillin	2.41	.39–50
Cefaclor	1.35	.18–6.25
Erythromycin	≤.39	≤.39, all strains
Sulfisoxazole	19.30	3.12–>800
Sulfamethoxazole	16.2	3.12–>800
Trimethoprim	>25	≥25, all strains

Potentially useful drug combinations were tested in ratios (by weight) that approximated their concentrations in body fluids during therapeutic use. The combinations tested were trimethoprim plus sulfamethoxazole and ampicillin in combination with either of the beta-lactamase inhibitors, clavulanic acid and sulbactam.

RESULTS

Minimal inhibitory concentrations for the 20 beta-lactamase–producing strains (BL+) are shown in Table 1. Erythromycin was the most active drug tested. Ampicillin had much less activity against BL+ strains than against BL− strains (BL− strains had MIC ≤ 0.006 mcg/m). Cefaclor was significantly less active against BL+ than against BL− strains when tested both by tube dilution and disk diffusion methods; the differences were less marked than for ampicillin. All strains were resistant to trimethoprim. Most strains were sensitive to sulfonamides, but three highly resistant isolates were identified (MIC > 800 mcg/ml for each).

Three drug combinations that are in clinical use for otitis media were tested. Equal concentrations (by weight) of either of two beta-lactamase inhibitors, clavulanic acid and sulbactam, produced more than a twenty-fold reduction in the concentration of ampicillin required to inhibit BL+ strains (Table 2).

Trimethoprim similarly reduced the MIC for sulfamethoxazole by 56 (Table 3). This was also documented for the sulfonamide-resistant strains. Synergistic bacterial killing was also documented with each of these drug combinations.

DISCUSSION

Beta-lactamase–producing strains of *B. catarrhalis* are common etiologic agents of AOM. Such strains are resistant to ampicillin and have intermediate susceptibility to cefaclor. Similar results have been reported by others.[3] Clinical studies are needed to define the importance of these findings for therapy of AOM. Sulfonamide resistance has not previously been described in this organism and may be relevant to the use of sulfonamides for prevention of AOM.

This study was supported by Biomedical Research Support grant # RR05410 awarded to the Case Western Reserve University School of Medicine and by the Perinatal Clinical Research Center, Cleveland Metropolitan General Hospital, NIH USPHS grant # 5M01-RR00210.

TABLE 2 In Vitro Susceptibility of Beta-Lactamase–Producing Strains of *Branhamella catarrhalis* to Ampicillin and to the Beta-Lactamase Inhibitors Clavulanic Acid and Sulbactam

	Minimal Inhibitory Concentrations (mcg/ml)		
Drug	*Geometric Mean*	*Range*	*Fold Reduction in Mean Ampicillin MIC*
Ampicillin	2.5	1.6–6.3	—
Clavulanic acid	6.3	6.3–6.3	—
Sulbactam	12.5	12.5–12.5	—
Ampicillin + clavulanic acid (1:1)	.098	.049–.39	26
Ampicillin + sulbactam (1:1)	.11	.049–.39	23

Note: Six strains tested in microtiter tube dilution assay.

TABLE 3 In Vitro Susceptibility of Beta-Lactamase–Producing Strains of *Branhamella catarrhalis* to Trimethoprim and Sulfamethoxazole

Drug	*Minimal Inhibitory Concentrations (mcg/ml)*		*Fold Reduction in Mean Sulfamethoxazole MIC*
	Geometric Mean	*Range*	
Trimethoprim	—	All > 25	—
Sulfamethoxazole	16.2	3.12–>800	—
Trimethoprim + sulfamethoxazole (1:19.5)	0.29	.08–1.32	56

Note: Seven strains tested in microtiter tube dilution assay.

REFERENCES

1. Kovatch AL, Wald ER, Michaels RH: β-Lactamase-producing *Branhamella catarrhalis* causing otitis media in children. J Pediatr 102:261, 1983
2. Shurin PA, Marchant CD, Kim CH, et al: Emergence of beta-lactamase-producing strains of *Branhamella catarrhalis* as important agents of acute otitis media. Pediatr Infect Dis 2:34, 1983
3. Wald E, Kovatch A, Rohn D, et al: Antimicrobial susceptibility of beta-lactamase-producing otic strains of *Branhamella catarrhalis*. Presented at the Third International Symposium on Recent Advances in Otitis Media with Effusion, Fort Lauderdale, May 1983

ANTIMICROBIAL THERAPY FOR CHRONIC OTITIS MEDIA WITH EFFUSION

GERALD B. HEALY, M.D.

Otitis media with effusion (OME) is the most common cause of hearing loss in children and is one of the most perplexing medical problems of infancy and childhood.[1]

Many terms, including "chronic secretory otitis media" and "serous otitis media," have been used to describe this process. More recently, the Committee on the Classification of Otitis Media proposed that the term "otitis media with effusion" be adopted in an effort to standardize nomenclature.[2] The disease itself, however, continues to elude efforts to establish a consistently effective treatment regimen.

Traditionally, otitis media with effusion has been thought to be a sterile process. Recently, however, several studies have identified, in the middle ear aspirants of children with chronic otitis media with effusion, bacteria similar to those found in acute otitis media.[3,4] In view of these studies it seemed appropriate to undertake a controlled clinical trial to evaluate the efficacy of antimicrobial therapy for chronic otitis media with effusion.

MATERIALS AND METHODS

The study was undertaken over a 12-month period between September 1, 1981, and August 31, 1982. Children between the ages of 2 and 5 years, referred to the author for treatment of chronic otitis media with effusion, were considered for the study.

Patients were not eligible for entry if any of the following conditions existed: prior history of tonsillectomy, adenoidectomy, and/or tympanostomy tube insertion; a middle ear abnormality, such as adhesive otitis media, tympanic membrane perforation, or cholesteatoma; facial anomalies or congenital syndromes (for example, Down's syndrome); a systemic illness, such as cystic fibrosis; acute suppurative otitis media; sinusitis; or a history of having received medical therapy for their middle ear effusion within the prior four weeks, including treatment with sympathomimetic amines, antihistamines, or antibiotics.

A complete history was taken from each patient and a careful examination of the head and neck was performed. The same examiner, who is a validated otoscopist,[5] evaluated all patients in the study. Pneumatic otoscopy was performed on each patient, as were tympanometry and middle ear muscle reflex testing. Air-conduction and bone-conduction thresholds were determined as well. The patients were re-evaluated six weeks later and, if an effusion was still present, the patient was randomized either to receive antimicrobial therapy for four weeks or to serve as a control. Patients were re-evaluated at the end of the fourth week and data collected. The investigation was not blinded as to whether treatment was given or withheld.

Drug Administration and Compliance

Trimethoprim-sulfamethoxazole (8 and 40 mg/kg, respectively, per 24 hours in two divided doses) was administered in a liquid preparation to the antimicrobial group for four weeks. Parents were required to record administration of the medication on a daily calendar and to return all bottles of medication used during the four weeks at the follow-up examination.

RESULTS

Two hundred patients were entered and randomized. There were 63 males and 37 females in the antimicrobial group and 58 males and 42 females in the observation group. Eighty-one patients in the antibiotic group had bilateral effusions at entry, while 19 had unilateral effusion, for a total of 181 ears with effusion. Seventy-six patients in the control group had bilateral effusions at entry, while 24 had unilateral involvement, for a total of 176 ears with effusion.

At the completion of the four-week period of treatment or observation, 96 patients in the antibiotic group and 93 patients in the observation group were evaluated. Two patients in the antibiotic group had acute suppurative otitis media during the four-week treatment period and two patients failed to return for follow-up. Five patients in the observation group had acute suppurative otitis media during the trial period and two patients failed to return for follow-up.

Compliance was determined from both medication calendars and from measurement of medication remaining in the bottles. More medication use was reported by the measurement method than by the calendar method. According to the calendar method, 89 percent of patients received at least 85 percent of the prescribed medication.

Fifty-six patients (58 percent) in the antibiotic group were free of middle ear effusion after four weeks, while nine patients had unilateral effusions. This represented 121 ears free of effusion. Thirty-one patients in this group had bilateral effusions at four weeks. When this number is combined with the nine patients who had unilateral effusion, there was a total of 71 ears with effusion in the antibiotic group (Table 1). Six patients (6 percent) in the observation group were free of effusion after the four-week follow-up period. When combined with the 22 patients who had unilateral fluid-free ears, this makes a total of 34 ears free of effusion, out of 176 ears with effusion at the beginning of the study. In this group 65 patients had bilateral effusion after four weeks of observation, while 22 had unilateral effusion, which makes a total of 152 ears with effusion after the observation period (Table 1). Normalization of middle ear status was determined by pneumatic otoscopy and tympanometry.

The proportion of subjects who became free of effusion by four weeks was significantly larger in the antibiotic group (58 percent) compared with the observation group (6 percent; $p < 0.0001$). Sixty-three percent of the treated ears were free of effusion at four weeks compared with 18 percent

TABLE 1 Results of Antimicrobial Therapy Trial

			With Fluid at 4 Weeks	
	Patients	*Free at 4 Weeks*	*Unilateral*	*Bilateral*
Antibiotic group	96	56 (58%)	9	31
Observation group	93	6 (6%)	22	65

of the untreated ears ($p < 0.0001$). The *chi*-square statistic with continuity correction was used to assess the statistical significance of differences between proportions.

DISCUSSION

The finding of viable bacteria in otitis media with effusion is well documented.[3,4] Use of antimicrobials for therapy of this common medical problem has not been employed in a controlled clinical trial until this time. This study indicates that antimicrobial agents might have a definite therapeutic role in the treatment of this widespread disease entity.

Use of other medical forms of therapy, such as topical nasal or oral decongestants and antihistamines, should be discouraged in the light of recent controlled clinical trails.[6] Although limited success has been reported with the use of short-term corticosteroids in the treatment of this disorder, large-scale clinical trials have yet to be undertaken.[7]

It would appear from this trial that antimicrobial agents have a definite role to play in the treatment of longstanding otitis media with effusion. Further clinical investigation is encouraged, however, to confirm or refute the findings of this study.

REFERENCES

1. Healy GB, Smith HG: Current concepts in the management of otitis media with effusion. Am J Otolaryngol 2:138, 1981
2. Senturia BH, Bluestone CD, Klein JO, et al: Report of the Ad Hoc Committee on Definition and Classification of Otitis Media and Otitis Media with Effusion. Ann Otol Rhinol Laryngol Suppl 68:3, 1980
3. Healy GB, Teele DW: The microbiology of chronic middle ear effusions in children. Laryngoscope 87:1472, 1977
4. Riding KH, Bluestone CD, Michaels RH, et al: Microbiology of recurrent and chronic otitis media with effusion. J Pediatr 93:739, 1978
5. Bluestone CD, Cantekin EI: Design factors in the characterization and identification of otitis media and certain related conditions. Ann Otol Rhinol Laryngol Suppl 60:13, 1979
6. Cantekin EI, Mandel EM, Bluestone CD, et al: Lack of efficacy of a decongestant-antihistamine combination for otitis media with effusion (''secretory'' otitis media) in children. New Engl J Med 308:297, 1983
7. Schwartz RH, Puglese J, Schwartz DM: Use of a short course of prednisone for treating middle ear effusion: A double-blind crossover study. Ann Otol Rhinol Laryngol 89(Suppl 68):296, 1980

CEFACLOR VERSUS AMOXICILLIN IN THE TREATMENT OF ACUTE OTITIS MEDIA

G. SCOTT GIEBINK, M.D., PAUL B. BATALDEN, M.D., JOYCE N. RUSS, M.D., and CHAP T. LE, M.D.

Ampicillin and amoxicillin have been commonly used for treating acute otitis media because the three most commonly encountered bacteria in the middle ear (*Streptococcus pneumoniae*, *Hemophilus influenzae*, and *Streptococcus pyogenes*) are usually susceptible to these antibiotics. However, an increasing prevalence of acute otitis media due to ampicillin-resistant strains of *H. influenzae* has been reported.[1] In addition, *Branhamella catarrhalis* has been isolated with increasing frequency from middle ear effusions of children with acute otitis media, and Shurin and colleagues found that 79 percent of these strains were resistant to ampicillin.[2–5] The problem of increasing ampicillin resistance has led to the search for more effective antimicrobial agents. One such agent is the cephalosporin cefaclor. To evaluate this drug in treating acute otitis media, we compared cefaclor with amoxicillin in a randomized clinical trial of 72 children with acute otitis media.

MATERIALS AND METHODS

All 72 children had signs and symptoms of acute unilateral or bilateral otitis media and had tympanocentesis performed on the most severely affected ear to obtain effusion for culture. Thirty-seven children were randomized to receive a 14-day course of cefaclor, and 35 received a 14-day course of amoxicillin; both antibiotics were given at a dosage of 40 mg/kg per day divided into three doses. Compliance was measured by a daily medication and temperature log kept by the parents.

Six patients treated with cefaclor and four patients treated with amoxicillin were excluded from analysis. Five of these ten patients were lost to follow-up. One cefaclor- and one amoxicillin-treated patient had worsening symptoms, and treatment was changed within 48 hours. One patient had a *H. influenzae* isolate resistant to both cefaclor and amoxicillin, necessitating a change in treatment. Two children had possible adverse drug reactions.

Treatment response was measured by otoscopy and tympanometry within seven days of discontinuing the antibiotic, at which time the presence or absence of effusion was documented using a previously validated algorithm.[6] Acute otitis media with effusion (OME) was defined as the presence of effusion plus symptoms (fever, irritability, otalgia, or otorrhea) or signs of inflammation (red and opaque or yellow-orange and opaque tympanic membrane).

RESULTS

The distribution of patients by age, sex, and prior history of otitis media was evenly balanced between the two treatment groups. Fifty-five percent of the 62 analyzed subjects were younger than 3 years, 69 percent were male, and 40 percent had previously experienced more than three otitis media episodes.

Of the 62 ears on which tympanocentesis was performed, 42 contained a purulent effusion, six contained a serous effusion, 13 contained mucoid effusion, and no effusion could be obtained from one ear. Seventy-one percent of purulent effusions, 50 percent of serous effusions, and 92 percent of mucoid effusions were culture positive.

Forty-one of the 62 cases (66 percent) cultured a known pathogen from the middle ear effusion sample, including *S. pneumoniae* (29 percent), nontype b *H. influenzae* (13 percent), and *B. catarrhalis* (7 percent). Four effusion samples yielded only presumed nonpathogens, including *Staphylococcus epidermidis, Corynebacterium,* and nonhemolytic streptococci. The distribution of bacterial species cultured was quite even between the cefaclor and amoxicillin treatment groups. Sixteen effusion samples were sterile.

Amoxicillin and cefaclor susceptibility testing was performed on 50 of the bacterial isolates. Resistance was defined as a minimum inhibitory concentration of 4 μg/ml or greater. Four percent of the isolates were resistant to amoxicillin, and 18 percent were resistant to cefaclor ($p = 0.007$).

Twenty-two percent of the cefaclor-treated patients and 13 percent of amoxicillin-treated patients had acute OME in the aspirated ear at the conclusion of treatment and therefore were treatment failures. Persistent OME without signs or symptoms of acute inflammation was noted in 28 percent of the aspirated ears in the cefaclor group and in 50 percent of the aspirated ears in the amoxicillin group. OME had resolved in the aspirated ear in 50 percent of patients in the cefaclor group and in 37 percent of patients in the amoxicillin group. The Wilcoxon test was applied to measure significance of these differences because the response was ordered. No significant difference ($p = 0.65$) was noted between the two treatment regimens for the aspirated ear.

Fifty percent of the cefaclor-treated patients and 57 percent of the amoxicillin-treated patients had unilateral acute OME on enrollment. Thus, approximately one-half of the nonaspirated ears were normal at the time treatment was started. Thirteen percent of the patients in both groups had acute OME in the nonaspirated ear when treatment was completed.

The response was scored by averaging the response for both of the patient's ears before and after treatment. Each ear was scored "2" if acute OME was diagnosed, "1" if OME without signs of acute inflammation was noted, and "0" if the ear was normal. The average score for both ears after treatment was subtracted from the average score for both ears before treatment to obtain the average response. Patients whose averaged response was less than "0" got worse with treatment, whereas patients whose averaged response was greater than "0" improved with treatment. Using these criteria, 13 percent of amoxicillin-treated patients and 6 percent of cefaclor-treated patients got worse with treatment (Table 1). How-

TABLE 1 Patient-Specific Treatment Response

	No. of Patients with Specified Response						
	−1.0	−0.5	0	0.5	1.0	1.5	2.0
	←WORSE		BETTER→				
Amoxicillin	2	1	4	7	10	4	2
Cefaclor	1	1	5	5	13	1	6

Note: $p = 0.48$

ever, the response was ordered, and the Wilcoxon test showed no significant difference in patient outcome between the amoxicillin- and cefaclor-treated groups.

Overall, considering both ears, 22 percent of cefaclor-treated patients and 17 percent of amoxicillin-treated patients failed to improve with treatment. Since this difference was not significant, the two treatment groups were combined to determine whether other factors affected the treatment response. Treatment failure was twice as common in children who entered with bilateral (32 percent failure rate) as opposed to unilateral (15 percent failures) acute otitis media. Twice as many patients with serous or mucoid effusion failed to improve with treatment (32 percent) compared with children who had purulent effusion (14 percent failure rate). Although none of the patients failed to improve with treatment because bacteria cultured from the aspirated ear were resistant to the antibiotic prescribed, treatment failure was twice as common in children with *H. influenzae* otitis media (50 percent failure rate) compared with those who had pneumococcal otitis media (22 percent). Treatment failure was three times as common in children 3 years and younger (29 percent failure rate) compared with children older than 3 years (8 percent).

Two children had adverse experiences during treatment. A 9-month-old boy developed a maculopapular rash, irritability, and symptoms suggestive of laryngeal stridor 24 hours after beginning cefaclor treatment. However, signs of upper airway obstruction could not be confirmed. Treatment was stopped and all symptoms disappeared within 48 hours. A 4-year-old child treated with cefaclor became extremely irritable, sleepless, and hyperactive two days after starting treatment. Treatment was stopped and symptoms disappeared. Identical symptoms developed when the child was rechallenged with the grape-flavored cefaclor vehicle several weeks later but disappeared when the material was discontinued.

All patients were re-examined two to eight weeks after discontinuing the study drug. Twenty-six of these patients (14 in the cefaclor group and 12 in the amoxicillin group) received no treatment after discontinuing the study drug. The patient-specific response during the period after discontinuing treatment was analyzed using the same averaged response for both ears previously described. There was no difference in the post-treatment outcome between the amoxicillin- and cefaclor-treated patients. In the amoxicillin group, five patients got worse, eight showed no change, and one improved. In the cefaclor group, five got worse, three stayed the same, and four improved ($p = 0.75$).

DISCUSSION

In summary, 19 percent of the 62 patients with acute otitis media with effusion failed to improve with amoxicillin or cefaclor treatment. While there was no significant difference in the ear-specific or patient-specific response between the amoxicillin- and cefaclor-treated groups, cefaclor-treated patients had a slightly greater rate of complete resolution in both the aspirated and nonaspirated ears, and a slightly lower rate of OME relapse during the two weeks after discontinuing antibiotics. These results, however, are paradoxical, since a significantly greater proportion of bacteria cultured from ear effusion were resistant to cefaclor compared with amoxicillin. Children who were 3 years of age and younger who had bilateral otitis, serous or mucoid effusion, or *H. influenzae* cultured from their effusion had a greater likelihood of treatment failure than did older children, those with unilateral otitis, purulent effusion, or cultures yielding other bacteria or sterile effusion.

Patients treated in this study had a poorer outcome than patients reported in other clinical trials using these antibiotics. Mandel and colleagues reported that only 5 percent of cefaclor-treated patients and 9 percent of amoxicillin-treated patients with acute OME had persistent or recurrent symptoms after treatment.[7] However, the frequency of complete OME resolution was similar in the two studies. Mandel and coworkers found that 59 percent of the ears that could be evaluated in the cefaclor group and 44 percent of ears in the amoxicillin group were effusion free after treatment.[7] Combining results for the aspirated and nonaspirated ears in our study, 64 percent of ears in the cefaclor group and 52 percent in the amoxicillin group were effusion free after treatment.

These results indicate that OME persists in a significant proportion of children two weeks after initiating treatment for acute OME, and acute OME relapse often occurs after discontinuing treatment. The increasing proportion of antibiotic-resistant bacteria cultured from acute middle ear effusions indicates that more effective therapeutic regimens than amoxicillin or cefaclor are required for treating children with this disease.

This study was supported in part by grant # NS-14538 from the National Institute of Neurological and Communicative Disorders and Stroke and by a grant from The Lilly Research Laboratories, Indianapolis, Indiana.

REFERENCES

1. Shurin PA, Pelton SI, Donner A, et al: Trimethoprim-sulfamethoxazole compared with ampicillin in the treatment of acute otitis media. J Pediatr 96:1081, 1980
2. Schwartz RH: Bacteriology of otitis media: A review. Otolaryngol Head Neck Surg 89:444, 1981
3. Lim DJ, Lewis DM, Schram JL, Birck HG: Antibiotic-resistant bacteria in otitis media with effusion. Ann Otol Rhinol Laryngol 98(Suppl 68):278, 1980
4. Shurin PA, Marchant CD, Kim CH, et al: Emergence of beta-lactamase-producing strains of *Branhamella catarrhalis* as important agents of acute otitis media. Pediatr Infect Dis 2:34, 1983
5. Kovatch AL, Wald ER, Michaels RH: Beta-lactamase-producing *Branhamella catarrhalis* causing otitis media in children. J. Pediatr 102:261, 1983
6. Cantekin EI, Bluestone CD, Fria TJ, et al: Identification of otitis media with effusion in children. Ann Otol Rhinol Laryngol 89(Suppl 68):190, 1980
7. Mandel EM, Bluestone CD, Cantekin EI, et al: Comparison of cefaclor and amoxicillin for acute otitis media with effusion. Ann Otol Rhinol Laryngol 90(Suppl 84):48, 1981

PANEL DISCUSSION: CONTROVERSIES IN ANTIMICROBIAL THERAPY FOR OTITIS MEDIA

PARTICIPANTS: CHARLES D. BLUESTONE, M.D. (MODERATOR), SYDNEY S. GELLIS, M.D., HANS RUNDKRANTZ, M.D., JOHN D. NELSON, M.D., JACK L. PARADISE, M.D., JENS THOMSEN, M.D., F.L. VAN BUCHEM, M.D.

THE PROBLEM

Even though there has been a dramatic reduction in the number of life-threatening complications from otitis media since the advent of the widespread availability of antimicrobial agents about 35 years ago, there remains a great deal of controversy concerning their use for this disease. A growing number of articles have appeared in the literature which raise serious doubts about the efficacy of antimicrobial treatment of every patient who has otitis media. It is the impression of some investigators that administration of antimicrobial agents early in the course of the disease may interfere with local or systemic immunity, which might then be responsible for the apparent increase in the number of children who have recurrent acute otitis media and chronic otitis media with effusion. The contention is that we have reduced the number of serious otitis-media–related suppurative complications but only at the price of "alarmingly" increasing the number of patients with recurrent and persistent disease, which has, in turn, led to an ever-increasing number of surgical procedures required to treat and prevent otitis media. In the United States the myringotomy and tympanostomy tube operation is the most common minor surgical procedure performed in children in which a general anesthesia is used; it has been estimated that about 1 million children have the operation annually. In addition, adenoidectomy with or without tonsillectomy remains the most common major surgical procedure performed in children in the United States, and many of these operations are for the treatment and prevention of otitis media. With these factors in mind, some investigators have suggested that treatment be given only to those patients with otitis media who are seriously ill or fail to improve without antimicrobial therapy.

In addition, many other aspects of treating otitis media with antimicrobial therapy arouse controversy. Thus, we have asked a group of clinicians from several countries to express their views concerning this problem. They have been chosen because of their recently published research addressing these questions or because of their expertise in antimicrobial therapy for infectious disease. The panel was asked by the moderator several specific questions designed to allow them to express their opinion based on their research findings, knowledge of the current literature and their clinical experience. Owing to time restraints, each panelist was instructed to limit his answer to only a few minutes. The following is a summary of the panel's discussion.

ARE ANTIMICROBIAL AGENTS INDICATED FOR THE TREATMENT OF ACUTE OTITIS MEDIA?

All but one of the panelists agreed that, until convincing clinical trials are published to the contrary, an antimicrobial agent *is* indicated initially for all patients who have acute otitis media. The moderator defined the disease as the acute onset of otalgia and fever in a patient who has a bulging, erythematous, opaque, and immobile tympanic membrane. Dr. Van Buchem from the Netherlands dissented. He stated that based on his studies, which have followed his controversial article recently published in the *Lancet,*[1] antimicrobial agents can be withheld in almost all children with acute otitis media and given only to those who have an "irregular course," that is, persistent otalgia or fever or both, and to those who continue to have an aural discharge after two weeks. However, he prescribes analgesics and nose drops for his patients. For those few children who have an "irregular course," he performs a myringotomy in addition to prescribing an antimicrobial agent (amoxicillin). He reported that following the institution of this method of management in approximately 4800 children, only two subsequently developed mastoiditis for which mastoid surgery was not necessary because antimicrobial therapy was successful. Dr. Nelson considered this incidence rate of mastoiditis to be unacceptable in the "antibiotic era" and not the rate experienced in the United States, where antimicrobial agents are given at the onset of illness. Drs. Rundkrantz and Thomsen also stated that in certain areas of their countries myringotomy was the only initial treatment and that antimicrobial agents were prescribed only in the patients who failed to improve rapidly following the procedure. The panelists concluded that there may be some merit in withholding antimicrobial therapy in selected patients who have acute otitis media, but the criteria for identifying patients for whom this type of management will be safe have not been defined. They recommended that clinical trials be conducted which are thoughtfully designed to answer this important question. Dr. Gellis strongly recommended that, at present, an antimicrobial agent is indicated for the treatment of acute otitis media.

WHICH ANTIMICROBIAL AGENTS ARE INDICATED FOR THE TREATMENT OF ACUTE OTITIS MEDIA?

Drs. Rundkrantz and Thomsen stated that penicillin V is initially used for the treatment of acute otitis media in Scandinavian countries. However, Drs. Nelson and Paradise indicated that ampicillin, or rather its analogue, amoxicillin, is the drug of choice in the United States. They cited clinical and laboratory studies that indicate that penicillin V alone is not as effective as ampicillin in cases of acute otitis media in which *Hemophilus influenzae* is the etiologic agent. Since the incidence of *H. influenzae* otitis media is approximately 20 percent in both Scandinavia and the United States, they would recommend treatment with penicillin V only when a bacterium has been isolated from a middle ear aspirate (or discharge) against which penicillin would be effective, such as *Streptococcus pneumoniae*. In response to this recommendation, the panelists from Scandinavia stated that they prescribe a higher daily dose of penicillin V than is given in the United States. They cited in vitro and clinical studies showing that a higher blood and middle ear concentration of penicillin V will eradicate *H. influenzae*. They also expressed concern that the widespread use of ampicillin and amoxicillin in the United States has been responsible for the rising incidence of beta-lactamase–producing strains of *H. influenzae*.*

---

*Moderator's note: There is no scientific proof that the use of the aminopenicillins is a factor in bacteria developing drug resistance. In addition, studies by Howie and Ploussard[2] have shown that ampicillin is superior to penicillin V in sterilizing middle ear infection caused by *H. influenzae* (non-beta-lactamase–producing).

WHAT IS THE PREFERRED MANAGEMENT OF PATIENTS WITH PERSISTENCE OR RECURRENCE OF SYMPTOMS AFTER ONSET OF INITIAL TREATMENT?

Even though Dr. Van Buchem would initially withhold antimicrobial therapy, he would recommend a myringotomy and treatment with amoxicillin for those children who have persistent otalgia or fever or both. Drs. Rundkrantz and Thomsen stated they would also perform a myringotomy and would change from penicillin to amoxicillin therapy in a patient who had persistent or recurrent symptoms while on penicillin V therapy. Drs. Paradise and Nelson agreed that a myringotomy would be the ideal management option for patients who have persistence or recurrence of signs and symptoms of acute infection while on ampicillin or amoxicillin therapy and stressed that a middle ear aspirate should be obtained and cultured in an attempt to identify a possible resistant organism. When initial treatment with amoxicillin is not successful and a middle ear effusion culture is not performed, they recommend a change of the antimicrobial agent to either erythromycin in combination with a sulfonamide, trimethoprim-sulfamethoxazole, or cefaclor.

WHAT IS THE RECOMMENDED DURATION OF THERAPY

There was no consensus among the panelists on the recommended duration of antimicrobial therapy, since there have been no convincing clinical trials reported that have been definitive. Dr. Thomsen stated that, based on his studies, even two days of antimicrobial therapy may be sufficient, but Drs. Paradise, Nelson, and Gellis recommended a 10- to 14-day course, based not on clinical trials of patients with otitis media but on the trials conducted on patients treated with penicillin who had streptococcal pharyngitis. Dr. Nelson stated that large, controlled trials will be needed to demonstrate that shorter periods of therapy are as effective.

IS ANTIMICROBIAL PROPHYLAXIS INDICATED FOR RECURRENT ACUTE OTITIS MEDIA?

Drs. Nelson and Paradise stated they would consider prophylaxis with a daily low dose of an antimicrobial agent, such as penicillin G (Dr. Paradise), amoxicillin or sulfisoxazole (Dr. Nelson) for those children who have frequently recurring episodes of acute otitis media and have no middle ear effusion between attacks. However, Drs. Thomsen, Rundkrantz, and Van Buchem would not advise chemoprophylaxis but would favor performing a myringotomy and tympanostomy tube insertion to prevent recurrent acute otitis media.

CONCLUSION

The moderator summarized the discussion and then recommended that carefully controlled studies of the efficacy of antimicrobial therapy for the treatment of acute otitis media are indicated. Clinical trials should be conducted to determine (1) whether antimicrobial therapy can be withheld in selected patients, (2) the most safe and efficacious agents, (3) the duration of therapy required to eliminate the infection, and (4) whether antimicrobial prophylaxis is safe and effective in patients who have frequently recurring attacks of acute otitis media.

REFERENCES

1. Van Buchem FL, Dunk JHM, Van't Hof MA: Therapy of acute otitis media: Myringotomy, antibiotics, or neither? A double-blind study in children. Lancet 2:883, 1981
2. Howie VM, Ploussard JH: The "in vivo" sensitivity test—bacteriology of middle ear exudate. Pediatrics 44:940, 1969

SURGICAL MANAGEMENT

SURGICAL MANAGEMENT OF OTITIS MEDIA WITH EFFUSION: STATE OF THE ART

CHARLES D. BLUESTONE, M.D.

None of the surgical methods of managing acute, recurrent acute or chronic otitis media with effusion has been proved effective in acceptable clinical trials. However, myringotomy is recommended for selected cases of acute otits media. Myringotomy with insertion of a tympanostomy tube is a common method of management for chronic otitis media with effusion. Adenoidectomy, with or without tonsillectomy—alone or in combination with a myringotomy—and with or without tympanostomy tube insertion also is commonly used. Tympanomastoidectomy has been advocated for children with chronic otitis media with effusion that appears to be resistant to myringotomy and tympanostomy tube insertion.[1] However, this procedure should be reserved for those children in whom cholesteatoma is suspected, since almost all chronic effusions are eliminated, at least temporarily, following tympanostomy tube insertion.

MYRINGOTOMY

Myringotomy became increasingly popular until the 1940s, when antimicrobial agents came into widespread use. Nowadays, myringotomy alone is reserved for selected cases and performed primarily by otolaryngologists and a handful of primary care physicians; cases are usually limited to those children who have severe otalgia or suppurative complications, or both. However, in the face of an apparent recent increase in the prevalence and incidence of acute and chronic otitis media with effusion, considerably more effort has been made to study the efficacy of myringotomy in the management of otitis media. The potential benefits from more liberal use of the procedure in cases of acute otitis media might be relief of otalgia and a decrease in persistence and recurrence rates. When chronic otitis media with effusion is present, myringotomy may be as effective in eliminating the middle ear effusion as when the procedure is followed by the insertion of a tympanostomy tube, with its attendant complications and sequelae, assuming a surgical procedure is indicated at all.

The results of studies conducted in the past to determine the efficacy of myringotomy in managing acute otitis media are shown in Table 1.[2–7] Unfortunately, all of these studies had design and methodologic flaws that make interpretation of their results difficult; the question of the value of myringotomy for acute otitis media therefore remains unanswered. In spite of the lack of convincing evidence to support the routine use of myringotomy for all children with acute otitis media, there are certain indications for its use on which there is general consensus at present:

Suppurative Complications

Whenever a child has acute mastoiditis, labyrinthitis, facial paralysis, or one or more of the intracranial suppurative complications, such as meningitis, myringotomy and aspiration should be performed as an emergency procedure. Tympanocentesis should precede the myringotomy to identify the causative organisms. In addition, in such cases the insertion of a tympanostomy tube should be attempted to provide prolonged drainage.

Severe Otalgia Requiring Immediate Relief

Even though some studies have failed to show that myringotomy alleviated earache,[8] Roddey and colleagues did show that acute pain was relieved in children who received myringotomy.[2] Culture of the effusion is reasonable, since the middle ear is being opened, but is not absolutely necessary if there is no reason to suspect an unusual organism.

TABLE 1 Percentage of Persistent Middle Ear Effusion Following Initial Myringotomy and Antimicrobial Therapy Compared with Antimicrobial Therapy Alone for Acute Otitis Media

Investigators	Procedure*	No. of Subjects	Percentage with Persistent Effusion After: 10–14 Days	4 Weeks	6 Weeks	Statistical Significance Achieved
Roddey et al[2]	AB	121	35	7	2	No
	AB&M	94	24	9	1	
Herberts et al[3]	AB	81	10	—	—	No
	AB&M	91	18	—	—	
Lorentzen and Haugsten[4]	AB	190	16	6		No
	AB&M	164	20 (est.)	6	—	
Puhakka et al[5]	AB	90	78	29	—	Yes
	AB&M	68	29	10	—	
Qvarnberg and Palva[6]	AB	151	50	—	—	Yes
	AB&M	97	28	—	—	
Schwartz and Schwartz[7]	AB	361	47	—	—	No
	AB&M	415	51	—	—	

*AB, Antibiotic; AB&M, antibiotic and myringotomy
From Bluestone CD, Stool SE (eds): *Pediatric Otolaryngology*. Philadelphia: WB Saunders Co, 1983, Chapter 16

Microbiologic Diagnosis

When severe otalgia or suppurative complications are present in a child with acute otitis media myringotomy is clearly indicated, since drainage of the middle ear–mastoid air cell system is provided. Although not as compelling as the above indications, whenever a diagnostic tympanocentesis is indicated, a myringotomy for drainage may follow the needle aspiration, especially when a copious amount of middle ear effusion is identified by the tympanocentesis. Myringotomy may then reasonably follow a tympanocentesis when acute otitis media is present and (1) the child is critically ill; (2) there is persistent or recurrent otalgia or fever or both, in spite of adequate and appropriate antimicrobial therapy; (3) the acute otitis media occurs during the course of antimicrobial therapy given for another infection and the agent is effective against the most common organisms causing otitis, for example, amoxicillin or ampicillin; (4) the patient is a neonate; or (5) the patient is immunologically compromised.

Complications and Sequelae

The complications of performing a myringotomy properly are minimal. The persistent otorrhea that follows the procedure and is the most common finding after a myringotomy can hardly be considered a complication, since it is the desired outcome; however, the discharge may become profuse and cause an eczematoid external otitis. Dislocation of the incudostapedial joint, severing of the facial nerve, and puncturing of an exposed jugular bulb are dreaded complications but are so rare in experienced hands that they should not deter the trained practitioner from employing the procedure when indicated. The most common sequelae of the procedure are persistent perforation, atrophic scar, or tympanosclerosis at the site of the incision. Even though the incidence of these conditions has not been systematically studied in a prospective manner, the risk of any or all occurring should not outweigh the benefits of the myringotomy when indicated. The incidence of these sequelae occurring would be greater in children who require repeated myringotomy.

Tympanostomy Tubes

Myringotomy with insertion of tympanostomy tubes currently is the most common surgical procedure performed in children that requires general anesthesia. The use of tympanostomy tubes was first suggested by Politzer over 100 years ago,[9] but the tubes did not become readily available until their reintroduction by Armstrong in 1954. Since then they have become increasingly popular: In 1976 an estimated two million tubes were manufactured and presumably inserted in more than one million patients.[10]

Several studies have addressed the efficacy of myringotomy and insertion of tympanostomy tubes for treatment of otitis media with effusion. The ones discussed below are the most widely cited.

Shah performed a myringotomy and aspiration in one ear and a myringotomy with insertion of a tympanostomy tube on the opposite ear of children with bilateral "mucoid otitis media with effusion." Adenoidectomies were performed on all of these children at the time the ear surgery was performed. He found the hearing in the ears into which the tympanostomy tubes had been inserted was better than the hearing in the other ears six to twelve months after the procedures.

Kilby and associates also performed bilateral myringotomy, inserting a tympanostomy tube into only one ear in a series of children, but they did not perform an adenoidectomy at the same time.[12] These investigators found no difference in the hearing in the two ears after surgery when all of the tubes had been extruded.

Mawson and Fagan performed adenoidectomy and myringotomy with insertion of tympanostomy tubes in a number of children and found the degree of hearing loss and number of tympanic membrane abnormalities (such as tympanosclerosis) increased the longer the children were followed.[13] They reported that 76 percent of the children in their study required insertion of another tympanostomy tube within four years of the initial treatment.

Kokko compared findings in the ears of children who had undergone adenoidectomy and myringotomy plus insertion of tympanostomy tubes with the findings in the ears of those who had undergone adenoidectomy and myringotomy without insertion of tubes.[14] He found no differences in the pathologic factors present in the tympanic membranes or in the degree of hearing loss present in the two groups four and a half years after the procedures.

Tos and Poulsen performed adenoidectomy and myringotomy with insertion of tympanostomy tubes in 108 children.[15] During the five- to eight-year follow-up period, they reported that only 2.5 percent of the children into whose ears tympanostomy tubes had been placed had hearing losses, but that scarring was a frequently observed abnormality.

Yagi compared 100 children who underwent adenoidectomy and myringotomy with insertion of a tympanostomy tube with 100 children who underwent only adenoidectomy.[16] There were no significant differences between the two groups in (1) the number of children whose hearing problems were "cured" without further surgery, (2) the number of children requiring insertion of tubes due to recurrence of problems after initial treatment, (3) the number of patients having abnormal tympanic membranes; or (4) the number of patients with more than a 20 dB hearing loss 18 months after treatment.

Marshak and Neriah did a retrospective study on 58 children, half of whom had undergone adenoidectomy and myringotomy for chronic otitis media with effusion, and half who had had tympanostomy tubes inserted.[17] Only 20.7 percent of the adenoidectomized children had normal hearing and aerated middle ears during a two-year follow-up, whereas 59 percent of the children who had had tympanostomy tubes inserted had normal hearing and aerated middle ears during the same period.

Lildholdt performed a myringotomy with insertion of a tympanostomy tube on one ear and left the contralateral ear untouched in 150 children with bilateral otitis media with effusion (of uncertain duration) and at the same time performed an adenoidectomy.[18] Early in the postoperative period the hearing was better in the ear with the tympanostomy tube, but there was no difference in hearing three months after the procedure. In addition, there was significantly more scarring in the ear with the tube, as compared with the "control" ear. However, the study included some children who also received a tonsillectomy and the duration of the effusion was not documented.

Smyth and coworkers performed a prospective study of myringotomy versus myringotomy with insertion of tympanostomy tube in 18 children.[19] In one ear myringotomy and aspiration was performed, and in the opposite ear a tympanostomy tube was inserted.

Gebhart studied the efficacy of myringotomy and tubes in children who had recurrent otitis media and reported less ear disease when tubes were in place.[20]

Data are also sparse concerning complications of these surgical procedures. Common complications of myringotomy with insertion of tympanostomy tube include scarring of the tympanic membrane (tympanosclerosis) and localized or diffuse membrane atrophy and persistent or recurrent otorrhea (Table 2). Much less commonly, a perforation may remain at the insertion site following extrusion of the tube, or, more rarely, an implantation cholesteatoma may develop.

These studies demonstrate the problems with myringotomy and myringotomy with insertion of a tympanostomy tube. No acceptable randomized

TABLE 2 Incidence of Complications and Sequelae Following Tympanostomy Tube Insertion for Otitis Media with Effusion in Children

Investigators	No. of Subjects (Ears)*	Follow-Up (Yrs.)	Tympano-sclerosis	Percentage of Incidence: Otorrhea	Percentage of Incidence: Persistent Perforation	Percentage of Incidence: Choles-teatoma
Kilby et al[12]	52 (52)	2	28†	NA	1.9	0
Brown et al[21]	55 (55)	5	42†	NA	0	0
Draf and Schultz[22]	677 (876)	NA	NA‡	12.5	0.1	1.6
Münker[23]	631 (1060)	NA	50	15	2.5	0.9
Barfoed and Rosborg[24]	102 (173)	7	61	34	3	0
Lildholdt[18]	150 (150)	5	52†	30	0	0

*Numbers in parentheses indicate ears
†In contralateral ears in which no tympanostomy tubes had been inserted, incidence was 21 percent (Kilby et al[12]), 0 percent (Brown et al[21]), and 11.3 percent (Lildholdt[18]).
‡NA, not available (modified after Bluestone et al[25]).

clinical trials of the efficacy of myringotomy or myringotomy with insertion of a tympanostomy tube have been reported.

Tonsillectomy and Adenoidectomy

Adenoidectomy performed either separately or in conjunction with tonsillectomy is the most common major surgical procedure employed to prevent otitis media. Myringotomy with tympanostomy tube insertion is the most common minor surgical procedure performed for otitis media with effusion. Table 3 shows that in 1972 tonsillectomy and adenoidectomy was the most common operation performed in all age groups, and in 1979 it ranked below only the common obstetric and gynecologic procedures. Tonsillectomy and adenoidectomy still is the most common major operation performed on children; approximately one-fourth undergo this surgery. Such operations account for about 50 percent of all major surgical operations performed on children, 25 percent of all hospital admissions, and 10 percent of hospital bed days.

The decrease in the total number of tonsil and adenoid operations may be related to a change in demography, since there was approximately a 20 percent reduction during the same period in the number of children in that age group. Although the number of adenoidectomies without tonsillectomy remained relatively small in comparison with the number of tonsillectomies performed either separately or in combination with adenoidectomy, it represented a more than twofold increase. Also, there appears to be great regional variation in the performance of these operations; the rates for adenoidectomy vary the most widely.[26] However, there are no data available on the indications for which the operations were performed. Certainly otitis media was one, and in many instances the only, indication for adenoidectomy, either with or without tonsillectomy.

Previous Clinical Trials

Despite its frequent use, it has never been established through controlled scientific studies that the benefits of tonsil and adenoid surgery for otitis media justify its cost in any age group of children. There have been only a few prospective clinical trials of tonsillectomy and adenoidectomy. The first randomized clinical trial was reported by McKee.[27] During the first year of the trial, the mean incidence of otitis media among control subjects was twice as high as among children who had tonsillectomy and adenoidectomy, but during the second year there was no difference in incidence of otitis media in the operated and control groups. In a second study, McKee attempted to distinguish the effects of tonsillectomy from those of adenoidectomy: the mean incidence of otitis media in each of the two surgical groups was approximately the same.[28] He concluded from these two studies that otitis media occurred infrequently after adenoidectomy, or after tonsillectomy and adenoidectomy, and that the combined operation did not offer any particular advantages in the prevention of the disease. However, Mawson and associates found no apparent difference in the incidence of otalgia or otitis media between children who did and did not undergo the procedure.[29] Roydhouse

TABLE 3 Most Frequent Operative Procedures, 1972 and 1979*

1972			*1979*		
Procedure	*No. (× 1000)*	*Rate/1000*	*Procedure*	*No. (× 1000)*	*Rate/1000*
Tonsillectomy and adenoidectomy	917	4.5	D&C	935	4.3
D&C	866	4.2	Hysterectomy	639	3.0
Hysterectomy	649	3.2	Tubal ligation	610	2.8
Hernia repair	510	2.5	Cesarean section	499	2.8
Cholecystectomy	399	2.0	Tonsillectomy and adenoidectomy	500	2.3
Oophorectomy	378	1.9	Hernia repair	500	2.3

*From American College of Surgeons.

in a study in New Zealand, reported reduction in the incidence of otitis media in the first year after tonsillectomy and adenoidectomy, but this difference was not maintained in the second year.[30] In a second clinical trial, Roydhouse randomly divided 100 children with persistent otitis media who had not responded to nonsurgical treatment into two groups.[31] One received adenoidectomy with tympanostomy tube insertion and the other, tympanostomy tube insertion alone. He compared these two groups to a third group of 69 children who had had otitis media but were free of middle ear effusion following nonsurgical management. The cure rate was similar in each of the groups operated on, with a greater relapse rate in the nonadenoidectomy group, which required 9 percent more tympanostomy tube insertions. Radiographs showed that the group cured without surgery had somewhat smaller adenoids; however, the relapse rate in the nonadenoidectomy surgical group was independent of the size of the adenoids. The study failed to show a favorable outcome following adenoidectomy.

Unfortunately, all of these studies had one or more of the following limitations in experimental design: (1) entry into the study was based on the occurrence of a sore throat and not on the presence of otitis media; (2) objective evidence of otitis media was not documented by tympanometry or audiometry; (3) no other surgical procedures that could have been performed (such as myringotomy or tympanostomy tube insertion) were reported; (4) the technique of adenoidectomy (for example, "midline sweep" or thorough removal of adenoid tissue from the fossa of Rosenmüller) was not described, nor was evidence of complete removal of the adenoids documented; and (5) nasal and eustachian tube functions were not assessed objectively.

Children's Hospital of Pittsburgh Clinical Trial

An ongoing prospective randomized controlled trial of the efficacy of adenoidectomy for otitis media currently is being conducted at the Children's Hospital of Pittsburgh. Preliminary analyses of data suggest that (1) adenoidectomy does not eliminate the problem of recurrent otitis media, and (2) it is not clear whether adenoidectomy somewhat reduces the rate, severity, or duration of recurrent episodes.[32] The effects of the following variables on the outcome of adenoidectomy for otitis media with effusion are being examined: age, sex, race, allergy, adenoid size, and eustachian tube function.

This study does not address the question of whether tonsillectomy and adenoidectomy are more effective in the prevention of otitis media with effusion than adenoidectomy alone, nor will it answer the question of the relative value of adenoidectomy, with or without tonsillectomy, for children who have not received myringotomy and insertion of tympanostomy tubes in the past. These questions are being addressed in another randomized clinical trial currently being conducted at the same institution.

Impact on Health Care

As estimated two billion dollars are spent annually on medical and surgical treatment of otitis media in the United States. Included in this figure are the estimated one million children who receive tympanostomy tubes and more than 600,000 who undergo tonsillectomy and adenoidectomy procedures, many primarily for the prevention of otitis media. The myringotomy and tube procedure is the most common minor surgical operation performed under general anesthesia, and tonsillectomy and adenoidectomy the most common major operation performed on children.

This study was supported in part by grant #5P01 NS 16337 from the National Institute of Neurological and Communicative Disorders and Stroke.

The author would like to thank Sandra Arjona for editorial assistance and preparation of the manuscript.

REFERENCES

1. Proud GO, Duff WE: Mastoidectomy and epitympanotomy. Ann Otol Rhinol Laryngol 85(25):289, 1976
2. Roddey OF Jr, Earle R Jr, Haggerty R: Myringotomy in acute otitis media: A controlled study. JAMA 197:849, 1966
3. Herberts G, Jeppson PH, Nylén O, Branefors-Helander P: Acute otitis media: Etiological and therapeutical aspects of acute otitis media. Prac Otol Rhinol Laryngol 33:191, 1971
4. Lorentzen P, Haugsten P: Treatment of acute suppurative otitis media. J Laryngol Otol 91:331, 1977
5. Puhakka H, Virolainen E, Aantaa E, et al: Myringotomy in the treatment of acute otitis media in children. Acta Otolaryngol (Stockh) 88:122, 1979
6. Qvarnberg Y, Palva T: Active and conservative treatment of acute otitis media: Prospective studies. Ann Otol Rhinol Laryngol 89(68):269, 1980
7. Schwartz RH, Schwartz DM: Acute otitis media: Diagnosis and drug therapy. Drugs 19:107, 1980
8. Schwartz RH, Rodriguez WJ, Schwartz DM: Office myringotomy for acute otitis media: Its value in preventing middle ear effusion. Laryngoscope. 91:616, 1981
9. Politzer A: Lehrbuch der Ohrenheilkunde. 5. Auflage, vol I. Stuttgart: F Enke, 1865, 1869
10. Paradise JL: On tympanostomy tubes: Rationale, results, reservations, and recommendations. Pediatrics 60:86, 1969
11. Shah N: Use of grommets in "glue" ears. J Laryngol Otol 85:283, 1971
12. Kilby D, Richards SH, Hart G: Grommets and glue ears. Two year results. J Laryngol Otol 86:881, 1972
13. Mawson SR, Fagan P: Tympanic effusions in children: Long-term results of treatment by myringotomy, aspiration, and in-dwelling tubes (grommets). J Laryngol Otol 86:105, 1972
14. Kokko E: Chronic secretory otitis media in children: A clinical study. Acta Otolaryngol (Stockh) Suppl 327:7, 1974
15. Tos M, Poulsen G: Secretory otitis media: Late results of treatment with grommets. Arch Otolaryngol 102:672, 1976
16. Yagi HA: The surgical treatment of secretory otitis media in children. Hearing in cleft palate patients. Arch Otolaryngol 91:267, 1977
17. Marshak G, Neriah ZB: Adenoidectomy versus tympanostomy in chronic secretory otitis media. Ann Otol Rhinol Laryngol 89(68):316, 1981
18. Lildholdt T: Ventilation tubes in secretory otitis media. Acta Otolaryngol (Stockh), in press
19. Smyth GDL, Patterson CC, Hall S: Tympanostomy tubes: Do they significantly benefit the patient? Otolaryngol Head Neck Surg 90:783, 1982
20. Gebhart DE: Tympanostomy tubes in the otitis media prone child. Laryngoscope 91:849, 1981
21. Brown MJ, Richards SH, Ambegaokar AG: Grommets and glue ear: A five year follow-up of a controlled trial. J R Soc Med 71:353, 1978
22. Draf W, Schulz P: Insertion of ventilation tubes into the middle ear: Results and complications—a seven-year review. Ann Otol Rhinol Laryngol 89(68):303, 1980
23. Münker G: Results after treatment of otitis media with effusion. Ann Otol Rhinol Laryngol 89(68):308, 1980
24. Barfoed C, Rosborg J: Secretory otitis media: Long-term observations after treatment with grommets. Arch Otolaryngol 106:553, 1980
25. Bluestone CD, Klein JO, Paradise JL, et al: Workshop on effects of otitis media on the child. Pediatrics 71:639, 1983
26. National Center for Health Statistics: Surgical Operations in Short-Stay Hospitals: United States, 1971. US Dept of Health, Education and Welfare Publication No. HRA-75-1769, Rockville, Md, 1974
27. McKee WJE: A controlled study of the effects of tonsillectomy and adenoidectomy in children. Br J Prev Soc Med 17:49, 1963
28. McKee WJE: The part played by adenoidectomy in the combined operation of tonsillectomy with adenoidectomy: Second part of a controlled study in children. Br J Prev Soc Med 17:133, 1963
29. Mawson SR, Adlington R, Evans M: A controlled study evaluation of adenotonsillectomy in children. J Laryngol Otol 81:777, 1967
30. Roydhouse N: A controlled study of adenotonsillectomy. Arch Otolaryngol 92:611, 1970
31. Roydhouse N: Adenoidectomy for otitis media with mucoid effusion. Ann Otol Rhinol Laryngol 89(68):312, 1980
32. Paradise JL, Bluestone CD, Rodgers KD, et al: Efficacy of adenoidectomy in recurrent otitis media: Historical overview and preliminary results from a randomized, controlled trial. Ann Otol Rhinol Laryngol 89(68):319, 1980

CHRONIC OTITIS MEDIA WITH EFFUSION AND ADENOTONSILLECTOMY: A PROSPECTIVE RANDOMIZED CONTROLLED STUDY

A. RICHARD MAW, M.B., F.R.C.S.

Otitis media with effusion (OME) is one of the most common chronic otologic conditions of childhood. As a result of eustachian tube malfunction, serous or mucoid fluid accumulates within the middle ear cleft where there is a negative pressure. It is especially prevalent in children with cleft palate and frequently occurs in association with upper respiratory infection and generalized nasal and sinus mucosal disorders, such as allergic rhinitis and ultrastructural cilial abnormalities.

Treatment of the condition varies widely; it is directed to the ears in the form of myringotomy and aspiration with or without grommet insertion, to the nose and sinuses by eradication of infection and control of allergy, and to the postnasal space and oropharynx in the form of adenoidectomy and, less frequently, tonsillectomy. If adenoidectomy is recommended, it is either the size of the adenoids or their role as a focus of ascending eustachian tube infection that is the main indication for surgery. The potential source of infection from the tonsils is similarly implicated. However, removal of the tonsils is often advised with adenoidectomy on grounds that on their own merit, might not prove valid for tonsillectomy. It is removal of the adenoids and tonsils that is mainly responsible for the morbidity and mortality attached to the treatment of chronic OME.

The arguments for[1–3] and against[4–7] adenoidectomy and adenotonsillectomy for all types of middle ear diseases have been reported and discussed at length.[8–11] It seems that the long-held belief that adenoidectomy relieves recurrent acute suppurative otitis media has been upheld without convincing supportive evidence as grounds for the management of OME. Considering the number of these operations performed for this condition it is remarkable that so few have been evaluated to substantiate their efficacy. The present study was started prospectively in September 1979 with the specific objective of evaluating randomly the effect of adenoidectomy and adenotonsillectomy, along with the effect of no treatment on established cases of OME.

MATERIALS AND METHODS

Approval was granted by the District Ethical Committee. A pilot study was undertaken to assess interobserver agreement and observer accuracy for the diagnosis of OME.[12] The definitive study involved 103 children between the ages of 2 and 12 (mean, 5.25 years), 60 percent were boys. Diagnosis was confirmed by otoscopy using Siegle's pneumatic speculum in addition to tympanometry and pure-tone audiometry. Only children with bilateral OME were included, and following the first appointment medical treatment with an antihistamine/sympathomimetic amine mixture (Dimotapp elixir) in an appropriate dosage for age was prescribed until the second appointment six weeks later. Repeat examination and investigation confirmed the presence of bilateral OME and for the following six weeks no treatment was prescribed. An identical review was done at 12 weeks, and if bilateral fluid was still present the child was admitted to the hospital within two weeks for operation. During this time a lateral cephalometric radiograph of the nasopharynx was taken. All of the surgery was performed by the investigator. Surgery on the tonsils and adenoids was randomized into three groups: (1) adenotonsillectomy (34 cases), (2) adenoidectomy (36 cases), (3) no surgery (33 cases). In addition unilateral myringotomy was performed in all cases on a randomly allocated basis, the middle ear fluid was assessed for quantity and type, and a Shepard-type Xomed grommet was inserted anteroinferiorly. The contralateral unoperated ear was examined using X6 magnification to confirm the presence of middle ear fluid but myringotomy was not performed. There was a similar distribu-

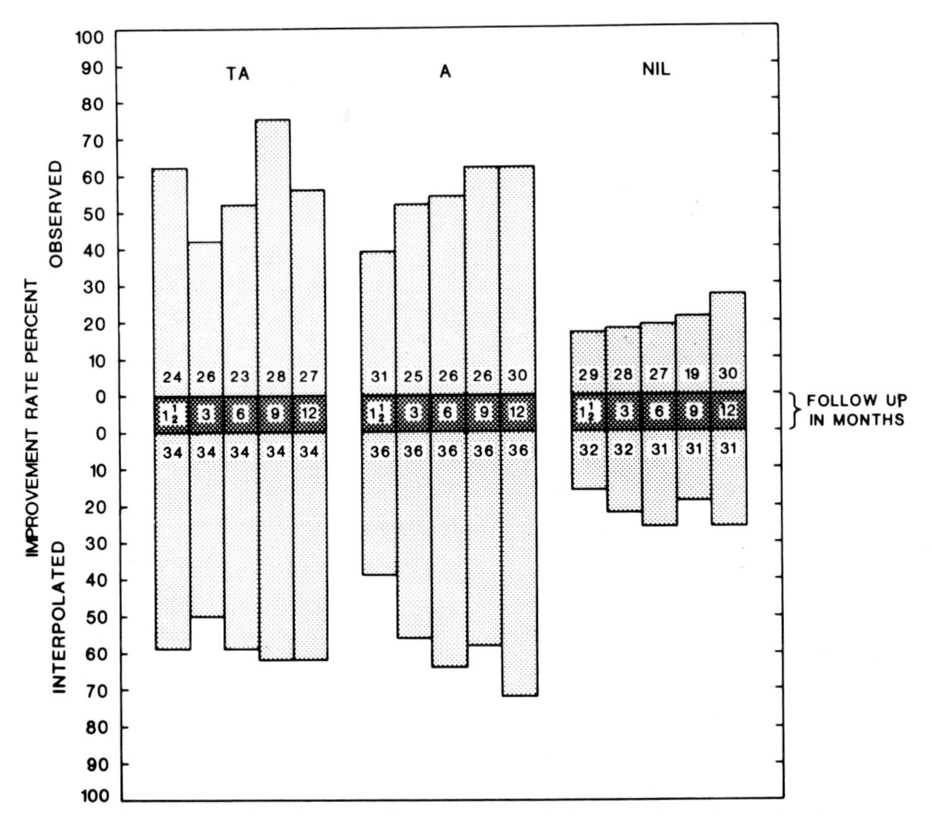

Figure 1 *Chi*-squared analysis shows no differences in any cells between observed and interpolated data.

tion of each treatment group within the seasonal divisions of the year, and there were no differences among the three treatment groups with respect to age, sex, and postnasal space airway measured on the lateral radiograph.

The children were re-examined six weeks, three months, six months, nine months, and one year following surgery. Similar examinations and investigations were performed and the unoperated ear was assessed for the presence or absence of middle ear fluid without prior examination of the pharynx or of the operation notes. As a result an improvement rate was calculated for each follow-up time based on the findings of the unoperated ear.

RESULTS

One case was lost to follow-up after three months. Not all of the children appeared for follow-up at their expected times. A comparison was therefore made between the rate of resolution of OME in the unoperated ear observed at the precise time of follow-up with an interpolated assessment at each selected follow-up time based on the middle ear findings at the next appointment. *Chi*-square analysis showed no difference in any of the cells between the observed and interpolated data, and therefore the larger numbers in the interpolated data were used for subsequent analysis (Fig. 1).

The group treated by adenoidectomy alone showed a rate of improvement increasing from 39 percent at six weeks to 56 percent at three months, 64 percent at six months, 58 percent at nine months, and 72 percent at a year. Following adenotonsillectomy the rate of improvement increased from 59 percent at six weeks to 50 percent at three months, 59 percent at six months, and 62 percent at nine months and one year. However, in the no-surgery control group, improvement rate increased from 16 percent at six weeks to 22 percent at three months, 26 percent at six months, 19 percent at nine months, and 26 percent at one year (Fig. 2). *Chi*-square analysis shows that, compared with the no-treatment group, the effect of adenoidectomy alone is significant at three months ($p < 0.05$) and at six and nine months ($p < 0.01$) and at one year

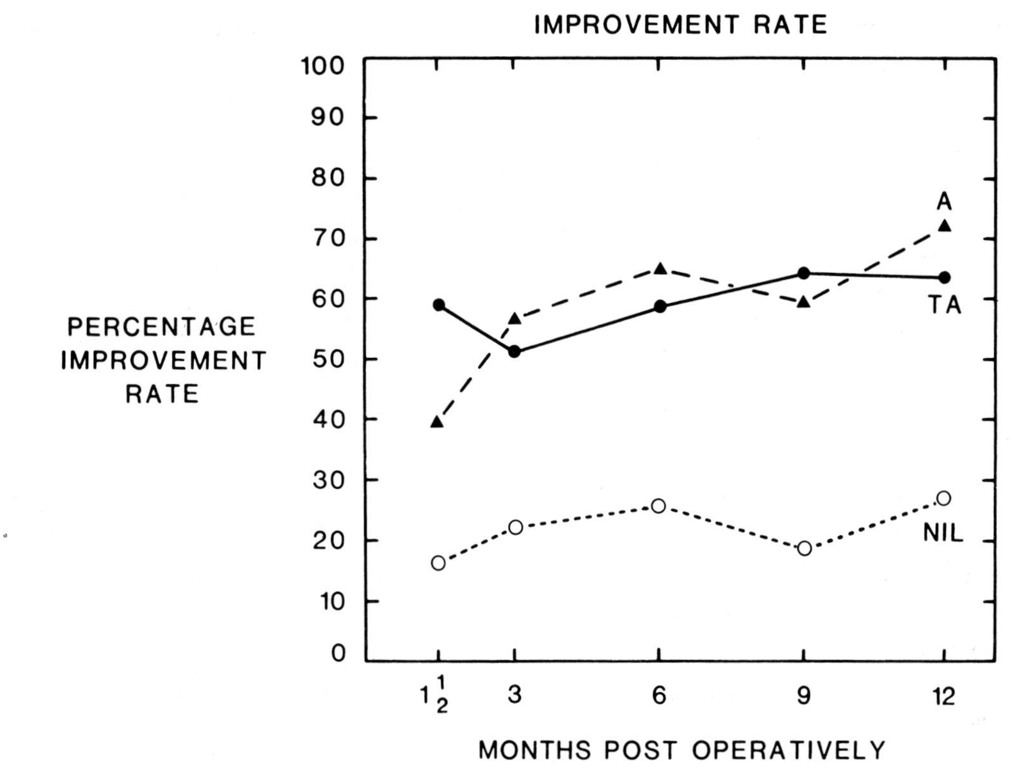

Figure 2 Percentage improvement rate of middle ear effusion following operation. A = Adenoidectomy. TA = Adenotonsillectomy. NIL = No surgery.

($p < 0.001$). Likewise there is a significant effect following adenotonsillectomy at six weeks ($p < 0.001$), at three and six months ($p < 0.05$), and at nine months and one year ($p < 0.01$). There was no significant difference between the adenoidectomy and adenotonsillectomy groups at any time following surgery.

DISCUSSION

Although adenotonsillectomy is less frequently recommended than adenoidectomy alone for the treatment of OME, only two prospective studies[4,13] investigated adenoidectomy alone for the treatment of middle ear disease. No properly controlled randomized study specific to OME has yet been reported. The natural history of nasopharyngeal and adenoid growth is poorly documented. Jeans reported disproportionate soft tissue growth in the postnasal space compared with the nasopharynx from 3 to 5½ years of age,[14] when there is reduction of the nasopharyngeal airway. Nasopharyngeal growth subsequently increases while the soft tissues remain relatively unchanged, and thus the airway increases. Equivocal results following adenoidectomy for acute suppurative otitis media have been reported,[15–17] and similar results have been found in relation to the management of OME.[5,6,18] The correlation between adenoid size, radiologically or volumetrically, and the presence or absence of OME is poor.[19] It is also accepted that there is a significant failure rate for adenoidectomy, particularly where allergy coexists, and in some cases otitis media worsens following adenoid removal.

A study designed to evaluate the effect of these operations on this condition must take into account inter- and intraobserver variability; the material must be homogeneous; and consideration must be given to the obvious variables of age, sex, degree of nasal obstruction, adenoid size, and allergy. The effect of seasonal variation and the known spontaneous improvement must also be considered.

The work presented here suggests that adenoidectomy has a significant therapeutic effect for up to 12 months in resolving the effusion in 36 to

46 percent of cases of OME established for at least three months. The effect is independent of age, sex, adenoid size, and the influence of any seasonal change on the condition. The study further suggests that the combination of tonsillectomy with adenoidectomy does not confer any additional therapeutic benefit. Finally, it demonstrates that without treatment 26 percent of these cases would resolve spontaneously during this period of time.

REFERENCES

1. Bateman GH: Secretory otitis media. J Laryngol Otol 71:261, 1959
2. Gottschalk GH: Serous otitis: A conservative approach to treatment. Arch Otolaryngol 96:110, 1972
3. Potsic WP: The role of adenoidectomy in secretory otitis media. In Snow JB (ed): *Controversy in Otolaryngology*. Philadelphia: WB Saunders, 1980, pp 154–159
4. Rynnel-Dagöö B, Ahlbom A, Schiratzki H: Effects of adenoidectomy: A controlled two-year follow-up. Ann Otol Rhinol Laryngol 87:272, 1978
5. Marshak G, Ben Neriah Z: Adenoidectomy versus tympanotomy in chronic secretory otitis media. Ann Otol Rhinol Laryngol 89(Suppl. 68):316, 1980
6. Sadé J: *Secretory Otitis Media and Its Sequelae*. New York: Churchill Livingstone, 1979
7. Roydhouse N: Adenoidectomy for otitis media with mucoid effusion. Ann Otol Rhinol Laryngol 89(Suppl 68):312, 1980
8. Lim DJ, Bluestone CD, Saunders WH, Senturia BH: Recent advances in middle ear effusions. Ann Otol Rhinol Laryngol 85(Suppl 125), 1976
9. Senturia BH, Bluestone CD, Lim DJ, Saunders WH: Recent advances in otitis media with effusion. Ann Otol Rhinol Laryngol 89(Suppl 68), 1980
10. Paradise JL: Paediatrician's view of middle ear effusions: More questions than answers. Ann Otol Rhinol Laryngol 85(Suppl 25):20, 1976
11. Snow JB: Role of tonsillectomy and adenoidectomy in the management of children with middle ear effusion. Ann Otol Rhinol Laryngol 1980
12. Maw AR, Jeans WD, Fernando DCJ: Interobserver variability in the clinical and radiological assessment of adenoid size and the correlation with adenoid volume. Clin Otolaryngol 6:317, 1981
13. McKee WJE: A controlled study of the effects of tonsillectomy and adenoidectomy in children. Br J Prev Soc Med 17:49, 1963
14. Jeans WD, Fernando DCJ, Maw AR, Leighton BC: A longitudinal study of the growth of the nasopharynx and its contents in normal children. Br J Radiol 54:117, 1981
15. McKee WJE: A controlled study of the effects of tonsillectomy and adenoidectomy in children. Br J Prev Soc Med 17:133, 1963
16. Roydhouse N: A controlled study of adenotonsillectomy. Arch Otolaryngol 92:611, 1970
17. Mawson SR, Adlington P, Evans A: A controlled evaluation of adenotonsillectomy in children. J Laryngol Otol 81:777, 1967
18. Fiellau-Nikolajsen M, Falbe-Hansen J. Knudstrup P: Adenoidectomy for middle ear disorders: A randomized controlled trial. Clin Otolaryngol 5:323, 1980
19. Hibbert J: The role of enlarged adenoids in the aetiology of serous otitis media. Clin Otolaryngol 7:253, 1982

ADENOIDECTOMY FOR EUSTACHIAN TUBE DYSFUNCTION: LONG-TERM RESULTS FROM A RANDOMIZED CONTROLLED TRIAL

MOGENS FIELLAU-NIKOLAJSEN, M.D., JENS ULRIK FELDING, M.D., and HANS HENRIK FISCHER, M.D.

Adenoidectomy—with or without tonsillectomy, paracentesis, or myringotomy—is among the most common surgical procedures in childhood. In Denmark we do this surgery in about 25,000 children a year,[1] and it has been calculated that up to 40 percent of the children in each Danish birth cohort will have one or more adenoidectomies before the age of 14. These figures are likely to be representative for other western countries as well. Our real knowledge of the effect of adenoidectomy is in glaring contrast to this frequency. Thus, in view of the widespread acceptance of adenoidectomy for treating persistent or recurrent eustachian tube dysfunction with or without middle ear effusion, it is surprising to find that until recently only eight prospective studies of the

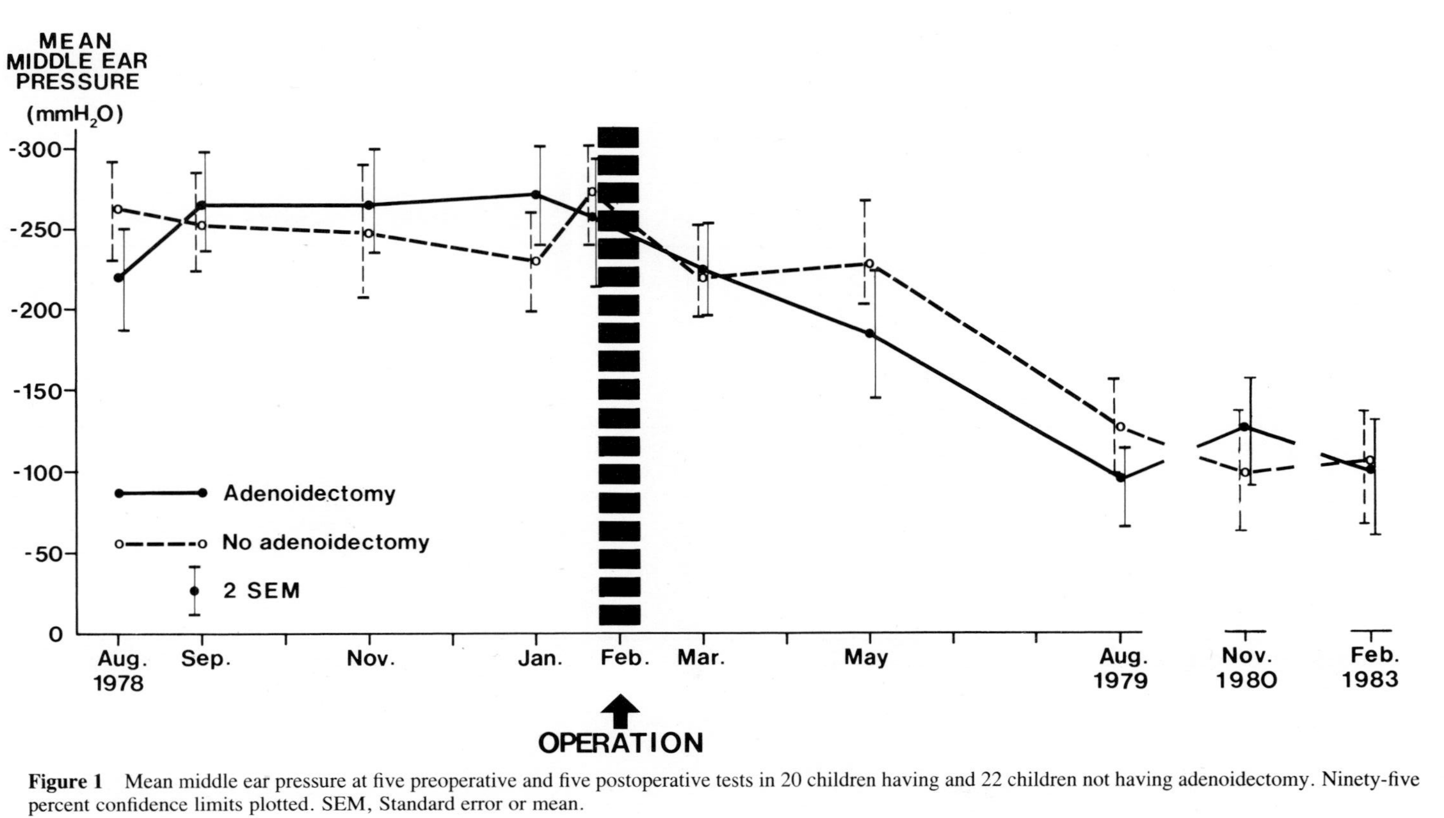

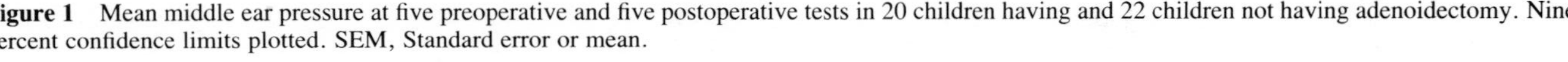

Figure 1 Mean middle ear pressure at five preoperative and five postoperative tests in 20 children having and 22 children not having adenoidectomy. Ninety-five percent confidence limits plotted. SEM, Standard error or mean.

TABLE 1 Adenoidectomy Trial: Pre- and Postoperative Distribution of Tympanogram Types According to Type of Treatment

	Preoperatively		*Postoperatively*									
	One-half Hour Prior to Surgery		*One Month (March 1979)*		*Three Months (May 1979)*		*Six Months (August 1979)*		*21 Months (November 1980)*		*48 Months (February 1983)*	
Tympanogram Type	*Adenoid-ectomy (N = 40)*	*No Adenoid-ectomy (N = 44)*	*Adenoid-ectomy (N = 40)*	*No Adenoid-ectomy (N = 44)*	*Adenoid-ectomy (N = 40)*	*No Adenoid-ectomy (N = 44)*	*Adenoid-ectomy (N = 40)*	*No Adenoid-ectomy (N = 44)*	*Adenoid-ectomy (N = 40)*	*No Adenoid-ectomy (N = 44)*	*Adenoid-ectomy (N = 38)*	*No Adenoid-ectomy (N = 39)†*
A	33	31	23	25	28	14	68	52	48	36	75	65
C_1	16	14	8	14	20	11	13	18	25	25	3	16
C_2	8	19	38	25	25	39	18	23	18	20	17	14
B	43	36	33	36	28	36	3	7	10	18*	5	5
p (chi-square test)	> 0.1		> 0.1		> 0.1		> 0.1		> 0.1		> 0.1	

Note: All numbers are percentages, not absolute figures.
*Two ears with grommets in situ included.
†One defective eardrum in 20 children excluded.

efficacy of adenoidectomy were on record,[2,3] and that collectively their results were conflicting.

In 1978 we initiated a study, which is still going on, with the object of investigating whether adenoidectomy actually influences eustachian tube dysfunction in young children. The short-term results from the study have been reported regularly, and details of the methods have been given explicitly.[6] In this chapter we report the results at follow-up 48 months after surgery.

MATERIALS AND METHODS

Of all 463 3-year-old children in a Danish municipality (population 37,500), 404 were examined by tympanometry and pneumatic otoscopy for the first time in August 1978 and again in September, in November, and finally in February 1979. Forty-two children who exhibited abnormal tympanometry, that is a flat curve (type B tympanogram) or a middle ear pressure of −100 mm H_2O (type C tympanogram), on all the four tests formed the material of the present study. The children were divided by randomized, blind allocation into one group of 20 subjected to myringotomy with adenoidectomy and another group of 22 subjected to myringotomy *without* adenoidectomy. The operations were carried out during the first two weeks of February 1979. All 42 were followed up by impedance audiometry, pure-tone audiometry, and otomicroscopy one month, three months, and six months postoperatively. These systematic and purely observational follow-up examinations were discontinued after the six-month test in August 1979, but all 42 children had long-term follow-ups in November 1980, 21 months after surgery,[5] and 39 of the children were examined again in February 1983, 48 months postoperatively.

RESULTS

The study failed to demonstrate any difference in middle ear status between the two groups during the first six months of postoperative observation (Fig. 1).[4,5] The tympanogram distribution in November 1980 and in February 1983 (Table 1) also afforded no support for a long-term effect of adenoidectomy on eustachian tube dysfunction. Similarly, the mean hearing loss and the percentage of children with sequelae to otitis media at follow-up in February 1983 were not significantly different in the two groups (Table 2).

TABLE 2 Results of Otomicroscopic Examination and Pure-tone/Speech Audiometry at Follow-up in February 1983 According to Type of Treatment

	Adenoidectomy (N = 38)	*No Adenoidectomy (N = 40)*
Otomicroscopy:		
Sequelae	55%	60%
No sequelae	45%	40%
Mean air conduction loss, TC (dB)	10.56 (2 SEM:3.52)	8.28 (2 SEM:1.66)

SEM, standard error or mean

DISCUSSION

As previously discussed in detail,[6] the present study and its conclusions are open to several criticisms. Still, we feel safe in saying that any real efficacy of adenoidectomy in improving eustachian tube dysfunction and in clearing middle ear effusion could at best be very slight, as this series of 42 children was not large enough to disclose it. Accordingly, the liberal indications for adenoidectomy as the primary or only "treatment" of eustachian tube dysfunction with or without middle ear effusion cannot be maintained. Large-scale studies are urgently needed for removing an ever-increasing suspicion that we at present perform much unnecessary surgery in this field.

REFERENCES

1. Pedersen CB, Elbrønd O: Frequency of adenoidectomy in Denmark. Dansk Otolaryngologisk Selskabs Forhandlinger 80:12, 1979
2. Paradise JL, Bluestone CD, Rogers K, et al: Efficacy of adenoidectomy in recurrent otitis media. Ann Otol Rhinol Laryngol 89 (Suppl 68):319, 1980
3. Roydhouse N: Adenoidectomy for otitis media with mucoid effusion. Ann Otol Rhinol Laryngol 89 (Supp 68):312, 1980
4. Fiellau-Nikolajsen M, Falbe-Hansen J, Knudstrup P: Adenoidectomy for middle ear disorders: A randomized controlled trial. Clin Otolaryngol 5:323, 1980
5. Fiellau-Nikolajsen M, Højslet PE, Felding JU: Adenoidectomy for eustachian tube dysfunction: Long-term results from a randomized controlled trial. Acta Otolaryngol Suppl 386:129, 1982
6. Fiellau-Nikolajsen M: Tympanometry and secretory otitis media. Acta Otolaryngol Suppl 394, 1983

VENTILATION TUBES IN THE PEDIATRIC POPULATION

MARK W. VOGELGESANG, M.D., and HERBERT G. BIRCK, M.D.

Tympanostomy tube insertion is the most common surgical procedure performed on children in the United States. It was first suggested by Politzer for the treatment of serous otitis in 1894, but he found the incidence of complications too high. The method was abandoned for almost 60 years and reintroduced by Armstrong in 1952. Since then the rate of failure and complications has apparently reached an acceptable level with the use of antibiotics and improved tube design. We hope that this chapter, based on a series of 4043 procedures, will contribute to an understanding and improved prognosis of otitis media with effusion.

MATERIALS AND METHODS

Between 1975 and 1980 1691 children were treated. All the patients were treated medically for a minimum of three months before their first tube insertion. One standard procedure was used by the same surgeon on all patients. Under general anesthesia a small anterior-superior radial myringotomy and a large inferior crescent myringotomy were made. Middle ear fluid, if present, was aspirated through the inferior incision and a Teflon arrow tube coated with an antibiotic ointment was inserted into the anterior-superior incision. The patients were seen three weeks postoperatively and thereafter at six-month intervals. Complications required more frequent visits. Antibiotics were given only when pus was aspirated at the time of surgery.

RESULTS

There were 1691 children in this study, for a total of 4043 ear procedures. Their ages varied from 3 months to 19 years. There were 722 females and 969 males (42.7 percent versus 57.3 percent). Bilateral procedures were done in 1622 patients. There were 34 tube insertions on the right side and 35 on the left.

The patient population included 1344 normal patients (no known associated problems), 268 allergic patients, 71 cleft palate patients, and 8 patients with Down's syndrome.

Looking at the age distribution for the first tube insertion, we found a sharp decrease at age 8. The majority of the patients were 1, 4, 5, or 6 years old. Both females and males followed this pattern. By age 7, 91.5 percent of the females and 90.9 percent of the males had had a tube insertion. The majority of patients—83 percent of the males and 78.6 percent of the females—required only one procedure. A second procedure was required in 11.2 percent of the females and 12.5 percent of the males.

In the allergic population the males were clearly in the majority, almost double the number of females, in a ratio of 65.3 percent to 34.7 percent. The average number of tube insertions was 2.5 per patient. The eight Down's syndrome patients were equally divided between the sexes and they also averaged 2.5 tubes per patient. Fifty-five percent of the cleft palate patients were male. Their average number of insertions was slightly higher, at 3 tubes per child. The normal population had the lowest number of insertions, with 2.3 tubes per patient.

In studying the number of repeat surgical procedures based on patient classification, we found that 19.5 percent of the normal population needed repeat tube insertion. The Down's syndrome population was similar, with a 20 percent recurrence rate. Both the allergic and the cleft palate patients were more likely to need repeat tube insertions, with over 36 percent having a second procedure.

The normal population was, on the average, 2 years old at the time of their initial tube insertion. The child with cleft palate was usually older, averaging 3 years. The allergic child averaged 3.85 years old and the Down's syndrome child averaged

9.1 years old. Overall, the average age for tube insertion was 4.5 years.

The middle ear findings were classified as mucoid, serous, purulent, and negative (no fluid found). The most common category was negative, 44 percent of the total. Mucoid fluid was found in 37.1 percent. Serous fluid was found in 14.9 percent and purulent effusion in 4 percent. The type of effusion found at their first surgical procedure in both males and females was surprisingly similar.

No effusion was the most common finding in the normal, allergic, and Down's syndrome populations. The child with cleft palate was more likely to have mucoid effusion. Otherwise the patterns of middle ear findings were similar in the four patient categories.

The 967 complications were divided into infections, perforations lasting longer than six months, cholesteatomas, atelectasis and tympanosclerosis involving more than 50 percent of the tympanic membrane. Infection was by far the most common complication, occurring in 23 percent of all ears. The rest of the complications were uncommon. Tympanosclerosis and perforations were found in 1 percent each and cholesteatomas and atelectasis in 0.1 percent each.

The allergic patients had the highest rate of complications, 30.4 percent. Infections were most common, occurring in 28.9 percent. Perforations and tympanosclerosis were found in less than 1 percent of these ears. There were no cholesteatomas or atelectatic membranes among allergic patients.

The cleft palate population had a 25.1 percent incidence of complications. Infection occurred in 21.4 percent of the ears, perforations in 1.9 percent, tympanosclerosis in 1.4 percent, and cholesteatomas in 0.45 percent.

Down's syndrome patients had the lowest rate of complications, with 10 percent. The normal population had a 24.6 percent rate of complications.

We examined the effect of repeat surgery on the occurrence of complications in the normal population. After the first tube insertions, 24.6 percent of the ears had complications. A second surgical procedure slightly increased the incidence of complications to 26.9 percent. With the third tube insertion a downward trend started, with 20 percent of these ears developing a complication. The fourth surgery caused 13.1 percent and the fifth 16.7 percent.

After the first surgery, infection was the most common complication, found in 22.7 percent of the ears. Perforations, tympanosclerosis, cholesteatomas, and atelectatic membranes were each found in 1 percent or fewer of these ears. With the second surgery, the rate of infection decreased to 18.5 percent. Tympanosclerosis was present in 2 percent of the ears. The other types of complications all had incidences of 1.3 percent or less. The third tube insertion resulted in a still lower rate of infection—14.2 percent—while the rate of tympanosclerosis continued to increase gradually to 4 percent. Subsequent surgical procedures showed a decline in the various types of complications except for the rate of perforations, which rose to 2.6 percent of the ears having a fourth procedure and 16.7 percent of the ears requiring a fifth.

DISCUSSION

The middle ear findings were correlated with the incidence and types of complication. Infection was the number one problem. Purulent ears had a 70 percent chance of developing a postoperative infection. Mucoid ears had a 24.1 percent incidence, serous ears 21.9 percent, and negative ears (no fluid found) had the lowest rate of infections at 17.9 percent. Perforations were the second most common complication. Purulent fluid had the highest rate with 4.5 percent. Tympanosclerosis was the third most common complication. Ears with serous effusions were more likely to develop tympanosclerosis than ears with the other effusion types. Interestingly, no tympanosclerosis developed in purulent ears.

Patients with purulent effusion were also most likely to need repeat surgery. Thirty-six percent needed repeat tube insertion. Ears with serous effusion had a repeat insertion rate of 27 percent and mucoid fluid ears 24.7 percent. Negative ears had the lowest incidence with 16 percent.

REFERENCES

1. Alberti PW: Myringotomy and ventilating tubes in the 19th century. Laryngoscope 84:805, 1974
2. Armstrong BW: A new treatment for chronic secretory otitis media. Arch Otolaryngol 59:653, 1954
3. Pappas JJ: Middle ear ventilation tubes. Laryngoscope 84:1098, 1974

4. Hughes LA, Warder FR, Hudson WR: Complications of tympanostomy tubes. Arch Otolaryngol 100:151, 1974
5. Gebhart DE: Tympanostomy tubes in the otitis prone child. Laryngoscope 91:849, 1981
6. Birck HG, Mravek JJ: Myringostomy for middle ear effusion: results of a two-year study. Ann Otol Rhinol Laryngol 85(Suppl 25): 263, 1976
7. Luxford W, Sheehy J: Myringotomy and ventilation tubes: A report of 1568 ears. Laryngoscope 92:1293, 1983
8. MacKinnon DM: The sequel to myringotomy for exudative otitis media. J Laryngol Otol 85:773, 1971
9. Mawson, SR, Fagan P: Tympanic effusions in children: long-term results of treatment by myringotomy, aspiration and indwelling tubes (grommets). J Laryngol Otol 86:105, 1972
10. McLelland CA: Incidence of complications from use of tympanostomy tubes. Arch Otolaryngol 106: 97, 1980
11. Per-Lee JH: Long-term middle ear ventilation. Laryngoscope 91:1063, 1981

EFFICACY OF MYRINGOTOMY WITH AND WITHOUT TYMPANOSTOMY TUBE INSERTION IN THE TREATMENT OF CHRONIC OTITIS MEDIA WITH EFFUSION IN INFANTS AND CHILDREN: RESULTS FOR THE FIRST YEAR OF A RANDOMIZED CLINICAL TRIAL

ELLEN M. MANDEL, M.D., CHARLES D. BLUESTONE, M.D., JACK L. PARADISE, M.D., ERDEM I. CANTEKIN, Ph.D., HOWARD E. ROCKETTE, Ph.D., THOMAS J. FRIA, Ph.D., SYLVAN E. STOOL, M.D., and GABRIEL MARSHAK, M.D.

The goal of this randomized clinical trial was to compare the relative efficacy of myringotomy (M) and of myringotomy and tympanostomy tube insertion (M&T) in relation to a control group (No Surgery), in subjects between 7 months and 12 years of age who had chronic otitis media with effusion (OME).

MATERIALS AND METHODS

Subjects who had persistent OME of two months' duration or longer which was documented and unresponsive to pre-entry medical treatment (antibiotic plus a decongestant and antihistamine combination) were arbitrarily divided into two groups: those who had "significant" hearing loss (defined as a pure-tone average of > 20 dB bilaterally or > 40 dB unilaterally, or an SAT > 20 dB above the age appropriate level[1]) and/or symptoms that included otalgia and vertigo unresponsive to medical treatment, and those who had neither significant hearing loss nor symptoms. After subjects were so divided, they were randomly assigned a treatment within each group. The rationale for this arbitrary division of patients before being randomized was that it was considered possibly unethical to randomize a child with a significant hearing loss and/or symptoms into the No Surgery treatment option. Therefore, subjects with significant hearing loss and/or symptoms were randomly assigned to receive either M or M&T, whereas those without significant hearing loss and/or symptoms were randomly assigned to receive either M, M&T, or No Surgery. The random assignment was stratified according to the patient's age and duration of OME. Following entry into the study and initial treatment according to assignment, all patients were re-evaluated at monthly intervals for one year.

A standardized history was obtained for each subject, and the findings of a standardized ear, nose, and throat examination were recorded. The diagnosis of otitis media at entry and at each subsequent examination was based on a previously described decision-tree algorithm, which combined the independent findings obtained by a "validated" otoscopist with the results of tympanometry and of middle-ear muscle-reflex testing.[2] Hearing acuity was assessed monthly by determining air-conduction and bone-conduction thresholds at four frequencies, as well as speech reception or awareness thresholds.

Children in the study were followed throughout the year for persistence and recurrence of OME. No additional medical treatment was given for persistent disease, but recurrent OME (that is, OME observed following a visit at which there was no OME) was treated with a 14-day course of antibiotic plus a decongestant-antihistamine combination. Acute symptomatic OME, purulent upper respiratory tract infection, or any other illness requiring antimicrobial therapy was treated appropriately.

The following criteria for repeat treatment and for "treatment failure" were used: in M subjects, three consecutive visits with OME warranted a repeat M; if a third M became warranted within one year of entry, M&T was performed instead and the subject was considered a treatment failure. In M&T subjects, three consecutive visits with OME warranted a repeat M&T; if a third M&T became warranted within one year of entry, the subject was considered a treatment failure. For subjects in the No Surgery group, two consecutive visits with both OME and significant hearing loss warranted performance of M&T and categorization as a treatment failure.

RESULTS

Table 1 shows the distribution of subjects by treatment group and selected patient characteristics. One hundred twelve subjects were randomized; however, three subjects withdrew from the study before initial treatment. Of the remaining 109 subjects, 39 were in the M group, 41 in the

TABLE 1 Distribution of Selected Patient Characteristics According to Treatment Group

	Treatment Group					
	Without Hearing Loss and/or Symptoms			*With Hearing Loss and/or Symptoms*		
Characteristic	*M*	*M&T*	*NS*	*M*	*M&T*	*Total*
Age group						
7–23 mo	6	8	7	7	6	34
2–5 yr	14	17	17	3	4	55
6–12 yr	7	5	5	2	1	20
Duration of effusion at entry						
2–3 mo	11	12	9	5	4	41
4–5 mo	4	4	3	3	3	17
6–12 mo	2	4	4	2	3	15
> 12 mo	3	1	0	0	0	4
Unknown	7	9	13	2	1	32
Laterality of chronic effusion at entry						
Unilateral	9	9	12	2	1	33
Bilateral	18	21	17	10	10	76
Sex						
Male	12	20	22	10	9	73
Female	15	10	7	2	2	36
Race						
White	20	24	22	7	8	81
Black	7	6	7	5	3	28
Total	27	30	29	12	11	109

Note: M, myringotomy; M&T, myringotomy and tube; NS, no surgery.

TABLE 2 Distribution of Subjects by Treatment Group and Clinical Outcome

		Treatment Group (N = 102)			
		No Surgery (N = 25)	*M (N = 39)*	*M&T (N = 38)*	*Total*
No ear disease		1 (4%)	0	14 (37%)	15
Ear disease*	Mild (1–2 mo)	2	3	12	
	Moderate (3–6 mo)	3	6	6	
	Extreme (7–12 mo)	6	4	0	
	Total	11 (44%)	13 (33%)	18 (47%)	42
Repeat surgery	Early (< 6 mo)	—	4	2	
	Late (≥ 6 mo)	—	2	4	
	Total	—	6 (15%)	6 (16%)	12
Treatment failure	Initial†	8	12	0	
	Subsequent	4	5	0	
	Nonprotocol	1	3	0	
	Total	13 (52%)	20 (51%)	0	33

Note: M, myringotomy; M&T, myringotomy and tube.

*Ear disease included otitis media with effusion, acute otitis media, and otorrhea. This classification excludes children who had repeat surgery or were treatment failures.

†Initial treatment failure is arbitrarily defined as persistent ear disease for ≥ 2 months after entry in the No Surgery group, ≥ 4 months after entry in the myringotomy group.

M&T group, and 29 in the No Surgery group. There is a smaller number in the No Surgery group because only children without significant hearing loss or symptoms could receive this treatment assignment. Of the 109 subjects, 86 (79 percent) had no significant hearing loss or symptoms and were distributed relatively evenly among the three treatment groups. The remaining 23 children who had significant hearing loss and/or symptoms were similarly distributed evenly between the M and M&T groups. The distribution of the subjects within the two randomization strata—age and duration of OME—was similar for the three treatment groups, although a higher proportion of children with an unknown duration of OME were in the No Surgery group. Even though the subjects were not stratified according to sex, race, or which ear was affected by OME, the distributions of those characteristics in each of the treatment groups were similar. About half of the children were between the ages of 2 and 5 years. Most of the children had had either two or three months of OME before entry (38 percent) or had an unknown duration of OME (29 percent). On entry, 70 percent of the subjects had bilateral OME. Seventy-four percent were white and 26 percent were black.

Table 2 shows the distribution of subjects in each treatment group in relation to clinical outcome. Of the 109 subjects, 7 withdrew before the one-year end point and without becoming treatment failures, leaving 102 subjects for analysis. The outcomes were arbitrarily divided into four categories: (1) children who had no ear disease, which includes OME, acute symptomatic OME, and otorrhea, after entry or initial procedure; (2) children who had ear disease during the year but who neither required a repeat surgical procedure (in the case of M or M&T subjects) nor became treatment failures; (3) children in the M and M&T groups who required a repeat surgical procedure but were not treatment failures, and (4) children who became treatment failures. Only one of the 25 children in the No Surgery group and none of the 39 children in the M group had no ear disease during the year. However, of 38 subjects in the M&T group, 14 (37 percent) had no ear disease during the year. Eleven children in the No Surgery group had some ear disease during the year but did not become treatment failures; two of these 11 had mild disease (lasting one or two months), while the other nine had disease for three months or more. Similarly, 13 children in the M group and 18 children in the M&T group had ear disease but did not require a repeat surgical procedure or become treatment failures. Three of the 13 children in the M group had only one to two months of ear disease, as did 12 of the 18 in the M&T group, the rest of these children having ear disease for three months or more. Six children in the M group and six in the M&T group required repeat surgical procedures during the year but did not become treatment failures. Thirteen of the 25 children (52 percent) in the No Surgery group met the criteria for treatment failure during this one-year period, as did 20 of the 39 children (51 percent) in the M group. By contrast, none of the 38 children in the M&T group became treatment failures.

In an attempt to determine the characteristics of children who were treatment failures as compared with those who were not, the effect of age, duration of OME, sex, race, and which ear was affected were analyzed. Of these characteristics, only duration of OME appeared to be related to treatment failure in the M group. In children in whom the duration of OME was six months or greater, or unknown, the chance of treatment failure was significantly greater ($p < 0.01$) than when the duration was less than six months. None of these selected patient characteristics seemed to be related to the development of significant hearing loss and/or symptoms in the No Surgery group which resulted in treatment failure.

The length of time tympanostomy tubes remained in place was examined. A total of 68 tubes was inserted in the 38 children in the M&T group who were followed for one year, and 54 (79.4 percent) were still in place at the end of one year. Thirty children received bilateral M&T at entry, and of these, 19 (63 percent) still had both tympanostomy tubes in place at the one-year end point. Of the remaining 11 children, in one child both tubes were spontaneously extruded during the year, and one tube extruded in 10 children. Five children received a second (repeat) procedure before the 12-month end point. Of the eight children who received unilateral M&T at entry, six had the tube in place throughout the year, one child received a repeat M&T in the "entered" ear, and one did not require a second procedure within the year. However, five of these eight children developed OME in the opposite, "unentered" ear at some time during the year, but in none did the effusion persist long enough to result in M&T in those ears. This finding is important, since the surgeon frequently is confronted with the child who has only unilateral chronic OME.

Nearly all children entering the trial with chronic OME had a conductive hearing loss in at least one ear, but the degree of elevation in the air conduction threshold was approximately 10 dB greater in children classified as having significant hearing loss at entry. Hearing levels at entry in ears without significant hearing loss were comparable in all three treatment groups, and hearing levels were also comparable for ears with significant hearing loss that were assigned to the two surgical groups. The percentage of time during the year spent at various hearing levels is shown in Table 3. These data are for 91 children, including children who were treatment failures, who were followed for one entire year. A hearing impairment of 25 to 44 dB was least likely to occur in the M&T group (2.9 percent); the clear majority of children in this group maintained hearing well within normal limits for the 12 months of observation. The likelihood of mild hearing loss at a given follow-up month was higher for children in the M and No Surgery groups and probably would have been

TABLE 3 Hearing Status During One-Year Observation Period after Entry According to Treatment Group (N = 91)

Treatment Group*	*Average*		*Hearing Status†*		
	Months Observed	*Months Observed*	*% Time with 0–14 dB*	*% Time with 15–24 dB*	*% Time with 25–44 dB*
No surgery (N = 18)	189	10.5	67.4	22.4	10.1
M (N = 36)	393	10.9	71.2	19.2	9.4
M&T (N = 37)	389	10.5	89.1	7.9	2.9

*No Surgery and M groups included children who received tubes during one-year observation period due to treatment failure.

†Hearing status is based on the hearing level in the better ear of a given child as determined by pure-tone average or age-adjusted speech awareness threshold.

higher if M&T had not been performed on those children who were treatment failures. None of the children in any treatment group had a hearing loss of 45 dB or poorer in the better ear.

There was no apparent relationship between the recovery of significant bacterial isolates obtained at the surgical procedures and the outcome in the three treatment groups. No significant complications or sequelae were observed during the year following entry into the study.

DISCUSSION

Within the limitations of the study's design, M&T permitted the child less time with ear disease and hearing loss during a one-year period than did either M or No Surgery. However, one of the important outcome measures, namely, the complications and sequelae of M&T, such as chronic perforation and myringosclerosis, could not be fully assessed in this study, since most of the tympanostomy tubes were still in place at the one-year end point. For this reason, children in this study are being followed for an additional two years. In an effort to correct some of the problems imposed by the design of this study, a second clinical trial is now in progress in which the criteria for entry into the three treatment groups are uniform, the duration of OME required for repeat surgery is four consecutive months of bilateral OME or six consecutive months of unilateral OME, and the criteria for treatment failure are uniform for all three groups.

It is estimated that approximately one million children have tympanostomy tubes inserted each year at an annual cost of about one billion dollars. It is important to determine if these commonly employed surgical treatments are helpful, so that children who stand to benefit may be treated and children who are not likely to benefit may be spared the risks, discomforts, inconvenience, and cost of treatment.

This study was supported in part by grant # MC-J-420434 from the Maternal and Child Health Research Grants Program and grant # NS16337 from the National Institute of Neurological and Communicative Disorders and Stroke.

REFERENCES

1. Wilbur LA: Threshold measurement methods and special consideration. In Rintelmann WF (eds): Hearing Assessment. Baltimore: University Park Press, 1979, p 20
2. Cantekin EI, Bluestone CD, Fria TJ, et al: Identification of otitis media and certain related conditions. Ann Otol Rhinol Laryngol 68:190, 1980

INFLAMMATORY EFFECTS OF OTIC DROPS ON THE MIDDLE EAR

ROBERT G. ANDERSON, M.D., CHARLES G. WRIGHT, Ph.D., and WILLIAM L. MEYERHOFF, M.D., Ph.D.

Topical otic preparations containing antibiotics, steroids, and carrier vehicles are frequently used to treat otitis media when tympanostomy tubes are in place or tympanic membrane perforations exist. These otic drops have also occasionally been used in normal middle ears following water exposure in patients with tympanostomy tubes or following traumatic tympanic membrane perforations.[1] Recent clinical experience and animal experimentation have suggested that under such conditions certain otic preparations may be toxic to the membranous labyrinth, resulting in sensorineural hearing loss.[2,3] It has thus been recommended that otic drops be used with caution in the presence of a tympanic membrane perforation without middle ear inflammatory disease. In addition, an inflammatory reaction of the middle ear mucosa has been suggested to result from the use of these same otic drops. The present study was designed to evaluate this possibility in experimental animal middle ears exposed to a topical otic preparation.

MATERIALS AND METHODS

Twelve young adult chinchillas weighing 350 to 500 gm each were used in this study. Bilateral tympanostomy tubes were inserted in each animal under ketamine anesthesia. Approximately 1 ml of Cortisporin Otic Suspension was instilled in the right external auditory canal of each animal daily for seven consecutive days. Three days later, on the tenth postoperative day, the animals were killed by transcardiac perfusion of a 2 percent glutaraldehyde, 2 percent paraformaldehyde fixative in phosphate buffer (pH 7.3). Immediately after whole-body intravital perfusion, the temporal bones were removed and placed in fresh fixative solution. The specimens were subsequently decalcified in EDTA, embedded in celloidin, and sectioned on a sliding microtome at 15 to 20 μ. The sections were stained with hematoxylin and eosin and studied by bright-field light microscopy.

RESULTS

Although all animals demonstrated some degree of granulation tissue, effusion, and focal hemorrhage in the ear subjected to Cortisporin Otic Suspension (Figs. 1, 2), two of the 12 ears had marked involvement in the inferior bullae, periannular middle ear air cells, and epitympanum around the head of the malleus and body of the incus (Fig. 3). The most common site of involvement was the middle ear air cells, followed by the inferior bulla, and epitympanum. The contralateral, control ears were normal in all animals. None of the ears demonstrated clinical or histologic evidence of acute otitis media or otitis externa.

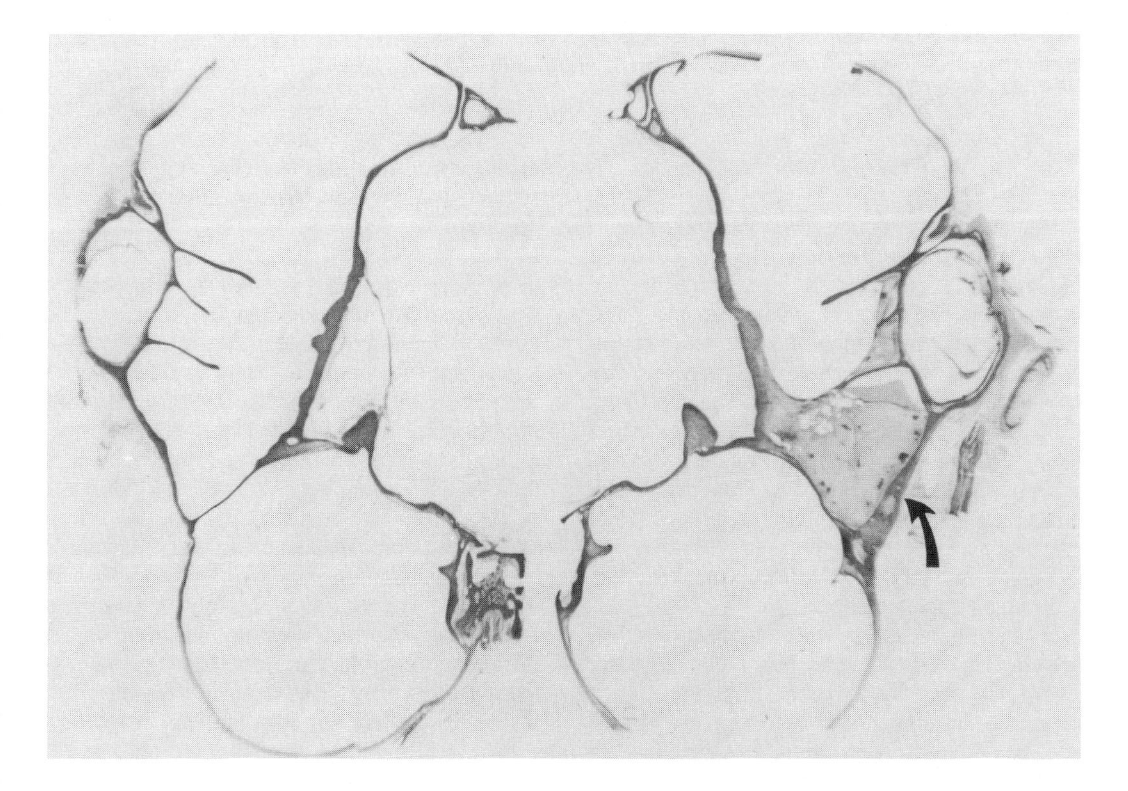

Figure 1 Cross-section of chinchilla skull showing left (control) and right (Cortisporin-treated) bullae. Note the accumulation of granulation tissue and effusion on the right (arrow).

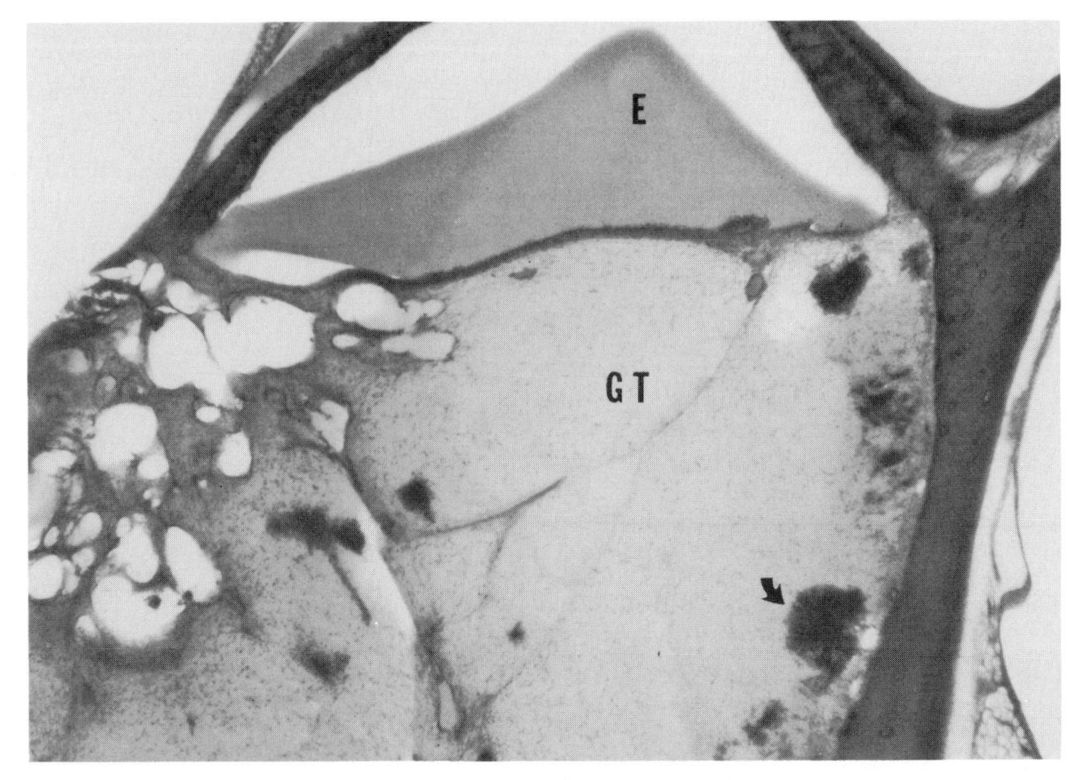

Figure 2 Higher-power view of area shown in Figure 1. Several areas of focal hemorrhage are seen, one of which is indicated by arrow. E, effusion; GT, granulation tissue.

DISCUSSION

Dumas and colleagues carefully studied eight cases of sensorineural hearing loss that occurred following the use of topical aminoglycoside otic drops in the presence of perforated tympanic membranes.[2] They concluded that the observed hearing loss was due, at least in part, to the antibiotic otic drops and noted that the risk of such a complication increased if the middle ear mucosa was not inflamed. Meyerhoff and colleagues confirmed this conclusion in an animal study by demonstrating a high-frequency sensorineural hearing loss and cochlear hair cell loss in chinchilla ears subjected to neomycin otic drops instilled into the middle ears through tympanostomy tubes.[3]

In addition to its known ototoxic properties, neomycin also causes a cutaneous hypersensitivity reaction. Although this hypersensitivity reaction is thought to occur clinically in 6 to 8 percent of patients, using a maximization skin test almost 25 percent of humans are found to be sensitive to topical neomycin.[4] Rodents, on the other hand, appear to be more sensitive to neomycin than humans, and approximately 75 percent of guinea pigs subjected to the same maximization skin test demonstrate hypersensitivity.[5]

Histologically it is extremely difficult to distinguish the cutaneous inflammatory response of a hypersensitivity reaction from that of a topical irritant or infection. Although the former is characterized by eosinophils and perivascular round cell infiltration and the latter two by varying numbers of polymorphonuclear leukocytes, the major histologic findings in all three conditions include epithelial and subepithelial edema, extravasated erythrocytes and fibrosis.[6] Although up to 75 percent of rodents may demonstrate a cutaneous hypersensitivity to neomycin on the maximization skin test, this does not adequately explain the uniformity of focal middle ear inflammation observed in this study of ears subjected to neomycin-containing otic drops. Based on the frequency with which the middle ear inflammatory response occurred in ears exposed to the otic drops, it is concluded that the demonstrated inflammatory response was due to a topical irritant in the otic preparation itself. It is possible, although unlikely,

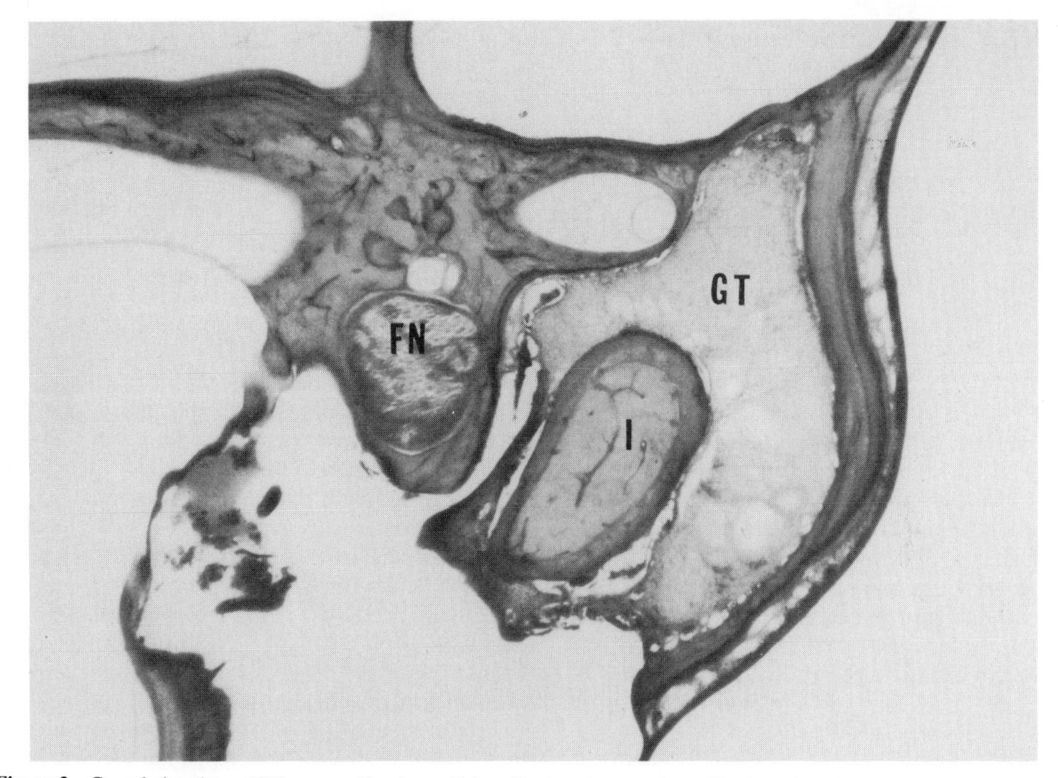

Figure 3 Granulation tissue (GT) surrounding incus (I) in a Cortisporin-treated ear. The lateral semicircular canal is seen immediately above the incus. FN, facial nerve.

that a topical irritant or infectious agent was carried from the external auditory canal to the middle ear by the otic drops.

Combination topical otic preparations are justifiably the mainstay in the treatment of many infections of the middle ear and external auditory canal. With their use, however, must come the recognition that there are potential adverse reactions of topical hypersensitivity and irritation resulting in local inflammatory responses and ototoxicity. Continued research in this area is necessary to develop a preparation with beneficial clinical effects in the absence of potentially morbid side effects.

This work was supported in part by the Jimmie Shiu Research Fund.

REFERENCES

1. Jaffe BF: Are water and tympanostomy tubes compatible? Laryngoscope 91:563, 1981
2. Dumas G, Bessard G, Gavend M, Charachon R: Risque de surdite par instillations de gouttes auricularies contenant des aminosides. Therapie 35:357, 1980
3. Meyerhoff WL, Morizono T, Wright CG, et al: Tympanostomy tubes and otic drops. Laryngoscope, 93:1022, 1983.
4. Kligman AM: The identification of contact allergies by human assay. J Invest Dermatol 43:393, 1966
5. Magnusson B, Kligman AM: The identification of contact allergins by animal assay: The guinea pig maximization test. J Invest Dermatol 52:268, 1969
6. Ackerman AB: *Histologic Diagnosis of Inflammatory Skin Diseases*. Philadelphia: Lea & Febiger, 1978

COMPLICATIONS AND SEQUELAE

COMPLICATIONS AND SEQUELAE OF OTITIS MEDIA: STATE OF THE ART

MICHAEL M. PAPARELLA, M.D. and PATRICIA A. SCHACHERN, M.D.

In discussing complications or sequelae of otitis media, it is just as important to understand the definitions of terms as to discuss otitis media itself. Considerations of pathogenesis are as important in understanding and classifying sequelae and complications as in understanding and classifying the clinical forms of otitis media from which they occur. Contemporary dictionary definitions are somewhat, but not entirely, helpful. ''Complication'' is defined as ''a disease or diseases concurrent with another disease,'' while ''sequela'' is defined as ''any lesion or affection following or caused by an attack of disease.''[1]

In this review, the term ''complications'' refers to those *serious* diseases occurring concurrently with or resulting from acute or chronic suppurative otitis media. They occur either in the temporal bone or in the intracranial spaces. The complications of suppurative otitis media have been described in classic textbooks of otology since before the time of Politzer. ''Sequelae'' herein refers to the more *subtle* (relating to dysfunction) and less serious (relating to life and death) affections following otitis media with effusion (OME). They include both active (infectious) and inactive (noninfectious) clinical pathologic results and developmental and behavioral problems. These ''sequelae'' have received deserved research attention only in recent years.

COMPLICATIONS OF OTITIS MEDIA

Complications occur within the temporal bone or within the intracranial spaces and are due to acute purulent (suppurative) otitis media (POM) or chronic suppurative otitis media (COM). Complications are discussed in standard textbooks of otology.[2,3] A scholarly discussion of this subject can be found in the text by Mawson and Ludman.[4]

Complications develop in cases of both POM and COM, especially in those patients with cholesteatoma. However, complications can and do occur more commonly than is generally thought in cases of COM with granulation tissue.[5] In COM, complications usually occur as a result of bony breakdown and erosion and of the direct spread of infection to involved structures. In POM, complications usually result from osteothrombophlebitis, through intact bone or through preformed pathways, but also from breakdown of bone and direct spread of infection.

Complications can occur inside or outside the temporal bone. Complications within the temporal bone include those of the inner ear (cochlear and vestibular labyrinths), the facial nerve, the mastoid, and petrous bone. Outside the temporal bone the disease can involve extracranial or intracranial parts. Extracranial complications of POM result from formation of subperiosteal abscess and can occur below the auricle (Bezold's abscess), behind the auricle (postauricular abscess), or anterosuperior to the auricle (zygomatic abscess). Bloodborne spread of infection in POM, or septicemia, can lead to involvement of distant structures by septic emboli. Our emphasis here is on intracranial complications.

There are clinical variants of otitis media that may produce unique features of sequelae and complications.[4] They include: (1) tuberculous otitis media, (2) syphilitic otitis media, (3) acute necrotizing otitis media, (4) type III pneumococcal otitis media, (5) hemorrhagic otitis media, (6) recurrent POM in infants and children, (7) pre-existing perforation of tympanic membrane, and (8) failure of antibiotic therapy. Space does not permit a detailed discussion of complications. Table 1 includes a classification of complications both in the temporal bone and intracranially. Detailed descriptions of these entities can be found in the literature.[2–4]

TABLE 1 Complications of Otitis Media

Temporal Bone	*Intracranial*
Facial paralysis	Extradural abscess
Petrositis (Gradenigo's)	Subdural abscess
Labyrinthitis	Brain abscess
Serous or suppurative (localized or generalized)	Meningitis (localized or generalized)
Acute mastoiditis and masked mastoiditis	Lateral sinus thrombophlebitis
Brain hernia (encephalocele)	Otitic hydrocephalus

TABLE 2 Sequelae of Otitis Media

Clinicopathologic Sequelae
- Active
  - Frequent recurrent attacks of POM and OME
  - Chronic OME
  - Continuum: OME (POM–SOM–MOM) → COM (granulation tissue, cholesterol granuloma, cholesteatoma)
- Inactive
  - Hearing loss (conductive, sensorineural)
  - Atelectasis
  - Tympanosclerosis
  - Otopathologic findings

Developmental and Behavioral Sequelae

SEQUELAE OF OTITIS MEDIA

Complications occurring from suppurative otitis media can be life threatening and were more common in the United States before the use of antibiotics. Otitis media with effusion (including serous otitis media [SOM] and mucoid otitis media [MOM], appears to be more common *since* the widespread use of antibiotics. Is this because of the greater frequency of OME, or because of better recognition of it? Sequelae occur from all clinical forms of otitis media, including OME, and thus involve large numbers of patients, have more subtle clinical manifestations, and are associated with significant cases of dysfunction and behavioral alterations. Sequelae of otitis media are classified in Table 2.

Clinicopathologic Sequelae of Active Otitis Media

Certain active (infectious) forms of otitis media can lead to other clinically active occurrences of otitis media. For example, one bout of POM or OME can be followed by frequently occurring bouts, as often as every week or month in some infants and children. Otitis media with effusion can occur as an acute disease that resolves spontaneously or under treatment, or a chronic form (sequela) can ensue. Transudative or serous otitis media is more apt to resolve than is secretory or mucoid otitis media, which is more likely to persist in a chronic state. Pathogenetic research on these clinical concepts requires controlled clinical studies (of both middle ear and eustachian tube) and bacteriologic, immunologic, and genetic studies.

The various clinical forms of otitis media can occur along a continuum; that is, one form can be followed by another. For example, in OME, POM can lead to SOM, to MOM, or to seromucinous OM (more common in children).[6,7] In turn, OME in children can lead to sequelae characterized by granulation tissue, cholesteatoma, or cholesterol granuloma later in life,[7–9] resulting in COM. *Cholesteatoma* is described as occurring from either migration of epithelial cells or metaplasia of mucosal cells or both. Granulation tissue can be seen to develop in the subepithelial space in animals with experimentally induced OME leading to COM.[10] COM characterized by cholesterol granuloma has been developed in monkeys[11] and in cats[12] consistently in a continuum from experimental OME. Cholesterol granuloma has been described after longstanding SOM,[13] and its pathologic factors and pathogenesis in humans have been discussed.[14,15]

Medical and surgical therapy have influenced pathogenesis and pathologic processes in individual patients, especially since the advent of antibiotics, and, it can be assumed, will do so in generations of patients who follow. Individual and epidemiologic studies are necessary to assess the effects of therapy on otitis media and its sequelae.

Sequelae of Inactive Otitis Media

The most important sequela of otitis media for most patients is hearing loss. *Conductive hearing loss* is well documented and common and is usually caused by various pathologic changes in the middle ear, including ossicular disruption or fixation.[16] Ossicular damage in otitis media results from inflammation (not necrosis from pressure) and has been studied by many.[17–20] Stapedial fixation can also occur as a sequela to otitis media.[21,22] *Sensorineural hearing loss* occurring from acute or chronic suppurative otitis media is not generally considered, but should be. Since our earlier studies of such cochlear losses,[23,24] other studies have followed to corroborate this finding.[25–29] It seems likely that temporary threshold shift occurs from serous labyrinthitis in the basal turn of the cochlea, leading to permanent threshold shift in the presence of active infection in the vicinity of the round window.[23,24,28,30]

Atelectasis may or may not be associated with other significant pathologic processes of the middle ear or with a hearing loss, but it often is and may require surgical correction.[31] Atelectasis and *retraction pockets* occurring after OME have recently been described.[32,33] *Tympanosclerosis* (hyalinized collagen) is seen very often in intact tympanic membranes of patients with normal hearing and with previous histories of otitis media. Occasionally, tympanosclerosis can involve the ossicles and mucoperiosteum of the promontory and region of the oval window, causing ossicular fixation and conductive deafness. In such advanced symptomatic cases of tympanosclerosis, calcification and formation of bone usually occur. The pathogenesis of this disorder has received little attention to date but its study is important.[34]

There are a number of otopathologic lesions of the middle ear cleft which follow previous otitis media and which may or may not be associated with dysfunctional hearing or with an active disease process. These lesions are often observed during otoscopy or surgery on the ear. Naturally, they are commonly seen in active otitis media. They include tympanosclerosis (as above), *perforation of the tympanic membrane, atrophic tympanic membrane* (healed perforation, retraction pockets), *ossicular discontinuity* (erosion) or *fixation,* adhesions or scar tissue, thickened granular mucoperiosteum, and osteolysis or osteoneogenesis.

Developmental and Behavioral Sequelae

In recent years interest has been aroused in developmental and behavioral sequelae resulting from otitis media in children. It can be assumed, in most cases, that an undetected hearing loss occurring in children from 1 to 3 years old with OME is a root cause of these problems. These disorders can be manifested as problems with hearing, speech, or language, or as problems in reading, learning, or psychosocial achievement. Impairments of speech and language associated with hearing losses from otitis media have received recent attention.[35–41] Impaired learning and intellectual sequelae presumably related to impairment of hearing and speech have also been described.[39–47] Behavioral or psychosocial sequelae resulting from childhood otitis media also loom as possible serious problems.[37,46,48]

Animal studies suggest critical and sensitive periods early in the development of the brain, during which time sensory (auditory) deprivation can apparently result in either permanently impaired cortical function or abnormal morphogenesis of brain cells, or both.[49,50,51] Whether such findings result from mild to moderate conductive losses, as seen in OME, is questionable. Although developmental impairments of a lasting nature can likely be attributed to otitis media in children,[42,43,52] a recent study challenges the legitimacy of earlier observations and data in this regard.[53]

SUMMARY

Complications and sequelae associated with or resulting from otitis media and its various clinical forms are classified and discussed. Complications occur inside or outside (intracranial) the temporal bone from acute (POM) or chronic (COM) purulent otitis media, and the term "complications" refers to life-threatening diseases more prevalent before the introduction of antibiotics in the United States. The term "sequelae" refers to active and inactive (burned-out) forms of otitis media that have led to conductive and sensorineural hearing losses and perhaps to developmental and behavioral impairment.

This study was supported by NIH grant NS-14538.

REFERENCES

1. Dorland WA: *Medical Dictionary,* 26th ed. Philadelphia: WB Saunders, 1981
2. Shambaugh GE, Glasscock ME: *Surgery of the Ear.* Philadelphia: WB Saunders, 1980
3. Paparella MM, Shumrick DA: *Otolaryngology.* Otology, Vol II. Philadelphia: WB Saunders, 1980
4. Mawson SR, Ludman H: *Diseases of the Ear: A Textbook of Otology,* 4th ed. Chicago, Ill: Year Book Medical Publishers, Inc, 1979
5. Paparella MM, Meyerhoff WL: Clinical significance of granulation tissue in chronic otitis media. In Sadé J (ed): *Cholesteatoma and Mastoid Surgery.* Amsterdam: Kugler Publications, 1982
6. Paparella MM, Hiraide F, Juhn SK, Kaneko Y: Cellular events involved in middle ear fluid production. Ann Otol Rhinol Laryngol 79:766, 1970

7. Juhn SK, Paparella MM, Kim CS, et al: Pathogenesis of otitis media. Ann Otol Rhinol Laryngol 86:481, 1977
8. Palva T, Kokko E: Middle ear effusions—complications of disease and treatment. J Otolaryngol 5:459, 1976
9. Tos M: Upon the relationship between secretory otitis in childhood and chronic otitis and its sequelae in adults. J Laryngol Otol 95:1011, 1981
10. Paparella MM, Schachern PA, Shea D: Genesis of granulation tissue in animals. In Sadé J (ed): *Cholesteatoma and Mastoid Surgery*. Amsterdam: Kugler Publications, 1982
11. Main TS, Shimada T, Lim DJ: Experimental cholesterol granuloma. Arch Otolaryngol 91:356, 1970
12. Goycoolea MV, Paparella MM, Carpenter AM, Juhn SK: A longitudinal study of cellular changes in experimental otitis media. Otolaryngol Head Neck Surg 87:685, 1979
13. Paparella MM, Lim DJ: Pathogenesis and pathology of the "idiopathic" blue ear drum. Arch Otolaryngol 85:35, 1967
14. Friedmann I, Graham MD: The ultrastructure of cholesterol granuloma of the middle ear: An electron microscope study. J Laryngol Otol 93:433, 1979
15. Sadé J, Teitz A: Cholesterol in cholesteatoma and in the otitis media syndrome. Am J Otol 3:203, 1982
16. Paparella MM, Koutroupas S: Exploratory tympanotomy revisited. Laryngoscope 92:531, 1982
17. Gantz BJ, Maynard J: Ultrastructural evaluation of biochemical events of bone resorption in human chronic otitis media. Am J Otol 3:279, 1982
18. Sadé J, Berco E, Buyanover D, Brown M: Ossicular damage in chronic middle ear inflammation. Acta Otolaryngol 92:273, 1981
19. Kärjä J, Jokinen K, Seppälä A: Destruction of ossicles in chronic otitis media. J Laryngol Otol 90:509, 1976
20. Thomsen J, Bretlau P, Jørgensen MB: Bone resorption in chronic otitis media. The role of cholesteatoma, a must or an adjunct? Clin Otolaryngol 6:179, 1981
21. Shea M: Postinflammatory osteogenic fixation of the stapes. Laryngoscope 87:2056, 1977
22. Adkins WY, Gussen R: Nonotosclerotic ankylosis of the stapedial footplate. South Med J 71:78, 1978
23. Paparella MM, Brady DR, Hoel R: Sensori-neural hearing loss in chronic otitis media and mastoiditis. Trans Am Acad Ophthalmol Otol 74:108, 1969
24. Paparella MM, Oda M, Hiraide F, Brady DR: Pathology of sensorineural hearing in otitis media. Ann Otol Rhinol Laryngol 81:632, 1972
25. English GM, Northern JL, Fria TJ: Chronic otitis media as a cause of sensorineural hearing loss. Arch Otolaryngol 98:18, 1973
26. Arnold W, Ganzer U, Kleinman H: Sensorineural hearing loss in mucous otitis. Arch Otorhinolaryngol 215:91, 1977
27. Moore DC, Best GF: A sensorineural component in chronic otitis media. Laryngoscope 90:1360, 1980
28. Münker G: Inner ear hearing loss in acute and chronic otitis media. Adv Otorhinolaryngol 27:138, 1981
29. Walby PA, Barrera A, Schuknecht HF: Cochlear pathology in chronic suppurative otitis media. Ann Otol Rhinol Laryngol 92 (Suppl 103):3, 1983
30. Morizono T, Giebink S, Sikora MA, Paparella MM: Sensorineural hearing loss in an animal model of purulent otitis media. Ann Otol Rhinol Laryngol, in press
31. Paparella MM, Jung TTK: Experience with tympanoplasty for atelectatic ears. Laryngoscope 91:1472, 1981
32. Sadé J, Berco E, Saba K: Atelectasis and secretory otitis media. Ann Otol Rhinol Laryngol 85 (Suppl 25):66, 1976
33. Tos M, Poulsen G: Attic retractions following secretory otitis. Acta Otolaryngol 89:479,1980
34. Schiff M, Poliquin JF, Catanzaro A, Ryan AF: Tympanosclerosis: A theory of pathogenesis. Ann Otol Rhinol Laryngol 89 (Suppl 70):1, 1980
35. Needleman H: Effects of hearing loss from early recurrent otitis media on speech and language development. In Jaffe B (ed): *Hearing Loss in Children.* Baltimore: University Park Press, 1977, pp 640–649
36. Katz J: The effects of conductive hearing loss on auditory function. ASHA 20:879, 1978
37. Gottlieb MI, Zinkus PW, Thompson A: Chronic middle ear disease and auditory perceptual deficits. Clin Pediatr 18:725, 1979
38. Lehmann MD, Charron K, Kummer A: The effects of chronic middle ear effusion on speech and language development: A descriptive study. Int J Pediatr Otorhinolaryngol 1:137, 1979
39. Cass R, Kaplan P: Middle ear disease and learning problems: A school system's approach to early detection. J Sch Health 49:557, 1979
40. Howie VM: Developmental sequelae of chronic otitis media: A review. J Dev Behav Pediatr 1:34, 1980
41. Zinkus PW, Gottlieb MI: Patterns of perceptual and academic deficits related to early chronic otitis media. Pediatrics 66:246, 1980
42. Downs MP: The expanding imperatives of early identification. In Bess FH (ed): *Childhood Deafness.* New York: Grune & Stratton, 1977, pp 95–106
43. Howie VM: Acute and recurrent otitis media. In Jaffe B (ed): *Hearing Loss in Children.* Baltimore: University Park Press, 1977, pp 421–429
44. Zinkus PW, Gottlieb MI, Schapiro M: Developmental and psychoeducational sequelae of chronic otitis media. Am J Dis Child 132:1100, 1978
45. Northern JL: Advanced techniques for measuring middle ear function. Pediatrics 61:761, 1978
46. Hersher L: Minimal brain dysfunction and otitis media. Percept Mot Skills 47:723, 1978
47. Howie VM, Jensen NJ, Fleming JW: The effect of early onset of otitis media and educational achievement. Int J Pediatr Otorhinolaryngol 1:151, 1979
48. McGee R, Silvia PA, Stewart IA: Behaviour problems and otitis media with effusion: A report from the Dunedin Multidisciplinary Child Development Study. NZ Med J 95:655, 1982
49. Greenough WE: Experiential modification of the developing brain. Am Sci 63:37, 1975
50. Webster DB, Webster M: Neonatal sound deprivation affects brain stem auditory nuclei. Arch Otolaryngol 102:387, 1976
51. Webster DB, Webster M: Effects of neonatal conductive hearing loss on brain stem auditory nuclei. Ann Otol Rhinol Laryngol 88:684, 1979
52. Paradise JL: Otitis media during early life: How hazardous to development? A critical review of the evidence. Pediatrics 68:869, 1981
53. Bluestone CD, Eichenwald H, Downs MP, et al: Special article: Workshop on effects of otitis media on the child. Pediatrics 71:639, 1983

THE EFFECT OF OTITIS MEDIA WITH EFFUSION ("SECRETORY" OTITIS MEDIA) ON HEARING SENSITIVITY IN CHILDREN

THOMAS J. FRIA, Ph.D., ERDEM I. CANTEKIN, Ph.D.,
JOHN A. EICHLER, B.Sc., ELLEN M. MANDEL, M.D.,
and CHARLES D. BLUESTONE, M.D.

This chapter summarizes the results of hearing tests performed in a large cohort of infants and children with otitis media with effusion (OME), that is, "secretory" otitis media. These children were enrolled in a clinical trial evaluating the efficacy of oral decongestant/antihistamine treatment for the disease. The findings of this clinical trial and the demographic characteristics of the study population are described in detail elsewhere.[1] The uniqueness of the audiologic data described here can be attributed to the prospective, well-controlled nature of the trial. The diagnosis of OME was made according to a uniform criterion, and hearing was assessed with a rigid protocol. Consequently, the data are important to the clinician as well as to the investigator interested in the effect of otitis media on hearing sensitivity.

MATERIALS AND METHODS

The population consisted of 553 children who received audiometric tests as part of the clinical trial. The group comprised 160 7- to 23-month-old children, 268 2- to 5-year-olds, and 125 6- to 12-year-olds. In all, 160 had unilateral OME and 393 had the disease in both ears. The diagnosis of OME was based on a decision tree algorithm[2] similar to that used in a previous study.[3] The approach incorporated the findings of otoscopy, tympanometry, and the acoustic middle ear muscle reflex. The sensitivity and specificity of this approach to the diagnosis of OME were about 97 and 90 percent, respectively.

Hearing tests and acoustic impedance measurements were conducted on entry into the study and one month later at an end-point visit. The behavioral audiometric technique was varied to suit the age of the child. Speech awareness thresholds were determined in the sound field for the children up to 36 months of age, play audiometry under earphones was used for children between 3 and 5 years of age, and the oldest group was tested with conventional audiometry. Three clinically certified audiologists were responsible for the hearing tests during the three-year course of the study.

RESULTS

Table 1 summarizes hearing sensitivity as determined by air and bone conduction tests for ears with and without OME at entry. The data for the infants and very young subjects include only the speech awareness threshold (SAT, adjusted to age-appropriate minimum response levels), since reliable pure-tone thresholds could not be obtained. Ears with the disease had an average loss of roughly 30 dB at all test frequencies except 2000 Hz, where thresholds were about 10 dB better. Ears not having OME—the uninvolved ears of children with unilateral disease—did not have completely normal acuity, although the average hearing levels were better than ears with OME. The speech reception threshold (SRT) and the pure-tone average (PTA) threshold at 500, 1000, 2000, and 4000 Hz were very similar for both groups, but the SAT of the infants was, on the average, 5 dB better than the SRT's of the older children. The typical 5- to 8-dB advantage for detection versus reception thresholds is probably reflected in this difference; moreover, the bilateral

TABLE 1 Summary of Hearing Sensitivity as Determined by Air and Bone Conduction Tests

	Test Frequency (Hz)						
	500	*1000*	*2000*	*4000*	*PTA*	*SRT*	*SAT*
Air Conduction Thresholds							
No OME							
Mean	15.3	12.1	8.6	12.2	12.2	11.0	—
Median	14.6	11.3	7.4	11.0	11.1	10.0	—
S.D.	9.5	7.4	7.2	8.8	7.2	8.1	—
No.	106	108	109	106	110	127	—
OME							
Mean	28.8	28.4	21.2	28.8	27.0	24.6	19.0
Median	27.7	27.8	20.4	27.5	26.1	24.4	17.7
S.D.	12.1	12.3	12.5	15.2	11.8	10.5	14.4
No.	650	667	661	630	669	779	101
Bone Conduction Thresholds							
No OME							
Mean	4.5	5.3	4.4	4.9	—	—	—
Median	3.9	4.6	3.9	3.8	—	—	—
S.D.	4.9	5.1	4.7	5.7	—	—	—
No.	86	87	87	85	—	—	—
OME							
Mean	4.2	6.2	7.5	8.4	—	—	—
Median	3.0	5.6	7.0	6.0	—	—	—
S.D.	5.3	5.7	6.4	8.0	—	—	—
No.	593	588	587	572	—	—	—

Note: Mean, median, and standard deviation (S.D.) values in dB; No. represents the number of children, not ears.

Key: PTA, pure-tone average thresholds for 500, 1000, 2000, and 4000 Hz; SRT, speech reception threshold; SAT, speech awareness threshold (adjusted to age-appropriate minimum response levels).

nature of the SAT determined in the free field and the consequent contribution of the better ear of the infant cannot be overlooked.

Bone conduction acuity was approximately the same for ears with and without OME, and the levels were mostly normal. However, there was a slight tendency for these thresholds to be elevated at 2000 and 4000 Hz for ears with OME.

Figure 1 shows cumulative frequency curves that represent the distribution of air conduction thresholds for pure tones. Only the ears with OME at entry are represented. As shown in the left frame, fewer ears presented with any degree of loss at 2000 Hz; that is, thresholds were distributed about 10 dB lower than the other three test frequencies. Clearly, not all ears had a mild to moderate conductive loss. In fact, the PTA data in the right frame show that approximately two-thirds (65.8 percent) of ears had hearing levels poorer than 20 dB; conversely, about one-third had levels equal to or better than 20 dB. Slightly more than half (51.8 percent) of the ears had PTAs poorer than 25 dB, and just over one-third (38.7 percent) were worse than 30 dB.

An additional set of cumulative frequency distributions is shown in Figure 2. The curves represent the SRTs, and the PTAs, for the better ears of children with unilateral and bilateral OME. These distributions illustrate the effect of the disease on the hearing acuity of "children" rather than of individual ears. It is apparent from these data that, as a group, children with unilateral OME had better hearing levels than children having the disease in both ears. About 60 percent of children with unilateral OME had an SRT of better than 10 dB, whereas only 20 percent of children with bilateral disease had similar SRT values. Overall, these SRT and PTA curves reveal that children with bilateral OME had an impairment at least 15 dB greater than that observed for children with unilateral disease.

The entire data set (that is, all pertinent observations across all children) was examined to determine the influence of various demographic and clinical characteristics on hearing sensitivity. At entry, acuity was not related to the previous duration of OME, the age of the child, or whether the child had previously received antibiotic therapy.

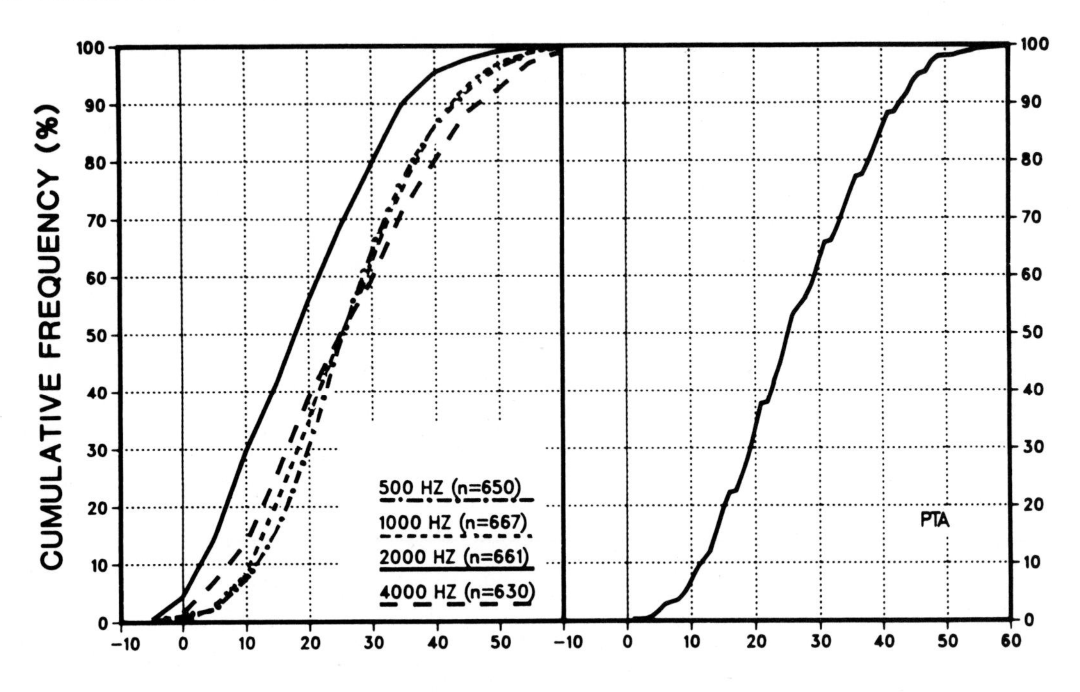

Figure 1 Cumulative frequency distribution of air conduction thresholds according to test frequency (left frame), and the pure-tone average (PTA) of thresholds at 500, 1000, 2000, and 4000 Hz (right frame) for ears having OME at entry.

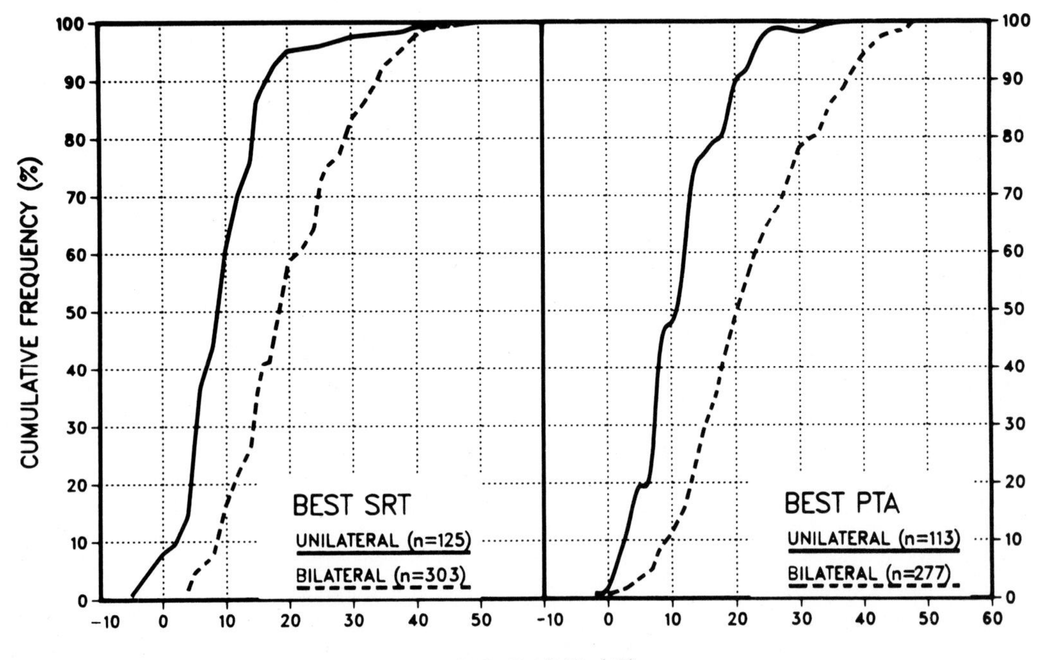

Figure 2 Cumulative frequency distribution of the speech reception threshold (SRT, left frame) and the pure-tone average (PTA, right frame) of thresholds at 500, 1000, 2000, and 4000 Hz for the better ears of children entering with unilateral and bilateral OME. In this figure, n represents the number of children.

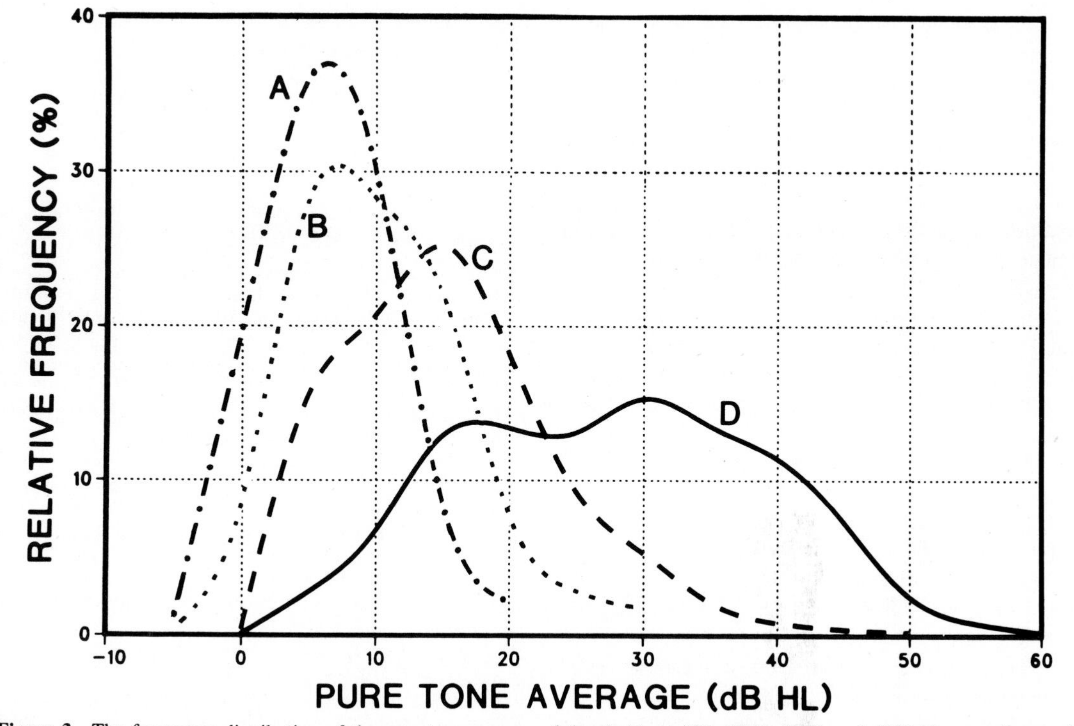

Figure 3 The frequency distribution of the pure-tone average of thresholds at 500, 1000, 2000, and 4000 Hz according to the outcome of the algorithm used to diagnose OME. The four curves represent (A) no OME and a normal tympanogram (N = 92), (B) no OME and an abnormal tympanogram (N = 280), (C) OME and otoscopic evidence of an air/fluid level and/or bubbles behind the tympanic membrane (N = 246), and (D) OME without otoscopic evidence of an air/fluid level and/or bubbles behind the tympanic membrane (N = 910). In each case, N represents the number of ears.

Pursuant to the lack of entirely normal thresholds in the uninvolved ears of children with unilateral disease, we found that only 20 percent of the variance in acuity for these ears could be attributed to the middle ear pressure determined by tympanometry (r = 0.44, N = 373 paired observations).

Thresholds for all ears (with and without OME) across all observations could not reasonably be predicted on the basis of the slope of the tympanogram (r = 0.15, N = 1523 paired observations). However, as shown in Figure 3, the distribution of hearing levels was associated with the clinical features inherent in the algorithm used to diagnose OME, namely, the relative "normalcy" of the tympanogram and otoscopic evidence of bubbles or an air/fluid level behind the tympanic membrane. In this context, a "normal" tympanogram was characterized by peak compliance occurring at 0 to 4.5 arbitrary units (roughly half- to full-scale deflection) and at +50 to −100 mm H_2O pressure. As the figure shows, when the algorithm indicated no OME, hearing was best for ears having a normal tympanogram (mean PTA 7.5 dB ± 6.9 dB) and slightly poorer for ears with an abnormal curve (mean PTA 11.9 dB ± 6.9 dB). Alternatively, when the algorithm indicated OME, hearing was better if an air/fluid level or bubbles behind the tympanic membrane were observed (mean PTA 17.8 dB ± 8.9 dB versus 28.6 dB ± 11.5 dB).

DISCUSSION

A clear understanding of the effect of OME on hearing acuity is mandated by the ubiquitous nature of the disease and its reputed association with linguistic function and child development. To date, our knowledge of hearing loss attendant on secretory otitis media has been based on a few reports of a relatively small number of subjects. Moreover, there was no agreement regarding the protocol used to diagnose the disease. Consequently, a report by Kokko[4] on 161 cases of "chronic" OME may not describe the same manifestation of the disease as depicted by Cohen and Sadé,[5] who reported only the "worst" audiograms observed in their patients. For similar reasons review articles, such as that of Bess published in a monograph by Bluestone and associates,[6] are seemingly no more informative. The data summarized here represent the most homogeneous set available to date. The diagnostic criteria and evaluation protocol were the same for all cases, and conventional audiometry was used by a limited number of examiners. The major findings can be summarized as follows:

On the average, a given ear with OME presented with a mild (approximately 30 dB) conductive hearing loss affecting all frequencies to the same degree except 2000 Hz, where acuity was about 10 dB better.

The pure-tone average was poorer than 20 dB in about two-thirds of ears with OME, poorer than 25 dB in half, and poorer than 30 dB in approximately one-third.

Acuity was minimally impaired for children having unilateral OME because of the hearing in the better ear.

The pure-tone average was associated with the general normalcy of the tympanogram and with the otoscopic evidence of an air/fluid level or bubbles, but not with the middle ear pressure or the slope of the tympanogram.

This clinical trial was funded by NINCDS contract NS-8-2384.

REFERENCES

1. Cantekin EI, Mandel EM, Bluestone CD, et al: Lack of efficacy of a decongestant-antihistamine combination for otitis media with effusion ("secretory" otitis media) in children. Results of a double-blind, randomized trial. N Engl J Med 308:297, 1983
2. Cantekin EI: Algorithm for the diagnosis of otitis media with effusion. In: Stool SE, Bluestone CD (eds): *Studies in Otitis Media:* Pittsburgh Otitis Media Research Center Progress Report, 1982. Ann Otol Rhinol Laryngol 92(107):6, 1983
3. Cantekin EI, Bluestone CD, Fria TJ, et al: Identification of otitis media with effusion in children. Ann Otol Rhinol Laryngol 89(68):190, 1980
4. Kokko E: Chronic secretory otitis media in children. Acta Otolaryngol Suppl 327:7, 1974
5. Cohen D, Sadé J: Hearing in secretory otitis media. Can J Otolaryngol 1:27, 1972
6. Bluestone C, Klein JO, Paradise J, et al: Workshop on effects of otitis media on the child. Pediatrics 71(4):639, 1983

NATURAL HISTORY OF ACUTE AND SEROUS OTITIS MEDIA DURING THE FIRST TWO YEARS OF LIFE

JULIETTE THOMPSON, M.S.N., PETER F. WRIGHT, M.D., JOHN W. GREENE, M.D., CLAUDIA S. ANDREWS, M.D., WILLIAM K. VAUGHN, Ph.D., ANN SITTON, M.S., KATHRYN B. McCONNELL, B.A., SARAH H. SELL, M.D., and FRED H. BESS, Ph.D.

Much of the natural history and epidemiology of otitis media remains to be defined.[1] For this reason, a group of 210 normal children were followed prospectively in a single comprehensive health care practice from birth to 2 years of age.

MATERIALS AND METHODS

Middle ear status was judged by pneumatic otoscopy and impedance tympanometry at each visit, whether the child was sick or well. Nasopharyngeal cultures for bacteria were collected at most visits. Viral nasal washings were obtained from most episodes of otitis media and febrile respiratory illnesses as well.

The clinical diagnosis of acute otitis media was based on finding an inflamed, immobile, bulging tympanic membrane with or without other associated clinical findings. Resolving otitis media was diagnosed at follow-up visits for acute otitis media as a condition in which inflammation had resolved but one or more of the following had not returned to normal: mobility, landmarks, or light reflex. Serous otitis media was defined by an immobile or poorly mobile tympanic membrane with evidence of retraction or persistent middle ear fluid.

Impedance tympanometry was performed by the standard method. Tympanograms were classified A (normal middle ear function), B (middle ear effusion) and C and As (intermediate curves indicating scarring, partial vacuum, or small amounts of fluid).[2] Diagnosis and tympanometry were assessed independently in a double-blind fashion. All episodes of acute otitis media were treated with the generally accepted oral antibiotic regimens for ten to 14 days with follow-up evaluation three weeks after therapy had been initiated. Antihistamines and decongestants were not used in the treatment of acute otitis media and only rarely in serous otitis. Very few tympanocenteses were performed and only three of 210 children had ventilation tubes inserted during the study period.

The 210 children were equally divided between males and females. and there were 130 white and 80 black children. A third of the children had older siblings, and the majority of the children were from the two lower social classes based on the Hollingshead Two-Factor Index. Motivation for participation in the clinic was measured in part by a 72 percent appointment compliance for all visits.

All children participated in the evaluation of either an octavalent or 14-valent pneumococcal vaccine. Vaccination did not significantly alter nasopharyngeal carriage, as demonstrated by 33 percent carriage rate in 140 of those vaccinated and 38 percent in 70 controls. Likewise, the mean number of episodes of acute otitis media was equal in vaccinated children and controls.

RESULTS

There were 3864 patient visits in the 210 children under 2 years of age. Acute otitis media was diagnosed 563 times, accounting for 15 percent of all visits. Further characterization of otitis revealed that 62 percent of all upper respiratory visits were accompanied by acute otitis media. Seventy-seven percent had one or more episodes of acute otitis media and 38 percent had three or more. Fifty-seven percent of all episodes were bilateral. No major infectious complications of acute otitis media were seen, and only one child, who had pneumatic tubes, had a perforation by age 2. One hundred seventy-eight cases of serous otitis were diagnosed, representing 47 percent of the children; 10 percent had otitis on three or more visits.

The incidence of otitis media peaked between 7 and 9 months of age, with a sharp decline up to 24 months of age. Serous otitis peaked between 10 and 15 months of age. The incidence of both acute and serous otitis media in white children was more than twice that in black children. No differences were observed between the sexes. The averaged seasonal incidence showed two to three times more otitis during the winter months.

One thousand seven bacterial cultures of the nasopharynx were done during visits when the children were well, 237 at visits with uncomplicated coryza, and 318 at visits with acute otitis media. Both pneumococcus and nontypable *Hemophilus influenzae* were seen frequently. However, because of the high asymptomatic carriage rates (26 percent with pneumococcus and 16 percent with *H. influenzae*) nasopharyngeal cultures were not helpful in determining the presence of otitis. Viral cultures were positive as often in children with acute otitis media as in children with uncomplicated coryza (28 percent of the time). There was no specific viral agent associated with otitis.

Care was taken that clinicians fully visualized the tympanic membrane and characterized the factors previously described. Among the three primary clinicians there was only a 2 percent difference in assessment of acute otitis media and normal ears. This close agreement supports the view that, with established criteria and careful observations, the diagnosis of acute otitis media can be consistent among observers. Correlation of individual examiners with results of impedance tympanometry in otoscopically normal ears showed a 92 to 95 percent agreement among examiners for ears judged to be normal with A tympanograms. The overall correlation of A tympanograms with otoscopically normal ears was 95 percent. However, noncompliant B tympanograms were frequently seen in ears judged to be normal by otoscopy. B tympanograms were infrequent during the first 3 months of life, peaked at 13 to 15 months of age, and by 2 years of age 23 percent of the tympanograms were type B. Correlation of B curves with abnormal ears was poorest beyond 15 months of age, suggesting that B curves at this time represent measurement of residual changes from the peak incidence of serous otitis. B curves in normal ears were more likely to occur in children with upper respiratory infection or contralateral otitis.

DISCUSSION

This population of normal children, followed longitudinally from birth to 2 years of age and without known predisposition to middle ear disorders, is a representative sample of the natural history of otitis. The role of viruses and bacteria in the pathogenesis of otitis media remains unclear. Tympanograms are helpful in screening for normality of the middle ear space; however, B tympanograms not associated with overt middle ear pathologic findings are frequently seen. This study emphasizes the very early age of the peak incidence of otitis, with a rapid decline in the second year of life, and suggests that this factor be taken into consideration when contemplating more aggressive treatment strategies.

REFERENCES

1. Klein JO: Persistent middle ear effusion: Natural history and morbidity. Ped Infect Dis Suppl 5:54, 1982
2. Jerger J: Clinical experience with impedance audiometry. Arch Otolaryngol 92:311, 1970

TYMPANOMETRIC PREDICTION OF HEARING LOSS IN SECRETORY OTITIS MEDIA

M. FIELLAU-NIKOLAJSEN, M.D., Ph.D.

The hearing loss associated with secretory otitis media (SOM) varies widely from case to case, and in the same patient from test to test. In 222 patients with SOM Cohen and Sadé[1] found an average hearing loss of 28 dB (range, 0 to 50 dB). The explanation for this fluctuation in hearing remains essentially unexplored, although to the clinician the magnitude of hearing loss often is the most important factor, for example, in deciding when and how to treat a young child with SOM. Therefore, it would be quite valuable to arrive at a handy, objective, and reasonably accurate method for estimating the actual amount of hearing impairment from SOM in the young child, in whom the degree of hearing loss probably is of quite particular significance, but unfortunately at the same time is most difficult to establish. With that in mind, the aim of the present study was to investigate any relationship between hearing and tympanometry in a very homogeneous population of preschool children.

MATERIALS AND METHODS

In 44 3-year-old children with chronic eustachian tube dysfunction selected by repeated tympanometric screenings from among all 3-year-olds in a Danish region, the results from impedance audiometry and pure-tone/speech audiometry were prospectively and blindly compared with the findings at paracentesis. Details of the methods, namely, series, selection, age range, equipment employed, surgical procedure, and so on, have been given elswhere,[2,3] as have the complete results.[4] Some main features of the method are listed in Table 1.

RESULTS

The gradient of the tympanogram[3]* and the magnitude of hearing loss separately correlated to the amount of middle ear effusion (Fig. 1) but not to the viscosity of the effusion. From Figure 2 it can be seen that no ear with a gradient of 0.1 or less had a mean hearing threshold better than 20 dB (HL), and no ear with a gradient of 0.2 or greater had a mean hearing threshold worse than 25 dB (HL).

---

*Editor's note: According to the author in a previous publication,[3] the relative gradient is the ratio of AG/AC, in which AC signifies the maximal height of the tympanogram, and AG (absolute gradient) is the distance from the peak of the tympanogram to a horizontal line intersecting the tympanogram in such a way that the distance between the points of intersection (x,y) is 100 mm H_2O.

DISCUSSION

In accordance with these findings, Bluestone and colleagues[5] found no relationship between the viscosity of middle ear effusion and the hearing loss, but these aspects have been only sparingly illustrated in man. Wiederhold and associates[6] arrived at the same conclusions after inducing middle ear effusion in cats that were examined by repeated auditory nerve response to broad-band clicks, tympanometry, and tympanocentesis. Furthermore, they concluded that there is a significant positive relationship between the size of hearing loss and the volume of fluid present in the middle ear. Renvall and colleagues[7] administered increasing quantities of fluid to the middle ear cavities of human temporal bone preparations, while doing tympanometry simultaneously. They observed that the tympanogram became rounded (that is, the gradient was reduced) when the level of fluid reached the umbo level of the eardrum and that it *gradually flattened* until the cavities became impacted with fluid. In the light of these two studies[6,7] combined, the present empiric demonstration of a reverse proportional relationship between the gradient and hearing loss (Figs. 1 and 2) is not surprising, although other factors, such as the thickness of the tympanic membrane and the position of the head during paracentesis/tympanometry/audiometry, might be imagined to play a role.

Table 1 Summary of Materials and Methods

Forty-four 3-year-old children in the series
Narrow age range (3.5 to 4.5 years)
Admission to the study exclusively based on preset, serial tympanometric results
Δ|TC–SRT| > 10 dB not considered
Audiometry within 24 hours and tympanometry within 0.5 hours prior to surgery
Same type of surgery
All operations done within a two-week period
One of two senior otologists performing all operations
No nitrous oxide in the general anesthesia
Findings at paracentesis recorded preoperatively
Investigator-blinded evaluation
No eardrum showing sequelae of otitis included

Because the frequency of low gradients unrelated to the presence of fluid in the middle ear increases through childhood,[8] the close relationship

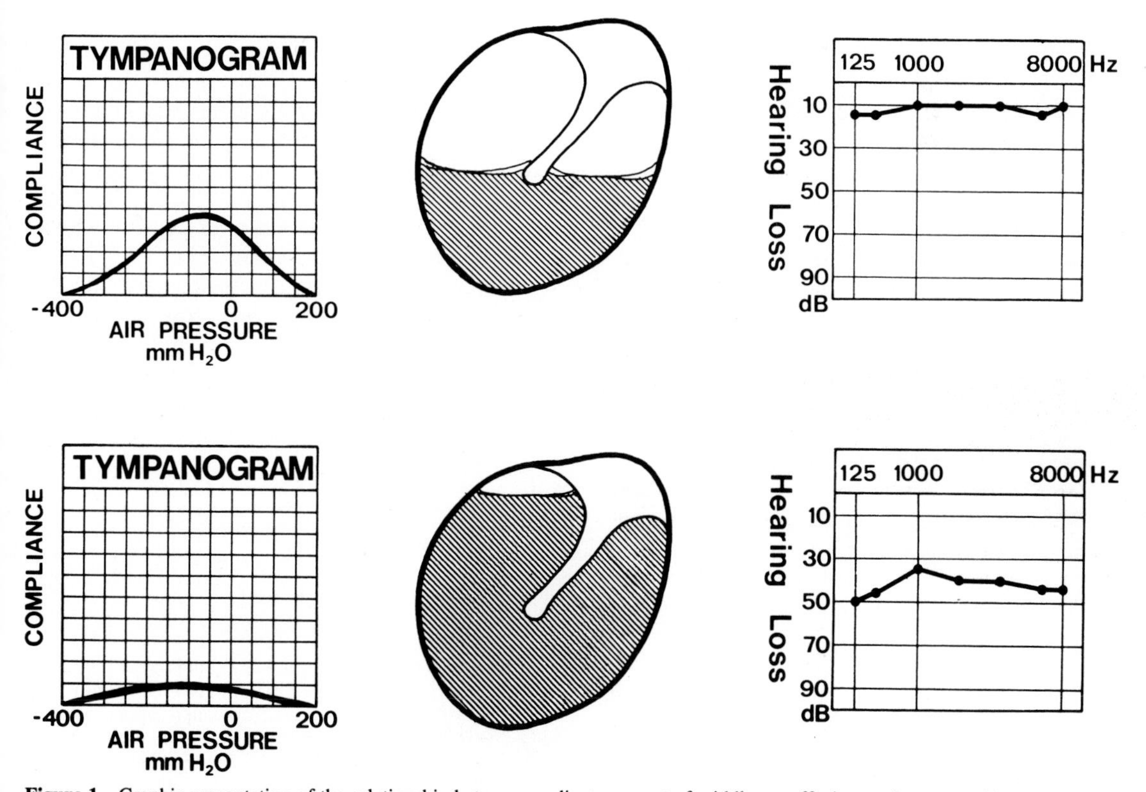

Figure 1 Graphic presentation of the relationship between gradient, amount of middle ear effusion, and amount of hearing loss.

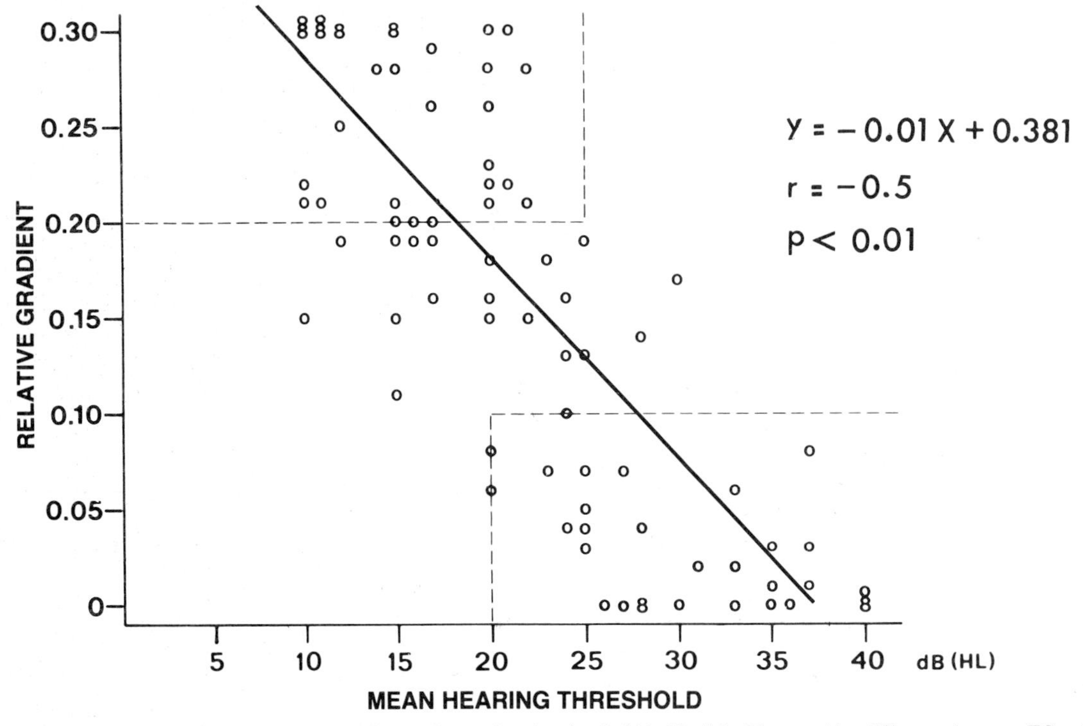

Figure 2 Relationship between relative gradient and mean hearing threshold in 79 of the 88 ears with a difference between TC and SRT less than 10 dB (HL).

between gradient, quantity of fluid, and amount of hearing loss may not apply directly to older children. Also, the irreversible changes of the tympanic membrane and ossicular chain resulting in changes of compliance at the drum, which often will be the case in children with longstanding histories of middle ear disease, will tend to obscure the demonstrated relationship in an ENT clinic clientele (see page 320). And indeed, it is among the youngest children with "primary" SOM—in whom a reliable recording of hearing cannot be obtained—that new possibilities of estimating the magnitude of hearing loss are most needed.

Among the additional studies needed in this field is a way to define the audiologically most appropriate borderline values of the gradient, but data so far indicate that a relative gradient of 0.1 or less pinpoints the majority of children having considerable conductive losses due to the effusion (Fig. 2).

The gradient concept should be incorporated in classification of tympanograms. Thus, the definition of the flat tympanogram as a curve having a relative gradient of 0.1 will eliminate the subjective element in deciding what is flat, and in almost 100 percent of young children the flat tympanogram correlates with middle ear effusion.[3] According to this definition, moreover, the flat tympanogram will not include cases of SOM in which the hearing impairment is minor (Fig. 2).

Because it has previously been shown that almost all preschool children can cooperate during tympanometry,[3] the present observations may delineate a badly needed, objective method of separating SOM *with* from SOM *without* major hearing loss in young children, who cannot cooperate to allow valid, conventional tone-audiometric testing.

REFERENCES

1. Cohen D, Sadé J: Hearing in secretory otitis media. Can J Otolaryngol 1:26, 1972
2. Fiellau-Nikolajsen M: Tympanometry and middle ear effusion: A cohort-study in three-year-old children. Int J Ped Otolaryngol 2:39, 1980

3. Fiellau-Nikolajsen M: Tympanometry and secretory otitis media. Acta Otolaryngol Suppl 394, 1983
4. Fiellau-Nikolajsen M: Tympanometric prediction of the magnitude of hearing loss in preschool children with secretory otitis media. Scand Audiol Suppl 17:68, 1982
5. Bluestone C, Beery Q, Paradise JL: Audiometry and tympanometry in relation to middle ear effusions in children. Laryngoscope 83:594, 1973
6. Wiederhold M, Zajtchuk J, Vap J, et al: Hearing loss in relation to physical properties of middle ear effusion. Ann Otol Rhinol Laryngol Suppl 69:185, 1980
7. Renvall U, Lidén G, Björkman G: Experimental tympanometry in human temporal bones. Scand Audiol 4:135, 1975
8. Brooks DN: The use of the electro-acoustic bridge in the assessment of middle ear function. Int Audiol 8:563, 1969

SOME DEVELOPMENTAL CHARACTERISTICS ASSOCIATED WITH OTITIS MEDIA WITH EFFUSION

IAN STEWART, M.B., Ch.B., F.R.C.S., CORALIE KIRKLAND, Dip.H.Sc., ANNE SIMPSON, M.B., Ch.B., PHIL SILVA, M.A., Ph.D., and SHEILA WILLIAMS, B.Sc.

The Dunedin Multidisciplinary Child Development Study sample, composed of children followed from ages 3 to 9, is described on page 25. This chapter examines the relationship between otitis media with effusion (OME) and various measurements of speech, language, and intelligence.

MATERIALS AND METHODS

Children were divided into somewhat different groups for analysis of developmental results. Those with sensorineural loss or severe mental retardation were excluded (N = 3). Results from 959 children were analyzed in the following groups (groups defined on page 26):

1. Bilateral tympanostomy tubes on one or more occasions for OME with hearing loss (descriptive group A, B, n = 52)
2. Bilateral persistent OME, with or without tympanostomy tubes but with no evidence of significant hearing loss (descriptive group C, D, n = 45)
3. Unilateral persistent OME, with or without tympanostomy tubes (descriptive group F, G, n = 26)
4. Transient unilateral or bilateral OME (descriptive group E, H, n = 118)
5. No evidence of OME but scar tissue present in tympanic membrane (descriptive group I, n = 136)
6. C tympanogram on at least one occasion but no OME, or a B tympanogram (descriptive group K, n = 449)
7. Always A tympanogram in both ears on assessment, OME never detected, no scar in tympanic membranes (descriptive group J, n = 133)

Analysis of variance was used to test for significant differences among the group means, followed by post hoc comparisons if the significance level was $p < 0.05$. A $p < 0.05$ significance level was also used for the post hoc comparisons.

At ages 3 and 5, language was assessed by the Reynell Developmental Language Scales.[1] Intelligence at age 3 was assessed by means of the Peabody Vocabulary Test[2] and at age 5 by the Stanford-Binet Intelligence Scale.[3]

At age 7, verbal comprehension and expression were assessed by the Illinois Test of Psycholinguistic Abilities[4] and intelligence by the Wechsler Intelligence Scale for Children (Revised).[5] Speech articulation was assessed by the Dunedin Articulation Check[6,7] and reading by the Burt Word Reading Test.[8] At age 9, the same measurements were used as at age 7, with the addition of a spelling test.[9]

TABLE 1 Developmental Measurements at Ages 3 and 5 (Means and Error Root Mean Square)

	Group									
	1	*2*	*3*	*4*	*5*	*6*	*7*	*ERMS*	*Significance*	*Significantly Different Groups by Post Hoc Comparisons*
Age 3										
Verbal comprehension	29.8	30.9	32.6	34.3	34.2	36.1	36.4	8.34	$p < 0.05$	1 & 7, 1 & 6, 2 & 7, 2 & 6
Verbal expression	32.7	31.7	34.9	35.7	34.2	36.9	37.3	8.06	$p < 0.05$	2 & 7, 2 & 6, 1 & 6
Peabody	20.5	20.5	21.8	22.9	22.5	24.3	25.2	9.42	$p < 0.05$	None
Age 5										
Verbal comprehension	49.6	48.1	50.6	51.1	50.9	51.2	52.0	4.76	$p < 0.05$	None
Verbal expression	48.6	46.3	50.8	51.3	49.8	50.7	50.4	6.38	$p < 0.05$	2 & 4, 2 & 6, 2 & 7
Stanford Binet IQ	99.3	95.6	103.0	107.5	105.2	107.2	108.6	16.00	$p < 0.05$	2 & 6, 2 & 4, 2 & 7, 1 & 7
Dunedin articulation screening scale	17.6	16.6	16.5	16.7	17.9	17.7	17.8	3.92	NS	

NS, not significant

RESULTS

There were no significant differences among the groups in socio-economic status,[10] maternal intelligence,[11] or in childhood experiences (a measure of environmental stimulation).[12] This indicates that the groups having OME were not disadvantaged in these respects, so it may reasonably be assumed that differences among the groups were due to OME rather than to these possibly confounding factors.

At age 3, none of the children had had tympanostomy tubes inserted. By age 5, 2.8 percent of the sample had had surgical intervention. The results at ages 3 and 5 are shown in Table 1.

At age 3, the groups with bilateral OME (1 and 2) were significantly disadvantaged in terms of verbal comprehension and expression. At age 5, these groups were also significantly disadvantaged in intelligence.

By age 7, 10 percent of the children had had surgical intervention. The results at age 7 are shown in Table 2.

At age 7, the groups with bilateral OME (1 and 2) were significantly disadvantaged in verbal expression, verbal IQ, and full scale IQ, but not in performance IQ. No other differences were significant.

By age 9, few children had active, continuing problems with OME. The results of tests at age 9 are shown in Table 3. The IQ and language differences between the groups were no longer significant but group 1 was still significantly disadvantaged in speech articulation.

DISCUSSION

Otitis media with effusion appears to be associated with significant disadvantages in speech articulation, verbal comprehension and expression,

TABLE 2 Developmental Measurements at Age 7 (Means and Error Root Mean Square)

	Group									
	1	*2*	*3*	*4*	*5*	*6*	*7*	*ERMS*	*Significance*	*Significantly Different Groups by Post Hoc Comparisons*
ITPA comprehension	26.4	26.0	29.3	29.5	29.4	29.0	30.0	8.02	NS	
ITPA expression	25.7	25.4	27.8	29.8	28.7	30.6	30.6	8.39	$p < 0.05$	2 & 6, 2 & 5, 1 & 6
Verbal IQ	98.7	102.1	104.7	106.4	105.0	106.5	107.8	14.73	$p < 0.05$	1 & 6, 1 & 7
Performance IQ	100.3	103.9	105.4	106.5	107.3	107.7	107.9	14.18	NS	
Full scale IQ	100.3	103.2	105.4	107.2	106.6	107.8	108.7	14.14	$p < 0.05$	1 & 7
Dundedin articulation check	13.2	13.3	13.4	13.8	14.4	14.7	15.2	3.61	$p < 0.05$	None
Reading	23.5	26.0	26.8	28.4	28.8	30.5	31.2	13.23	$p < 0.05$	None

NS, not significant

TABLE 3 Developmental Measurements at Age 9 (Means and Error Root Mean Square)

	Group								
	1	*2*	*3*	*4*	*5*	*6*	*7*	*ERMS*	*Significance*
ITPA comprehension	33.6	32.0	35.6	34.2	33.9	35.3	36.2	7.67	NS
ITPA expression	33.7	35.0	34.8	34.2	34.2	36.0	36.6	9.02	NS
Verbal IQ	97.2	101.2	98.2	101.9	102.0	104.4	104.5	15.72	NS
Performance IQ	100.7	103.5	105.2	105.0	104.5	106.1	106.0	14.93	NS
Full scale IQ	98.6	102.2	101.7	103.5	103.6	105.7	105.6	15.21	NS
Reading	47.0	51.7	51.2	52.7	52.5	54.6	56.5	18.9	NS
Spelling	8.1	10.2	9.9	9.9	10.2	10.4	10.9	6.16	NS
Dunedin articulation check	14.8	15.5	15.8	15.8	16.4	16.0	17.0	3.05	$p < 0.05$*

NS, not significant
*Post hoc comparisons showed Groups 1 and 7 differed significantly ($p < 0.05$).

and IQ for the first seven years of life. With increasing age and falling prevalence of OME, associated with an active treatment program, these disadvantages tend to disappear, although delayed speech articulation is still evident at the age of 9. Further research is required to address the major unanswered question of whether available intervention measures are effective in overcoming these developmental disadvantages associated with OME.

The Dunedin Multidisciplinary Research and Development Unit is supported by the Medical Research Council of New Zealand, the National Children's Health Research Foundation, The McKenzie Education Foundation, and the Departments of Education and Health of the New Zealand Government. The otologic research has also been supported by The Deafness Research Foundation.

REFERENCES

1. Reynell J: *Reynell Developmental Language Scales.* London: National Foundation for Educational Research, 1969
2. Dunn L: *The Peabody Picture Vocabulary Test.* Minneapolis: American Guidance Service, 1965
3. Terman LM, Merrill MR: *Stanford-Binet Intelligence Scale.* Boston: Houghton Mifflin, 1960
4. Kirk SA, McCarthy JJ, Kirk WD: *The Illinois Test of Psycholinguistic Abilities* (Revised ed). Urbana, IL: The University of Illinois Press, 1968
5. Wechsler D: *The Wechsler Intelligence Scale for Children* (revised). New York: The Psychological Corporation, 1974
6. Silva PA: *The Dunedin Articulation Screening Scale.* Dunedin: Otago Speech Therapy Association, 1980
7. Silva PA, McGee RO, Williams SM: *From Birth to Seven: Child Development in Dunedin: A Multidisciplinary Study.* Unpublished report available from the University of Otago Medical Library, 1981
8. Scottish Council for Educational Research: *The Burt Word Reading Test,* (1974 revision). London: Hodder and Stoughton, 1976
9. Smith CTW, Pearce DW: Testing spelling: Attainment norms and comparisons for pupils from 9–13 years. National Education April 1, p. 117, 1966
10. Elley WR, Irving JC: Revised socio-economic index for New Zealand. NZ J Educ Studies 11:433, 1976
11. Thurstone TJ, Thurstone LL: *The SRA Verbal Form.* Chicago: Science Research Associates, 1973
12. Silva PA: Experiences, activities and the preschool child: A report from the Dunedin Multidisciplinary Child Development Study. Aust J Early Childhood 5:13, 1980

OTITIS MEDIA WITH EFFUSION DURING THE FIRST THREE YEARS OF LIFE AND DEVELOPMENT OF SPEECH AND LANGUAGE

JEROME O. KLEIN, M.D., DAVID W. TEELE, M.D., RONNI MANNOS, M.A., PAULA MENYUK, Ph.D., and BERNARD A. ROSNER, Ph.D.

To determine the association of infections of the middle ear and time spent with middle ear effusion (MEE) with development of speech and language, we studied 205 white children of varying socioeconomic strata (SES) from Greater Boston. The children were selected from a cohort of children who have been followed from birth in five health centers with regular examination of the middle ear at each visit to office or clinic, whether for illness or routine care. The study was prospective, used uniform criteria for diagnosis of otitis media and MEE, and tested children from all SES.

MATERIAL AND METHODS

In July 1975, pediatricians and nurse practitioners in five health centers who formed the Greater Boston Collaborative Otitis Media Study Group began to enroll each newborn infant coming to their offices for care. Over the next two years they enrolled 2568 consecutive children, all of whom were first seen before the age of 3 months. At each visit practitioners examined the children's ears using a standard sealed pneumatic otoscope. Diminished or absent mobility was required for the diagnosis of MEE. To ensure interobserver reliability, one of the investigators (J. O. K. or D. W. T.) assessed the diagnostic skills of the pediatricians and nurse practitioners using a specially designed doubled-headed pneumatic otoscope.

Since daily observation to establish precise onset and end of MEE was not possible, we had to make certain assumptions about time spent with MEE. For the purposes of this analysis, we assumed that unless documented to be shorter each episode of MEE lasted 29 days. We based this estimate on the observation that the median duration of MEE after first diagnosis of acute otitis media was 23 days (based on over 700 such episodes).

We selected 205 children for testing at age 3 years, including children who had no more than one episode of acute otitis media by age 2 years and children who had had at least three episodes of acute otitis media by age 2 years. We excluded children whose primary language was not English, who were nonwhite, or who had a history of cleft palate, developmental delay, or seizures.

Tests of speech and language administered at the third birthday, plus or minus three months, included the Peabody Picture Vocabulary Test (a test of comprehension of vocabulary), the Zimmerman Pre-School Language Scale (a test of both early receptive and expressive language), the Fisher-Logemann/Goldman-Fristoe Test of Articulation (a test of production of speech sounds), estimate of intelligibility, measurements of number of grammatical transformations (a test of complexity of language structure), and measurements of mean length of utterance in a collected sample of speech. Each child underwent a screening audiogram before being tested to ensure that loss of hearing would not affect the results of the tests. No child was found to have sufficiently impaired hearing to be excluded.

For each score from tests of speech and language, we used a one-way analysis of variance to compare children who had spent less than 30 days with MEE during the first three years of life with those who had spent 30 to 129 days with MEE during the first three years of life and with those who had spent 130 or more days with MEE during the first three years of life. We performed a similar analysis for the first six months of life to compare children who had spent less than 30 days with those who had spent 30 to 59 days and with those who had spent 60 or more days with MEE.

RESULTS

Scores on selected tests for children from all five health centers were lower for children with prolonged time with MEE than for children who had spent little or no time with MEE, but the differences were significant only for the Peabody Picture Vocabulary Test at 130 or more days spent with MEE. For children from private practice, a high SES group, scores in all three tests for those who spent 130 or more days with MEE were significantly lower than for those who had spent little or no time with MEE (Table 1). No significant differences were found for children from a single large, urban health center, a low SES group. Results of other tests, including connected discourse intelligibility, number of grammatic transformations, mean length of utterance, and test of articulation, showed no association with time with MEE.

Increased time with MEE during the first six months of life was associated with lower scores on the Peabody Picture Vocabulary Test, Auditory Comprehension Quotient, and Verbal Ability Quotient. These findings were most significant for children from private practice. No consistent significant associations were found for other periods of six or 12 months after the first six months of life. In addition, no significant associations were found when we examined results for the period from 7 to 36 months of age.

DISCUSSION

These data showed that children who suffered from recurrent acute otitis media with prolonged time with MEE scored less well on standard tests of language administered at 3 years of age than did children who had little or no middle ear disease. Children from higher SES who suffered from otitis media and persistent MEE were at greatest risk for poor performance. Within the first three years of life, disease of the middle ear during the first six to 12 months appeared to be most important. This association appeared to be independent of later experience with MEE. Thus, children who spent little time with MEE during the first six months and then spent much time with MEE during the next 30 months had scores similar to children who had spent little time with MEE during the entire first three years of life.

This study in Greater Boston was prospective and included a large number of children who were

TABLE 1 Association Between Time with MEE During First Three Years of Life and Scores on Tests of Speech and Language

Time with MEE* in First 3 Years	Entire Group				Private Practice				Urban Neighborhood Health Center			
	No.	*Mean*	*S.D.*	*P*†	*No.*	*Mean*	*S.D.*	*P*	*No.*	*Mean*	*S.D.*	*P*
					Peabody Picture Vocabulary Test							
< 30 days	52	101.4	17.1	—	20	113.5	12.3	—	18	92.2	14.2	—
30–129 days	58	99.4	16.5	NS‡	18	108.5	14.8	NS	28	94.0	14.0	NS
130+ days	80	96.4	15.3	.044	27	104.2	12.3	.01	35	92.8	15.4	NS
					Auditory Comprehension Quotient							
< 30 days	54	123.4	21.7	—	20	135.0	19.3	—	20	111.6	15.3	—
30–129 days	63	120.1	20.3	NS	20	126.6	17.3	.07	30	113.2	20.0	NS
130+ days	88	119.9	18.6	NS	29	120.4	17.2	.003	38	116.9	18.6	NS
					Verbal Ability Quotient							
< 30 days	53	120.6	23.7	—	20	130.0	26.1	—	19	108.8	16.4	—
30–129 days	62	116.0	22.4	NS	19	114.4	19.4	.015	30	114.1	23.5	NS
130+ days	86	116.0	24.6	NS	28	112.4	20.0	.004	37	115.8	26.1	NS

*MEE, middle ear effusion, either unilateral or bilateral

†Obtained from one-tailed *t*-tests within the context of a one-way analysis of variance. Each group compared with those children with less than 30 days with MEE.

‡NS, not significant

screened for significant loss of hearing at the time of administration of tests of speech and language. Confounding variables, such as SES, race, birth order and patterns of day care, were either controlled for or excluded as having any significant effects. We were unable to avoid other deficiencies: Selection of subjects was based on most and least severely affected children and thus was not random; audiologic assessment was not available during every episode of MEE; data about the quality of parental-child stimulation was not available; nor did we investigate the effects of chronic illness on such stimulation.

Although these results show a significant association between time with MEE and scores on certain tests of speech and language, they do not show if such an association leads to permanent impairment. Current studies with the same cohort of children (now 7 years of age and older) should yield information to help provide an answer to this question.

This study was supported in part by Contract #NO1 A1 5253 from the National Institute of Allergy and Infectious Diseases.

INFLUENCE OF EARLY OTITIS MEDIA WITH EFFUSION ON READING ACHIEVEMENT: A FIVE-YEAR PROSPECTIVE CASE-CONTROL STUDY

JØRGEN LOUS, M.D., and MOGENS FIELLAU-NIKOLAJSEN, M.D.

Otitis media with effusion and tubal dysfunction may result in permanent changes of the eardrum and middle ear, and it may cause permanent hearing loss and have developmental consequences.

In this study we tried to ascertain, by a prospective investigation, whether a substantiated long duration of otitis media with effusion and tubal dysfunction in 3-year-old children had affected their reading achievement five years later.

MATERIALS AND METHODS

All 523 3-year-old children in a Danish provincial municipality were invited for impedance screening in January 1976. One thousand five ears (96.1 percent) in 504 children, all white, were fully examined according to the plan.[1] Ears exhibiting abnormal tympanometry, that is, type B (relative gradient less than 0.1), type C_1 (middle ear pressure -100 to -199 mm H_2O), or type C_2 (pressure -200 mm H_2O or less) were retested at one, three, and six months or until spontaneous normalization had occurred.[2]

The equipment employed for the impedance tests was a Madsen impedance meter (ZO-72) connected to an X-Y writer.

Five years later, in February 1981, a Silent Reading Test (OS-400) was done on all children in the second grade in the municipality of Hjørring. In this reading test, given to a whole class at a time, each pupil was to identify as many as possible of the 400 test words presented in writing. The result is stated as the number of correct word/drawing pairs achieved in 15 minutes (range 0 to 400 points). The test has been standardized in 4,77[illegible] pupils on 11 different occasions during the fir[illegible] three years of school. The test has a great test-retest reliability (Person's r, 0.7–0.8) within three to six months and a good validity (Person's r, 0.6[illegible] 0.7) in the correlation with the teachers' opinion a[illegible] to the pupils' ability to understand a written text.

Case Pupils

Forty-six children—27 boys and 19 girls—had had abnormal tympanometry results in at least one ear at each test by the age of 3 years. Thirty

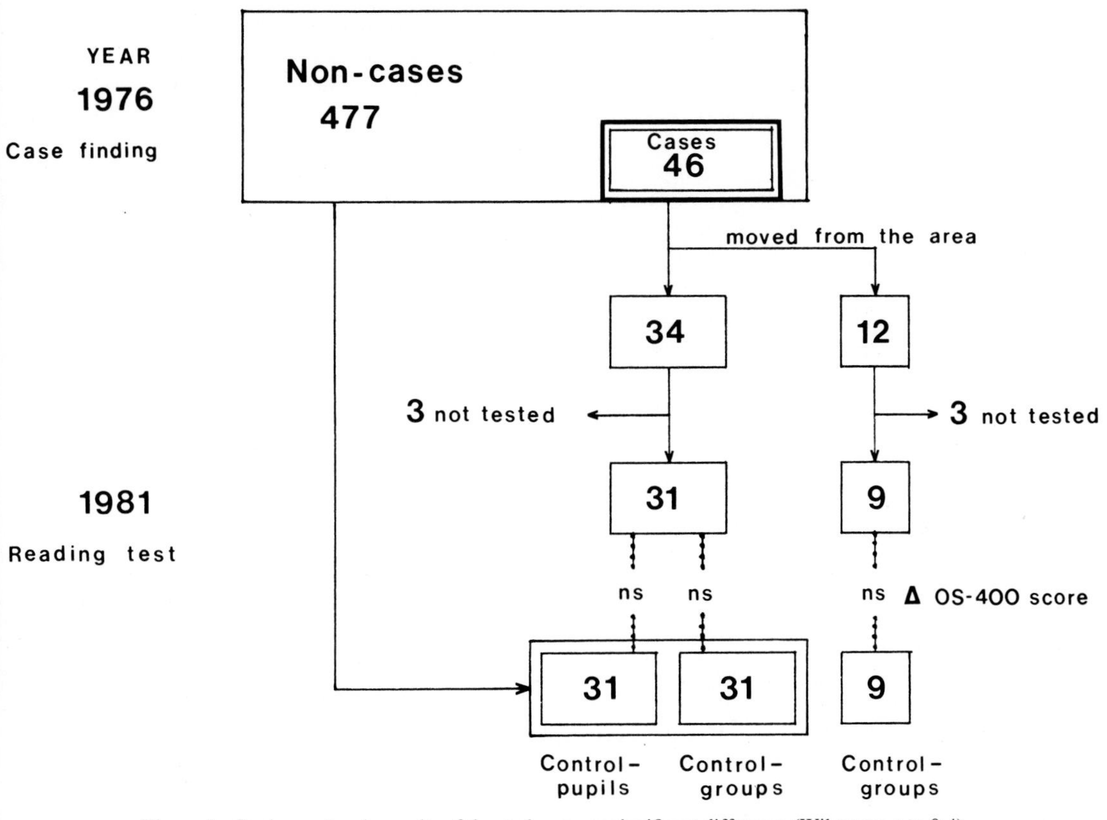

Figure 1 Design and main results of the study. ns, no significant difference (Wilcoxon, $p > 0.4$).

three of the 46 had had abnormal tympanograms in both ears at each test and ten more at three of the four tests. None of the 46 children had had a normal tympanogram in one ear on all four occasions. Of all 368 tympanograms from the four tests only 5 percent were type A and 12 percent type C_1, and more than half of the tympanograms were type B. Twenty-three of the 46 had bilateral otitis media with effusion at the paracentesis one to eight days after the last test in July. Ninety-seven percent of the ears with type B and 59 percent of the ears with type C_2 tympanograms had middle ear effusion.[4]

During the period from July 1976 to February 1981 12 case pupils left the municipality (Fig. 1), but nine of them were subjected to the reading test (OS-400) in their new schools. Of the 34 case pupils who were residents of the Hjørring municipality on February 1, 1981, three were not in the classes corresponding to their age and therefore had not had the reading test (OS-400) at the time of analysis.

Control Pupils

Prior to the reading test (OS-400) each of the 31 case pupils still residing in the municipality of Hjørring and in the second class of school was matched with a classmate whose tympanogram had been bilaterally normal (type A) in January 1976 at 3 years of age and who was of the same sex and came from a family of the same social stratum. We used the classification of the Danish National Institute of Social Research[5] with 5 social strata in four groups. If more than one in the class met the matching criteria, the classmate whose birthday was nearest to the case pupil's was selected as control pupil. Exact matching by social stratum was possible in all but one case.

Control Groups

All 40 reading-tested case pupils were compared as to OS-400 score, each with his control group, which comprised all classmates of the same sex and not of the case group. One of the nine extramunicipal case pupils was one year younger than his control classmates. There were 34 different control groups, totaling 286 pupils, because in some classes there was more than one case pupil. The distribution on social strata was the same in case pupils and in the control groups tested in Hjørring. The middle ear status and the social strata in the nine control groups tested elsewhere were unknown.

Thus, we used two different control materials, namely, individually matched control pupils and matched control groups. The individual control pupils were of same race, sex, age and social stratum and were from the same classroom as their matching case pupils, and all the control pupils had had bilaterally normal middle ears (type A tympanograms) at the age of 3. The control groups were of the same sex and from the same classroom as their matching case pupils.

Statistical Method

In comparing case pupils with their control pupils or with the control group, we used a two-sided, paired, nonparametric method (Wilcoxon's matched pairs signed rank test[6]) so that the results of the individual reading tests would be regarded as being placed on a rank scale rather than on an interval scale. The significance limit was considered to be 5 percent.

RESULTS

Of the 46 pupils with histories of long-lasting middle ear pathologic conditions at 3 years of age (the case group), two were in a class below that corresponding to their age, one in a class ahead of his age, and one pupil was attending a special class in the normal school. These findings correspond closely with those for the whole of the Hjørring municipality.

At the reading test (OS-400) in the second class in Feburary 1981 the mean score was 196 points (S.D., 85) for the municipality as a whole (N = 489). The girls had statistically significantly higher OS-400 scores than the boys, as did the two highest social groups as compared with the lowest one.

In the case-control analysis of the 31 pairs from the municipality of Hjørring tested in February 1981 (second class), there was no difference in reading achievement (Wilcoxon, $t = 0.2, p > 0.8$) Fig. 2). Separate analysis of 15 pairs of children in which the case pupil had constantly shown a bilateral middle ear pathologic condition and had had bilateral otitis media with effusion at paracentesis after the six-months follow-up at 3 years of age also revealed no difference between the case and the control pupils (Wilcoxon, $t = 1.5, p > 0.1$). There was even a slight tendency for the case pupils to be a bit better at reading than the control pupils.

The case-control group analysis, comparing each case pupil with an average of eight classmates, also failed to demonstrate a statistically significant difference between the case pupils and their control groups (Fig. 3). This applied to the 31 pupils still living in Hjørring (Wilcoxon, $t = 0.8$, $p > 0.4$) as well as to the nine who had moved (Wilcoxon, $t = 0.2, p > 0.8$). Separate analysis of the 18 case pupils with histories of bilateral, chronic middle ear pathologic conditions and bilateral otitis media with effusion at the age of 3 and their control groups also showed no difference (Wilcoxon, $t = 0.6, p > 0.5$).

An overall finding was the very wide range in average reading achievement among the groups tested in the municipality of Hjørring (Fig. 3). For the school classes as a whole, the range was 131 to 236 points. This difference in average reading achievement between the best and poorest class of around 100 points corresponded to a whole year of school for this age group.

DISCUSSION

In reviews on middle ear pathologic conditions and impaired learning, Ventry[7] and Paradise[8] pointed out that all studies on this problem so far have been inconclusive for various reasons.

The present study too has its weak points. Only a few of the factors influencing the children's learning ability were taken into consideration, namely, race, sex, age, social stratum, and classroom. According to several investigations, sex and age are important to reading achievement. The most important, and often overlooked, factor is without a doubt the classroom factor, as the difference between the control groups having the lowest and the highest averages in the reading test in Hjørring (Fig. 3) corresponded to a whole year of

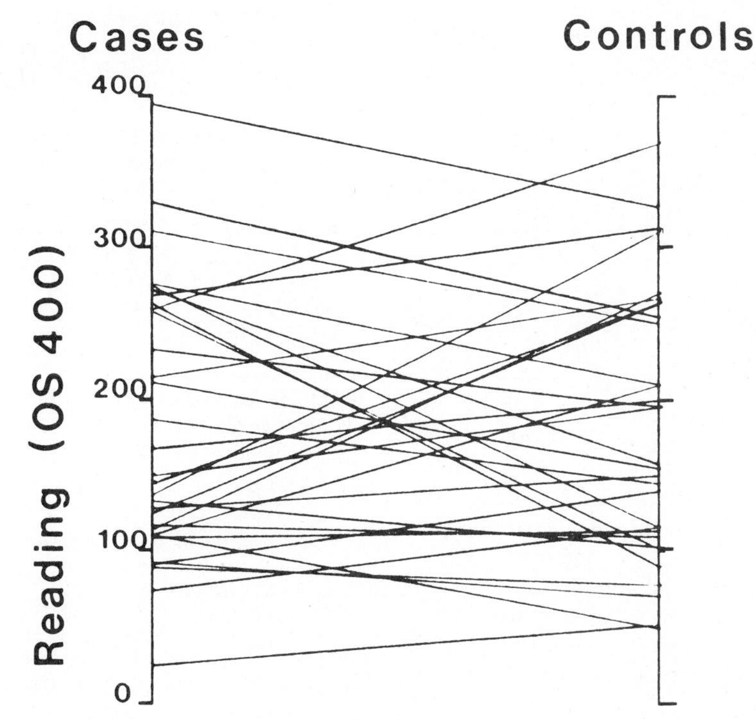

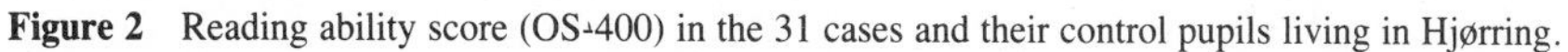

Figure 2 Reading ability score (OS-400) in the 31 cases and their control pupils living in Hjørring.

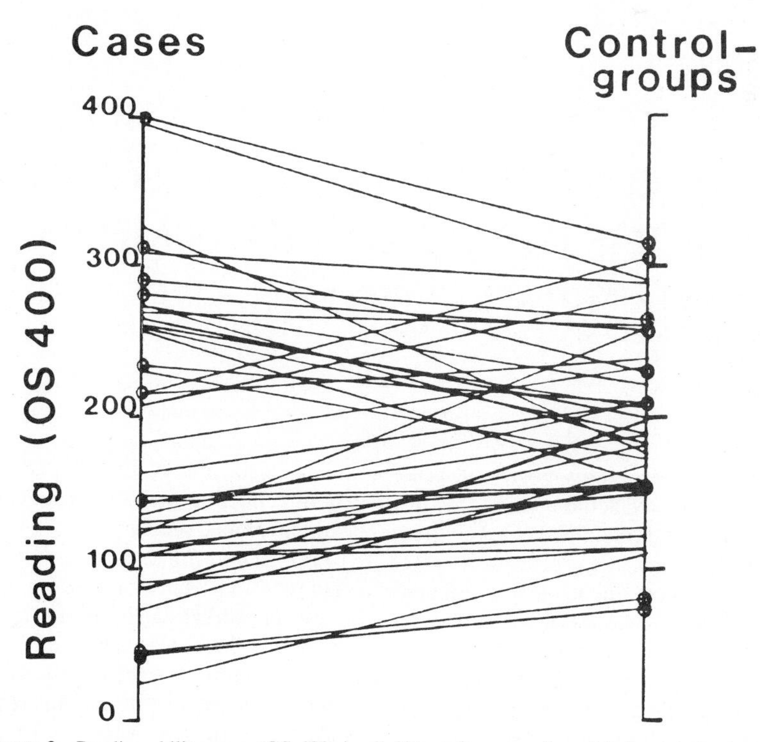

Figure 3 Reading ability score (OS-400) in all 40 tested case pupils and their control groups.

school, and this was found after only about a year and a half of school training.

Only in another two studies[9,10] has an attempt been made to match for this very important "pedagogic factor," but this has not been done consistently by matching for the classroom. These authors could not find any difference in reading achievement between case pupils and control pupils.

This study revealed no difference in school class level between the 46 children (9 percent) of the cohort who had for six months had constant middle ear pathologic conditions at the age of 3 years and the rest of the cohort. In the Silent Reading Test (OS-400), the case pupils' results did not differ from those for the other pupils in the municipality nor from other pupils of same sex in the same classroom, nor from individual control pupils matched by sex, social stratum, and classroom.

Considering the high frequency of otitis media with effusion during childhood and the divergent views on its influence on learning, further research in this field is needed before it can be established how important it is to diagnose and treat asymptomatic otitis media with effusion.

REFERENCES

1. Fiellau-Nikolajsen M, Lous J, Pedersen SV, Schousboe HH: Tympanometry in 3-year-old children I. Scand Audiol 6:199, 1977
2. Fiellau-Nikolajsen M, Lous J: Prospective tympanometry in 3-year-old children. Arch Otolaryngol 105:461, 1979
3. Søegaard A, Petersen SPB, Hansen M: *Ordstillelæsningsprøve OS 400 ord.* København: Dansk Psykologisk Forlag, 1974
4. Fiellau-Nikolajsen M, Lous J: Tympanometry in three-year-old children. A cohort study on the prognostic value of tympanometry and operative findings in middle ear effusion. ORL 41:11, 1979
5. Hansen EJ: Hvordan man indplacerer personer i Socialforskningsinstituttets socialgrupper (Udkast). (Form. D. 8561). København: Socialforskningsinstituttet, 1974
6. Andersen B: Nogle statistiske metoder. In Pedersen J, Havsteen B (eds): *Lægevidenskabelig forskning, en introduktion.* København: FADLs forlag, 1973, pp 103–159
7. Ventry IM: Effects of conductive hearing loss: Facts or fiction. J Speech Hear Dis 45:143, 1980
8. Paradise JL: Otitis media during early life: How hazardous to development? A critical review of the evidence. Pediatrics 68:869, 1981
9. Howie VM, Jensen NJ, Flemming JW, et al. The effect of early onset of otitis media on educational achievement. Int J Ped Otorhinolaryngol 1:151, 1979
10. Brandes PJ, Ehinger DM: The effect of early middle ear pathology on auditory perception and academic achievement. J Speech Hear Dis 46:301, 1981

AUDIOLOGIC AND SPEECH EVALUATION OF A PROSPECTIVELY FOLLOWED COHORT OF NORMAL CHILDREN: THE IMPACT OF OTITIS MEDIA

PETER F. WRIGHT, M.D., JULIETTE THOMPSON, M.S.N.,
KATHRYN B. McCONNELL, B.A., ANN B. SITTON, M.S., and FRED H. BESS, Ph.D.

Among the major problems posed by acute otitis media and its sequelae is the hearing loss that may attend middle ear effusion. With recurrent bouts of otitis media, middle ear effusion is often present for long periods of time in early childhood. The recurrent otitis and resultant effusion may result in delayed speech and language development. The postulation that recurrent otitis media leads to hearing loss, language delay, and even subsequent learning disability could magnify the impact of childhood otitis media even further. Proof of the causal relationship between otitis media and subsequent audiologic, linguistic, and scholastic deficiencies is not available, particularly in popula tions reflecting the current levels of health care ir the developed world.

MATERIALS AND METHODS

In an attempt to clarify the relationships be tween recurrent otitis and hearing and speech, 21(normal children were followed prospectivel through the first two years of life, with pneumati otoscopy and impedance tympanometry performe at virtually all visits to the doctor, whether th child was sick or well. The clinical and epidemiologic picture of otitis media in these children has been described. The hearing and speech of 160 of the children were tested at approximately 24 months of age at the Bill Wilkerson Hearing and Speech Center. A subset of 36 of the children had further follow-up testing between 3 and 4 years of age. The accumulated data were then analyzed with respect to their past histories of otitis media.

RESULTS

Hearing could be successfully tested in 156 children at 2 years of age. The number of episodes of acute otitis media showed a direct correlation with hearing loss at ≥30 dB at all frequencies (Table 1). The same significant correlations were seen when data were analyzed according to the total number of bilaterally abnormal tympanograms, but tympanograms had no greater predictive value for hearing loss than otoscopy. Mean hearing loss associated with 3 or more episodes of otitis was 2 to 3 dB when compared with otitis-free children. These differences were not significant. However, the observation that 18 percent of children with recurrent otitis have a mild to moderate hearing loss at 2 years of age implies a large reservoir of conductive hearing loss related to otitis media.

TABLE 1 Sound Field Hearing Loss of ≥30 dB in Two-Year-Old Children

	No. of Episodes of Acute Otitis Media		
Frequency	*0*	*1–2*	*≥3*
250 Hz	0/28 (0%)	9/55* (16%)	19/64† (30%)
500 Hz	1/30 (3%)	8/55 (15%)	13/71* (18%)
1000 Hz	1/30 (3%)	5/55 (9%)	13/71* (18%)
2000 Hz	1/30 (3%)	5/55 (9%)	13/71* (18%)
4000 Hz	2/29 (6%)	5/54 (9%)	12/70* (17%)

*$p \leq 0.05$ by children when compared to group without otitis.

†$p \leq 0.01$ by children when compared to group without otitis.

Speech and language development at 24 months of age proved to be highly variable and probably dependent on many factors. A racial difference in speech and language acquisition at 1 to 3 months was reflected in the 66 white and 44 nonwhite children in the study. Other variables, such as stimulation in the home environment, presence of siblings, and innate intelligence, quite likely influence speech and language development. To analyze the influence of recurrent otitis, data were examined for three groups of children: those with no otitis, those with one to four episodes of otitis, and those with five or more episodes of otitis (Fig. 1).

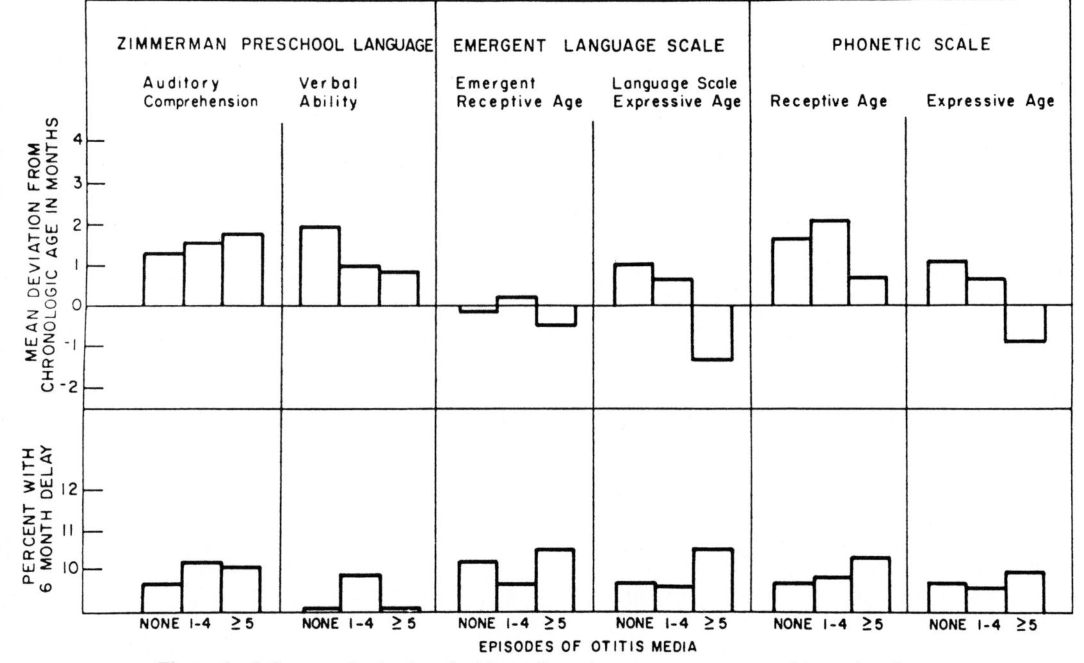

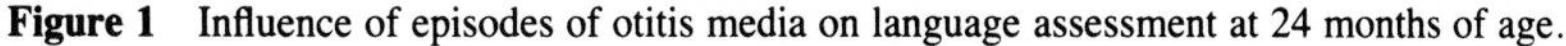

Figure 1 Influence of episodes of otitis media on language assessment at 24 months of age.

Although a mean one- to two-month delay in language and speech development in children with multiple episodes of otitis was evident in five of six assays, no significant differences in mean deviation from chronologic age were present nor were six-month delays in speech and language significantly more frequent in those with recurrent otitis. The number of tympanograms in the first two years of life did not influence speech and language testing results at 24 months.

In an effort to improve the discrimination of the testing, a thirty-minute language sample was recorded for each of the remaining 50 children. The language sample approach proved extremely difficult to transcribe and analyze and ultimately could not be utilized in assessing speech and language development.

A subgroup of 36 children between the ages of 36 and 48 months was retested at the Bill Wilkerson Center. Sixteen of these children could be defined as otitis prone, that is, having six or more episodes of both acute and serous otitis, with a mean number of 11.1 episodes. Twenty of the children had had six or fewer episodes of otitis, with a mean number of 2.8 episodes.

Hearing evaluation at 3 to 4 years of age was strikingly different than at age 2. Each of nine children with a >25-dB loss at a frequency between 250 and 4000 Hz at age 2 had normal hearing by age 3 to 4. One child had apparently acquired a mild hearing deficit between age 2 and 3. Whereas hearing loss at age 2 was clearly associated with otitis—eight of 16 children with frequent otitis had hearing loss as opposed to one of 20 without otitis—by age 3 to 4 years that association was gone.

Speech evaluation at 3 to 4 years of age could not be compared with the same earlier speech and language battery, as all of these children had taken part in the experimental 30-minute language sample. However, no correlation of speech or language development with frequency of otitis media was present.

A prospectively followed group of 160 normal children who had careful documentation of their middle ear status by tympanometry and otoscopy through the first two years of life was evaluated for their auditory and linguistic development at 24 months of age. Chronic or recurrent middle ear effusion was associated with a significant degree of mild to moderate hearing loss in 18 percent of children so affected. This finding alone suggests that audiologic screening of all children with recurrent otitis would be indicated to detect this relatively high incidence of hearing loss. If our population is representative, however, 45 percent of normal children would require audiologic screening based on this clinical parameter.

Although only 36 children could be retested at 3 to 4 years of age, each of the nine children in that group with hearing loss at 2 years had normal hearing at age 3 to 4 years. Several explanations for the reversal of this hearing deficit are possible: (1) The hearing deficit at 2 years was a transient result of middle ear effusion at the time of testing. This did not seem to be the case in most children in whom neither abnormal otoscopy nor tympanometry was present. (2) The accuracy of testing hearing acuity had increased in the older children. (3) The decreased auditory acuity at age 2 was a residue of recurrent middle ear infection, but it resolved in older children as the frequency of otitis media continued to decrease. We favor the last explanation, which thus suggests that hearing screening at 2 years may detect only a temporary defect that will correct itself without intervention.

Language testing in early childhood proved difficult. No consensus exists on what tests of articulation, expression, or reception are optimal. Nor are well-defined normative standards available for most of the assays. Furthermore, the language development is clearly a function of many influences on the young child, of which mild decreases in auditory acuity may be only one. Our sample size did not allow us to control for each of these variables. Within the sample as a whole the battery of language tests utilized did not implicate recurrent otitis in speech delay.

DISCUSSION

The primary conclusion to be drawn may be that, for any study to succeed in documenting such an association, the testing tools must be improved, the study size must be very large, and control and documentation of the variables of language development must be achieved. The public health implications of acute otitis media and its sequelae are profound and will remain so until effective prevention of this illness is achieved. All intervention must be viewed against the natural history of the disease. Increasingly this is being done with medical and surgical intervention. The same critical analysis will have to be applied to audiologic and linguistic screening and intervention.

SENSORINEURAL HEARING LOSS IN AN ANIMAL MODEL OF PURULENT OTITIS MEDIA

TETSUO MORIZONO, M.D., G. SCOTT GIEBINK, M.D., MICHAEL A. SIKORA, and MICHAEL M. PAPARELLA, M.D.

Sensorineural hearing loss (SNHL) has been described clinically following chronic otitis media with effusion (OME),[1–5] but no experimental studies, as far as we know, have demonstrated SNHL in an animal model of otitis media. In the present study, we present evidence of SNHL in chinchillas following an induced bout of purulent otitis media with effusion (POME).

MATERIALS AND METHODS

The right bullae of 29 animals were inoculated with 20 type 7F *Streptococcus pneumoniae* after both ears were confirmed to be otoscopically normal and to have normal type A tympanograms.[6,7] Both ears were examined otoscopically and tympanometrically daily until the animals were killed. When OME was confirmed by these methods, a culture of the middle ear effusion was collected by an epitympanic fenestra to confirm infection. At this time a daily regimen of penicillin (100,000 U/kg) for five consecutive days was initiated. Resolution of the effusion and infection was confirmed by tympanometry and by bacterial culture. Some animals were killed in midinfection (Group I).

Before they were killed, the animals were anesthetized (20 mg ketamine HCl, 45 mg/kg sodium pentobarbital i.m.), and inner ear function was evaluated bilaterally with measurements of compound action potential (AP).[8] Core temperature was maintained at 37°C and the animals were mechanically ventilated with room air. A closed acoustic system with probe microphone was used to deliver asynchronous tonebursts (1 ms rise/fall, 10 ms plateau) at 12, 8, 4, and 2 kHz, at a pulse rate of 12/sec. Through a fenestra made in the auditory bulla overlying the round window, a thin, Teflon-coated silver wire with exposed ball tip was placed either on the round window of the animals with resolved POME animals or on the niche overhang on animals tested midinfection. The niche overhang placement was used bilaterally when even a small amount of effusion was present to avoid the leakage current artifact present when recording from "moist" round windows. The biological signal was amplified, filtered, and fed to a mini-computer, which averaged 100 time-locked responses to the stimuli. The sound pressure level (SPL) to elicit a 10 μV AP response was determined at such frequency by interpolation.

RESULTS

Of the 29 animals used in the study, the physiologic findings in only 14 are reported here. The remaining animals were excluded for one of the following reasons: (1) death of the animal before testing, (2) observation of ataxia, (3) development of sterile OME in the inoculated ear, or (4) development of pneumococcal or sterile OME in the uninoculated ear.

Of the 14 animals reported here, four were killed five to six days postinoculation (Group I), and ten were sacrificed two to five weeks postinoculation (Group II). Observation with an operating microscope of the middle ear cavity prior to AP testing revealed a small amount of clear, nonviscous fluid in the Group I animals. The Group II animals had no fluid present at this time, and the tympanic membrane and round window appeared normal. Tympanograms taken just before AP testing in Group I animals were classed B+ or C; Group II animals all had normal A tympanograms. The uninoculated ears revealed normal tympanograms throughout testing.

In Table 1A the mean AP threshold SPL of the inoculated ears of Groups I and II is presented, along with mean threshold SPL of a group of normal chinchillas. Both Groups I and II were signifi-

TABLE 1 Compound Action Potential Threshold (10 μV) in dB SPL ($\overline{X}$ ± S.D.) in Normal Animals in Inoculated and Uninoculated Ears Tested at 5–6 Days (Group I) or 2–5 Weeks (Group II) Postinoculation

	2 kHz	*4 kHz*	*8 kHz*	*12 kHz*
Normal (N = 22)	23.4 ± 5.1	20.4 ± 6.7	23.8 ± 5.7	28.7 ± 8.5
A. *Inoculated (right)*				
Group I* (N = 4)	54.1 ± 25.5	56.8 ± 23.3	72.0 ± 19.4	78.4 ± 21.6
Group II (N = 10)	39.9 ± 22.4 $p < 0.005$	36.3 ± 17.3 $p < 0.001$	52.6 ± 25.7 $p < 0.001$	52.8 ± 27.6 $p < 0.001$
B. *Uninoculated (left)*				
Group I* (N = 4)	33.5 ± 11.5	30.4 ± 5.2	37.2 ± 4.5	43.6 ± 11.4
Group II (N = 10)	23.8 ± 5.8 N.S.†	23.8 ± 7.3 N.S.	35.8 ± 14.9 $p < 0.002$	43.8 ± 26.9 $p < 0.05$
C. *Interaural difference (right–left)*				
Normal (N = 16)	−1.7 ± 5.2	−0.5 ± 2.8	−0.1 ± 7.5	−3.4 ± 7.5
Group I (N = 4)	20.6 ± 28.6 $p < 0.01$	26.4 ± 27.7 $p < 0.001$	34.7 ± 19.6 $p < 0.001$	34.8 ± 29.7 $p < 0.001$

Note: Significance measured using *t*-test comparing group to normal.
*Statistical test not performed. Different electrode placement used than in normal group (see text).
†N.S., not significantly different from normal.

cantly different from the normal group at all frequencies. It should be noted that the Group I AP thresholds were obtained with an electrode placement less sensitive* than Group II thresholds; thus, the threshold elevation is exaggerated. The elevation in threshold in Group I does appear to be real, as the interaural AP threshold difference† is significantly elevated when compared with interaural differences in the normal animal (Table 1C) obtained with a round window electrode. Conduction losses cannot be ruled out in Group I animals, however, owing to the abnormal tympanograms obtained here. Our experience with artificial effusion (Ringer's) and conductive loss limits this contribution to no more than 10 dB at the test frequencies used in the ventilated and aspirated bullae.

*The dB difference ($\overline{X}$ ± S.D.) between electrode placement in normal chinchillas (N = 12): 12 kHz, 11.1 ± 2.1; 8 kHz, 8.5 ± 1.7; 4 kHz, 12.1 ± 2.9; 2 kHz, 14.2 ± 2.6.

†In both groups, the interaural difference was calculated as the first ear measured minus the second ear. In the experimental group, the inoculated ear was tested first; thus, the expressed interaural difference is a conservative measure, in light of any possible preparation deterioration.

Table 1B presents the AP thresholds obtained from the uninoculated ears of both groups. Group I thresholds, obtained with an overhang electrode, are problematic, as described above, although no conductive element is present. Most interesting are the Group II uninoculated ears. While these ears showed no clinical (tympanometric or otoscopic) signs of infection or effusion at any time and were all observed to have normal middle ears when the animals were killed, significant threshold elevations were observed at 12 and 8 kHz.

Further analysis of the Group II uninoculated ears is presented in Tables 2B and 3B. The ten ears are divided into two groups in two different ways. If we look at the duration of effusion in the inoculated ear it appears that persistent effusion may effect the uninoculated ear at the higher frequencies, as shown in Table 2B. The inoculated ear, analyzed in the same manner, shows significant threshold elevation compared with normal ears at all test frequencies in both subgroups, as seen in Table 2A. In the inoculated ears, the subgroup with an extended duration of effusion has a mean AP threshold approximately 20 dB greater than the

TABLE 2 Effect of Duration of Effusion on Compound Action Potential Threshold (10 μV) of Group II Animals' Inoculated and Uninoculated Ears in dB SPL ($\overline{X}$ ± S.D.)

	2 kHz	*4 kHz*	*8 kHz*	*12 kHz*
A. *Inoculated ear (right)*				
13 days (N = 5)	43.8 ± 30.4 $p < 0.005$	37.7 ± 23.8 $p < 0.01$	63.9 ± 32.6 $p < 0.001$	62.6 ± 36.9 $p < 0.001$
7–12 days (N = 5)	35.9 ± 12.9 $p < 0.002$	34.8 ± 10.1 $p < 0.001$	41.3 ± 10.0 $p < 0.001$	42.9 ± 10.2 $p < 0.005$
B. *Uninoculated ear (left)*				
13 days (N = 5)	22.3 ± 7.7 N.S.*	19.9 ± 8.6 N.S.	44.0 ± 17.4 $p < 0.001$	58.4 ± 32.3 $p < 0.001$
7–12 days (N = 5)	25.4 ± 3.1 N.S.	27.7 ± 2.9 $p < 0.05$	27.6 ± 5.6 N.S.	29.2 ± 7.1 N.S.

Note: Significance measured using *t*-test comparing group to normal animals (N = 22) in Table 1.
*N.S., not significantly different.

short duration subgroup at 8 kHz and 12 kHz, but the difference between the two subgroups is not statistically significant.

The same set of data may be analyzed in a different way, as shown in Table 3. Here it appears that the time between resolution of effusion and AP testing may be inversely related to threshold elevation in the inoculated and uninoculated ears. Since the present data do not allow differentiation between these two possibilities, and because we are not able to control the duration of effusion, further studies with the animal model of POME should be designed, keeping the time between resolution of effusion and electrophysiologic testing constant.

We can only speculate at this time as to why the uninoculated ear would have a high-frequency hearing loss. Two possibilities are: (1) a susceptibility in infected animals to the anesthetics being used for AP testing, leading to a degenerating preparation; and (2) an unlikely ototoxic effect of penicillin. An intriguing third possibility is that we are looking at an animal model of "silent otitis media" in the uninoculated ear.[9] Further control experiments are necessary to distinguish between these possibilities.

TABLE 3 Effect of Time from Resolution of Effusion to Test Compound Action Potential Threshold (10 μV) of Group II Animals' Inoculated and Uninoculated Ears in dB SPL ($\overline{X}$ ± S.D.)

	2 kHz	*4 kHz*	*8 kHz*	*12 kHz*
A. *Inoculated ear (right)*				
0 days (N = 6)	41.1 ± 30.0 $p < 0.02$	37.7 ± 21.3 $p < 0.002$	60.0 ± 30.7 $p < 0.001$	58.9 ± 34.2 $p < 0.001$
4–38 days (N = 4)	38.1 ± 13.8 $p < 0.005$	34.2 ± 11.5 $p < 0.002$	41.4 ± 11.5 $p < 0.001$	43.6 ± 11.6 $p < 0.01$
B. *Uninoculated ear (left)*				
0 days (N = 6)	22.9 ± 7.1 N.S.*	21.2 ± 8.3 N.S.	41.1 ± 17.0 $p < 0.001$	52.2 ± 32.7 $p < 0.01$
4–38 days (N = 4)	25.2 ± 3.5 N.S.	27.7 ± 3.4 $p < 0.05$	27.8 ± 6.5 N.S.	31.3 ± 6.1 N.S.

Note: Significance measured using *t*-test comparing group to normal animals (N = 22) in Table 1.
*N.S., not significantly different.

In summary, we have found a significant sensorineural hearing loss in an animal model of purulent otitis media with effusion. This supports clinical observations of permanent hearing losses seen in some patients with otitis media.

This study was supported by grant #NS14538 from the National Institutes of Health.

REFERENCES

1. Paparella MM, Goycoolea MV, Meyerhoff WL: Inner ear pathology and otitis media—a review. Ann Otol Rhinol Laryngol 89(Suppl 68):249, 1980
2. English GM, Northern JL, Fria TJ: Chronic otitis media as a cause of sensorineural hearing loss. Arch Otolaryngol 98:18, 1973
3. Prado S, Paparella MM: Sensorineural hearing loss secondary to bacterial infection. Otolaryngol Clin North Am 11:35, 1978
4. Aviel A, Ostfeld E: Acquired irreversible sensorineural hearing loss associated with otitis media with effusion. Am J Otolaryngol 3:217, 1982
5. Walby AP, Barrera A, Schuknecht HF: Cochlear pathology in chronic suppurative otitis media. Ann Otol Rhinol Laryngol 92(Suppl 103), 1983
6. Giebink GS, Payne EE, Mills EL, et al: Experimental otitis media due to *Streptococcus pneumoniae:* Immunopathogenic response in the chinchilla. J Infect Dis 134:595, 1976
7. Giebink GS, Heller KA, Harford ER: Tympanometric configuration and middle ear findings in experimental otitis media. Ann Otol Rhinol Laryngol 91:20, 1982
8. Morizono T, Sikora MA: The ototoxicity of topically applied povidone-iodine preparations. Arch Otolaryngol 108:210, 1982
9. Paparella MM, Shea D, Meyerhoff WL, Goycoolea MV: Silent otitis media. Laryngoscope 90:1089, 1980

CONDUCTIVE LOSS AFFECTS AUDITORY NEURONAL SOMA SIZE ONLY DURING A SENSITIVE POSTNATAL PERIOD

DOUGLAS B. WEBSTER, Ph.D.

In normal postnatal development, the neurons of the CBA/J mouse auditory brain stem reach adult soma size by 12 days after birth, coincident with the inception of hearing.[1] However, mice that undergo either auditory deprivation or experimentally produced conductive losses extending from four to 45 days after birth have significantly smaller than normal auditory brain stem neurons. If auditorily deprived mice are returned to a normal acoustic environment at 45 days, they retain these smaller than normal neurons.[3] On the other hand, soma size is not affected in mice raised normally until 45 days and then either auditorily deprived or given a conductive loss until 90 days after birth.[5] Taken together, these data demonstrate that there is a time period, somewhere between four and 45 days after birth, during which adequate sound stimulation is necessary to maintain normal auditory brain stem neuronal soma size. The present study defines this sensitive period.

MATERIALS AND METHODS

Nine groups of CBA/J mice (seven mice per group) were given unilateral conductive hearing losses of about 50 dB by removing the left cartilaginous external auditory meatus and associated epithelium; these groups differed only in the ages at onset of conductive loss and of sacrifice (Table 1). Their brain stems were serially sectioned at 15 μm in the transverse plane and stained with cresyl violet. Quantitative analyses were performed on the globular and large spherical cells of the ventral cochlear nucleus, the principal cells of the medial nucleus of the trapezoid body of the superior olivary complex, and the principal bitufted cells of the central nucleus of the inferior colliculus. The cross-sectional soma areas of 30 cells of each neuronal type were measured from both right and left sides in each brain stem, and statistical analyses of size differences between sides and between groups were performed.

RESULTS

The quantitative data are given in Table 1. As previously reported,[1] neurons of the mouse auditory brain stem have attained adult soma size by 12 days after birth. In this experiment it was found that with conductive losses extending from 12 to 24 days after birth, the left globular cells, left large spherical cells, right medial nucleus of trapezoid body cells, and right inferior colliculus cells were significantly smaller ($p > 0.01$) than comparable cells on the opposite side. This same effect was seen from conductive losses of four to 24, four to 45, and four to 90 days after birth. There were no significant differences ($p > 0.05$) between right and left cell sizes from conductive losses of four to 12 or 24 to 45 days after birth. There were significant right/left cell size differences ($p > 0.01$) when the conductive loss was four to 18, 12 to 18, or 18 to 24 days, but these differences were smaller than when the conductive loss covered the full 12- to 24-day period (Table 1).

DISCUSSION

These data demonstrate a sensitive period from 12 to 24 days after birth during which CBA/J mice require adequate sound stimulation to maintain normal neuronal soma size in their auditory brain stems. Since these neuronal somas have normally grown to adult size by 12 days, a conductive loss between 12 and 24 days actually results in their shrinking. The only data we have on the functional significance of reduced brain stem neuronal sizes is that mice so affected have shorter than normal auditory brain stem response latencies.[6]

It remains to be demonstrated whether these CBA/J mouse data relate directly to other species. One must be particularly cautious in applying these data to the possible effects of chronic otitis media in children, for there are several important differ-

TABLE 1 Results of Quantitative Analyses on CBA/J Mouse Cells

Age (Days after Birth)		*Soma Size* (μm^2) $\pm$ *1 S.D.*		
Left EAM Removed	*Killed*	*Left*	*Right*	*P*
Large Spherical Cells of the Ventral Cochlear Nucleus				
4	12	148 ± 18	147 ± 18	> 0.05
4	18	123 ± 17	149 ± 18	< 0.01
4	24	114 ± 15	144 ± 18	< 0.01
4	45	116 ± 18	143 ± 21	< 0.01
4	90	120 ± 15	149 ± 18	< 0.01
12	18	135 ± 16	148 ± 15	< 0.01
12	24	120 ± 14	148 ± 18	< 0.01
18	24	125 ± 16	146 ± 14	< 0.01
24	45	147 ± 17	147 ± 15	> 0.05
Globular Cells of the Ventral Cochlear Nucleus				
4	12	177 ± 22	174 ± 22	> 0.05
4	18	158 ± 22	174 ± 23	< 0.01
4	24	140 ± 18	177 ± 25	< 0.01
4	45	149 ± 18	177 ± 20	< 0.01
4	90	150 ± 19	178 ± 23	< 0.01
12	18	153 ± 18	178 ± 21	< 0.01
12	24	143 ± 19	177 ± 23	< 0.01
18	24	158 ± 16	176 ± 21	< 0.01
24	45	174 ± 20	175 ± 22	> 0.05
Principal Cells of the Medial Nucleus of the Trapezoid Body				
4	12	178 ± 18	181 ± 18	> 0.05
4	18	184 ± 24	162 ± 21	< 0.01
4	24	182 ± 22	148 ± 18	< 0.01
4	45	186 ± 25	156 ± 22	< 0.01
4	90	190 ± 20	155 ± 22	< 0.01
12	18	189 ± 22	157 ± 22	< 0.01
12	24	184 ± 21	149 ± 19	< 0.01
18	24	191 ± 25	160 ± 21	< 0.01
24	45	185 ± 23	184 ± 25	> 0.05
Principal Bitufted Cells of the Central Nucleus of the Inferior Colliculus				
4	12	104 ± 14	100 ± 13	> 0.05
4	18	104 ± 15	85 ± 12	< 0.01
4	24	104 ± 13	86 ± 11	< 0.01
4	45	102 ± 13	86 ± 12	< 0.01
4	90	104 ± 16	86 ± 14	< 0.01
12	18	100 ± 14	92 ± 14	< 0.01
12	24	107 ± 18	91 ± 11	< 0.01
18	24	102 ± 18	87 ± 15	< 0.01
24	45	104 ± 18	104 ± 17	> 0.05

Note: EAM, external auditory meatus; *P*, probability that left and right populations are not different

ences. For one thing, the conductive loss given the mice is about 50 dB—much greater than that usually present in cases of otitis media. Moreover, the loss is chronic, rather than fluctuating. Finally, the demonstrated sensitive period starts at the inception of hearing, which occurs postnatally in mice but prenatally in humans. Nonetheless, the fact that early auditory restriction has a profound effect on the central auditory system in one mammal must arouse concern about possible related effects in humans.

This work was supported by grant #NS-11647 from the National Institutes of Health. The technical support of Ms. Sandra Blanchard and Ms. Jennifer Powell is appreciated. Molly Webster edited the manuscript. Equipment important to the study was provided by Zenetron, Inc. and The Louisiana Lions Eye Foundation.

REFERENCES

1. Webster DB, Webster M: Mouse brainstem auditory nuclei development. Ann Otol Rhinol Laryngol 89(Suppl 68):254, 1980
2. Webster DB, Webster M: Neonatal sound deprivation affects brainstem auditory nuclei. Arch Otolaryngol 103:392, 1977
3. Webster DB, Webster M: Effects of neonatal conductive hearing loss on brain stem auditory nuclei. Ann Otol Rhinol Laryngol 88:684, 1979
4. Webster DB: Auditory neuronal sizes after a unilateral conductive hearing loss. Exp Neurol 79:130, 1983
5. Webster DB: Auditory deprivation initiated at puberty does not affect brainstem auditory neuron soma size. Abstracts, Sixth Midwinter ARO Meeting, 1983, p 4
6. Evans WJ, Webster DB, Cullen JK Jr: Auditory brainstem responses in neonatally sound deprived CBA/J mice. Hearing Res 10:269, 1983

HISTORY OF TREATED PERSISTENT OTITIS MEDIA WITH EFFUSION

GEORGE A. GATES, M.D., CHRISTINE A. WACHTENDORF, M.D., G. RICHARD HOLT, M.D., and ERWIN M. HEARNE III, Ph.D.

The natural history of otitis media is difficult to determine because most patients receive treatment of one sort or another. Therefore, if the treatment is standardized, an opportunity exists to record the subsequent clinical course in a manner that should make possible certain inferences about the biological responses of the middle ear.

MATERIALS AND METHODS

Our study is based on the assumption that persistent otitis media with effusion (POME) is a stage in the continuum of otitis media and is related temporally and etiologically to acute otitis media with effusion. Therefore, all patients admitted to our treatment protocol received standardized medical treatment prior to randomization for surgical therapy to ensure that each patient had received adequate medical therapy and to select out the self-limited cases. In most instances this constituted "repeat" medical therapy. We then determined the rate of resolution of the middle ear effusion 30 and 60 days later.

If the effusion persisted, the child was evaluated in detail; stratified according to age, sex, race, and prior treatment history; and then randomized into one of four surgical treatment groups. Eligibility criteria were: POME, unilateral or bilateral; age 4 to 8 years; absence of systemic disease; control of any allergic condition; no prior tonsil or adenoid surgery; and no middle ear surgery for otitis media within the past two years. Medical therapy consisted of a ten-day course of a fixed preparation of erythromycin ethylsuccinate and sulfisoxazole (Pediazole) and a 30-day course of decongestant preparation (Novafed). Diagnosis of POME was made by an algorithm based on pneumotoscopy by validated observers and tympanometry.[1] Clearance of the effusion was determined by reversal of the findings.

Surgical treatment was given to 185 children with preoperative diagnoses of POME in 343 ears. Treatment groups were (1) myringotomy, (2) tympanostomy tubes, (3) adenoidectomy and myringotomy, and (4) adenoidectomy and tympanostomy tubes. Both ears received the same treatment regardless of whether the fluid had cleared or not, except for the 5 percent of children with solely unilateral disease. Postoperatively the children were examined every six weeks by otoscopy and tympanometry, and every 12 weeks an audiogram was also done.

TABLE 1 Effectiveness of "Repeat" Medical Therapy (E/S + D)*

	POME Cases			*Ears*
	Unilateral No. (%)	*Bilateral No. (%)*		
Total	*414*	*611*		*1636*
		Both Ears	*One Ear*	
Cleared:				
1st month	196 (47)	100 (16)	77 (13)	473 (29)
2nd month	131 (32)	67 (11)	54 (9)	319 (19)
Total cleared [494 (48)]	327 (79)	167 (27)	131 (22)	792 (48)

*E/S, erythromycin ethylsuccinate and sulfisoxazole (Pediazole); D, decongestant (Novafed).

RESULTS

The one- and two-month clearance rates for 1025 medically treated children with POME in 1636 ears are displayed in Table 1. The variables of age, sex, race, and prior treatment did not correlate with outcome. Time of year (by quarter) in which the "repeat" course of medical therapy was begun influenced the outcome significantly ($p = 0.0001$) (Table 2) using the *Chi*-square (3df) test.

The outcome of the surgical therapy for the entire group is noted in Table 3. Inasmuch as the study has not been completed, the code has not been broken and therefore the results for each of the four groups are not available.

DISCUSSION

Because the standardized medical regimen was not compared with a control group it is not possible to separate the effects of the treatment from the effects of time. Because this aspect of the study simulates the real-world practice policies of many physicians, the finding that effusion in 40 percent of ears and 48 percent of patients resolves within 60 days should be of use in clinical decision-making. Our medical control rate is similar to that reported by Roydhouse,[2] who noted that in 42 percent of children (mean age 7.5 years) with POME treated medically effusion resolved in two months. Interestingly, his regimen did not include an antibiotic but concentrated on intensive nasal hygiene, nasal decongestant therapy, breathing exercises, diet, and health education.

The decrease over time in the proportion of children with effusion following treatment with an antibiotic in our sample parallels that noted by Teele and colleagues in infants and young children after an episode of acute otitis media,[3] except that fewer of our children (who were older) had clearing of effusion by two months (48 percent versus 80 percent). Also, they noted no relationship between duration of effusion and age or sex but did

TABLE 2 Time of Year at Treatment: Proportion of Children Clearing

	Quarter							
	1st		*2nd*		*3rd*		*4th*	
	1 mo	*2 mo*	*1 mo*	*2 mo*	*1 mo*	*2 mo*	*1 mo*	*2 mo*
One ear affected	.72	.68	.61	.79	.54	.32	.55	.51
Both ears affected	.38	.55	.59	.65	.25	.34	.38	.32

TABLE 3 Efficacy of Surgical Treatments of POME*

Outcome	*MEE†*		*Total (Ears)*
Number	(+256)	(−87)	(343)
Time to 1st recurrence	213 days	451 days	224 days
No relapse in 1 year	30%	50%	37%

*Surgical treatment was myringotomy, tubes, adenoidectomy plus myringotomy, or adenoidectomy plus tubes. Children were aged 4 to 8, with POME for 60 days after E/S + D treatment.

†MEE, middle ear effusion

find that the effusions of bottle-fed infants persisted longer.

The effect of time of the year on clearance rate is difficult to interpret with certainty. Common knowledge indicates that acute otitis media is more common in the winter months. It is our presumption that higher clearance rates in the winter months reflect the acute nature of many of the effusions seen during the school-related upper respiratory infection season. In contrast, those children with POME who are first seen in the third quarter probably have had truly chronic effusions that had persisted through the summer season and were presumably more resistant to medical therapy.

In the analysis of the preliminary overall surgical results it was found that only 36 percent of the children remained completely free of effusion during the first postoperative year. These results differed substantially depending on whether effusion was present at the time of surgery: The relapse rate for the "dry" ears was 50 percent and for those with effusion 70 percent. Therefore, the clinical diagnosis of POME, independent of clearance of the effusion in the period between diagnosis and operation, indicates a high likelihood of recurrent infection regardless of the type of surgery done.

This study was supported by NINCDS/NIH contract NS-NO-1-02328 and a grant in kind from Ross Laboratories.

REFERENCES

1. Wachtendorf CW, Hearne EM, Gates GA, Cooper JC: Evaluation of the Pittsburgh tympanogram typing system. Abstract presented at the Third International Symposium on Recent Advances in Otitis Media with Effusion, Fort Lauderdale, Florida, May 1983
2. Roydhouse N. Adenoidectomy for otitis media with mucoid effusion. Ann Otol Rhinol Laryngol 89(Suppl 68):312, 1980
3. Teele DW, Klein JO, Rosner BA: Epidemiology of otitis media in children. Ann Otol Rhinol Laryngol 89(Suppl 68):5, 1980

FINE MORPHOLOGY OF TYMPANOSCLEROSIS

BURKHARD HUSSL, M.D., and DAVID J. LIM, M.D.

Tympanosclerosis is a frequent sequela of chronic secretory otitis media (SOM)[1] and of chronic purulent otitis media (POM) with perforation. Following SOM it is mainly confined to the tympanic membrane,[1] but following POM it is found in the tympanic mucosa as well. The light microscopic histopathology has been described as consisting of hyalin degeneration and calcification of the connective tissue layer in the tympanic membrane and tympanic mucosa.[2–7] The pathogenesis of tympanosclerosis, however, is not yet fully understood. The prevailing hypothesis is that chronic inflammation leads to degenerative changes in the connective tissue layer. It has also been suggested that autoimmunity against collagenous fibers in the tympanic membrane and in the tympanic mucosa may be the underlying mechanism.[8] As to the mechanism of calcification, the fundamental role of extracellular membrane-bound structures (matrix vesicles) in the pathogenesis of this disease has been suggested, on the basis of electron microscopic observations.[9,10] The present study was undertaken to clarify the mechanism involved in the pathologic process in tympanosclerosis by investigating fine morphology of surgical specimens using electron microscopy.

MATERIALS AND METHODS

Seven specimens from the tympanic membrane and 20 biopsy specimens from the tympanic mucosa taken during middle ear surgery performed for chronic otitis media were used. They were processed for light microscopy using the methyl methacrylate (JB-4) embedding technique following EDTA decalcification or routine transmission electron microscopy and x-ray microanalysis using the epoxy embedding technique without decalcification.

RESULTS

Light microscopy of the tympanic membrane shows that the tympanosclerotic tissue occupies the lamina propria layer (Fig. 1A). It is formed by alternating layers of connective tissue that contain varying amounts of dark-blue–staining granules representing calcium deposits in undecalcified sections. This lamellation is responsible for the onionskin-like macroscopic appearance of tympanosclerotic tissue. Some scattered granular deposits are also present in the subepidermal and submucosal loose connective tissue layers.

At the ultrastructural level the lamina propria of the normal human tympanic membrane is formed of outer radial and inner circular fibers. The fibrils of these fibers are rectangular in cross-sectional view and are mixed with varying amounts of collagen fibrils as shown in Figure 1B and C.[11] In the tympanosclerotic tissue, degeneration of both rectangular (reticular) and collagen fibrils is evident. The fibrils have lost their normal texture and arrangement (Fig. 1D). Although some collagen fibrils have preserved the normal banding pattern, a motheaten appearance of collagen ground substance is apparent in other areas. At lower magnifications, distinct zones of calcification are noted that alternate with layers of noncalcified tissue.

In areas of connective tissue degeneration, fine granular deposits of electron-dense material can be seen in the ground substance of the connective tissue (Fig. 2A). One type is spindle-shaped deposits related to the ground substance (Fig. 2A). The other type is calcospherules, which are globular structures of varying sizes and electron densities. Some of them have well-defined smooth surfaces, while others have fuzzy surfaces covered with needle-shaped crystallites (Fig. 2A). Moreover, globular, electron-dense structures that resemble calcospherules with laminae limitantes as described by Friedmann and Galey[10] were also noted (Fig. 2A, insert).

In the ground substance of degenerated connective tissue, there are also scattered noncalcified, membrane-bound vesicles that may represent so-called matrix vesicles (Fig. 2B). In some areas outlines of lacunae resembling degenerated fibroblasts can be observed. They contain a large number of calcospherules, giving the impression that these calcospherules are possibly derived from degenerated and calcified cell organelles (Fig. 2C).

In advanced states of mineralization, the calcospherules have fused to form larger aggregations of calcified matter, through which only shadowlike outlines of degenerated connective tissue fibrils are discernible (Fig. 2D).

X-ray microanalysis of undecalcified tympanosclerotic tissue shows it to contain a high concentration of calcium and phosphorus.

DISCUSSION

The most consistent light microscopic finding in tympanosclerosis is thickening and "hyalinization" of the connective tissue layer. This term denotes a homogeneous translucent appearance of connective tissue fibers that show typical staining reactions with acid dyes. It is caused by the deposition of proteinaceous substances triggered by cellular damage due to inflammatory processes or vascular disturbances. It is a nonspecific process occurring in different connective tissues in the body, for example, in scars, certain tumors, or the reticulum of lymph nodes. In the hyalinized connective tissue, dystrophic calcification may occur.

At the ultrastructural level degeneration of collagen and reticulin fibrils and mineralization are the most prominent findings. The precise mechanisms of tissue mineralization in normal tissue

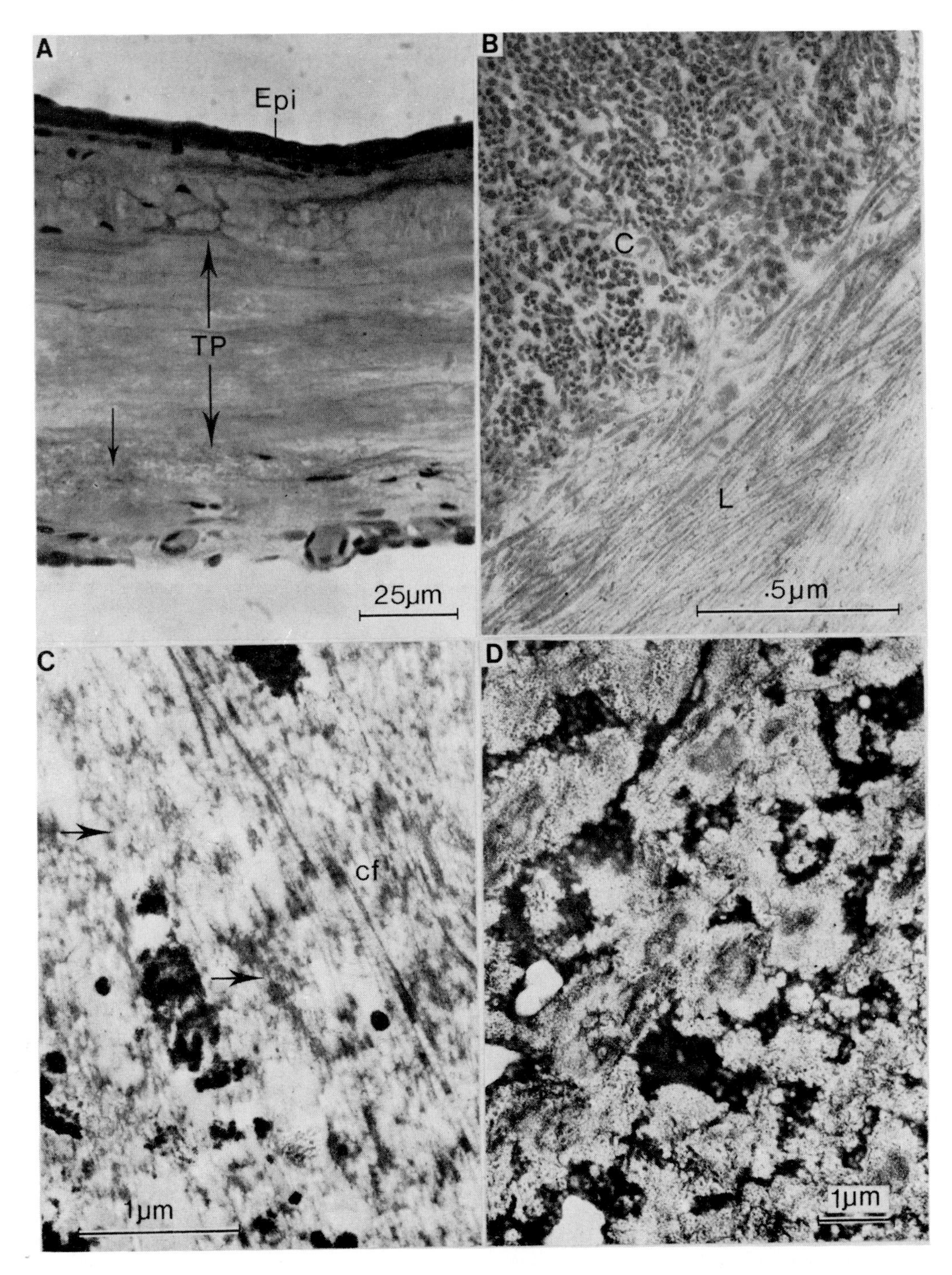

Figure 1 A, A light microscopic photograph of a tympanic membrane shows tympanosclerotic plaque (TP) in the middle fibrous layer. Fine granular deposits of calcium phosphate are scattered in the submucosal connective tissue (arrows). Epi, epidermis. B, A TEM photomicrograph shows the fibrillar texture of the collagenous fibers in cross-sectional (C) and longitudinal (L) sectioned view of a normal human tympanic membrane (pars tensa). C, Human tympanosclerotic tympanic membrane (pars tensa) in longitudinal section shows indistinct fiber arrangement (arrows) due to degeneration of collagen fibers (cf). D, Tympanosclerotic middle ear mucosa shows degenerated collagenous fibers which appear motheaten.

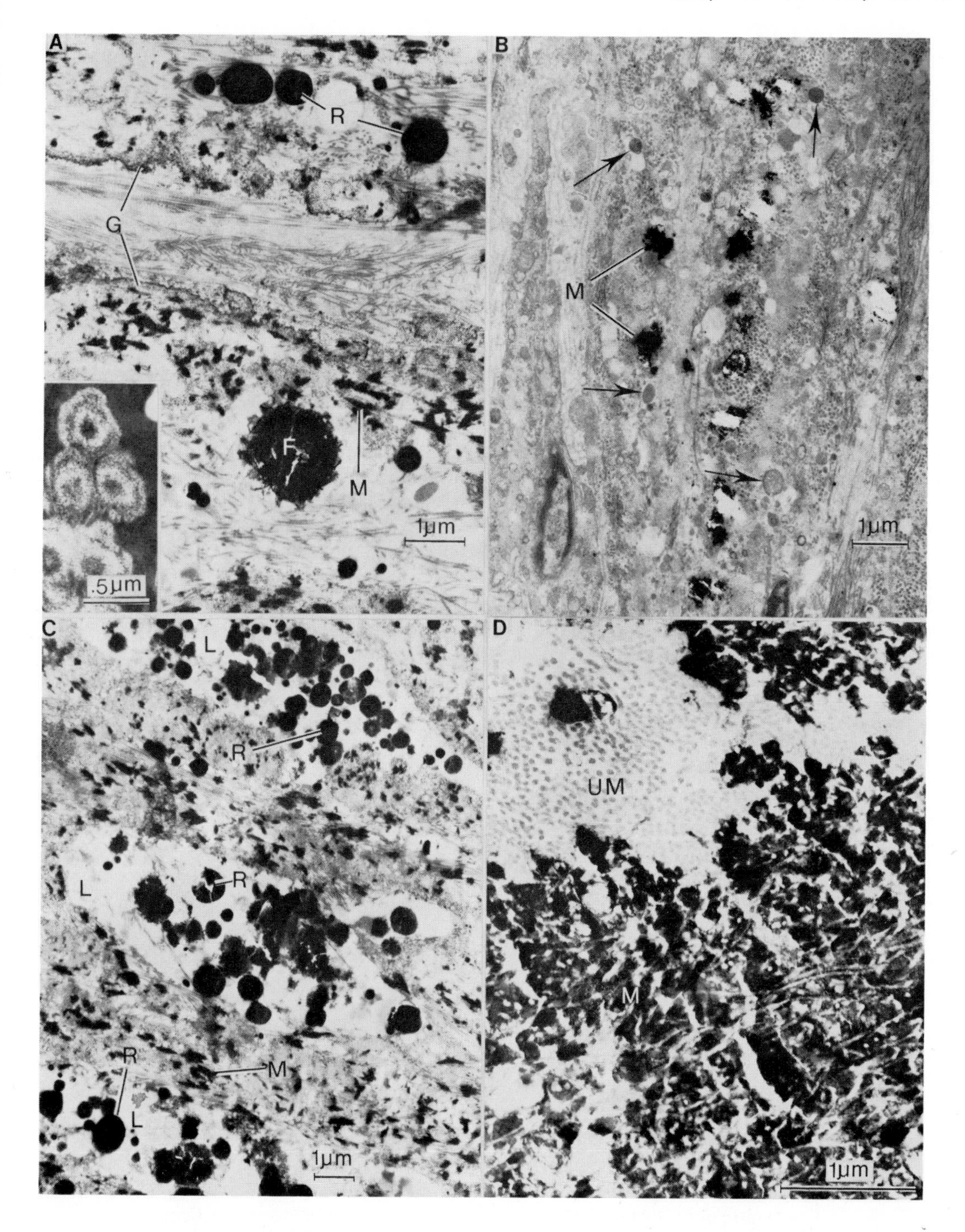

Figure 2 A, A tympanosclerotic plaque from the middle ear mucosa shows numerous round-surfaced (R) or fuzzy-surfaced (F) calcospherules. Fine aggregates of granular deposits (G) in the ground substance can also be observed. Some fine mineral deposits (M) appear to be related to this ground substance. An insert shows calcospherules with "lamina limitans." B, Membrane-bound vesicles (arrows) are found in the connective tissue near the small, irregular, osmiophilic mineral deposits (M). C, Concentration of round calcospherules (R) in the lacuna-shaped areas (L), which are suspected to be formed by the ghosts of degenerated fibroblasts. Also observe the irregular spindle-shaped mineral deposits in the connective tissue (M). D, A TEM photomicrograph shows highly mineralized (M) tympanosclerotic plaque with ghost images of collagen fibers. An unmineralized (UM) clear area with collagen fibers can also be seen.

(bone, cartilage, dentin) and under pathologic conditions are still controversial. One of the current hypotheses proposes a critical role for extracellular matrix vesicles for calcification. These vesicles are membrane-bound structures, 300 to 1500 Å in diameter, that contain a variety of enzymes, including alkaline phosphates and ATPase.[13–15] It has been suggested that the initial deposition of a solid phase of calcium phosphate in the extracellular spaces of mineralized tissue occurs in these matrix vesicles and that the solid mineral phase in these vesicles is directly responsible for the subsequent calcification of the remaining extracellular compartments.[13,16] Matrix vesicles have been identified in tympanosclerotic tissue[9,12] and, based on the above cited concept, were claimed to be the primary site of calcification in tympanosclerosis.[10] In our material, some membrane-bound vesicles that may represent matrix vesicles and numerous calcospherules of varying sizes, shapes, and electron densities were noted. However, we could not determine with certainty whether calcospherules derive from calcified matrix vesicles, although there is circumstantial evidence to suggest that the matrix vesicles are somehow related to the calcospherules. The vesicles similar to the matrix vesicles have also been observed in the nontympanosclerotic middle ear connective tissue (Lim, 1983). Furthermore, we noted numerous fine granular deposits of calcium phosphate in the ground substance of degenerated connective tissue. Mineralization seems, therefore, at least in part, derived from the degeneration of the collagenous component of connective tissue in the absence of matrix vesicles.

Recently, Landis and Glimcher also questioned the proposed role of calcification of matrix vesicles in tissue mineralization.[7] They failed to detect a mineral phase in matrix vesicles in undecalcified, unfixed, and unstained thin sections of rat growth plate cartilage but identified heterodispersed particles as the initial solid phase of calcium phosphate in the extracellular matrix. They interpret the presence of electron-dense particles in matrix vesicles treated with aqueous methods as an artifact of preparation. However, they ascribe a possible indirect role in mineralization to matrix vesicles, inasmuch as they could act as calcium and/or phosphorus pumps into the extracellular fluid or could function by certain biochemical action such as by degradation of proteoglycans that inhibit mineralization.

Based on the present data, it is apparent that the primary pathologic factor leading to tympano-

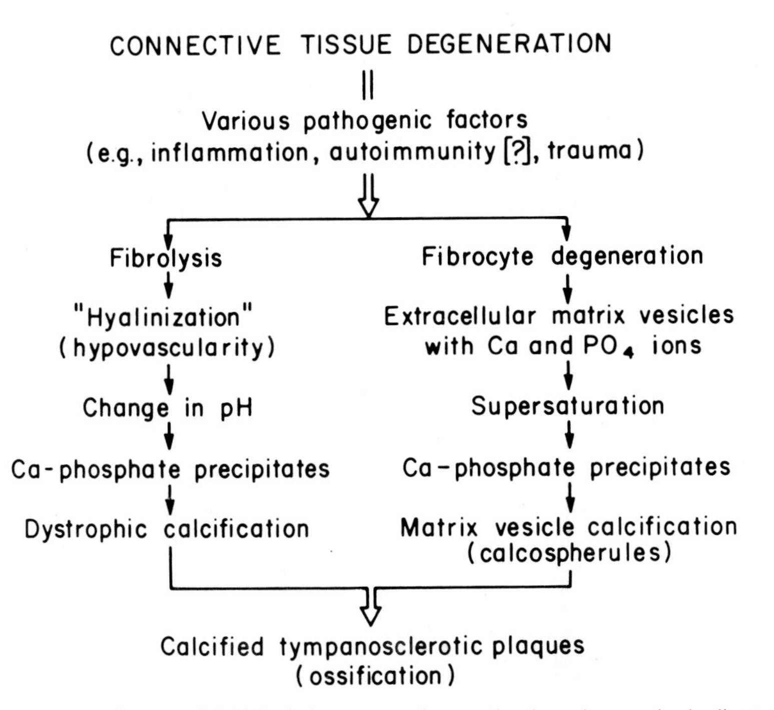

Figure 3 A schematic diagram of two possible biological sequences of connective tissue degeneration leading to tympanosclerosis.

sclerosis is degenerative processes in the connective tissue layer. This observation is consistent with the concept that tympanosclerosis occurs as a sequela of an inflammatory process in the middle ear cleft. Another factor contributing to tympanosclerosis may be trauma, which would explain the high incidence in cases of serous otitis media after insertion of ventilating tubes. Recently, Poliquin and colleagues produced tympanosclerosis in an animal model.[8] They isolated the lamina propria of the guinea pig tympanic membrane, prepared it as an antigen, and produced rabbit antiguinea pig tympanic membrane antibody. This antiserum was used to sensitize guinea pigs passively. When the tympanic membrane was traumatized in the sensitized guinea pigs, immunopathologic responses occurred at the site of injury to the tympanic membrane that resulted in tympanosclerosis. On this basis, Poliquin and colleagues suggested that an autoimmune process is yet another possibility to be considered in the pathogenesis of this condition.[8]

In conclusion, the present study confirmed that degeneration of connective tissue is a prerequisite for the formation of tympanosclerosis. The calcification appears to be initiated by formation of numerous dispersed microscopic mineral (calcium phosphate) deposits, as shown in Figure 3. The present study cannot substantiate the matrix vesicles as a primary mechanism in the mineralization process involved in tympanosclerosis. Further studies are needed to clarify these questions regarding the pathogenesis of tympanosclerosis.

This study was supported in part by grant #NS-08854 from NINCDS/NIH. We would like to thank Dr. William H. Saunders for providing some of the specimens; Ilija Karanfilov, Atha Ralston, and Roberta Arbaugh for technical assistance; Margaret Hawkins for photomicrography; Nancy Sally for illustration; and Katherine Adamson for manuscript preparation.

REFERENCES

1. Hussl B, Mueller G: Long-term results of tympanostomy in secretory otitis media. In *Physiology and Pathophysiology of Eustachian Tube and Middle Ear*. G. Münker, W. Arnold, eds. Stuttgart: Georg Thieme, 1980, pp 217–222
2. Beck C, Ebert B: Ein Beitrag zur Paukensklerose. Z Laryng Rhinol 43:404, 1964
3. House WF, Sheehy JL: Tympanosclerosis. Arch Otolaryngol 72:308, 1960
4. Igarashi M, Konishi S, Alford BR, Guilford FR. The pathology of tympanosclerosis. Laryngoscope 80:233, 1970
5. Soerensen H, True O: Histology of tympanosclerosis. Acta Otolaryngol (Stockh) 73:18, 1971
6. Weichselbaumer W, Pauler G: Zur Tympanosklerose. Laryng Rhinol 58:417, 1979
7. Makishima K, Toriya Y, Inue S, et al: Clinicopathologic studies in tympanosclerosis. Am J Otol 3:260, 1982
8. Poliquin JF, Catanzaro A, Robb J, Schiff M: Adaptive immunity of the tympanic membrane. Am J Otol 2:94, 1981
9. Mann W, Riede UN, Jonas I, Beck C: The role of matrix vesicles in the pathogenesis of tympanosclerosis. Acta Otolaryngol (Stockh) 89:43, 1980
10. Friedmann I, Galey FR: Initiation and stages of mineralization in tympanosclerosis. J Laryngol Otol 94:1215, 1980
11. Lim DJ: Human tympanic membrane: An ultrastructural observation. Acta Otolaryngol (Stockh) 70:176, 1970
12. Friedmann I, Galey FR, Odnert S: The ultrastructure of tympanosclerosis. The source of the matrix vesicles and the pattern of calcospherules. Am J Otol 3:144, 1981
13. Ali SY: Analysis of matrix vesicles and their role in the calcification of epiphyseal cartilage. Fed Proc 35:135, 1976
14. Anderson HC: Matrix vesicles calcification introduction. Fed Proc 35:105, 1976
15. Katchburian E: Membrane bound bodies as initiators of mineralization. J Anat 116:285, 1973
16. Bonucci E: The locus of initial calcification in cartilage and bone. Clin Orthop Rel Res 78:108, 1971
17. Landis W, Glimcher MJ: Electron optical and analytical observations of rat growth plate cartilage prepared by ultracryomicrotomy: The failure to detect a mineral phase in matrix vesicles and the identification of heterodispersed particles as the initial solid phase of calcium phosphate deposited in the extracellular matrix. J Ultrastruct Res 78:227, 1982

SECRETORY OTITIS MEDIA AND MIDDLE EAR CHOLESTEATOMA: AN EXPERIMENTAL STUDY

YOSHIO HONDA, M.D., TADAHITO MIZOROGI, M.D.,
and SHIRO ESAKI, M.D.

Ruedi's animal experiment[1] is a famous model explaining the origin of middle ear cholesteatoma. From the clinical standpoint, however, the cholesteatoma is a retraction of the tympanic membrane into the attic and mastoid cavity. Thus, Ruedi's hypothesis is difficult to accept.

We have conducted various experiments to establish an experimental model analogous to cholesteatoma in man. We assume that cholesteatoma in man originates from chronic otitis media with effusion during childhood. Based on this point of view, we produced a nonperforative chronic otitis media in animals and examined the morphologic changes in the tympanic membrane. We were able to produce a condition resembling retraction cholesteatoma originating in the pars flaccida of the tympanic membrane and performed further experiments, the results of which are reported here. The rabbit was used as the experimental animal.

EXPERIMENTAL OBSTRUCTION OF THE TYMPANIC ORIFICE OF THE EUSTACHIAN TUBE

The tympanic orifice of the eustachian tube was obstructed with pieces of muscle through the mastoid bulla without damaging the tympanic membrane. The experiment was performed on 117 ears. The rabbits were kept for 16 weeks from the third day after the operation, and then the specimens were prepared for observation.

The tympanic membrane was perforated by infection of the middle ear cavity in 62 of the 117 ears. Retention of effusion and infiltration of mildly inflammatory cells in the middle ear cavity were seen in the other 55 ears. Although there was no major change in the pars tensa of the tympanic membrane, cell division of the epithelial cells in the epidermal layer of the pars flaccida was profuse and growth of the middle layer was rapid. In nine ears the pars flaccida was retracted severely into the middle ear cavity (Fig. 1), and in two ears keratotic epithelium and exfoliative epithelium were retained in the retracted cavity, showing typical retraction cholesteatoma production (Fig. 2).

EXPERIMENTAL OBSTRUCTION OF THE PHARYNGEAL ORIFICE OF THE EUSTACHIAN TUBE

The purpose of this experiment was the same as for the experiment described above. It was performed on 70 ears, which were observed for 16 weeks after the operation. In this group the tympanic membrane did not become perforated until two weeks after the operation and the ears all had otitis media with effusion. In these cases, although the pars tensa was not changed, the epithelium of the epidermal layer of the pars flaccida became hyperplastic and proliferative. After two weeks had elapsed the middle ear became infected and the tympanic membrane became perforated. In one case, however, the ear was still not perforated at 16 weeks, and in this ear a typical retraction cholesteatoma originating in the pars flaccida was formed.

The following changes were found when the tympanic membrane had not been perforated in the two experiments in which the eustachian tube of the rabbit had been obstructed. That is, effusions were retained because of the negative pressure in the middle ear cavity. Mild inflammatory cell infiltration was also seen. When such a condition continued, no prominent change occurred in the pars tensa, but in some cases the epithelial cells in the epidermal layer of the pars flaccida grew to form retraction cholesteatoma.

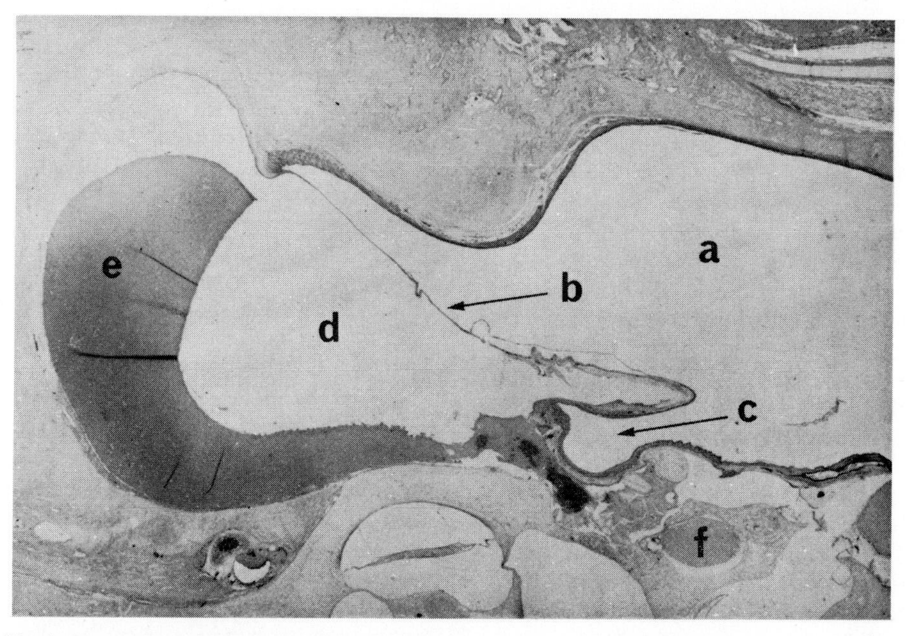

Figure 1 Histologic specimen at three weeks after tubal obstruction. Severe retraction is limited to the pars flaccida, as shown in this micrograph, and is not seen in the pars tensa. Key: a, external auditory canal; b, pars tensa; c, pars flaccida; d, middle ear cavity; e, effusion; and f, facial nerve.

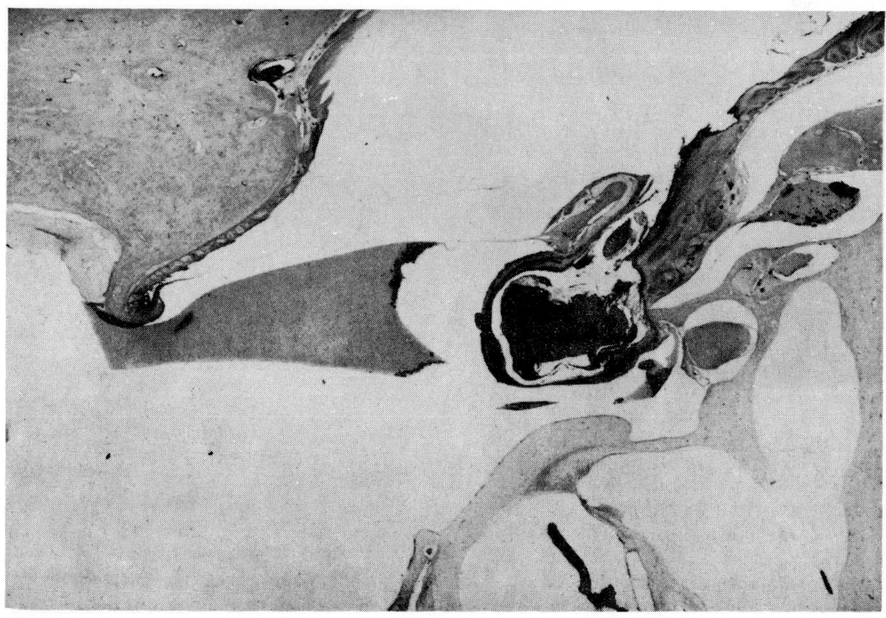

Figure 2 The retraction cholesteatoma originating from pars flaccida five weeks after tubal obstruction.

IN VITRO CULTURE OF EPITHELIAL CELLS OF EPIDERMAL LAYER OF TYMPANIC MEMBRANE

The epithelial cells of the epidermal layer of the pars flaccida and pars tensa of the tympanic membrane and the epithelial cells of the epidermal layer of the external ear canal of rabbits were cultured separately, and the growth rate of the cells was examined to confirm their differences.

We had previously found that hyaluronic acid is contained in large amounts in the periphery of the cholesteatoma tissue.[2] In the present experiment we added dilute hyaluronic acid to the culture vessel and examined the growth of the cells. The cell activity was measured by incorporation of uptake of H^3-thymidine and H^3-leucine.

The uptake of H^3-thymidine and H^3-leucine by the cells in the epithelium of the pars flaccida was greater than that by the epithelial cells of the pars tensa, and intake by pars flaccida epithelial cells was greatly changed by the addition of hyaluronic acid (Fig. 3).

Effect of hyaluronic acid on the incorporation of H^3-Leucine into the protein by PT, PF, and Ext.

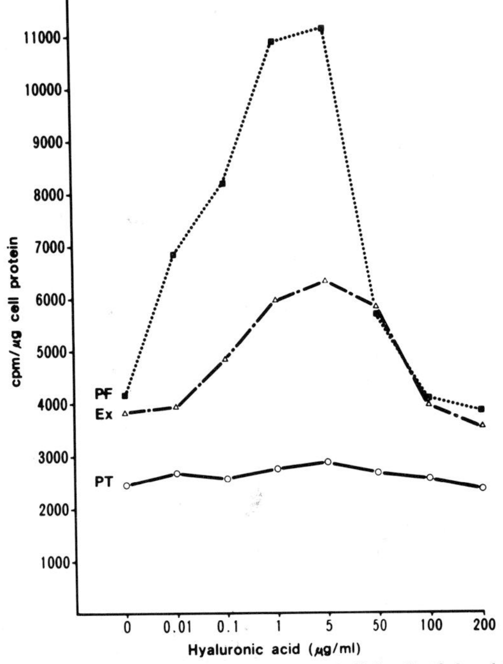

Figure 3 Proliferation rate of the epithelial cell of the skin. The vertical and horizontal lines indicate the incorporation of H^3-leucine and the consistency of hyaluronic acid respectively. Key: Ex, external auditory canal; PF, pars flaccida; PT, pars tensa.

The cell culture results showed that the growth potential of the epithelial cells of the epidermal layer of the pars flaccida is greater than that of the pars tensa in the rabbit. The growth and development of the epithelium of the pars flaccida were found to be greatly affected by hyaluronic acid, but those of the epithelium of the pars tensa were not.

CONCLUSIONS

When the eustachian tube is obstructed and otitis media with effusion is produced in the middle ear of rabbits, both the pars flaccida and pars tensa of the tympanic membrane are presumed to be stimulated similarly. But the epithelial cells of the epidermal layer in the pars flaccida respond more strongly than those of the pars tensa and result in rapid growth. This growth causes retraction of the pars flaccida owing to the negative pressure in the middle ear cavity, and as this condition progresses, it takes the form of retraction cholesteatoma.

This is presumed to happen because of the greater activity of the epithelial cells and the higher rate of growth in response to the stimulus in the epidermal layer of the pars flaccida than in that of the pars tensa. The high responsiveness of the epithelial cells in the pars flaccida is considered to be caused by the abundant connective tissue in the middle layer, but the epithelial cells in the pars tensa also seem to have enough activity to form cholesteatoma if appropriate conditions are maintained for an extended time.

The morphology of the middle ear and the type of otitis media with effusion in man differ from those in rabbits. The time course of occurrence of cholesteatoma is also different in man, but the above animal experiments may help us understand the origin of cholesteatoma in man.

REFERENCES

1. Ruedi L: Acquired cholesteatoma. Arch Otolaryngol 72:252, 1963
2. Sugita T: An experimental study on the proliferation of cholesteatoma epithelium in the middle ear. Otorhinolaryngology Tokyo 25 (Suppl):153, 1982

IMPEDANCE AS AN INDICATOR IN IRREVERSIBLE OTOPATHOLOGY AND HEARING LOSS IN NINE-YEAR-OLDS

JENS ULRIK FELDING, M.D., MOGENS FIELLAU-NIKOLAJSEN, M.D., and POUL ERIK HØJSLET, M.D.

This chapter presents the preliminary results of a study of impedance measurement as a tool for diagnosing irreversible sequelae in the tympanic membrane. In this study we give first importance to compliance, as that is the impedance parameter that has been most discussed in the literature.[1–5]

MATERIALS AND METHODS

An unselected group of 523 children, all born in 1972 and living in the municipality of Hjørring in Denmark, provided the material. Of these children 510, or 97.7 percent, attended; among them 501, representing 1001 ears, were subjected to all investigations. A total of 17 ears were excluded from the study because of poor cooperation by the patients,[4] grommets in situ,[8] perforation of the drum,[2] and congenital hearing loss.[3] Two ears had such a low compliance that impedance was not measured.

The method used was prospective screening, and the parameters consisted of audiometry and impedance measurement, which included tympanometry with measurement of middle ear pressure and gradient compliance, determination of the stapedial reflex ipsilaterally as well as contralaterally, and otomicroscopy.

According to the otomicroscopic findings, we described the various parts of the drum schematically, the pars flaccida by a modified Tos 0–4 classification[6] and mapping the various retractions. Then we described the pars tensa in two planes. The surface was divided into four squares in which we described atrophy with myringosclerosis, perforations, and grommets. In a plane passing down into the middle ear we described the findings according to van Baarle[7] and Sadé and colleagues[8] supported by pneumotomicroscopy in which we evaluated mobility, retractions, fixations, and atelectases. We also mapped the situation and extent of retraction pockets. A final otomicroscopic diagnosis was made, in this case a brief sequelae versus no sequelae determination (Table 1).

RESULTS

Sequelae were found in 9.7 percent of normal children. Like most, investigators who have discussed the effect of such sequelae on hearing, we found a difference in hearing when measured as the speech reception threshold.[4,9–11] In patients with no sequelae we found a mean hearing of 11.37 dB and in patients with sequelae a mean hearing of 13.03 dB. This is a small difference, but it is statistically significant within the 5 percent range.

Using the otomicroscopic findings we then analyzed, by a number of validity tests, the diagnostic value of increasing compliance values in predicting sequelae. In this analysis we calculated "the predictive value of a positive test" as no sequelae with high compliance rates, divided by the total number of high-compliance patients. We also calculated "the predictive value of a negative test" as being the total number of no sequelae with nor-

TABLE 1 Mean Hearing (SPL) in 1001 Ears of Nine-Year-Olds Grouped by Otomicroscopy

	No Sequelae	*Sequelae*
N	904	97 (9.7%)
$\bar{X}$	11.37 dB*	13.03 dB*
SEM†	0.04 dB	0.65 dB
Confidence	11.29 dB	11.73 dB
Limits	11.45 dB	14.33 dB

*$p < 0.05$
†SEM, standard error of the mean

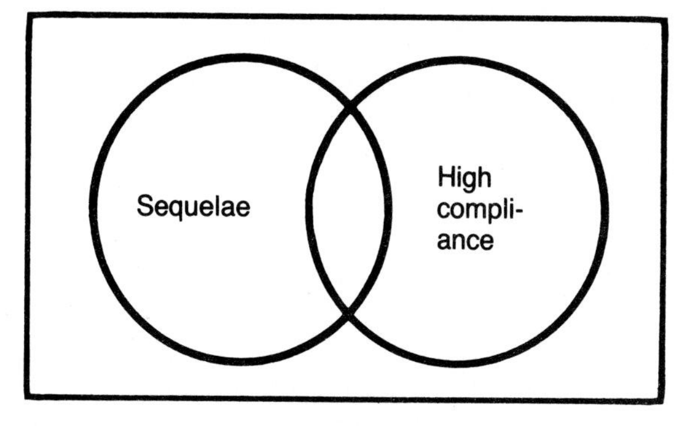

1. Predictive value of positive test = $\frac{\text{No. of Sequelae with High Compliance}}{\text{Total No. of High Compliances}}$

2. Predictive value of negative test = $\frac{\text{No. of No Sequelae with Normal Compliance}}{\text{Total No. of Normal Compliances}}$

3. Accuracy = 1 $\times$ 2

Figure 1 Principle analysis of the study.

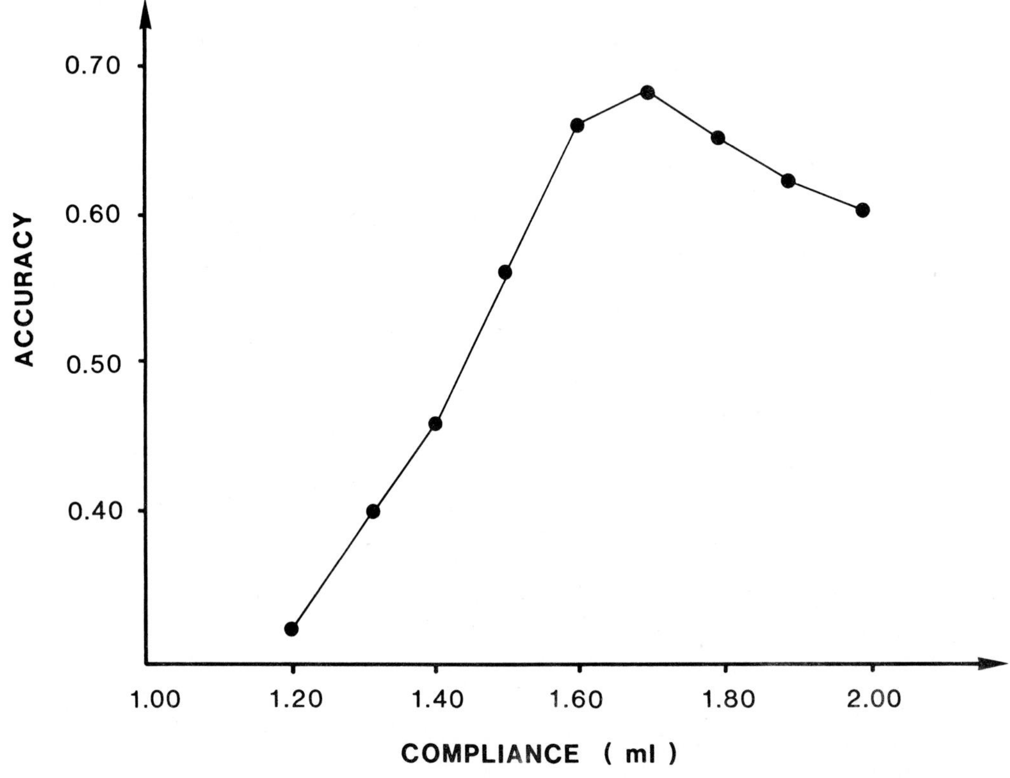

Figure 2 Accuracy of predicting sequelae to otitis media with increasing values of compliance.

mal compliance rates, divided by the total number of normal-compliance patients[12] (Fig. 1). On this basis, we defined the accuracy as 1 × 2.

The results are shown as a graph in Figure 2, in which we evaluated the compliance limits for 1.20, 1.40, 1.50, 1.60, 1.70, 1.80, 1.90, and 2.00. There is a distinct peak at 1.70, and thereafter the accuracy decreases. The rise is due to an increase in the predictive value of a positive test, while the predictive value of a negative test is practically constant.

DISCUSSION

Interest in the difference in hearing between ears with sequelae and ears with no sequelae is presumably going to increase in the years to come, especially because some investigations indicate that this difference does not become less important with increased time and because the prevalence of drum sequelae in groups of normal children has proved unexpectedly high, as demonstrated in the present study. Longitudinal studies are needed to provide the knowledge we now lack concerning the long-term consequences of the sequelae. For this purpose, simple diagnostic tests are of value, and our present study is one part of these efforts. In a future study we are going to combine the previously mentioned parameters—audiometry, middle ear pressure, gradient, and stapedial reflex—with compliance to obtain greater accuracy.

It can be concluded that 10 percent of normal 9-year-olds have drum sequelae and that this causes a slight, but statistically significant, hearing loss. A compliance of 1.70 ml appears to be a reasonable predictive limit between normal and abnormal values. Compliance as a diagnostic test affords an accuracy of 0.70 in predicting drum sequelae, and a combination of impedance parameters will no doubt increase this accuracy.

REFERENCES

1. Jerger J, Anthony L, Jerger S, Mauldin L: Studies in impedance audiometry. Arch Otolaryngol 99:165, 1974
2. Alberti P, Kristensen R: The clinical application of impedance audiometry: A preliminary appraisal of an electroacoustic impedance bridge. Laryngoscope 80:735, 1970
3. Brooks D: An objective method of detecting fluid in the middle ear. Int Aud 7:280, 1968
4. Brooks D: Possible long-term consequences of middle ear effusion. Ann Otol Rhinol Laryngol 89(Suppl 68):246, 1980
5. Feldmann AS: Eardrum abnormality and the measurement of middle ear function. Arch Otolaryngol 99:211, 1974
6. Tos M, Poulsen G: Attic retractions following secretory otitis. Acta Otolaryngol 89:479, 1980
7. van Baarle PWL: A documentation system for surgical treatment of chronic otitis media. Clin Otolaryngol 6:245, 1981
8. Sadé J, Avraham S, Brown M: Atelectasis, retraction pockets and cholesteatoma. Acta Otolaryngol 92:501, 1981
9. Mawson SR, Fagan P: Tympanic effusions in children. Long-term results of treatment by myringotomy aspiration and indwelling tubes. J Laryngol Otol 86:105, 1972
10. Barfoed C, Rosborg J: Secretory otitis media: Long-term observations after treatment with grommets. Arch Otolaryngol 106:553, 1980
11. Tos M, Poulsen G: Changes of pars tensa in secretory otitis. ORL 41:313, 1979
12. Wulff HR: *Rationel Klinik*. København: Munksgaard, 1973

COMPLICATIONS OF OTITIS MEDIA WITH EFFUSION IN JAPANESE CHILDREN

TOSHIO OHNISHI, M.D., MOTOHIRO MOCHIZUKI, M.D.,
and SATORU HONGO, M.D.

Characteristics of a disease are usually determined by the severity of its complications. Since frequencies and nature of complications of otitis media with effusion (OME) have already been described by many authors, we report here the complications in Japanese children for comparison with those in Western children.

MATERIALS AND METHODS

A total of 230 Japanese children (114 boys and 116 girls) with OME who had received tympanostomy tubes from 1972 to 1982 were examined once every two months with pure-tone audiometry and impedance tests until the disease subsided. A total of 288 tympanostomy tubes were inserted. A ventilating tube was inserted in 512 of the 576 ears that were examined under the operating microscope.

RESULTS

Complications of OME were classified into three groups according to the location of the main findings, for example, the tympanic membrane, middle ear, or inner ear.

Complications found in the tympanic membrane were granulation around the ventilating tube in 19 ears, or 3.7 percent, of 512 tube insertions; diffuse atrophy in 23 ears, or 5 percent; diffuse tympanosclerosis in ten ears, or 2 percent; and persisting perforation in five ears, or 1 percent of the 460 ears. The incidence of complications is shown in Table 1.

Complications of the middle ear were acute middle ear infection in 35 ears, or 8 percent of the 460 ears; atelectasis in 23 ears, or 5 percent, blue eardrum in eight ears, or 2 percent; adhesive otitis media in two ears, or 0.4 percent; ossicular disruption in one ear, or 0.2 percent; and cholesteatoma in one ear, or 0.2 percent.

Complication of the inner ear was bone conduction loss in four ears, or 1 percent of 460 ears.

DISCUSSION

The results of the present study indicate that there is no significant quality difference in the complications of OME between Japanese and Western children when compared with the data from Tos and colleagues,[1] Muenker[2] and Barfoed and Rosborg.[3] A quantitative difference is noted in the incidence of tympanosclerosis, which turned out to be considerably lower among Japanese children.

TABLE 1 Frequencies of Complications of OME in Japanese Children

Complications	*Incidence*	*Percent*	*Population*
Tympanic Membrane			
Granulation around tube	19	3.7	512 ears
Atrophy (diffuse)	23	5	460 ears
Tympanosclerosis (diffuse)	10	2	—
Perforation	5	1	—
Middle Ear			
Acute middle ear infection	35	8	—
Atelectasis	23	5	—
Blue eardrum	8	2	—
Adhesive otitis media	2	0.4	—
Chronic suppurative otitis media	0	0	
Ossicular disruption	1	0.2	—
Cholesteatoma	1	0.2	—
Inner Ear			
Bone conduction loss	4	1	—

The difference, however, does not seem to suggest any different implications for the prognosis of the disease in different races, because the presence of tympanosclerotic lesions rarely affects the hearing of the patients.

Among the listed complications, simple middle ear infection, atelectasis, tympanosclerosis, and blue eardrum are considered to be mild, because these changes are reversible or not detrimental to hearing. Such pathologic changes would be controlled by antibiotics and/or reventilation of the middle ear by insertion of a ventilating tube.

Although blue eardrum has sometimes been regarded as an independent pathologic change because of its specific manifestations, long-term observation of eight such cases revealed that the findings of blue eardrum and OME are interchangeable. It seemed that blue eardrum was a phase in various manifestations of OME and thus can and should be controlled without resorting to mastoidectomy.

Complications affecting hearing acuity include persistent perforation, adhesive otitis media, chronic suppurative otitis media, ossicular disruption, and cholesteatoma.

Retraction of the tympanic membrane and atelectasis are ubiquitous in OME. However, it is quite rare to see adhesions of the tympanic membrane to the promontory. Adhesive otitis media, ossicular adhesions, ossicular disruption, and cholesteatoma may not be attributable to OME per se. These changes can probably be ascribed to secondary infections in ears with OME.

The mucous membrane of the middle ear in OME, as we observe during tympanostomy tube insertion, is distinctly different from the one we see during tympanoplasty for chronic infections in that there is little or no granulation tissue in the middle ear.

We saw only a few cases of severe atrophy of the eardrum or atelectasis without effusion. Most of these ears had normal hearing in spite of marked thinning of the eardrum and atelectasis. It may be only those changes due to secondary infections that bring about irreversible changes in the middle ear resulting in various degrees of permanent hearing loss.

It is the authors' impression, based on a previous study[4] and on the present one, that OME is not a simple infectious disease but has its origin in immunologic problems.

Possible cochlear involvement and cholesteatoma are of major clinical significance. Besides the 11 ears with congenital sensorineural hearing loss seen in the present series, reproducible normal bone conduction thresholds worsened 15 to 20 dB in four ears during the observation period of three to seven years. In two of these ears the eardrum showed retraction and adhesions at the posterior part.

Bone conduction loss in otitis media with effusion is more frequently seen in adult cases, which are almost always associated with secondary infections accompanied by proliferation of granulation in the middle ear. Although it is highly possible that sensorineural hearing loss could occur in adult cases of secretory otitis media via the invasive inflammation through the round window, as was suggested by Paparella in cases with chronic otitis media,[5] bone conduction loss in childhood cases of OME may be due to proliferation of granulation tissue around or obliteration of the round window due to secondary infections.

A cholesteatoma developed in an ear with middle ear effusion after destruction of bone at the superior wall of the external auditory canal accompanied by proliferation of granulation in the canal skin overlying the lesions. The bone defect seemed to have induced an ingrowth of the epithelial cells into the attic and antrum without formation of a cholesteatoma mass. It appeared that inflammatory erosion or destruction of the bony canal wall can cause cholesteatoma to develop by inducing an ingrowth of the epithelial cells as a healing process regardless of the presence or absence of negative pressure within the middle ear, attic, or antrum.

In conclusion, we found that there was no significant difference in the quality of complications between Japanese and Western children and that OME was a benign condition, except for the hearing defect, with a high propensity to resolve on its own. Primary complications of OME characterized by atrophy of the tympanic membrane and atelectasis are usually not detrimental to hearing acuity.

Irreversible changes involving hearing would probably be the consequences of secondary infections in ears with OME. Such complications include granulation around the tube, chronic suppurative otitis media, adhesive otitis media, ossicular disruption, cholesteatoma, and bone conduction loss.

REFERENCES

1. Tos M, Holm-Jensen S, Sørensen CH, Mogensen C: Spontaneous course and frequency of secretory otitis in 4-year-old children. Arch Otolaryngol 108:4, 1982

2. Muenker G: Results after treatment of otitis media with effusion. Ann Otol Rhinol Laryngol 89 (Suppl 68):308, 1980
3. Barfoed C, Rosborg J: Secretory otitis media: Long-term observation after treatment with grommets. Arch Otolaryngol 106:553, 1980
4. Ohnishi T, Shirahata Y, Kamide Y, Watanabe K: Some predisposing factors to otitis media with effusion. ORL Tokyo 25:272, 1982
5. Paparella MM, Goycoolea MV, Meyerhoff WL: Inner ear pathology and otitis media: A review. Ann Otol Rhinol Laryngol 89 (Suppl 68): 249, 1980

INDEX

(Note: t following a page number indicates a table; f indicates a figure, and n indicates a footnote)

Ceclor®

cefaclor

Description: Ceclor is a semisynthetic cephalosporin antibiotic for oral administration. It is chemically designated as 3-chloro-7-D-(2-phenylglycinamido)-3-cephem-4-carboxylic acid. Ceclor is available in 250-mg and 500-mg Pulvules* and in a powder for oral suspension containing 125 or 250 mg/5 ml.

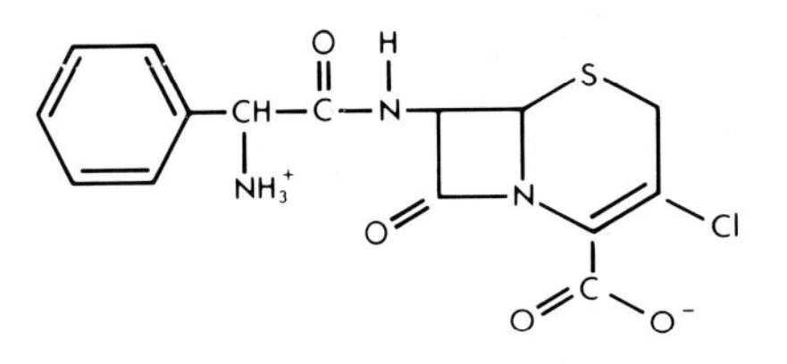

Clinical Pharmacology: Cefaclor is well absorbed after oral administration to fasting subjects. Total absorption is the same whether the drug is given with or without food; however, when it is taken with food, the peak concentration achieved is 50 to 75 percent of that observed when the drug is administered to fasting subjects and generally appears from three-fourths to one hour later. Following administration of 250-mg, 500-mg, and 1-g doses to fasting subjects, average peak serum levels of approximately 7, 13, and 23 mcg/ml respectively were obtained within 30 to 60 minutes. Approximately 60 to 85 percent of the drug is excreted unchanged in the urine within eight hours, the greater portion being excreted within the first two hours. During this eight-hour period, peak urine concentrations following the 250-mg, 500-mg, and 1-g doses were approximately 600, 900, and 1900 mcg/ml respectively. The serum half-life in normal subjects is 0.6 to 0.9 hour. In patients with reduced renal function, the serum half-life of cefaclor is slightly prolonged. In those with complete absence of renal function, the biologic half-life of the intact molecule is 2.3 to 2.8 hours. Excretion pathways in patients with markedly impaired renal function have not been determined. Hemodialysis shortens the half-life by 25 to 30 percent.

Microbiology—In vitro tests demonstrate that the bactericidal action of the cephalosporins results from inhibition of cell-wall synthesis. Cefaclor is usually active against the following organisms in vitro and in clinical infections:

- Staphylococci, including coagulase-positive, coagulase-negative, and penicillinase-producing strains
- *Streptococcus pyogenes* (group A beta-hemolytic streptococci)
- *S. pneumoniae* (formerly *Diplococcus pneumoniae*)
- *Escherichia coli*
- *Proteus mirabilis*
- *Klebsiella* species
- *Haemophilus influenzae*, including some beta-lactamase-producing ampicillin-resistant strains

Note: Pseudomonas species, *Acinetobacter calcoaceticus* (formerly *Mima* and *Herellea* species), and most strains of enterococci (*S. faecalis*, group D streptococci), *Enterobacter* species, indole-positive *Proteus*, and *Serratia* species are resistant to cefaclor. When tested by in vitro methods, staphylococci exhibit cross-resistance between cefaclor and methicillin-type antibiotics.

Disc Susceptibility Tests—Quantitative methods that require measurement of zone diameters give the most precise estimates of antibiotic susceptibility. One such procedure* has been recommended for use with discs for testing susceptibility to cephalothin. The currently accepted zone diameter interpretative criteria for the cephalothin disc are appropriate for determining bacterial susceptibility to cefaclor. With this procedure, a report from the laboratory of "resistant" indicates that the infecting organism is not likely to respond to therapy. A report of "intermediate susceptibility" suggests that the organism would be susceptible if the infection is confined to tissues and fluids (e.g., urine) in which high antibiotic levels can be obtained or if high dosage is used.

Indications and Usage: Ceclor is indicated in the treatment of the following infections when caused by susceptible strains of the designated microorganisms:

- Otitis media caused by *S. pneumoniae (D. pneumoniae), H. influenzae*, staphylococci, and *S. pyogenes* (group A beta-hemolytic streptococci)
- Lower respiratory infections, including pneumonia caused by *S. pneumoniae (D. pneumoniae), H. influenzae*, and *S. pyogenes* (group A beta-hemolytic streptococci)
- Upper respiratory infections, including pharyngitis and tonsillitis caused by *S. pyogenes* (group A beta-hemolytic streptococci)
  Note: Penicillin is the usual drug of choice in the treatment and prevention of streptococcal infections, including the prophylaxis of rheumatic fever. Ceclor is generally effective in the eradication of streptococci from the nasopharynx; however, substantial data establishing the efficacy of Ceclor in the subsequent prevention of rheumatic fever are not available at present.
- Urinary tract infections, including pyelonephritis and cystitis caused by *E. coli, P. mirabilis, Klebsiella* species, and coagulase-negative staphylococci
- Skin and skin-structure infections caused by *Staphylococcus aureus* and *S. pyogenes* (group A beta-hemolytic streptococci)

Appropriate culture and susceptibility studies should be performed to determine susceptibility of the causative organism to Ceclor.

Contraindication: Ceclor is contraindicated in patients with known allergy to the cephalosporin group of antibiotics.

Warnings: IN PENICILLIN-SENSITIVE PATIENTS, CEPHALOSPORIN ANTIBIOTICS SHOULD BE ADMINISTERED CAUTIOUSLY. THERE IS CLINICAL AND LABORATORY EVIDENCE OF PARTIAL CROSS-ALLERGENICITY OF THE PENICILLINS AND THE CEPHALOSPORINS, AND THERE ARE INSTANCES IN WHICH PATIENTS HAVE HAD REACTIONS, INCLUDING ANAPHYLAXIS, TO BOTH DRUG CLASSES.

Antibiotics, including Ceclor, should be administered cautiously to any patient who has demonstrated some form of allergy, particularly to drugs.

Pseudomembranous colitis has been reported with virtually all broad-spectrum antibiotics (including macrolides, semisynthetic penicillins, and cephalosporins); therefore, it is important to consider its diagnosis in patients who develop diarrhea in association with the use of antibiotics. Such colitis may range in severity from mild to life-threatening.

Treatment with broad-spectrum antibiotics alters the normal flora of the colon and may permit overgrowth of clostridia. Studies indicate that a toxin produced by *Clostridium difficile* is one primary cause of antibiotic-associated colitis.

Mild cases of pseudomembranous colitis usually respond to drug discontinuance alone. In moderate to severe cases, management should include sigmoidoscopy, appropriate bacteriologic studies, and fluid, electrolyte, and protein supplementation. When the colitis does not improve after the drug has been discontinued, or when it is severe, oral vancomycin is the drug of choice for antibiotic-associated pseudomembranous colitis produced by *C. difficile*. Other causes of colitis should be ruled out.

Precautions: *General Precautions*—If an allergic reaction to Ceclor occurs, the drug should be discontinued, and, if necessary, the patient should be treated with appropriate agents, e.g., pressor amines, antihistamines, or corticosteroids.

Prolonged use of Ceclor may result in the overgrowth of nonsusceptible organisms. Careful observation of the patient is essential. If superinfection occurs during therapy, appropriate measures should be taken.

Positive direct Coombs' tests have been reported during treatment with the cephalosporin antibiotics. In hematologic studies or in transfusion cross-matching procedures when antiglobulin tests are performed on the minor side or in Coombs' testing of newborns whose mothers have received cephalosporin antibiotics before parturition, it should be recognized that a positive Coombs' test may be due to the drug.

Ceclor should be administered with caution in the presence of markedly impaired renal function. Under such a condition, careful clinical observation and laboratory studies should be made because safe dosage may be lower than that usually recommended.

As a result of administration of Ceclor, a false-positive reaction for glucose in the urine may occur. This has been observed with Benedict's and Fehling's solutions and also with Clinitest* tablets but not with Tes-Tape* (Glucose Enzymatic Test Strip, USP, Lilly).

Broad-spectrum antibiotics should be prescribed with caution in individuals with a history of gastrointestinal disease, particularly colitis.

Usage in Pregnancy—Pregnancy Category B—Reproduction studies have been performed in mice and rats at doses up to 12 times the human dose and in ferrets given three times the maximum human dose and have revealed no evidence of impaired fertility or harm to the fetus due to Ceclor. There are, however, no adequate and well-controlled studies in pregnant women. Because animal reproduction studies are not always predictive of human response, this drug should be used during pregnancy only if clearly needed.

Nursing Mothers—Small amounts of Ceclor have been detected in mother's milk following administration of single 500-mg doses. Average levels were 0.18, 0.20, 0.21, and 0.16 mcg/ml at two, three, four, and five hours respectively. Trace amounts were detected at one hour. The effect on nursing infants is not known. Caution should be exercised when Ceclor is administered to a nursing woman.

Usage in Children—Safety and effectiveness of this product for use in infants less than one month of age have not been established.

Adverse Reactions: Adverse effects considered related to therapy with Ceclor are uncommon and are listed below:

Gastrointestinal symptoms occur in about 2.5 percent of patients and include diarrhea (1 in 70).

Symptoms of pseudomembranous colitis may appear either during or after antibiotic treatment. Nausea and vomiting have been reported rarely.

Hypersensitivity reactions have been reported in about 1.5 percent of patients and include morbilliform eruptions (1 in 100). Pruritus, urticaria, and positive Coombs' tests each occur in less than 1 in 200 patients. Cases of serum-sickness-like reactions (erythema multiforme or the above skin manifestations accompanied by arthritis/arthralgia and, frequently, fever) have been reported. These reactions are apparently due to hypersensitivity and have usually occurred during or following a second course of therapy with Ceclor. Such reactions have been reported more frequently in children than in adults. Signs and symptoms usually occur a few days after initiation of therapy and subside within a few days after cessation of therapy. No serious sequelae have been reported. Antihistamines and corticosteroids appear to enhance resolution of the syndrome.

Cases of anaphylaxis have been reported, half of which have occurred in patients with a history of penicillin allergy.

Other effects considered related to therapy included eosinophilia (1 in 50 patients) and genital pruritus or vaginitis (less than 1 in 100 patients).

Causal Relationship Uncertain—Transitory abnormalities in clinical laboratory test results have been reported. Although they were of uncertain etiology, they are listed below to serve as alerting information for the physician.

Hepatic—Slight elevations in SGOT, SGPT, or alkaline phosphatase values (1 in 40).

Hematopoietic—Transient fluctuations in leukocyte count, predominantly lymphocytosis occurring in infants and young children (1 in 40).

Renal—Slight elevations in BUN or serum creatinine (less than 1 in 500) or abnormal urinalysis (less than 1 in 200).

Dosage and Administration: Ceclor is administered orally.

Adults—The usual adult dosage is 250 mg every eight hours. For more severe infections (such as pneumonia) or those caused by less susceptible organisms, doses may be doubled. Doses of 4 g/day have been administered safely to normal subjects for 28 days, but the total daily dosage should not exceed this amount.

Children—The usual recommended daily dosage for children is 20 mg/kg/day in divided doses every eight hours, as indicated:

	Ceclor Suspension	
Child's Weight	125 mg/5 ml	250 mg/5 ml
9 kg	1/2 tsp t.i.d.	
18 kg	1 tsp t.i.d.	1/2 tsp t.i.d.

In more serious infections, otitis media, and infections caused by less susceptible organisms, 40 mg/kg/day are recommended, with a maximum dosage of 1 g/day.

Ceclor may be administered in the presence of impaired renal function. Under such a condition, the dosage usually is unchanged (*see* Precautions).

In the treatment of beta-hemolytic streptococcal infections, a therapeutic dosage of Ceclor should be administered for at least ten days.

How Supplied: For Oral Suspension, Ceclor* (cefaclor, Lilly), 125 mg/5 ml (strawberry flavor) and 250 mg/5 ml (grape flavor), in 75 and 150-ml-size packages.

Pulvules Ceclor, 250 and 500 mg, in bottles of 15 and 100 and in Identi-Dose* (unit dose medication, Lilly) in boxes of 100. [061782]

*Bauer, A. W., Kirby, W. M. M., Sherris, J. C., and Turck, M.: Antibiotic Susceptibility Testing by a Standardized Single Disk Method. Am. J. Clin. Pathol., *45*:493, 1966; Standardized Disc Susceptibility Test, Federal Register *39*:19182-19184, 1974.

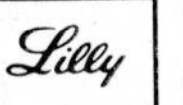

Eli Lilly Industries, Inc.
Carolina, Puerto Rico 00630
A Subsidiary of Eli Lilly and Company
Indianapolis, Indiana 46285